HEALTH CARE
R
2005

Health Care in the 50 United States

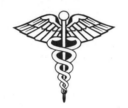

Kathleen O'Leary Morgan and Scott Morgan, Editors

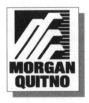

Morgan Quitno Press
© Copyright 2005, All Rights Reserved

512 East 9th Street, P.O. Box 1656
Lawrence, KS 66044-8656
USA
800-457-0742 or 785-841-3534
www.statestats.com
Thirteenth Edition

© Copyright 2005 by
Morgan Quitno Corporation
512 East 9th Street, P.O. Box 1656
Lawrence, Kansas 66044-8656

800-457-0742 or 785-841-3534
www.statetats.com

Cover Photo: comstock.com

ISBN: 0-7401-0941-3
ISSN: 1065-1403

Health Care State Rankings 2005 sells for $56.95 ($6 shipping) and is only available in paper binding. For those who prefer ranking information tailored to a particular state, we also offer *Health Care State Perspectives*, state-specific reports for each of the 50 states. These individual guides provide information on a state's data and rank for each of the categories featured in the national *Health Care State Rankings* volume. Perspectives sell for $19 or $9.50 if ordered with *Health Care State Rankings*. If crime statistics are your interest, please ask about our annual *Crime State Rankings* ($56.95 paper). If you are interested in city and metropolitan crime data, we offer *City Crime Rankings* ($44.95 paper). For a general view of the states, please ask about our annual *State Rankings* reference book ($56.95 paper) or our new annual *State Trends* ($59.95 paper). Also available is *Education State Rankings*. This view of preK-12 education at the state level is $49.95. All of our books are available on CD-ROM in PDF format (same price as printed book) or with both PDF format and data sets in various database formats ($99.95). Shipping and handling is $6 per order. For information, please visit our website at www.statestats.com.

Thirteenth Edition
Printed in the United States of America
March 2005

PREFACE

When asked to identify quality of life factors that matter the most, Americans choose the cost of and access to health care as one of their top concerns. As the price of health insurance coverage, prescription drugs and medical services continues to rise, access to reliable health care information is more important than ever.

This newly revised, 13th edition of *Health Care State Rankings* provides an extensive collection of state health care data. Births and reproductive health, deaths, disease, insurance and finance, health care providers, facilities and physical fitness are compared state-by-state. Find out how much workers in your state are paying in health insurance premiums, learn how your state's teen birth rate compares to others and discover what percentage of your state's citizens are overweight or obese. In all, more than 500 tables of state comparisons are provided, covering virtually every aspect of health care in the 50 United States.

Important Notes About *Health Care State Rankings 2005*

Health Care State Rankings 2005 presents information from government and private sector sources in one user-friendly volume. Our goal is to translate complicated and often convoluted health care data into easy-to-understand, meaningful state comparisons. As we revise this volume each year, we reexamine each table, update most, delete others and add new tables of interest to our readers.

We make every effort to present the data in *Health Care State Rankings 2005* as simply and straightforwardly as possible. Source information and other pertinent footnotes are clearly shown at the bottom of each page. National totals, rates and percentages are prominently displayed at the top of each table. Every other line is shaded in gray for easier reading. In addition, numerous information-finding tools are provided: a thorough table of contents, table listings at the beginning of each chapter, a roster of sources with addresses and phone numbers, a detailed index and a chapter thumb index.

For the ease of our readers, the numbers shown in *Health Care State Rankings* require no additional calculations to convert them from millions, thousands, etc. All states are ranked on a high to low basis, with any ties among the states listed alphabetically for a given ranking. Negative numbers are shown in parentheses "( )." For tables with national totals (as opposed to rates, per capitas, etc.) a separate column is included showing what percent of the national total each individual state's total represents. This column is headed by "% of USA." This percentage figure is particularly interesting when compared with a state's share of the nation's population for a particular year (provided in an appendix).

Those researchers who need information for just one state should check out our *Health Care State Perspective* series of publications. These 21-page comb bound reports feature data and ranking information for an individual state, as reported in *Health Care State Rankings 2005*. (For example *California Health Care in Perspective* features information about the state of California only.) These serve as handy, quick reference guides for those who do not want to page through the entire *Health Care State Rankings* volume searching for information for their particular state. *Health Care State Perspectives* sell for $19. When purchased with a copy of *Health Care State Rankings 2005*, these handy quick reference guides are just $9.50. For additional information, please call us toll-free at 1-800-457-0742.

Other Books From Morgan Quitno Press

In addition to *Health Care State Rankings 2005*, our company offers five other rankings reference books. *State Rankings* is our original rankings reference book, providing a general view of the states. Now in its 16th edition, *State Ranking 2005* provides easy-to-understand state statistics for categories ranging from agriculture to transportation, government finance to social welfare and crime to housing. *Education State Rankings 2004-2005* compares states in teachers' salaries, class sizes, graduation rates and more than 400 other categories relating to preK-12 education. *Crime State Rankings 2005* provides a huge collection of user-friendly state statistics regarding law enforcement personnel and expenditures, corrections, juvenile crime and delinquency, arrests and offenses. For crime information in communities, *City Crime Rankings* compares crime in all metropolitan areas and cities of 75,000 or more population (approx. 360 cities). Numbers of crimes, crime rates and changes in crime rates over one and five years are presented for all major crime categories reported by the FBI. Final 2003 crime data are featured in the most recent 11th edition. *State Trends* is the newest reference book in Morgan Quitno's collection. The most recent, first edition of this annual volume has earned rave reviews for providing a quick and easy way to track important quality of life changes in the 50 United States. One, five, 10 and 20-year trends are measured in health care, taxes, crime, education and more.

The information in all our books also is available on CD-ROM. These electronic editions provide a searchable PDF version of each book as well as the raw data in .dbf, Excel and ASCII formats. Additional information about all of our publications is available online at www.statestats.com or by calling 1-800-457-0742.

Finally, many thanks to the librarians, government and health care industry officials who help us year after year. Thanks also to you, our readers. We always welcome your thoughts and suggestions, so please give us a call, send us an e-mail or drop us a note with your ideas.

- THE EDITORS

WHICH STATE IS HEALTHIEST?

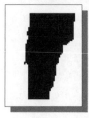

Vermont has reclaimed its title as the nation's Healthiest State. This year marks the fourth time in the 13 years of Morgan Quitno's Healthiest State Award that Vermont has ranked as the No. 1 state. Last year's winner, New Hampshire, slipped to second place, followed by Massachusetts, Minnesota and Maine.

At the opposite end of the rankings scale, Louisiana broke Mississippi's five-year string of last place finishes to earn the designation as the nation's least healthy state. The last time Louisiana ranked 50th was in 1999. Mississippi moved up to 49th and is preceded by New Mexico in 48th, Nevada in 47th and Oklahoma in 46th.

Methodology

The Healthiest State designation is awarded based on 21 factors chosen from the 2005 edition of our annual reference book, *Health Care State Rankings*. These factors reflect access to health care providers, affordability of health care and a generally healthy population (see box below.)

For this year's award, three factors were changed. Dropped due to a lack of updated

2005 HEALTHIEST STATE AWARD

RANK	STATE	SUM	04	RANK	STATE	SUM	04
1	Vermont	22.67	2	26	Ohio	3.12	24
2	New Hampshire	21.40	1	27	Colorado	1.61	27
3	Massachusetts	18.69	8	28	West Virginia	1.23	34
4	Minnesota	16.30	5	29	Maryland	0.77	32
5	Maine	16.06	9	30	Wyoming	(0.19)	16
6	Iowa	14.57	4	31	New York	(0.64)	33
7	Utah	14.19	6	32	Kentucky	(0.86)	29
8	Hawaii	13.71	3	33	North Carolina	(1.03)	30
9	Nebraska	12.82	7	34	Illinois	(1.17)	31
10	Connecticut	12.63	10	35	Delaware	(1.49)	44
11	North Dakota	11.47	12	36	Missouri	(2.89)	37
12	Rhode Island	10.51	18	37	Alaska	(4.98)	35
13	Washington	9.87	13	38	Tennessee	(5.00)	36
14	Wisconsin	8.07	21	39	Arizona	(5.78)	40
15	Kansas	7.85	17	40	Arkansas	(5.93)	38
16	New Jersey	7.71	11	41	Alabama	(9.97)	47
17	Virginia	6.74	22	42	Georgia	(10.00)	42
18	California	6.51	14	43	South Carolina	(10.63)	46
19	Oregon	5.92	15	44	Florida	(11.21)	41
20	Idaho	5.42	20	45	Texas	(11.85)	42
21	Pennsylvania	5.33	26	46	Oklahoma	(12.07)	39
22	South Dakota	5.29	19	47	Nevada	(13.37)	45
23	Michigan	3.73	25	48	New Mexico	(17.69)	49
24	Indiana	3.33	28	49	Mississippi	(18.43)	50
25	Montana	3.19	23	50	Louisiana	(20.95)	48

data were per capita personal health expenditures, health care expenditures as a percent of gross state product and the number of days in the past month when physical health was "not good." In their place, three new factors were added: the average annual health insurance premium for family coverage, the percent of children not covered by health insurance and the percent of adults who exercise vigorously. As in previous years, the 21 factors were divided into two groups: those that are "negative" for which a high ranking would be considered bad for a state, and those that are "positive" for which a high ranking would be considered good for a state. Rates for each of the 21 factors were processed through a formula that measures how a state compares to the national average for a given category. The positive and negative nature of each factor was taken into account as part of the formula. Once these computations were made, the factors then were weighted equally. These weighted scores then were added together to get a state's final score ("SUM" on the table above). This way, states are assessed based on how they stack up against the national average. The end result is that the farther below the national average a state's health ranking is, the lower (and less healthy) it ranks. The farther above the national average, the higher (and healthier) a state ranks. This same methodology is used for our Dangerous State and Safest/Dangerous City Awards.

The table above shows how each state fared in the 2005 Healthiest State Award as well as its placement in 2004. While we never claim our findings are indisputable, we do believe they provide an interesting statistical match-up of how states are doing with regard to health care. Congratulations to the citizens of Vermont for their healthy comeback!　　　　- THE EDITORS

POSITIVE (+) AND NEGATIVE (-) FACTORS CONSIDERED:

1. Births of Low Birthweight as a Percent of All Births (Table 13) -
2. Teenage Birth Rate (Table 32) -
3. Percent of Mothers Receiving Late or No Prenatal Care (Table 60) -
4. Age-Adjusted Death Rate (Table 84) -
5. Infant Mortality Rate (Table 88) -
6. Age-Adjusted Death Rate by Malignant Neoplasms (Table 149) -
7. Age-Adjusted Death Rate by Suicide (Table 173) -
8. Average Annual Family Coverage Health Insurance Premium (Table 234) -
9. Percent of Population Not Covered by Health Insurance (Table 238) -
10. Percent of Children Not Covered by Health Insurance (Table 242) -
11. Estimated Rate of New Cancer Cases (Table 318) -

12. AIDS Rate (Table 347) -
13. Sexually Transmitted Disease Rate (Table 384) -
14. Percent of Population Lacking Access to Primary Care (Table 410) -
15. Percent of Adults Who Are Binge Drinkers (Table 491) -
16. Percent of Adults Who Smoke (Table 492) -
17. Percent of Adults Obese (Table 498) -
18. Beds in Community Hospitals per 100,000 Population (Table 195) +
19. Percent of Children Aged 19-35 Months Immunized (Table 380) +
20. Percent of Adults Who Exercise Vigorously (Table 501) +
21. Safety Belt Usage Rate (Table 512) +

TABLE OF CONTENTS

I. Births and Reproductive Health

TABLE OF CONTENTS (continued)

Abortions

II. Deaths

TABLE OF CONTENTS (continued)

TABLE OF CONTENTS (continued)

TABLE OF CONTENTS (continued)

TABLE OF CONTENTS (continued)

V. Incidence of Disease

TABLE OF CONTENTS (continued)

VI. Providers

TABLE OF CONTENTS (continued)

TABLE OF CONTENTS (continued)

VII. Physical Fitness

VIII. Appendix

IX. Sources

X. Index

I. BIRTHS AND REPRODUCTIVE HEALTH

1   Births in 2003
2   Birth Rate in 2003
3   Percent Change in Birth Rate: 1994 to 2003
4   Ratio of Male to Female Births in 2002
5   Fertility Rate in 2003
6   Births to White Women in 2003
7   White Births as a Percent of All Births in 2003
8   Births to Black Women in 2003
9   Black Births as a Percent of All Births in 2003
10   Births to Hispanic Women in 2003
11   Hispanic Births as a Percent of All Births in 2003
12   Births of Low Birthweight in 2003
13   Births of Low Birthweight as a Percent of All Births in 2003
14   Births of Low Birthweight to White Women in 2003
15   Births of Low Birthweight to White Women as a Percent of All Births to White Women in 2003
16   Births of Low Birthweight to Black Women in 2003
17   Births of Low Birthweight to Black Women as a Percent of All Births to Black Women in 2003
18   Births of Low Birthweight to Hispanic Women in 2003
19   Births of Low Birthweight to Hispanic Women as a Percent of All Births to Hispanic Women in 2003
20   Births to Unmarried Women in 2003
21   Births to Unmarried Women as a Percent of All Births in 2003
22   Births to Unmarried White Women in 2003
23   Births to Unmarried White Women as a Percent of All Births to White Women in 2003
24   Births to Unmarried Black Women in 2003
25   Births to Unmarried Black Women as a Percent of All Births to Black Women in 2003
26   Births to Unmarried Hispanic Women in 2003
27   Births to Unmarried Hispanic Women as a Percent of All Births to Hispanic Women in 2003
28   Pregnancy Rate in 2001
29   Pregnancy Rate for 15 to 19 Year Old Women in 2001
30   Percent Change in Pregnancy Rate for 15 to 19 Year Old Women: 1997 to 2001
31   Births to Teenage Mothers in 2003
32   Teenage Birth Rate in 2003
33   Births to Teenage Mothers as a Percent of Births in 2003
34   Percent Change in Teenage Birth Rate: 1999 to 2003
35   Births to White Teenage Mothers in 2003
36   White Teenage Birth Rate in 2003
37   Births to White Teenage Mothers as a Percent of White Births in 2003
38   Births to Black Teenage Mothers in 2003
39   Black Teenage Birth Rate in 2003
40   Births to Black Teenage Mothers as a Percent of Black Births in 2003
41   Births to Young Teenagers: 2000 to 2002
42   Young Teen Birthrate: 2000 to 2002
43   Births to Women 35 to 54 Years Old in 2002
44   Births to Women 35 to 54 Years Old as a Percent of All Births in 2002
45   Births by Vaginal Delivery in 2003
46   Percent of Births by Vaginal Delivery in 2003
47   Births by Cesarean Delivery in 2003
48   Percent of Births by Cesarean Delivery in 2003
49   Percent Change in Rate of Cesarean Births: 1999 to 2003
50   Percent of Vaginal Births After a Cesarean (VBAC) in 2002
51   Assisted Reproductive Technology Procedures in 2001
52   Infants Born from Assisted Reproductive Technology Procedures in 2001
53   Percent of Assisted Reproductive Technology Procedures that Resulted in Live Births in 2001
54   Percent of Total Live Births Resulting from Assisted Reproductive Technology Procedures (ARTP) in 2001
55   Percent of Infants Born in Multiple-Birth Deliveries as a Percent of All Infants Born Through ARTP in 2001
56   Percent of Mothers Beginning Prenatal Care in First Trimester in 2003
57   Percent of White Mothers Beginning Prenatal Care in First Trimester in 2003
58   Percent of Black Mothers Beginning Prenatal Care in First Trimester in 2003
59   Percent of Hispanic Mothers Beginning Prenatal Care in First Trimester in 2003
60   Percent of Mothers Receiving Late or No Prenatal Care in 2002
61   Percent of White Mothers Receiving Late or No Prenatal Care in 2002
62   Percent of Black Mothers Receiving Late or No Prenatal Care in 2002
63   Percent of Hispanic Mothers Receiving Late or No Prenatal Care in 2002

I. BIRTHS AND REPRODUCTIVE HEALTH (CONTINUED)

Abortions

Births in 2003

National Total = 4,091,063 Live Births*

ALPHA ORDER

RANK	STATE	BIRTHS	% of USA
24	Alabama	59,621	1.5%
47	Alaska	10,122	0.2%
13	Arizona	91,005	2.2%
34	Arkansas	38,159	0.9%
1	California	540,995	13.2%
22	Colorado	69,363	1.7%
30	Connecticut	42,848	1.0%
45	Delaware	11,264	0.3%
4	Florida	212,286	5.2%
8	Georgia	136,012	3.3%
40	Hawaii	18,114	0.4%
38	Idaho	21,802	0.5%
5	Illinois	182,590	4.5%
14	Indiana	86,600	2.1%
33	Iowa	38,182	0.9%
32	Kansas	39,493	1.0%
26	Kentucky	55,281	1.4%
23	Louisiana	65,298	1.6%
42	Maine	13,861	0.3%
19	Maryland	74,856	1.8%
16	Massachusetts	80,250	2.0%
9	Michigan	130,937	3.2%
20	Minnesota	70,157	1.7%
31	Mississippi	42,362	1.0%
18	Missouri	77,079	1.9%
44	Montana	11,416	0.3%
37	Nebraska	25,924	0.6%
35	Nevada	33,644	0.8%
41	New Hampshire	14,393	0.4%
11	New Jersey	116,269	2.8%
36	New Mexico	27,845	0.7%
3	New York	254,187	6.2%
10	North Carolina	118,308	2.9%
48	North Dakota	7,975	0.2%
6	Ohio	151,983	3.7%
27	Oklahoma	50,484	1.2%
29	Oregon	45,975	1.1%
7	Pennsylvania	140,660	3.4%
43	Rhode Island	13,192	0.3%
25	South Carolina	55,658	1.4%
46	South Dakota	11,035	0.3%
17	Tennessee	78,901	1.9%
2	Texas	381,239	9.3%
28	Utah	49,870	1.2%
50	Vermont	6,591	0.2%
12	Virginia	101,226	2.5%
15	Washington	80,474	2.0%
39	West Virginia	20,908	0.5%
21	Wisconsin	70,053	1.7%
49	Wyoming	6,708	0.2%

RANK ORDER

RANK	STATE	BIRTHS	% of USA
1	California	540,995	13.2%
2	Texas	381,239	9.3%
3	New York	254,187	6.2%
4	Florida	212,286	5.2%
5	Illinois	182,590	4.5%
6	Ohio	151,983	3.7%
7	Pennsylvania	140,660	3.4%
8	Georgia	136,012	3.3%
9	Michigan	130,937	3.2%
10	North Carolina	118,308	2.9%
11	New Jersey	116,269	2.8%
12	Virginia	101,226	2.5%
13	Arizona	91,005	2.2%
14	Indiana	86,600	2.1%
15	Washington	80,474	2.0%
16	Massachusetts	80,250	2.0%
17	Tennessee	78,901	1.9%
18	Missouri	77,079	1.9%
19	Maryland	74,856	1.8%
20	Minnesota	70,157	1.7%
21	Wisconsin	70,053	1.7%
22	Colorado	69,363	1.7%
23	Louisiana	65,298	1.6%
24	Alabama	59,621	1.5%
25	South Carolina	55,658	1.4%
26	Kentucky	55,281	1.4%
27	Oklahoma	50,484	1.2%
28	Utah	49,870	1.2%
29	Oregon	45,975	1.1%
30	Connecticut	42,848	1.0%
31	Mississippi	42,362	1.0%
32	Kansas	39,493	1.0%
33	Iowa	38,182	0.9%
34	Arkansas	38,159	0.9%
35	Nevada	33,644	0.8%
36	New Mexico	27,845	0.7%
37	Nebraska	25,924	0.6%
38	Idaho	21,802	0.5%
39	West Virginia	20,908	0.5%
40	Hawaii	18,114	0.4%
41	New Hampshire	14,393	0.4%
42	Maine	13,861	0.3%
43	Rhode Island	13,192	0.3%
44	Montana	11,416	0.3%
45	Delaware	11,264	0.3%
46	South Dakota	11,035	0.3%
47	Alaska	10,122	0.2%
48	North Dakota	7,975	0.2%
49	Wyoming	6,708	0.2%
50	Vermont	6,591	0.2%
	District of Columbia	7,606	0.2%

Source: U.S. Department of Health and Human Services, National Center for Health Statistics
    "National Vital Statistics Reports" (Vol. 53, No. 9, November 23, 2004)
*Final data by state of residence.

Birth Rate in 2003

National Rate = 14.1 Live Births per 1,000 Population*

ALPHA ORDER

RANK ORDER

RANK	STATE	RATE	RANK	STATE	RATE
33	Alabama	13.2	1	Utah	21.2
6	Alaska	15.6	2	Texas	17.2
3	Arizona	16.3	3	Arizona	16.3
20	Arkansas	14.0	4	Idaho	16.0
7	California	15.2	5	Georgia	15.7
7	Colorado	15.2	6	Alaska	15.6
44	Connecticut	12.3	7	California	15.2
23	Delaware	13.8	7	Colorado	15.2
41	Florida	12.5	9	Nevada	15.0
5	Georgia	15.7	10	Nebraska	14.9
15	Hawaii	14.4	10	New Mexico	14.9
4	Idaho	16.0	12	Mississippi	14.7
15	Illinois	14.4	13	Kansas	14.5
20	Indiana	14.0	13	Louisiana	14.5
36	Iowa	13.0	15	Hawaii	14.4
13	Kansas	14.5	15	Illinois	14.4
29	Kentucky	13.4	15	Oklahoma	14.4
13	Louisiana	14.5	15	South Dakota	14.4
49	Maine	10.6	19	North Carolina	14.1
25	Maryland	13.6	20	Arkansas	14.0
41	Massachusetts	12.5	20	Indiana	14.0
36	Michigan	13.0	22	Minnesota	13.9
22	Minnesota	13.9	23	Delaware	13.8
12	Mississippi	14.7	24	Virginia	13.7
26	Missouri	13.5	25	Maryland	13.6
43	Montana	12.4	26	Missouri	13.5
10	Nebraska	14.9	26	New Jersey	13.5
9	Nevada	15.0	26	Tennessee	13.5
48	New Hampshire	11.2	29	Kentucky	13.4
26	New Jersey	13.5	29	South Carolina	13.4
10	New Mexico	14.9	29	Wyoming	13.4
33	New York	13.2	32	Ohio	13.3
19	North Carolina	14.1	33	Alabama	13.2
40	North Dakota	12.6	33	New York	13.2
32	Ohio	13.3	35	Washington	13.1
15	Oklahoma	14.4	36	Iowa	13.0
38	Oregon	12.9	36	Michigan	13.0
47	Pennsylvania	11.4	38	Oregon	12.9
44	Rhode Island	12.3	39	Wisconsin	12.8
29	South Carolina	13.4	40	North Dakota	12.6
15	South Dakota	14.4	41	Florida	12.5
26	Tennessee	13.5	41	Massachusetts	12.5
2	Texas	17.2	43	Montana	12.4
1	Utah	21.2	44	Connecticut	12.3
49	Vermont	10.6	44	Rhode Island	12.3
24	Virginia	13.7	46	West Virginia	11.5
35	Washington	13.1	47	Pennsylvania	11.4
46	West Virginia	11.5	48	New Hampshire	11.2
39	Wisconsin	12.8	49	Maine	10.6
29	Wyoming	13.4	49	Vermont	10.6
				District of Columbia	13.5

Source: U.S. Department of Health and Human Services, National Center for Health Statistics
    "National Vital Statistics Reports" (Vol. 53, No. 9, November 23, 2004)
*Final data by state of residence.

Percent Change in Birth Rate: 1994 to 2003

National Percent Change = 7.2% Decrease*

ALPHA ORDER

RANK	STATE	PERCENT CHANGE
32	Alabama	(8.3)
43	Alaska	(11.4)
27	Arizona	(6.3)
10	Arkansas	(1.4)
49	California	(16.0)
5	Colorado	2.7
44	Connecticut	(11.5)
26	Delaware	(6.1)
35	Florida	(8.8)
6	Georgia	0.0
46	Hawaii	(13.3)
3	Idaho	3.2
41	Illinois	(10.6)
16	Indiana	(2.8)
9	Iowa	(0.8)
7	Kansas	(0.7)
17	Kentucky	(2.9)
30	Louisiana	(7.6)
34	Maine	(8.6)
31	Maryland	(8.1)
39	Massachusetts	(10.1)
40	Michigan	(10.3)
10	Minnesota	(1.4)
28	Mississippi	(6.4)
17	Missouri	(2.9)
19	Montana	(3.9)
2	Nebraska	4.2
33	Nevada	(8.5)
48	New Hampshire	(15.8)
37	New Jersey	(9.4)
42	New Mexico	(10.8)
47	New York	(13.7)
10	North Carolina	(1.4)
29	North Dakota	(6.7)
22	Ohio	(5.0)
4	Oklahoma	2.9
23	Oregon	(5.1)
45	Pennsylvania	(12.3)
36	Rhode Island	(8.9)
25	South Carolina	(5.6)
10	South Dakota	(1.4)
20	Tennessee	(4.3)
14	Texas	(1.7)
1	Utah	5.5
50	Vermont	(16.5)
24	Virginia	(5.5)
38	Washington	(9.7)
14	West Virginia	(1.7)
21	Wisconsin	(4.5)
7	Wyoming	(0.7)

RANK ORDER

RANK	STATE	PERCENT CHANGE
1	Utah	5.5
2	Nebraska	4.2
3	Idaho	3.2
4	Oklahoma	2.9
5	Colorado	2.7
6	Georgia	0.0
7	Kansas	(0.7)
7	Wyoming	(0.7)
9	Iowa	(0.8)
10	Arkansas	(1.4)
10	Minnesota	(1.4)
10	North Carolina	(1.4)
10	South Dakota	(1.4)
14	Texas	(1.7)
14	West Virginia	(1.7)
16	Indiana	(2.8)
17	Kentucky	(2.9)
17	Missouri	(2.9)
19	Montana	(3.9)
20	Tennessee	(4.3)
21	Wisconsin	(4.5)
22	Ohio	(5.0)
23	Oregon	(5.1)
24	Virginia	(5.5)
25	South Carolina	(5.6)
26	Delaware	(6.1)
27	Arizona	(6.3)
28	Mississippi	(6.4)
29	North Dakota	(6.7)
30	Louisiana	(7.6)
31	Maryland	(8.1)
32	Alabama	(8.3)
33	Nevada	(8.5)
34	Maine	(8.6)
35	Florida	(8.8)
36	Rhode Island	(8.9)
37	New Jersey	(9.4)
38	Washington	(9.7)
39	Massachusetts	(10.1)
40	Michigan	(10.3)
41	Illinois	(10.6)
42	New Mexico	(10.8)
43	Alaska	(11.4)
44	Connecticut	(11.5)
45	Pennsylvania	(12.3)
46	Hawaii	(13.3)
47	New York	(13.7)
48	New Hampshire	(15.8)
49	California	(16.0)
50	Vermont	(16.5)

District of Columbia (22.4)

*Source: Morgan Quitno Press using data from U.S. Department of Health and Human Services
"National Vital Statistics Reports" (Vol. 53, No. 9, November 23, 2004)
"Monthly Vital Statistics Report" (Vol. 44, No. 11s, Supplement, June 24, 1996)*
Final data by state of residence.

Ratio of Male to Female Births in 2002

National Ratio = 1,047 Male Births for Every 1,000 Female Births*

ALPHA ORDER

RANK	STATE	RATIO
44	Alabama	1,041
14	Alaska	1,053
33	Arizona	1,046
18	Arkansas	1,050
33	California	1,046
14	Colorado	1,053
10	Connecticut	1,055
6	Delaware	1,057
30	Florida	1,047
47	Georgia	1,038
1	Hawaii	1,075
49	Idaho	1,035
37	Illinois	1,045
18	Indiana	1,050
23	Iowa	1,049
23	Kansas	1,049
9	Kentucky	1,056
30	Louisiana	1,047
6	Maine	1,057
37	Maryland	1,045
41	Massachusetts	1,042
17	Michigan	1,052
23	Minnesota	1,049
33	Mississippi	1,046
28	Missouri	1,048
48	Montana	1,037
46	Nebraska	1,040
6	Nevada	1,057
3	New Hampshire	1,063
14	New Jersey	1,053
50	New Mexico	1,030
18	New York	1,050
41	North Carolina	1,042
5	North Dakota	1,058
18	Ohio	1,050
10	Oklahoma	1,055
23	Oregon	1,049
33	Pennsylvania	1,046
2	Rhode Island	1,064
30	South Carolina	1,047
41	South Dakota	1,042
28	Tennessee	1,048
37	Texas	1,045
10	Utah	1,055
18	Vermont	1,050
40	Virginia	1,043
23	Washington	1,049
4	West Virginia	1,060
44	Wisconsin	1,041
13	Wyoming	1,054

RANK ORDER

RANK	STATE	RATIO
1	Hawaii	1,075
2	Rhode Island	1,064
3	New Hampshire	1,063
4	West Virginia	1,060
5	North Dakota	1,058
6	Delaware	1,057
6	Maine	1,057
6	Nevada	1,057
9	Kentucky	1,056
10	Connecticut	1,055
10	Oklahoma	1,055
10	Utah	1,055
13	Wyoming	1,054
14	Alaska	1,053
14	Colorado	1,053
14	New Jersey	1,053
17	Michigan	1,052
18	Arkansas	1,050
18	Indiana	1,050
18	New York	1,050
18	Ohio	1,050
18	Vermont	1,050
23	Iowa	1,049
23	Kansas	1,049
23	Minnesota	1,049
23	Oregon	1,049
23	Washington	1,049
28	Missouri	1,048
28	Tennessee	1,048
30	Florida	1,047
30	Louisiana	1,047
30	South Carolina	1,047
33	Arizona	1,046
33	California	1,046
33	Mississippi	1,046
33	Pennsylvania	1,046
37	Illinois	1,045
37	Maryland	1,045
37	Texas	1,045
40	Virginia	1,043
41	Massachusetts	1,042
41	North Carolina	1,042
41	South Dakota	1,042
44	Alabama	1,041
44	Wisconsin	1,041
46	Nebraska	1,040
47	Georgia	1,038
48	Montana	1,037
49	Idaho	1,035
50	New Mexico	1,030
	District of Columbia	1,037

Source: U.S. Department of Health and Human Services, National Center for Health Statistics
    "National Vital Statistics Reports" (Vol. 52, No. 19, May 10, 2004)
*Three-year average for years 2000 through 2002.

Fertility Rate in 2003

National Rate = 66.1 Live Births per 1,000 Women 15 to 44 Years Old*

ALPHA ORDER

RANK	STATE	RATE
34	Alabama	62.6
5	Alaska	72.7
2	Arizona	79.3
16	Arkansas	68.1
11	California	69.9
12	Colorado	69.5
43	Connecticut	59.6
24	Delaware	64.3
28	Florida	63.4
14	Georgia	69.3
6	Hawaii	72.3
4	Idaho	76.0
18	Illinois	67.0
19	Indiana	66.5
29	Iowa	63.3
12	Kansas	69.5
31	Kentucky	63.2
20	Louisiana	66.4
49	Maine	52.1
37	Maryland	62.3
45	Massachusetts	57.2
38	Michigan	61.6
25	Minnesota	64.2
17	Mississippi	67.9
26	Missouri	64.1
34	Montana	62.6
9	Nebraska	71.4
7	Nevada	72.2
48	New Hampshire	52.7
23	New Jersey	64.5
8	New Mexico	71.5
41	New York	61.1
21	North Carolina	65.8
38	North Dakota	61.6
27	Ohio	63.7
15	Oklahoma	69.2
36	Oregon	62.5
47	Pennsylvania	56.0
46	Rhode Island	56.5
33	South Carolina	63.0
10	South Dakota	70.8
32	Tennessee	63.1
3	Texas	78.3
1	Utah	92.2
50	Vermont	51.1
29	Virginia	63.3
40	Washington	61.2
44	West Virginia	58.1
42	Wisconsin	60.7
22	Wyoming	65.7

RANK ORDER

RANK	STATE	RATE
1	Utah	92.2
2	Arizona	79.3
3	Texas	78.3
4	Idaho	76.0
5	Alaska	72.7
6	Hawaii	72.3
7	Nevada	72.2
8	New Mexico	71.5
9	Nebraska	71.4
10	South Dakota	70.8
11	California	69.9
12	Colorado	69.5
12	Kansas	69.5
14	Georgia	69.3
15	Oklahoma	69.2
16	Arkansas	68.1
17	Mississippi	67.9
18	Illinois	67.0
19	Indiana	66.5
20	Louisiana	66.4
21	North Carolina	65.8
22	Wyoming	65.7
23	New Jersey	64.5
24	Delaware	64.3
25	Minnesota	64.2
26	Missouri	64.1
27	Ohio	63.7
28	Florida	63.4
29	Iowa	63.3
29	Virginia	63.3
31	Kentucky	63.2
32	Tennessee	63.1
33	South Carolina	63.0
34	Alabama	62.6
34	Montana	62.6
36	Oregon	62.5
37	Maryland	62.3
38	Michigan	61.6
38	North Dakota	61.6
40	Washington	61.2
41	New York	61.1
42	Wisconsin	60.7
43	Connecticut	59.6
44	West Virginia	58.1
45	Massachusetts	57.2
46	Rhode Island	56.5
47	Pennsylvania	56.0
48	New Hampshire	52.7
49	Maine	52.1
50	Vermont	51.1
	District of Columbia	53.8

Source: U.S. Department of Health and Human Services, National Center for Health Statistics
"National Vital Statistics Reports" (Vol. 53, No. 9, November 23, 2004)
*Final data by state of residence.

Births to White Women in 2003

National Total = 3,227,755 Live Births to White Women*

ALPHA ORDER

RANK	STATE	BIRTHS	% of USA
26	Alabama	40,912	1.3%
47	Alaska	6,491	0.2%
12	Arizona	78,966	2.4%
33	Arkansas	30,048	0.9%
1	California	438,035	13.6%
18	Colorado	63,189	2.0%
31	Connecticut	35,372	1.1%
45	Delaware	7,903	0.2%
4	Florida	158,053	4.9%
9	Georgia	88,085	2.7%
50	Hawaii	4,831	0.1%
38	Idaho	20,972	0.6%
5	Illinois	142,216	4.4%
13	Indiana	75,688	2.3%
30	Iowa	35,692	1.1%
32	Kansas	35,019	1.1%
22	Kentucky	49,457	1.5%
28	Louisiana	37,459	1.2%
41	Maine	13,371	0.4%
24	Maryland	45,780	1.4%
16	Massachusetts	66,061	2.0%
8	Michigan	103,042	3.2%
21	Minnesota	59,491	1.8%
35	Mississippi	23,575	0.7%
17	Missouri	63,814	2.0%
43	Montana	9,833	0.3%
36	Nebraska	23,382	0.7%
34	Nevada	27,693	0.9%
40	New Hampshire	13,646	0.4%
11	New Jersey	85,278	2.6%
37	New Mexico	23,306	0.7%
3	New York	184,059	5.7%
10	North Carolina	86,395	2.7%
46	North Dakota	6,893	0.2%
6	Ohio	125,476	3.9%
27	Oklahoma	39,578	1.2%
25	Oregon	41,590	1.3%
7	Pennsylvania	114,043	3.5%
42	Rhode Island	11,208	0.3%
29	South Carolina	36,266	1.1%
44	South Dakota	8,910	0.3%
19	Tennessee	60,982	1.9%
2	Texas	324,790	10.1%
23	Utah	47,338	1.5%
48	Vermont	6,413	0.2%
14	Virginia	71,900	2.2%
15	Washington	66,569	2.1%
39	West Virginia	20,005	0.6%
20	Wisconsin	60,256	1.9%
49	Wyoming	6,299	0.2%

RANK ORDER

RANK	STATE	BIRTHS	% of USA
1	California	438,035	13.6%
2	Texas	324,790	10.1%
3	New York	184,059	5.7%
4	Florida	158,053	4.9%
5	Illinois	142,216	4.4%
6	Ohio	125,476	3.9%
7	Pennsylvania	114,043	3.5%
8	Michigan	103,042	3.2%
9	Georgia	88,085	2.7%
10	North Carolina	86,395	2.7%
11	New Jersey	85,278	2.6%
12	Arizona	78,966	2.4%
13	Indiana	75,688	2.3%
14	Virginia	71,900	2.2%
15	Washington	66,569	2.1%
16	Massachusetts	66,061	2.0%
17	Missouri	63,814	2.0%
18	Colorado	63,189	2.0%
19	Tennessee	60,982	1.9%
20	Wisconsin	60,256	1.9%
21	Minnesota	59,491	1.8%
22	Kentucky	49,457	1.5%
23	Utah	47,338	1.5%
24	Maryland	45,780	1.4%
25	Oregon	41,590	1.3%
26	Alabama	40,912	1.3%
27	Oklahoma	39,578	1.2%
28	Louisiana	37,459	1.2%
29	South Carolina	36,266	1.1%
30	Iowa	35,692	1.1%
31	Connecticut	35,372	1.1%
32	Kansas	35,019	1.1%
33	Arkansas	30,048	0.9%
34	Nevada	27,693	0.9%
35	Mississippi	23,575	0.7%
36	Nebraska	23,382	0.7%
37	New Mexico	23,306	0.7%
38	Idaho	20,972	0.6%
39	West Virginia	20,005	0.6%
40	New Hampshire	13,646	0.4%
41	Maine	13,371	0.4%
42	Rhode Island	11,208	0.3%
43	Montana	9,833	0.3%
44	South Dakota	8,910	0.3%
45	Delaware	7,903	0.2%
46	North Dakota	6,893	0.2%
47	Alaska	6,491	0.2%
48	Vermont	6,413	0.2%
49	Wyoming	6,299	0.2%
50	Hawaii	4,831	0.1%
	District of Columbia	2,125	0.1%

Source: U.S. Department of Health and Human Services, National Center for Health Statistics
    "National Vital Statistics Reports" (Vol. 53, No. 9, November 23, 2004)
*Final data by state of residence. By race of mother.

White Births as a Percent of All Births in 2003

National Percent = 78.9% of Live Births*

ALPHA ORDER

RANK	STATE	PERCENT
43	Alabama	68.6
46	Alaska	64.1
15	Arizona	86.8
32	Arkansas	78.7
30	California	81.0
9	Colorado	91.1
25	Connecticut	82.6
42	Delaware	70.2
37	Florida	74.5
45	Georgia	64.8
50	Hawaii	26.7
3	Idaho	96.2
35	Illinois	77.9
14	Indiana	87.4
8	Iowa	93.5
13	Kansas	88.7
12	Kentucky	89.5
48	Louisiana	57.4
2	Maine	96.5
47	Maryland	61.2
27	Massachusetts	82.3
32	Michigan	78.7
21	Minnesota	84.8
49	Mississippi	55.7
23	Missouri	82.8
17	Montana	86.1
11	Nebraska	90.2
27	Nevada	82.3
6	New Hampshire	94.8
38	New Jersey	73.3
22	New Mexico	83.7
40	New York	72.4
39	North Carolina	73.0
16	North Dakota	86.4
25	Ohio	82.6
34	Oklahoma	78.4
10	Oregon	90.5
29	Pennsylvania	81.1
20	Rhode Island	85.0
44	South Carolina	65.2
31	South Dakota	80.7
36	Tennessee	77.3
19	Texas	85.2
5	Utah	94.9
1	Vermont	97.3
41	Virginia	71.0
24	Washington	82.7
4	West Virginia	95.7
18	Wisconsin	86.0
7	Wyoming	93.9

RANK ORDER

RANK	STATE	PERCENT
1	Vermont	97.3
2	Maine	96.5
3	Idaho	96.2
4	West Virginia	95.7
5	Utah	94.9
6	New Hampshire	94.8
7	Wyoming	93.9
8	Iowa	93.5
9	Colorado	91.1
10	Oregon	90.5
11	Nebraska	90.2
12	Kentucky	89.5
13	Kansas	88.7
14	Indiana	87.4
15	Arizona	86.8
16	North Dakota	86.4
17	Montana	86.1
18	Wisconsin	86.0
19	Texas	85.2
20	Rhode Island	85.0
21	Minnesota	84.8
22	New Mexico	83.7
23	Missouri	82.8
24	Washington	82.7
25	Connecticut	82.6
25	Ohio	82.6
27	Massachusetts	82.3
27	Nevada	82.3
29	Pennsylvania	81.1
30	California	81.0
31	South Dakota	80.7
32	Arkansas	78.7
32	Michigan	78.7
34	Oklahoma	78.4
35	Illinois	77.9
36	Tennessee	77.3
37	Florida	74.5
38	New Jersey	73.3
39	North Carolina	73.0
40	New York	72.4
41	Virginia	71.0
42	Delaware	70.2
43	Alabama	68.6
44	South Carolina	65.2
45	Georgia	64.8
46	Alaska	64.1
47	Maryland	61.2
48	Louisiana	57.4
49	Mississippi	55.7
50	Hawaii	26.7

District of Columbia 27.9

Source: Morgan Quitno Press using data from U.S. Dept. of Health and Human Services, Nat'l Center for Health Statistics
    "National Vital Statistics Reports" (Vol. 53, No. 9, November 23, 2004)
*Final data by state of residence. By race of mother.

Births to Black Women in 2003

National Total = 599,414 Live Births to Black Women*

ALPHA ORDER

RANK	STATE	BIRTHS	% of USA
17	Alabama	17,959	3.0%
41	Alaska	406	0.1%
29	Arizona	3,279	0.5%
22	Arkansas	7,307	1.2%
5	California	32,676	5.5%
30	Colorado	2,938	0.5%
25	Connecticut	5,184	0.9%
32	Delaware	2,883	0.5%
2	Florida	47,349	7.9%
3	Georgia	43,059	7.2%
40	Hawaii	519	0.1%
47	Idaho	108	0.0%
6	Illinois	31,602	5.3%
20	Indiana	9,387	1.6%
35	Iowa	1,287	0.2%
33	Kansas	2,765	0.5%
26	Kentucky	4,859	0.8%
8	Louisiana	26,328	4.4%
44	Maine	184	0.0%
9	Maryland	24,776	4.1%
21	Massachusetts	8,606	1.4%
12	Michigan	22,574	3.8%
24	Minnesota	5,378	0.9%
15	Mississippi	18,367	3.1%
19	Missouri	11,163	1.9%
50	Montana	51	0.0%
34	Nebraska	1,467	0.2%
31	Nevada	2,905	0.5%
43	New Hampshire	244	0.0%
14	New Jersey	20,120	3.4%
39	New Mexico	533	0.1%
1	New York	48,098	8.0%
7	North Carolina	27,170	4.5%
46	North Dakota	109	0.0%
10	Ohio	23,059	3.8%
27	Oklahoma	4,568	0.8%
37	Oregon	1,024	0.2%
13	Pennsylvania	21,333	3.6%
36	Rhode Island	1,260	0.2%
16	South Carolina	18,345	3.1%
45	South Dakota	122	0.0%
18	Tennessee	16,250	2.7%
4	Texas	42,245	7.0%
42	Utah	384	0.1%
48	Vermont	54	0.0%
11	Virginia	22,605	3.8%
28	Washington	4,029	0.7%
38	West Virginia	722	0.1%
23	Wisconsin	6,496	1.1%
49	Wyoming	53	0.0%

RANK ORDER

RANK	STATE	BIRTHS	% of USA
1	New York	48,098	8.0%
2	Florida	47,349	7.9%
3	Georgia	43,059	7.2%
4	Texas	42,245	7.0%
5	California	32,676	5.5%
6	Illinois	31,602	5.3%
7	North Carolina	27,170	4.5%
8	Louisiana	26,328	4.4%
9	Maryland	24,776	4.1%
10	Ohio	23,059	3.8%
11	Virginia	22,605	3.8%
12	Michigan	22,574	3.8%
13	Pennsylvania	21,333	3.6%
14	New Jersey	20,120	3.4%
15	Mississippi	18,367	3.1%
16	South Carolina	18,345	3.1%
17	Alabama	17,959	3.0%
18	Tennessee	16,250	2.7%
19	Missouri	11,163	1.9%
20	Indiana	9,387	1.6%
21	Massachusetts	8,606	1.4%
22	Arkansas	7,307	1.2%
23	Wisconsin	6,496	1.1%
24	Minnesota	5,378	0.9%
25	Connecticut	5,184	0.9%
26	Kentucky	4,859	0.8%
27	Oklahoma	4,568	0.8%
28	Washington	4,029	0.7%
29	Arizona	3,279	0.5%
30	Colorado	2,938	0.5%
31	Nevada	2,905	0.5%
32	Delaware	2,883	0.5%
33	Kansas	2,765	0.5%
34	Nebraska	1,467	0.2%
35	Iowa	1,287	0.2%
36	Rhode Island	1,260	0.2%
37	Oregon	1,024	0.2%
38	West Virginia	722	0.1%
39	New Mexico	533	0.1%
40	Hawaii	519	0.1%
41	Alaska	406	0.1%
42	Utah	384	0.1%
43	New Hampshire	244	0.0%
44	Maine	184	0.0%
45	South Dakota	122	0.0%
46	North Dakota	109	0.0%
47	Idaho	108	0.0%
48	Vermont	54	0.0%
49	Wyoming	53	0.0%
50	Montana	51	0.0%
	District of Columbia	5,223	0.9%

Source: U.S. Department of Health and Human Services, National Center for Health Statistics
    "National Vital Statistics Reports" (Vol. 53, No. 9, November 23, 2004)
*Final data by state of residence. By race of mother.

Black Births as a Percent of All Births in 2003

National Percent = 14.7% of Live Births*

ALPHA ORDER

RANK	STATE	PERCENT
6	Alabama	30.1
35	Alaska	4.0
36	Arizona	3.6
12	Arkansas	19.1
31	California	6.0
34	Colorado	4.2
20	Connecticut	12.1
7	Delaware	25.6
9	Florida	22.3
5	Georgia	31.7
39	Hawaii	2.9
49	Idaho	0.5
14	Illinois	17.3
22	Indiana	10.8
38	Iowa	3.4
30	Kansas	7.0
27	Kentucky	8.8
2	Louisiana	40.3
44	Maine	1.3
3	Maryland	33.1
23	Massachusetts	10.7
16	Michigan	17.2
29	Minnesota	7.7
1	Mississippi	43.4
19	Missouri	14.5
50	Montana	0.4
32	Nebraska	5.7
28	Nevada	8.6
42	New Hampshire	1.7
14	New Jersey	17.3
41	New Mexico	1.9
13	New York	18.9
8	North Carolina	23.0
43	North Dakota	1.4
17	Ohio	15.2
26	Oklahoma	9.0
40	Oregon	2.2
17	Pennsylvania	15.2
24	Rhode Island	9.6
4	South Carolina	33.0
45	South Dakota	1.1
11	Tennessee	20.6
21	Texas	11.1
46	Utah	0.8
46	Vermont	0.8
9	Virginia	22.3
33	Washington	5.0
37	West Virginia	3.5
25	Wisconsin	9.3
46	Wyoming	0.8

RANK ORDER

RANK	STATE	PERCENT
1	Mississippi	43.4
2	Louisiana	40.3
3	Maryland	33.1
4	South Carolina	33.0
5	Georgia	31.7
6	Alabama	30.1
7	Delaware	25.6
8	North Carolina	23.0
9	Florida	22.3
9	Virginia	22.3
11	Tennessee	20.6
12	Arkansas	19.1
13	New York	18.9
14	Illinois	17.3
14	New Jersey	17.3
16	Michigan	17.2
17	Ohio	15.2
17	Pennsylvania	15.2
19	Missouri	14.5
20	Connecticut	12.1
21	Texas	11.1
22	Indiana	10.8
23	Massachusetts	10.7
24	Rhode Island	9.6
25	Wisconsin	9.3
26	Oklahoma	9.0
27	Kentucky	8.8
28	Nevada	8.6
29	Minnesota	7.7
30	Kansas	7.0
31	California	6.0
32	Nebraska	5.7
33	Washington	5.0
34	Colorado	4.2
35	Alaska	4.0
36	Arizona	3.6
37	West Virginia	3.5
38	Iowa	3.4
39	Hawaii	2.9
40	Oregon	2.2
41	New Mexico	1.9
42	New Hampshire	1.7
43	North Dakota	1.4
44	Maine	1.3
45	South Dakota	1.1
46	Utah	0.8
46	Vermont	0.8
46	Wyoming	0.8
49	Idaho	0.5
50	Montana	0.4

District of Columbia — 68.7

Source: Morgan Quitno Press using data from U.S. Dept. of Health and Human Services, Nat'l Center for Health Statistics "National Vital Statistics Reports" (Vol. 53; No. 9, November 23, 2004)
*Final data by state of residence. By race of mother.

Births to Hispanic Women in 2003

National Total = 912,256 Live Births to Hispanic Women*

ALPHA ORDER

RANK	STATE	BIRTHS	% of USA
34	Alabama	2,907	0.3%
41	Alaska	776	0.1%
6	Arizona	39,798	4.4%
32	Arkansas	3,307	0.4%
1	California	268,867	29.5%
8	Colorado	21,398	2.3%
19	Connecticut	7,547	0.8%
40	Delaware	1,369	0.2%
4	Florida	54,864	6.0%
9	Georgia	18,266	2.0%
35	Hawaii	2,619	0.3%
33	Idaho	2,940	0.3%
5	Illinois	42,486	4.7%
21	Indiana	6,764	0.7%
36	Iowa	2,521	0.3%
26	Kansas	5,443	0.6%
38	Kentucky	1,964	0.2%
39	Louisiana	1,684	0.2%
48	Maine	167	0.0%
22	Maryland	6,296	0.7%
16	Massachusetts	9,809	1.1%
18	Michigan	7,666	0.8%
27	Minnesota	4,937	0.5%
44	Mississippi	461	0.1%
30	Missouri	3,480	0.4%
45	Montana	381	0.0%
31	Nebraska	3,449	0.4%
13	Nevada	12,207	1.3%
43	New Hampshire	527	0.1%
7	New Jersey	26,504	2.9%
11	New Mexico	14,856	1.6%
3	New York	55,340	6.1%
10	North Carolina	16,084	1.8%
47	North Dakota	168	0.0%
25	Ohio	5,444	0.6%
23	Oklahoma	5,654	0.6%
17	Oregon	8,440	0.9%
14	Pennsylvania	10,494	1.2%
37	Rhode Island	2,514	0.3%
29	South Carolina	3,587	0.4%
46	South Dakota	340	0.0%
28	Tennessee	4,934	0.5%
2	Texas	184,912	20.3%
20	Utah	7,072	0.8%
50	Vermont	59	0.0%
15	Virginia	10,389	1.1%
12	Washington	13,307	1.5%
49	West Virginia	99	0.0%
24	Wisconsin	5,539	0.6%
42	Wyoming	666	0.1%

RANK ORDER

RANK	STATE	BIRTHS	% of USA
1	California	268,867	29.5%
2	Texas	184,912	20.3%
3	New York	55,340	6.1%
4	Florida	54,864	6.0%
5	Illinois	42,486	4.7%
6	Arizona	39,798	4.4%
7	New Jersey	26,504	2.9%
8	Colorado	21,398	2.3%
9	Georgia	18,266	2.0%
10	North Carolina	16,084	1.8%
11	New Mexico	14,856	1.6%
12	Washington	13,307	1.5%
13	Nevada	12,207	1.3%
14	Pennsylvania	10,494	1.2%
15	Virginia	10,389	1.1%
16	Massachusetts	9,809	1.1%
17	Oregon	8,440	0.9%
18	Michigan	7,666	0.8%
19	Connecticut	7,547	0.8%
20	Utah	7,072	0.8%
21	Indiana	6,764	0.7%
22	Maryland	6,296	0.7%
23	Oklahoma	5,654	0.6%
24	Wisconsin	5,539	0.6%
25	Ohio	5,444	0.6%
26	Kansas	5,443	0.6%
27	Minnesota	4,937	0.5%
28	Tennessee	4,934	0.5%
29	South Carolina	3,587	0.4%
30	Missouri	3,480	0.4%
31	Nebraska	3,449	0.4%
32	Arkansas	3,307	0.4%
33	Idaho	2,940	0.3%
34	Alabama	2,907	0.3%
35	Hawaii	2,619	0.3%
36	Iowa	2,521	0.3%
37	Rhode Island	2,514	0.3%
38	Kentucky	1,964	0.2%
39	Louisiana	1,684	0.2%
40	Delaware	1,369	0.2%
41	Alaska	776	0.1%
42	Wyoming	666	0.1%
43	New Hampshire	527	0.1%
44	Mississippi	461	0.1%
45	Montana	381	0.0%
46	South Dakota	340	0.0%
47	North Dakota	168	0.0%
48	Maine	167	0.0%
49	West Virginia	99	0.0%
50	Vermont	59	0.0%
	District of Columbia	954	0.1%

Source: U.S. Department of Health and Human Services, National Center for Health Statistics
   "National Vital Statistics Reports" (Vol. 53, No. 9, November 23, 2004)
*Final data by state of residence. By race of mother. Persons of Hispanic origin may be of any race.

Hispanic Births as a Percent of All Births in 2003

National Percent = 22.3% of Live Births*

ALPHA ORDER

RANK	STATE	PERCENT
38	Alabama	4.9
31	Alaska	7.7
4	Arizona	43.7
27	Arkansas	8.7
2	California	49.7
6	Colorado	30.8
13	Connecticut	17.6
22	Delaware	12.2
7	Florida	25.8
20	Georgia	13.4
15	Hawaii	14.5
19	Idaho	13.5
8	Illinois	23.3
30	Indiana	7.8
34	Iowa	6.6
17	Kansas	13.8
41	Kentucky	3.6
45	Louisiana	2.6
47	Maine	1.2
28	Maryland	8.4
22	Massachusetts	12.2
37	Michigan	5.9
33	Minnesota	7.0
48	Mississippi	1.1
39	Missouri	4.5
43	Montana	3.3
21	Nebraska	13.3
5	Nevada	36.3
40	New Hampshire	3.7
9	New Jersey	22.8
1	New Mexico	53.4
10	New York	21.8
18	North Carolina	13.6
46	North Dakota	2.1
41	Ohio	3.6
24	Oklahoma	11.2
12	Oregon	18.4
32	Pennsylvania	7.5
11	Rhode Island	19.1
35	South Carolina	6.4
44	South Dakota	3.1
36	Tennessee	6.3
3	Texas	48.5
16	Utah	14.2
49	Vermont	0.9
25	Virginia	10.3
14	Washington	16.5
50	West Virginia	0.5
29	Wisconsin	7.9
26	Wyoming	9.9

RANK ORDER

RANK	STATE	PERCENT
1	New Mexico	53.4
2	California	49.7
3	Texas	48.5
4	Arizona	43.7
5	Nevada	36.3
6	Colorado	30.8
7	Florida	25.8
8	Illinois	23.3
9	New Jersey	22.8
10	New York	21.8
11	Rhode Island	19.1
12	Oregon	18.4
13	Connecticut	17.6
14	Washington	16.5
15	Hawaii	14.5
16	Utah	14.2
17	Kansas	13.8
18	North Carolina	13.6
19	Idaho	13.5
20	Georgia	13.4
21	Nebraska	13.3
22	Delaware	12.2
22	Massachusetts	12.2
24	Oklahoma	11.2
25	Virginia	10.3
26	Wyoming	9.9
27	Arkansas	8.7
28	Maryland	8.4
29	Wisconsin	7.9
30	Indiana	7.8
31	Alaska	7.7
32	Pennsylvania	7.5
33	Minnesota	7.0
34	Iowa	6.6
35	South Carolina	6.4
36	Tennessee	6.3
37	Michigan	5.9
38	Alabama	4.9
39	Missouri	4.5
40	New Hampshire	3.7
41	Kentucky	3.6
41	Ohio	3.6
43	Montana	3.3
44	South Dakota	3.1
45	Louisiana	2.6
46	North Dakota	2.1
47	Maine	1.2
48	Mississippi	1.1
49	Vermont	0.9
50	West Virginia	0.5

District of Columbia   12.5

Source: Morgan Quitno Press using data from U.S. Dept. of Health and Human Services, Nat'l Center for Health Statistics "National Vital Statistics Reports" (Vol. 53, No. 9, November 23, 2004)
*Final data by state of residence. By race of mother. Persons of Hispanic origin may be of any race.

Births of Low Birthweight in 2003

National Total = 323,194 Live Births*

<u>ALPHA ORDER</u>

RANK	STATE	BIRTHS	% of USA
21	Alabama	5,962	1.8%
47	Alaska	607	0.2%
17	Arizona	6,461	2.0%
29	Arkansas	3,396	1.1%
1	California	35,706	11.0%
18	Colorado	6,243	1.9%
31	Connecticut	3,214	1.0%
42	Delaware	1,059	0.3%
4	Florida	18,044	5.6%
7	Georgia	12,241	3.8%
39	Hawaii	1,558	0.5%
40	Idaho	1,417	0.4%
5	Illinois	15,155	4.7%
16	Indiana	6,755	2.1%
35	Iowa	2,520	0.8%
32	Kansas	2,922	0.9%
25	Kentucky	4,809	1.5%
14	Louisiana	6,987	2.2%
43	Maine	901	0.3%
15	Maryland	6,812	2.1%
20	Massachusetts	6,099	1.9%
9	Michigan	10,737	3.3%
27	Minnesota	4,420	1.4%
24	Mississippi	4,829	1.5%
19	Missouri	6,166	1.9%
45	Montana	776	0.2%
38	Nebraska	1,789	0.6%
34	Nevada	2,725	0.8%
44	New Hampshire	892	0.3%
11	New Jersey	9,418	2.9%
36	New Mexico	2,367	0.7%
3	New York	20,081	6.2%
10	North Carolina	10,648	3.3%
49	North Dakota	518	0.2%
6	Ohio	12,615	3.9%
28	Oklahoma	3,887	1.2%
33	Oregon	2,804	0.9%
8	Pennsylvania	11,112	3.4%
41	Rhode Island	1,148	0.4%
22	South Carolina	5,566	1.7%
46	South Dakota	728	0.2%
13	Tennessee	7,417	2.3%
2	Texas	30,118	9.3%
30	Utah	3,242	1.0%
50	Vermont	468	0.1%
12	Virginia	8,301	2.6%
23	Washington	4,909	1.5%
37	West Virginia	1,798	0.6%
26	Wisconsin	4,764	1.5%
48	Wyoming	597	0.2%

<u>RANK ORDER</u>

RANK	STATE	BIRTHS	% of USA
1	California	35,706	11.0%
2	Texas	30,118	9.3%
3	New York	20,081	6.2%
4	Florida	18,044	5.6%
5	Illinois	15,155	4.7%
6	Ohio	12,615	3.9%
7	Georgia	12,241	3.8%
8	Pennsylvania	11,112	3.4%
9	Michigan	10,737	3.3%
10	North Carolina	10,648	3.3%
11	New Jersey	9,418	2.9%
12	Virginia	8,301	2.6%
13	Tennessee	7,417	2.3%
14	Louisiana	6,987	2.2%
15	Maryland	6,812	2.1%
16	Indiana	6,755	2.1%
17	Arizona	6,461	2.0%
18	Colorado	6,243	1.9%
19	Missouri	6,166	1.9%
20	Massachusetts	6,099	1.9%
21	Alabama	5,962	1.8%
22	South Carolina	5,566	1.7%
23	Washington	4,909	1.5%
24	Mississippi	4,829	1.5%
25	Kentucky	4,809	1.5%
26	Wisconsin	4,764	1.5%
27	Minnesota	4,420	1.4%
28	Oklahoma	3,887	1.2%
29	Arkansas	3,396	1.1%
30	Utah	3,242	1.0%
31	Connecticut	3,214	1.0%
32	Kansas	2,922	0.9%
33	Oregon	2,804	0.9%
34	Nevada	2,725	0.8%
35	Iowa	2,520	0.8%
36	New Mexico	2,367	0.7%
37	West Virginia	1,798	0.6%
38	Nebraska	1,789	0.6%
39	Hawaii	1,558	0.5%
40	Idaho	1,417	0.4%
41	Rhode Island	1,148	0.4%
42	Delaware	1,059	0.3%
43	Maine	901	0.3%
44	New Hampshire	892	0.3%
45	Montana	776	0.2%
46	South Dakota	728	0.2%
47	Alaska	607	0.2%
48	Wyoming	597	0.2%
49	North Dakota	518	0.2%
50	Vermont	468	0.1%
	District of Columbia	829	0.3%

Source: Morgan Quitno Press using data from U.S. Dept. of Health and Human Services, Nat'l Center for Health Statistics "National Vital Statistics Reports" (Vol. 53, No. 9, November 23, 2004)
*Preliminary data by state of residence. Births of less than 2,500 grams (5 pounds 8 ounces).

Births of Low Birthweight as a Percent of All Births in 2003

National Percent = 7.9% of Live Births*

ALPHA ORDER

RANK	STATE	PERCENT
3	Alabama	10.0
50	Alaska	6.0
34	Arizona	7.1
11	Arkansas	8.9
39	California	6.6
8	Colorado	9.0
32	Connecticut	7.5
5	Delaware	9.4
17	Florida	8.5
8	Georgia	9.0
15	Hawaii	8.6
42	Idaho	6.5
19	Illinois	8.3
29	Indiana	7.8
39	Iowa	6.6
33	Kansas	7.4
13	Kentucky	8.7
2	Louisiana	10.7
42	Maine	6.5
7	Maryland	9.1
31	Massachusetts	7.6
21	Michigan	8.2
46	Minnesota	6.3
1	Mississippi	11.4
25	Missouri	8.0
37	Montana	6.8
36	Nebraska	6.9
23	Nevada	8.1
47	New Hampshire	6.2
23	New Jersey	8.1
17	New Mexico	8.5
26	New York	7.9
8	North Carolina	9.0
42	North Dakota	6.5
19	Ohio	8.3
30	Oklahoma	7.7
48	Oregon	6.1
26	Pennsylvania	7.9
13	Rhode Island	8.7
3	South Carolina	10.0
39	South Dakota	6.6
5	Tennessee	9.4
26	Texas	7.9
42	Utah	6.5
34	Vermont	7.1
21	Virginia	8.2
48	Washington	6.1
15	West Virginia	8.6
37	Wisconsin	6.8
11	Wyoming	8.9

RANK ORDER

RANK	STATE	PERCENT
1	Mississippi	11.4
2	Louisiana	10.7
3	Alabama	10.0
3	South Carolina	10.0
5	Delaware	9.4
5	Tennessee	9.4
7	Maryland	9.1
8	Colorado	9.0
8	Georgia	9.0
8	North Carolina	9.0
11	Arkansas	8.9
11	Wyoming	8.9
13	Kentucky	8.7
13	Rhode Island	8.7
15	Hawaii	8.6
15	West Virginia	8.6
17	Florida	8.5
17	New Mexico	8.5
19	Illinois	8.3
19	Ohio	8.3
21	Michigan	8.2
21	Virginia	8.2
23	Nevada	8.1
23	New Jersey	8.1
25	Missouri	8.0
26	New York	7.9
26	Pennsylvania	7.9
26	Texas	7.9
29	Indiana	7.8
30	Oklahoma	7.7
31	Massachusetts	7.6
32	Connecticut	7.5
33	Kansas	7.4
34	Arizona	7.1
34	Vermont	7.1
36	Nebraska	6.9
37	Montana	6.8
37	Wisconsin	6.8
39	California	6.6
39	Iowa	6.6
39	South Dakota	6.6
42	Idaho	6.5
42	Maine	6.5
42	North Dakota	6.5
42	Utah	6.5
46	Minnesota	6.3
47	New Hampshire	6.2
48	Oregon	6.1
48	Washington	6.1
50	Alaska	6.0
	District of Columbia	10.9

Source: U.S. Department of Health and Human Services, National Center for Health Statistics "National Vital Statistics Reports" (Vol. 53, No. 9, November 23, 2004)
*Preliminary data by state of residence. Births of less than 2,500 grams (5 pounds 8 ounces).

Births of Low Birthweight to White Women in 2003

National Total = 222,715 Live Births*

ALPHA ORDER

RANK	STATE	BIRTHS	% of USA
23	Alabama	3,273	1.5%
49	Alaska	370	0.2%
13	Arizona	5,449	2.4%
32	Arkansas	2,284	1.0%
1	California	26,720	12.0%
14	Colorado	5,434	2.4%
30	Connecticut	2,441	1.1%
44	Delaware	609	0.3%
4	Florida	11,222	5.0%
10	Georgia	6,254	2.8%
50	Hawaii	329	0.1%
39	Idaho	1,363	0.6%
5	Illinois	9,813	4.4%
12	Indiana	5,450	2.4%
33	Iowa	2,249	1.0%
31	Kansas	2,416	1.1%
19	Kentucky	4,055	1.8%
26	Louisiana	2,884	1.3%
41	Maine	869	0.4%
24	Maryland	3,205	1.4%
17	Massachusetts	4,756	2.1%
8	Michigan	7,110	3.2%
22	Minnesota	3,450	1.5%
35	Mississippi	2,004	0.9%
18	Missouri	4,531	2.0%
43	Montana	649	0.3%
38	Nebraska	1,543	0.7%
34	Nevada	2,049	0.9%
42	New Hampshire	832	0.4%
11	New Jersey	5,969	2.7%
36	New Mexico	1,981	0.9%
3	New York	12,516	5.6%
9	North Carolina	6,307	2.8%
48	North Dakota	434	0.2%
6	Ohio	9,285	4.2%
27	Oklahoma	2,850	1.3%
29	Oregon	2,454	1.1%
7	Pennsylvania	7,869	3.5%
40	Rhode Island	908	0.4%
28	South Carolina	2,756	1.2%
45	South Dakota	579	0.3%
16	Tennessee	4,879	2.2%
2	Texas	23,060	10.4%
25	Utah	3,077	1.4%
47	Vermont	455	0.2%
15	Virginia	4,889	2.2%
20	Washington	3,794	1.7%
37	West Virginia	1,700	0.8%
21	Wisconsin	3,615	1.6%
46	Wyoming	561	0.3%

RANK ORDER

RANK	STATE	BIRTHS	% of USA
1	California	26,720	12.0%
2	Texas	23,060	10.4%
3	New York	12,516	5.6%
4	Florida	11,222	5.0%
5	Illinois	9,813	4.4%
6	Ohio	9,285	4.2%
7	Pennsylvania	7,869	3.5%
8	Michigan	7,110	3.2%
9	North Carolina	6,307	2.8%
10	Georgia	6,254	2.8%
11	New Jersey	5,969	2.7%
12	Indiana	5,450	2.4%
13	Arizona	5,449	2.4%
14	Colorado	5,434	2.4%
15	Virginia	4,889	2.2%
16	Tennessee	4,879	2.2%
17	Massachusetts	4,756	2.1%
18	Missouri	4,531	2.0%
19	Kentucky	4,055	1.8%
20	Washington	3,794	1.7%
21	Wisconsin	3,615	1.6%
22	Minnesota	3,450	1.5%
23	Alabama	3,273	1.5%
24	Maryland	3,205	1.4%
25	Utah	3,077	1.4%
26	Louisiana	2,884	1.3%
27	Oklahoma	2,850	1.3%
28	South Carolina	2,756	1.2%
29	Oregon	2,454	1.1%
30	Connecticut	2,441	1.1%
31	Kansas	2,416	1.1%
32	Arkansas	2,284	1.0%
33	Iowa	2,249	1.0%
34	Nevada	2,049	0.9%
35	Mississippi	2,004	0.9%
36	New Mexico	1,981	0.9%
37	West Virginia	1,700	0.8%
38	Nebraska	1,543	0.7%
39	Idaho	1,363	0.6%
40	Rhode Island	908	0.4%
41	Maine	869	0.4%
42	New Hampshire	832	0.4%
43	Montana	649	0.3%
44	Delaware	609	0.3%
45	South Dakota	579	0.3%
46	Wyoming	561	0.3%
47	Vermont	455	0.2%
48	North Dakota	434	0.2%
49	Alaska	370	0.2%
50	Hawaii	329	0.1%
	District of Columbia	138	0.1%

Source: Morgan Quitno Press using data from U.S. Dept. of Health and Human Services, Nat'l Center for Health Statistics "National Vital Statistics Reports" (Vol. 53, No. 9, November 23, 2004)
*Preliminary data by state of residence. Births of less than 2,500 grams (5 pounds 8 ounces).

Births of Low Birthweight to White Women
As a Percent of All Births to White Women in 2003
National Percent = 6.9% of Live Births to White Women*

<u>ALPHA ORDER</u>

RANK	STATE	PERCENT
8	Alabama	8.0
49	Alaska	5.7
27	Arizona	6.9
12	Arkansas	7.6
44	California	6.1
2	Colorado	8.6
27	Connecticut	6.9
10	Delaware	7.7
20	Florida	7.1
20	Georgia	7.1
33	Hawaii	6.8
38	Idaho	6.5
27	Illinois	6.9
17	Indiana	7.2
42	Iowa	6.3
27	Kansas	6.9
6	Kentucky	8.2
10	Louisiana	7.7
38	Maine	6.5
25	Maryland	7.0
17	Massachusetts	7.2
27	Michigan	6.9
48	Minnesota	5.8
3	Mississippi	8.5
20	Missouri	7.1
36	Montana	6.6
36	Nebraska	6.6
14	Nevada	7.4
44	New Hampshire	6.1
25	New Jersey	7.0
3	New Mexico	8.5
33	New York	6.8
16	North Carolina	7.3
42	North Dakota	6.3
14	Ohio	7.4
17	Oklahoma	7.2
47	Oregon	5.9
27	Pennsylvania	6.9
7	Rhode Island	8.1
12	South Carolina	7.6
38	South Dakota	6.5
8	Tennessee	8.0
20	Texas	7.1
38	Utah	6.5
20	Vermont	7.1
33	Virginia	6.8
49	Washington	5.7
3	West Virginia	8.5
46	Wisconsin	6.0
1	Wyoming	8.9

<u>RANK ORDER</u>

RANK	STATE	PERCENT
1	Wyoming	8.9
2	Colorado	8.6
3	Mississippi	8.5
3	New Mexico	8.5
3	West Virginia	8.5
6	Kentucky	8.2
7	Rhode Island	8.1
8	Alabama	8.0
8	Tennessee	8.0
10	Delaware	7.7
10	Louisiana	7.7
12	Arkansas	7.6
12	South Carolina	7.6
14	Nevada	7.4
14	Ohio	7.4
16	North Carolina	7.3
17	Indiana	7.2
17	Massachusetts	7.2
17	Oklahoma	7.2
20	Florida	7.1
20	Georgia	7.1
20	Missouri	7.1
20	Texas	7.1
20	Vermont	7.1
25	Maryland	7.0
25	New Jersey	7.0
27	Arizona	6.9
27	Connecticut	6.9
27	Illinois	6.9
27	Kansas	6.9
27	Michigan	6.9
27	Pennsylvania	6.9
33	Hawaii	6.8
33	New York	6.8
33	Virginia	6.8
36	Montana	6.6
36	Nebraska	6.6
38	Idaho	6.5
38	Maine	6.5
38	South Dakota	6.5
38	Utah	6.5
42	Iowa	6.3
42	North Dakota	6.3
44	California	6.1
44	New Hampshire	6.1
46	Wisconsin	6.0
47	Oregon	5.9
48	Minnesota	5.8
49	Alaska	5.7
49	Washington	5.7
	District of Columbia	6.5

Source: U.S. Department of Health and Human Services, National Center for Health Statistics
    "National Vital Statistics Reports" (Vol. 53, No. 9, November 23, 2004)
*Preliminary data by state of residence. Births of less than 2,500 grams (5 pounds 8 ounces).

Births of Low Birthweight to Black Women in 2003

National Total = 79,722 Live Births*

ALPHA ORDER			
RANK	STATE	BIRTHS	% of USA
16	Alabama	2,604	3.3%
42	Alaska	39	0.0%
32	Arizona	367	0.5%
21	Arkansas	1,067	1.3%
6	California	3,954	5.0%
28	Colorado	458	0.6%
26	Connecticut	617	0.8%
29	Delaware	412	0.5%
1	Florida	6,203	7.8%
4	Georgia	5,598	7.0%
40	Hawaii	67	0.1%
NA	Idaho**	NA	NA
5	Illinois	4,551	5.7%
20	Indiana	1,239	1.6%
34	Iowa	167	0.2%
33	Kansas	354	0.4%
24	Kentucky	656	0.8%
7	Louisiana	3,923	4.9%
NA	Maine**	NA	NA
9	Maryland	3,196	4.0%
22	Massachusetts	904	1.1%
10	Michigan	3,183	4.0%
27	Minnesota	549	0.7%
14	Mississippi	2,792	3.5%
19	Missouri	1,485	1.9%
NA	Montana**	NA	NA
34	Nebraska	167	0.2%
31	Nevada	381	0.5%
43	New Hampshire	26	0.0%
17	New Jersey	2,535	3.2%
39	New Mexico	83	0.1%
2	New York	5,772	7.2%
8	North Carolina	3,858	4.8%
NA	North Dakota**	NA	NA
11	Ohio	3,113	3.9%
25	Oklahoma	630	0.8%
37	Oregon	119	0.1%
13	Pennsylvania	2,816	3.5%
36	Rhode Island	155	0.2%
15	South Carolina	2,752	3.5%
NA	South Dakota**	NA	NA
18	Tennessee	2,405	3.0%
3	Texas	5,745	7.2%
41	Utah	58	0.1%
NA	Vermont**	NA	NA
12	Virginia	2,893	3.6%
30	Washington	407	0.5%
38	West Virginia	87	0.1%
23	Wisconsin	883	1.1%
NA	Wyoming**	NA	NA

RANK ORDER			
RANK	STATE	BIRTHS	% of USA
1	Florida	6,203	7.8%
2	New York	5,772	7.2%
3	Texas	5,745	7.2%
4	Georgia	5,598	7.0%
5	Illinois	4,551	5.7%
6	California	3,954	5.0%
7	Louisiana	3,923	4.9%
8	North Carolina	3,858	4.8%
9	Maryland	3,196	4.0%
10	Michigan	3,183	4.0%
11	Ohio	3,113	3.9%
12	Virginia	2,893	3.6%
13	Pennsylvania	2,816	3.5%
14	Mississippi	2,792	3.5%
15	South Carolina	2,752	3.5%
16	Alabama	2,604	3.3%
17	New Jersey	2,535	3.2%
18	Tennessee	2,405	3.0%
19	Missouri	1,485	1.9%
20	Indiana	1,239	1.6%
21	Arkansas	1,067	1.3%
22	Massachusetts	904	1.1%
23	Wisconsin	883	1.1%
24	Kentucky	656	0.8%
25	Oklahoma	630	0.8%
26	Connecticut	617	0.8%
27	Minnesota	549	0.7%
28	Colorado	458	0.6%
29	Delaware	412	0.5%
30	Washington	407	0.5%
31	Nevada	381	0.5%
32	Arizona	367	0.5%
33	Kansas	354	0.4%
34	Iowa	167	0.2%
34	Nebraska	167	0.2%
36	Rhode Island	155	0.2%
37	Oregon	119	0.1%
38	West Virginia	87	0.1%
39	New Mexico	83	0.1%
40	Hawaii	67	0.1%
41	Utah	58	0.1%
42	Alaska	39	0.0%
43	New Hampshire	26	0.0%
NA	Idaho**	NA	NA
NA	Maine**	NA	NA
NA	Montana**	NA	NA
NA	North Dakota**	NA	NA
NA	South Dakota**	NA	NA
NA	Vermont**	NA	NA
NA	Wyoming**	NA	NA

District of Columbia — 674 — 0.8%

Source: Morgan Quitno Press using data from U.S. Dept. of Health and Human Services, Nat'l Center for Health Statistics
    "National Vital Statistics Reports" (Vol. 53, No. 9, November 23, 2004)
*Preliminary data by state of residence. Births of less than 2,500 grams (5 pounds 8 ounces).
**Not available. Fewer than 20 births of low birthweight to black women.

Births of Low Birthweight to Black Women
As a Percent of All Births to Black Women in 2003
National Percent = 13.3% of Live Births to Black Women*

<table>
<tr><td colspan="3">ALPHA ORDER</td><td colspan="3">RANK ORDER</td></tr>
<tr><td>RANK</td><td>STATE</td><td>PERCENT</td><td>RANK</td><td>STATE</td><td>PERCENT</td></tr>
<tr><td>9</td><td>Alabama</td><td>14.5</td><td>1</td><td>Colorado</td><td>15.6</td></tr>
<tr><td>43</td><td>Alaska</td><td>9.7</td><td>1</td><td>New Mexico</td><td>15.6</td></tr>
<tr><td>38</td><td>Arizona</td><td>11.2</td><td>3</td><td>Mississippi</td><td>15.2</td></tr>
<tr><td>8</td><td>Arkansas</td><td>14.6</td><td>3</td><td>Utah</td><td>15.2</td></tr>
<tr><td>32</td><td>California</td><td>12.1</td><td>5</td><td>South Carolina</td><td>15.0</td></tr>
<tr><td>1</td><td>Colorado</td><td>15.6</td><td>6</td><td>Louisiana</td><td>14.9</td></tr>
<tr><td>35</td><td>Connecticut</td><td>11.9</td><td>7</td><td>Tennessee</td><td>14.8</td></tr>
<tr><td>11</td><td>Delaware</td><td>14.3</td><td>8</td><td>Arkansas</td><td>14.6</td></tr>
<tr><td>22</td><td>Florida</td><td>13.1</td><td>9</td><td>Alabama</td><td>14.5</td></tr>
<tr><td>24</td><td>Georgia</td><td>13.0</td><td>10</td><td>Illinois</td><td>14.4</td></tr>
<tr><td>26</td><td>Hawaii</td><td>12.9</td><td>11</td><td>Delaware</td><td>14.3</td></tr>
<tr><td>NA</td><td>Idaho**</td><td>NA</td><td>12</td><td>North Carolina</td><td>14.2</td></tr>
<tr><td>10</td><td>Illinois</td><td>14.4</td><td>13</td><td>Michigan</td><td>14.1</td></tr>
<tr><td>20</td><td>Indiana</td><td>13.2</td><td>14</td><td>Oklahoma</td><td>13.8</td></tr>
<tr><td>24</td><td>Iowa</td><td>13.0</td><td>15</td><td>Texas</td><td>13.6</td></tr>
<tr><td>28</td><td>Kansas</td><td>12.8</td><td>15</td><td>Wisconsin</td><td>13.6</td></tr>
<tr><td>17</td><td>Kentucky</td><td>13.5</td><td>17</td><td>Kentucky</td><td>13.5</td></tr>
<tr><td>6</td><td>Louisiana</td><td>14.9</td><td>17</td><td>Ohio</td><td>13.5</td></tr>
<tr><td>NA</td><td>Maine**</td><td>NA</td><td>19</td><td>Missouri</td><td>13.3</td></tr>
<tr><td>26</td><td>Maryland</td><td>12.9</td><td>20</td><td>Indiana</td><td>13.2</td></tr>
<tr><td>40</td><td>Massachusetts</td><td>10.5</td><td>20</td><td>Pennsylvania</td><td>13.2</td></tr>
<tr><td>13</td><td>Michigan</td><td>14.1</td><td>22</td><td>Florida</td><td>13.1</td></tr>
<tr><td>41</td><td>Minnesota</td><td>10.2</td><td>22</td><td>Nevada</td><td>13.1</td></tr>
<tr><td>3</td><td>Mississippi</td><td>15.2</td><td>24</td><td>Georgia</td><td>13.0</td></tr>
<tr><td>19</td><td>Missouri</td><td>13.3</td><td>24</td><td>Iowa</td><td>13.0</td></tr>
<tr><td>NA</td><td>Montana**</td><td>NA</td><td>26</td><td>Hawaii</td><td>12.9</td></tr>
<tr><td>37</td><td>Nebraska</td><td>11.4</td><td>26</td><td>Maryland</td><td>12.9</td></tr>
<tr><td>22</td><td>Nevada</td><td>13.1</td><td>28</td><td>Kansas</td><td>12.8</td></tr>
<tr><td>39</td><td>New Hampshire</td><td>10.7</td><td>28</td><td>Virginia</td><td>12.8</td></tr>
<tr><td>30</td><td>New Jersey</td><td>12.6</td><td>30</td><td>New Jersey</td><td>12.6</td></tr>
<tr><td>1</td><td>New Mexico</td><td>15.6</td><td>31</td><td>Rhode Island</td><td>12.3</td></tr>
<tr><td>33</td><td>New York</td><td>12.0</td><td>32</td><td>California</td><td>12.1</td></tr>
<tr><td>12</td><td>North Carolina</td><td>14.2</td><td>33</td><td>New York</td><td>12.0</td></tr>
<tr><td>NA</td><td>North Dakota**</td><td>NA</td><td>33</td><td>West Virginia</td><td>12.0</td></tr>
<tr><td>17</td><td>Ohio</td><td>13.5</td><td>35</td><td>Connecticut</td><td>11.9</td></tr>
<tr><td>14</td><td>Oklahoma</td><td>13.8</td><td>36</td><td>Oregon</td><td>11.6</td></tr>
<tr><td>36</td><td>Oregon</td><td>11.6</td><td>37</td><td>Nebraska</td><td>11.4</td></tr>
<tr><td>20</td><td>Pennsylvania</td><td>13.2</td><td>38</td><td>Arizona</td><td>11.2</td></tr>
<tr><td>31</td><td>Rhode Island</td><td>12.3</td><td>39</td><td>New Hampshire</td><td>10.7</td></tr>
<tr><td>5</td><td>South Carolina</td><td>15.0</td><td>40</td><td>Massachusetts</td><td>10.5</td></tr>
<tr><td>NA</td><td>South Dakota**</td><td>NA</td><td>41</td><td>Minnesota</td><td>10.2</td></tr>
<tr><td>7</td><td>Tennessee</td><td>14.8</td><td>42</td><td>Washington</td><td>10.1</td></tr>
<tr><td>15</td><td>Texas</td><td>13.6</td><td>43</td><td>Alaska</td><td>9.7</td></tr>
<tr><td>3</td><td>Utah</td><td>15.2</td><td>NA</td><td>Idaho**</td><td>NA</td></tr>
<tr><td>NA</td><td>Vermont**</td><td>NA</td><td>NA</td><td>Maine**</td><td>NA</td></tr>
<tr><td>28</td><td>Virginia</td><td>12.8</td><td>NA</td><td>Montana**</td><td>NA</td></tr>
<tr><td>42</td><td>Washington</td><td>10.1</td><td>NA</td><td>North Dakota**</td><td>NA</td></tr>
<tr><td>33</td><td>West Virginia</td><td>12.0</td><td>NA</td><td>South Dakota**</td><td>NA</td></tr>
<tr><td>15</td><td>Wisconsin</td><td>13.6</td><td>NA</td><td>Vermont**</td><td>NA</td></tr>
<tr><td>NA</td><td>Wyoming**</td><td>NA</td><td>NA</td><td>Wyoming**</td><td>NA</td></tr>
<tr><td></td><td></td><td></td><td></td><td>District of Columbia</td><td>12.9</td></tr>
</table>

Source: U.S. Department of Health and Human Services, National Center for Health Statistics
      "National Vital Statistics Reports" (Vol. 53, No. 9, November 23, 2004)
Preliminary data by state of residence. Births of less than 2,500 grams (5 pounds 8 ounces).
**Not available. Fewer than 20 births of low birthweight to black women.*

Births of Low Birthweight to Hispanic Women in 2003

National Total = 61,121 Live Births*

ALPHA ORDER

RANK ORDER

RANK	STATE	BIRTHS	% of USA		RANK	STATE	BIRTHS	% of USA
35	Alabama	195	0.3%		1	California	16,132	26.4%
42	Alaska	40	0.1%		2	Texas	12,944	21.2%
5	Arizona	2,746	4.5%		3	New York	4,151	6.8%
34	Arkansas	205	0.3%		4	Florida	3,786	6.2%
1	California	16,132	26.4%		5	Arizona	2,746	4.5%
8	Colorado	1,776	2.9%		6	Illinois	2,719	4.4%
17	Connecticut	649	1.1%		7	New Jersey	1,908	3.1%
40	Delaware	107	0.2%		8	Colorado	1,776	2.9%
4	Florida	3,786	6.2%		9	New Mexico	1,292	2.1%
10	Georgia	1,041	1.7%		10	Georgia	1,041	1.7%
31	Hawaii	220	0.4%		11	North Carolina	997	1.6%
36	Idaho	191	0.3%		12	Pennsylvania	881	1.4%
6	Illinois	2,719	4.4%		13	Nevada	854	1.4%
22	Indiana	399	0.7%		14	Massachusetts	814	1.3%
37	Iowa	156	0.3%		15	Washington	745	1.2%
26	Kansas	332	0.5%		16	Virginia	655	1.1%
39	Kentucky	120	0.2%		17	Connecticut	649	1.1%
38	Louisiana	135	0.2%		18	Michigan	506	0.8%
NA	Maine**	NA	NA		19	Utah	495	0.8%
20	Maryland	447	0.7%		20	Maryland	447	0.7%
14	Massachusetts	814	1.3%		20	Oregon	447	0.7%
18	Michigan	506	0.8%		22	Indiana	399	0.7%
28	Minnesota	252	0.4%		23	Ohio	392	0.6%
44	Mississippi	33	0.1%		24	Wisconsin	343	0.6%
32	Missouri	212	0.3%		25	Oklahoma	339	0.6%
43	Montana	35	0.1%		26	Kansas	332	0.5%
33	Nebraska	210	0.3%		27	Tennessee	301	0.5%
13	Nevada	854	1.4%		28	Minnesota	252	0.4%
46	New Hampshire	31	0.1%		29	South Carolina	233	0.4%
7	New Jersey	1,908	3.1%		30	Rhode Island	226	0.4%
9	New Mexico	1,292	2.1%		31	Hawaii	220	0.4%
3	New York	4,151	6.8%		32	Missouri	212	0.3%
11	North Carolina	997	1.6%		33	Nebraska	210	0.3%
NA	North Dakota**	NA	NA		34	Arkansas	205	0.3%
23	Ohio	392	0.6%		35	Alabama	195	0.3%
25	Oklahoma	339	0.6%		36	Idaho	191	0.3%
20	Oregon	447	0.7%		37	Iowa	156	0.3%
12	Pennsylvania	881	1.4%		38	Louisiana	135	0.2%
30	Rhode Island	226	0.4%		39	Kentucky	120	0.2%
29	South Carolina	233	0.4%		40	Delaware	107	0.2%
45	South Dakota	32	0.1%		41	Wyoming	58	0.1%
27	Tennessee	301	0.5%		42	Alaska	40	0.1%
2	Texas	12,944	21.2%		43	Montana	35	0.1%
19	Utah	495	0.8%		44	Mississippi	33	0.1%
NA	Vermont**	NA	NA		45	South Dakota	32	0.1%
16	Virginia	655	1.1%		46	New Hampshire	31	0.1%
15	Washington	745	1.2%		NA	Maine**	NA	NA
NA	West Virginia**	NA	NA		NA	North Dakota**	NA	NA
24	Wisconsin	343	0.6%		NA	Vermont**	NA	NA
41	Wyoming	58	0.1%		NA	West Virginia**	NA	NA
						District of Columbia	73	0.1%

Source: Morgan Quitno Press using data from U.S. Dept. of Health and Human Services, Nat'l Center for Health Statistics
"National Vital Statistics Reports" (Vol. 53, No. 9, November 23, 2004)
*Preliminary data by state of residence. Births of less than 2,500 grams (5 pounds 8 ounces). Hispanic can be of
any race.
**Not available. Fewer than 20 births of low birthweight to Hispanic women.

Births of Low Birthweight to Hispanic Women
As a Percent of All Births to Hispanic Women in 2003
National Percent = 6.7% of Live Births to Hispanic Women*

ALPHA ORDER

ALPHA ORDER

RANK	STATE	PERCENT
23	Alabama	6.7
45	Alaska	5.2
21	Arizona	6.9
29	Arkansas	6.2
38	California	6.0
9	Colorado	8.3
6	Connecticut	8.6
12	Delaware	7.8
21	Florida	6.9
42	Georgia	5.7
7	Hawaii	8.4
25	Idaho	6.5
27	Illinois	6.4
40	Indiana	5.9
29	Iowa	6.2
33	Kansas	6.1
33	Kentucky	6.1
11	Louisiana	8.0
NA	Maine**	NA
17	Maryland	7.1
9	Massachusetts	8.3
24	Michigan	6.6
46	Minnesota	5.1
14	Mississippi	7.2
33	Missouri	6.1
2	Montana	9.2
33	Nebraska	6.1
18	Nevada	7.0
40	New Hampshire	5.9
14	New Jersey	7.2
4	New Mexico	8.7
13	New York	7.5
29	North Carolina	6.2
NA	North Dakota**	NA
14	Ohio	7.2
38	Oklahoma	6.0
44	Oregon	5.3
7	Pennsylvania	8.4
3	Rhode Island	9.0
25	South Carolina	6.5
1	South Dakota	9.4
33	Tennessee	6.1
18	Texas	7.0
18	Utah	7.0
NA	Vermont**	NA
28	Virginia	6.3
43	Washington	5.6
NA	West Virginia**	NA
29	Wisconsin	6.2
4	Wyoming	8.7

RANK ORDER

RANK	STATE	PERCENT
1	South Dakota	9.4
2	Montana	9.2
3	Rhode Island	9.0
4	New Mexico	8.7
4	Wyoming	8.7
6	Connecticut	8.6
7	Hawaii	8.4
7	Pennsylvania	8.4
9	Colorado	8.3
9	Massachusetts	8.3
11	Louisiana	8.0
12	Delaware	7.8
13	New York	7.5
14	Mississippi	7.2
14	New Jersey	7.2
14	Ohio	7.2
17	Maryland	7.1
18	Nevada	7.0
18	Texas	7.0
18	Utah	7.0
21	Arizona	6.9
21	Florida	6.9
23	Alabama	6.7
24	Michigan	6.6
25	Idaho	6.5
25	South Carolina	6.5
27	Illinois	6.4
28	Virginia	6.3
29	Arkansas	6.2
29	Iowa	6.2
29	North Carolina	6.2
29	Wisconsin	6.2
33	Kansas	6.1
33	Kentucky	6.1
33	Missouri	6.1
33	Nebraska	6.1
33	Tennessee	6.1
38	California	6.0
38	Oklahoma	6.0
40	Indiana	5.9
40	New Hampshire	5.9
42	Georgia	5.7
43	Washington	5.6
44	Oregon	5.3
45	Alaska	5.2
46	Minnesota	5.1
NA	Maine**	NA
NA	North Dakota**	NA
NA	Vermont**	NA
NA	West Virginia**	NA

District of Columbia   7.7

Source: U.S. Department of Health and Human Services, National Center for Health Statistics
    "National Vital Statistics Reports" (Vol. 53, No. 9, November 23, 2004)
Final data by state of residence. Births of less than 2,500 grams (5 pounds 8 ounces). Hispanic can be of any race.
**Not available. Fewer than 20 births of low birthweight to Hispanic women.*

Births to Unmarried Women in 2003

National Total = 1,415,508 Live Births*

ALPHA ORDER

RANK	STATE	BIRTHS	% of USA
23	Alabama	20,867	1.5%
47	Alaska	3,502	0.2%
11	Arizona	37,767	2.7%
30	Arkansas	14,500	1.0%
1	California	181,233	12.8%
28	Colorado	18,520	1.3%
33	Connecticut	12,897	0.9%
41	Delaware	4,731	0.3%
4	Florida	84,702	6.0%
7	Georgia	51,821	3.7%
39	Hawaii	6,050	0.4%
40	Idaho	4,862	0.3%
5	Illinois	64,454	4.6%
13	Indiana	32,129	2.3%
35	Iowa	11,416	0.8%
34	Kansas	12,440	0.9%
26	Kentucky	18,685	1.3%
14	Louisiana	31,082	2.2%
43	Maine	4,657	0.3%
18	Maryland	26,050	1.8%
21	Massachusetts	22,310	1.6%
9	Michigan	45,435	3.2%
25	Minnesota	19,433	1.4%
24	Mississippi	19,698	1.4%
17	Missouri	27,440	1.9%
45	Montana	3,676	0.3%
37	Nebraska	7,699	0.5%
32	Nevada	13,121	0.9%
46	New Hampshire	3,569	0.3%
12	New Jersey	34,299	2.4%
31	New Mexico	13,477	1.0%
3	New York	92,778	6.6%
10	North Carolina	41,763	3.0%
48	North Dakota	2,281	0.2%
6	Ohio	54,866	3.9%
27	Oklahoma	18,629	1.3%
29	Oregon	14,574	1.0%
8	Pennsylvania	47,684	3.4%
42	Rhode Island	4,696	0.3%
20	South Carolina	22,987	1.6%
44	South Dakota	3,774	0.3%
16	Tennessee	29,351	2.1%
2	Texas	130,384	9.2%
36	Utah	8,578	0.6%
50	Vermont	1,971	0.1%
15	Virginia	30,773	2.2%
19	Washington	23,177	1.6%
38	West Virginia	7,234	0.5%
22	Wisconsin	21,296	1.5%
49	Wyoming	2,187	0.2%

RANK ORDER

RANK	STATE	BIRTHS	% of USA
1	California	181,233	12.8%
2	Texas	130,384	9.2%
3	New York	92,778	6.6%
4	Florida	84,702	6.0%
5	Illinois	64,454	4.6%
6	Ohio	54,866	3.9%
7	Georgia	51,821	3.7%
8	Pennsylvania	47,684	3.4%
9	Michigan	45,435	3.2%
10	North Carolina	41,763	3.0%
11	Arizona	37,767	2.7%
12	New Jersey	34,299	2.4%
13	Indiana	32,129	2.3%
14	Louisiana	31,082	2.2%
15	Virginia	30,773	2.2%
16	Tennessee	29,351	2.1%
17	Missouri	27,440	1.9%
18	Maryland	26,050	1.8%
19	Washington	23,177	1.6%
20	South Carolina	22,987	1.6%
21	Massachusetts	22,310	1.6%
22	Wisconsin	21,296	1.5%
23	Alabama	20,867	1.5%
24	Mississippi	19,698	1.4%
25	Minnesota	19,433	1.4%
26	Kentucky	18,685	1.3%
27	Oklahoma	18,629	1.3%
28	Colorado	18,520	1.3%
29	Oregon	14,574	1.0%
30	Arkansas	14,500	1.0%
31	New Mexico	13,477	1.0%
32	Nevada	13,121	0.9%
33	Connecticut	12,897	0.9%
34	Kansas	12,440	0.9%
35	Iowa	11,416	0.8%
36	Utah	8,578	0.6%
37	Nebraska	7,699	0.5%
38	West Virginia	7,234	0.5%
39	Hawaii	6,050	0.4%
40	Idaho	4,862	0.3%
41	Delaware	4,731	0.3%
42	Rhode Island	4,696	0.3%
43	Maine	4,657	0.3%
44	South Dakota	3,774	0.3%
45	Montana	3,676	0.3%
46	New Hampshire	3,569	0.3%
47	Alaska	3,502	0.2%
48	North Dakota	2,281	0.2%
49	Wyoming	2,187	0.2%
50	Vermont	1,971	0.1%
	District of Columbia	4,069	0.3%

Source: Morgan Quitno Press using data from U.S. Dept. of Health and Human Services, Nat'l Center for Health Statistics
"National Vital Statistics Reports" (Vol. 53, No. 9, November 23, 2004)
*Preliminary data by state of residence.

Births to Unmarried Women as a Percent of All Births in 2003

National Percent = 34.6% of Live Births*

<table>
<tr><td colspan="3">ALPHA ORDER</td><td colspan="3">RANK ORDER</td></tr>
<tr><td>RANK</td><td>STATE</td><td>PERCENT</td><td>RANK</td><td>STATE</td><td>PERCENT</td></tr>
<tr><td>20</td><td>Alabama</td><td>35.0</td><td>1</td><td>New Mexico</td><td>48.4</td></tr>
<tr><td>23</td><td>Alaska</td><td>34.6</td><td>2</td><td>Louisiana</td><td>47.6</td></tr>
<tr><td>5</td><td>Arizona</td><td>41.5</td><td>3</td><td>Mississippi</td><td>46.5</td></tr>
<tr><td>10</td><td>Arkansas</td><td>38.0</td><td>4</td><td>Delaware</td><td>42.0</td></tr>
<tr><td>30</td><td>California</td><td>33.5</td><td>5</td><td>Arizona</td><td>41.5</td></tr>
<tr><td>47</td><td>Colorado</td><td>26.7</td><td>6</td><td>South Carolina</td><td>41.3</td></tr>
<tr><td>38</td><td>Connecticut</td><td>30.1</td><td>7</td><td>Florida</td><td>39.9</td></tr>
<tr><td>4</td><td>Delaware</td><td>42.0</td><td>8</td><td>Nevada</td><td>39.0</td></tr>
<tr><td>7</td><td>Florida</td><td>39.9</td><td>9</td><td>Georgia</td><td>38.1</td></tr>
<tr><td>9</td><td>Georgia</td><td>38.1</td><td>10</td><td>Arkansas</td><td>38.0</td></tr>
<tr><td>31</td><td>Hawaii</td><td>33.4</td><td>11</td><td>Tennessee</td><td>37.2</td></tr>
<tr><td>49</td><td>Idaho</td><td>22.3</td><td>12</td><td>Indiana</td><td>37.1</td></tr>
<tr><td>18</td><td>Illinois</td><td>35.3</td><td>13</td><td>Oklahoma</td><td>36.9</td></tr>
<tr><td>12</td><td>Indiana</td><td>37.1</td><td>14</td><td>New York</td><td>36.5</td></tr>
<tr><td>39</td><td>Iowa</td><td>29.9</td><td>15</td><td>Ohio</td><td>36.1</td></tr>
<tr><td>35</td><td>Kansas</td><td>31.5</td><td>16</td><td>Missouri</td><td>35.6</td></tr>
<tr><td>28</td><td>Kentucky</td><td>33.8</td><td>16</td><td>Rhode Island</td><td>35.6</td></tr>
<tr><td>2</td><td>Louisiana</td><td>47.6</td><td>18</td><td>Illinois</td><td>35.3</td></tr>
<tr><td>29</td><td>Maine</td><td>33.6</td><td>18</td><td>North Carolina</td><td>35.3</td></tr>
<tr><td>21</td><td>Maryland</td><td>34.8</td><td>20</td><td>Alabama</td><td>35.0</td></tr>
<tr><td>45</td><td>Massachusetts</td><td>27.8</td><td>21</td><td>Maryland</td><td>34.8</td></tr>
<tr><td>22</td><td>Michigan</td><td>34.7</td><td>22</td><td>Michigan</td><td>34.7</td></tr>
<tr><td>46</td><td>Minnesota</td><td>27.7</td><td>23</td><td>Alaska</td><td>34.6</td></tr>
<tr><td>3</td><td>Mississippi</td><td>46.5</td><td>23</td><td>West Virginia</td><td>34.6</td></tr>
<tr><td>16</td><td>Missouri</td><td>35.6</td><td>25</td><td>South Dakota</td><td>34.2</td></tr>
<tr><td>33</td><td>Montana</td><td>32.2</td><td>25</td><td>Texas</td><td>34.2</td></tr>
<tr><td>41</td><td>Nebraska</td><td>29.7</td><td>27</td><td>Pennsylvania</td><td>33.9</td></tr>
<tr><td>8</td><td>Nevada</td><td>39.0</td><td>28</td><td>Kentucky</td><td>33.8</td></tr>
<tr><td>48</td><td>New Hampshire</td><td>24.8</td><td>29</td><td>Maine</td><td>33.6</td></tr>
<tr><td>42</td><td>New Jersey</td><td>29.5</td><td>30</td><td>California</td><td>33.5</td></tr>
<tr><td>1</td><td>New Mexico</td><td>48.4</td><td>31</td><td>Hawaii</td><td>33.4</td></tr>
<tr><td>14</td><td>New York</td><td>36.5</td><td>32</td><td>Wyoming</td><td>32.6</td></tr>
<tr><td>18</td><td>North Carolina</td><td>35.3</td><td>33</td><td>Montana</td><td>32.2</td></tr>
<tr><td>44</td><td>North Dakota</td><td>28.6</td><td>34</td><td>Oregon</td><td>31.7</td></tr>
<tr><td>15</td><td>Ohio</td><td>36.1</td><td>35</td><td>Kansas</td><td>31.5</td></tr>
<tr><td>13</td><td>Oklahoma</td><td>36.9</td><td>36</td><td>Virginia</td><td>30.4</td></tr>
<tr><td>34</td><td>Oregon</td><td>31.7</td><td>36</td><td>Wisconsin</td><td>30.4</td></tr>
<tr><td>27</td><td>Pennsylvania</td><td>33.9</td><td>38</td><td>Connecticut</td><td>30.1</td></tr>
<tr><td>16</td><td>Rhode Island</td><td>35.6</td><td>39</td><td>Iowa</td><td>29.9</td></tr>
<tr><td>6</td><td>South Carolina</td><td>41.3</td><td>39</td><td>Vermont</td><td>29.9</td></tr>
<tr><td>25</td><td>South Dakota</td><td>34.2</td><td>41</td><td>Nebraska</td><td>29.7</td></tr>
<tr><td>11</td><td>Tennessee</td><td>37.2</td><td>42</td><td>New Jersey</td><td>29.5</td></tr>
<tr><td>25</td><td>Texas</td><td>34.2</td><td>43</td><td>Washington</td><td>28.8</td></tr>
<tr><td>50</td><td>Utah</td><td>17.2</td><td>44</td><td>North Dakota</td><td>28.6</td></tr>
<tr><td>39</td><td>Vermont</td><td>29.9</td><td>45</td><td>Massachusetts</td><td>27.8</td></tr>
<tr><td>36</td><td>Virginia</td><td>30.4</td><td>46</td><td>Minnesota</td><td>27.7</td></tr>
<tr><td>43</td><td>Washington</td><td>28.8</td><td>47</td><td>Colorado</td><td>26.7</td></tr>
<tr><td>23</td><td>West Virginia</td><td>34.6</td><td>48</td><td>New Hampshire</td><td>24.8</td></tr>
<tr><td>36</td><td>Wisconsin</td><td>30.4</td><td>49</td><td>Idaho</td><td>22.3</td></tr>
<tr><td>32</td><td>Wyoming</td><td>32.6</td><td>50</td><td>Utah</td><td>17.2</td></tr>
<tr><td></td><td></td><td></td><td></td><td>District of Columbia</td><td>53.5</td></tr>
</table>

Source: U.S. Department of Health and Human Services, National Center for Health Statistics
    "National Vital Statistics Reports" (Vol. 53, No. 9, November 23, 2004)
*Preliminary data by state of residence.

Births to Unmarried White Women in 2003

National Total = 948,960 Live Births*

ALPHA ORDER

RANK	STATE	BIRTHS	% of USA
34	Alabama	8,264	0.9%
49	Alaska	1,551	0.2%
8	Arizona	30,876	3.3%
33	Arkansas	8,774	0.9%
1	California	150,246	15.8%
18	Colorado	16,303	1.7%
32	Connecticut	9,232	1.0%
44	Delaware	2,655	0.3%
4	Florida	51,683	5.4%
11	Georgia	22,902	2.4%
50	Hawaii	1,246	0.1%
39	Idaho	4,551	0.5%
5	Illinois	39,678	4.2%
10	Indiana	24,750	2.6%
30	Iowa	10,101	1.1%
28	Kansas	10,156	1.1%
20	Kentucky	14,936	1.6%
26	Louisiana	10,676	1.1%
40	Maine	4,479	0.5%
25	Maryland	11,170	1.2%
17	Massachusetts	16,383	1.7%
9	Michigan	27,924	2.9%
22	Minnesota	14,218	1.5%
38	Mississippi	5,847	0.6%
14	Missouri	18,378	1.9%
43	Montana	2,665	0.3%
37	Nebraska	6,243	0.7%
29	Nevada	10,108	1.1%
42	New Hampshire	3,425	0.4%
13	New Jersey	20,808	2.2%
27	New Mexico	10,394	1.1%
3	New York	56,690	6.0%
12	North Carolina	22,463	2.4%
48	North Dakota	1,599	0.2%
6	Ohio	37,015	3.9%
24	Oklahoma	12,546	1.3%
23	Oregon	13,018	1.4%
7	Pennsylvania	30,906	3.3%
41	Rhode Island	3,587	0.4%
31	South Carolina	9,465	1.0%
45	South Dakota	2,201	0.2%
16	Tennessee	17,136	1.8%
2	Texas	102,634	10.8%
35	Utah	7,811	0.8%
47	Vermont	1,924	0.2%
19	Virginia	16,178	1.7%
15	Washington	18,173	1.9%
36	West Virginia	6,662	0.7%
21	Wisconsin	14,883	1.6%
46	Wyoming	1,953	0.2%

RANK ORDER

RANK	STATE	BIRTHS	% of USA
1	California	150,246	15.8%
2	Texas	102,634	10.8%
3	New York	56,690	6.0%
4	Florida	51,683	5.4%
5	Illinois	39,678	4.2%
6	Ohio	37,015	3.9%
7	Pennsylvania	30,906	3.3%
8	Arizona	30,876	3.3%
9	Michigan	27,924	2.9%
10	Indiana	24,750	2.6%
11	Georgia	22,902	2.4%
12	North Carolina	22,463	2.4%
13	New Jersey	20,808	2.2%
14	Missouri	18,378	1.9%
15	Washington	18,173	1.9%
16	Tennessee	17,136	1.8%
17	Massachusetts	16,383	1.7%
18	Colorado	16,303	1.7%
19	Virginia	16,178	1.7%
20	Kentucky	14,936	1.6%
21	Wisconsin	14,883	1.6%
22	Minnesota	14,218	1.5%
23	Oregon	13,018	1.4%
24	Oklahoma	12,546	1.3%
25	Maryland	11,170	1.2%
26	Louisiana	10,676	1.1%
27	New Mexico	10,394	1.1%
28	Kansas	10,156	1.1%
29	Nevada	10,108	1.1%
30	Iowa	10,101	1.1%
31	South Carolina	9,465	1.0%
32	Connecticut	9,232	1.0%
33	Arkansas	8,774	0.9%
34	Alabama	8,264	0.9%
35	Utah	7,811	0.8%
36	West Virginia	6,662	0.7%
37	Nebraska	6,243	0.7%
38	Mississippi	5,847	0.6%
39	Idaho	4,551	0.5%
40	Maine	4,479	0.5%
41	Rhode Island	3,587	0.4%
42	New Hampshire	3,425	0.4%
43	Montana	2,665	0.3%
44	Delaware	2,655	0.3%
45	South Dakota	2,201	0.2%
46	Wyoming	1,953	0.2%
47	Vermont	1,924	0.2%
48	North Dakota	1,599	0.2%
49	Alaska	1,551	0.2%
50	Hawaii	1,246	0.1%
	District of Columbia	227	0.0%

Source: Morgan Quitno Press using data from U.S. Dept. of Health and Human Services, Nat'l Center for Health Statistics "National Vital Statistics Reports" (Vol. 53, No. 9, November 23, 2004)
Preliminary data by state of residence. By race of mother.

Births to Unmarried White Women
As a Percent of All Births to White Women in 2003
National Percent = 29.4% of Live Births*

ALPHA ORDER

RANK	STATE	PERCENT
49	Alabama	20.2
44	Alaska	23.9
2	Arizona	39.1
19	Arkansas	29.2
4	California	34.3
35	Colorado	25.8
31	Connecticut	26.1
5	Delaware	33.6
8	Florida	32.7
33	Georgia	26.0
35	Hawaii	25.8
48	Idaho	21.7
25	Illinois	27.9
8	Indiana	32.7
23	Iowa	28.3
20	Kansas	29.0
16	Kentucky	30.2
22	Louisiana	28.5
6	Maine	33.5
42	Maryland	24.4
38	Massachusetts	24.8
27	Michigan	27.1
44	Minnesota	23.9
38	Mississippi	24.8
21	Missouri	28.8
27	Montana	27.1
30	Nebraska	26.7
3	Nevada	36.5
37	New Hampshire	25.1
42	New Jersey	24.4
1	New Mexico	44.6
15	New York	30.8
33	North Carolina	26.0
46	North Dakota	23.2
18	Ohio	29.5
11	Oklahoma	31.7
13	Oregon	31.3
27	Pennsylvania	27.1
10	Rhode Island	32.0
31	South Carolina	26.1
40	South Dakota	24.7
24	Tennessee	28.1
12	Texas	31.6
50	Utah	16.5
17	Vermont	30.0
47	Virginia	22.5
26	Washington	27.3
7	West Virginia	33.3
40	Wisconsin	24.7
14	Wyoming	31.0

RANK ORDER

RANK	STATE	PERCENT
1	New Mexico	44.6
2	Arizona	39.1
3	Nevada	36.5
4	California	34.3
5	Delaware	33.6
6	Maine	33.5
7	West Virginia	33.3
8	Florida	32.7
8	Indiana	32.7
10	Rhode Island	32.0
11	Oklahoma	31.7
12	Texas	31.6
13	Oregon	31.3
14	Wyoming	31.0
15	New York	30.8
16	Kentucky	30.2
17	Vermont	30.0
18	Ohio	29.5
19	Arkansas	29.2
20	Kansas	29.0
21	Missouri	28.8
22	Louisiana	28.5
23	Iowa	28.3
24	Tennessee	28.1
25	Illinois	27.9
26	Washington	27.3
27	Michigan	27.1
27	Montana	27.1
27	Pennsylvania	27.1
30	Nebraska	26.7
31	Connecticut	26.1
31	South Carolina	26.1
33	Georgia	26.0
33	North Carolina	26.0
35	Colorado	25.8
35	Hawaii	25.8
37	New Hampshire	25.1
38	Massachusetts	24.8
38	Mississippi	24.8
40	South Dakota	24.7
40	Wisconsin	24.7
42	Maryland	24.4
42	New Jersey	24.4
44	Alaska	23.9
44	Minnesota	23.9
46	North Dakota	23.2
47	Virginia	22.5
48	Idaho	21.7
49	Alabama	20.2
50	Utah	16.5
	District of Columbia	10.7

Source: U.S. Department of Health and Human Services, National Center for Health Statistics
   "National Vital Statistics Reports" (Vol. 53, No. 9, November 23, 2004)
*Preliminary data by state of residence. By race of mother.

Births to Unmarried Black Women in 2003

National Total = 408,800 Live Births*

ALPHA ORDER

ALPHA ORDER

RANK	STATE	BIRTHS	% of USA
17	Alabama	12,446	3.0%
40	Alaska	186	0.0%
29	Arizona	2,036	0.5%
21	Arkansas	5,539	1.4%
6	California	20,259	5.0%
33	Colorado	1,534	0.4%
25	Connecticut	3,421	0.8%
31	Delaware	2,018	0.5%
2	Florida	31,676	7.7%
3	Georgia	28,204	6.9%
42	Hawaii	138	0.0%
46	Idaho	43	0.0%
5	Illinois	24,112	5.9%
20	Indiana	7,153	1.7%
35	Iowa	958	0.2%
32	Kansas	1,891	0.5%
24	Kentucky	3,552	0.9%
7	Louisiana	20,009	4.9%
44	Maine	64	0.0%
12	Maryland	14,494	3.5%
23	Massachusetts	5,009	1.2%
10	Michigan	16,637	4.1%
27	Minnesota	3,022	0.7%
14	Mississippi	13,720	3.4%
19	Missouri	8,596	2.1%
50	Montana	27	0.0%
34	Nebraska	1,031	0.3%
30	Nevada	2,025	0.5%
43	New Hampshire	103	0.0%
16	New Jersey	12,776	3.1%
39	New Mexico	326	0.1%
1	New York	31,985	7.8%
8	North Carolina	18,014	4.4%
47	North Dakota	32	0.0%
9	Ohio	17,386	4.3%
26	Oklahoma	3,243	0.8%
37	Oregon	654	0.2%
11	Pennsylvania	15,829	3.9%
36	Rhode Island	814	0.2%
15	South Carolina	13,300	3.3%
45	South Dakota	56	0.0%
18	Tennessee	11,928	2.9%
4	Texas	26,445	6.5%
41	Utah	182	0.0%
48	Vermont	29	0.0%
13	Virginia	14,083	3.4%
28	Washington	2,075	0.5%
38	West Virginia	539	0.1%
22	Wisconsin	5,346	1.3%
49	Wyoming	28	0.0%

RANK ORDER

RANK	STATE	BIRTHS	% of USA
1	New York	31,985	7.8%
2	Florida	31,676	7.7%
3	Georgia	28,204	6.9%
4	Texas	26,445	6.5%
5	Illinois	24,112	5.9%
6	California	20,259	5.0%
7	Louisiana	20,009	4.9%
8	North Carolina	18,014	4.4%
9	Ohio	17,386	4.3%
10	Michigan	16,637	4.1%
11	Pennsylvania	15,829	3.9%
12	Maryland	14,494	3.5%
13	Virginia	14,083	3.4%
14	Mississippi	13,720	3.4%
15	South Carolina	13,300	3.3%
16	New Jersey	12,776	3.1%
17	Alabama	12,446	3.0%
18	Tennessee	11,928	2.9%
19	Missouri	8,596	2.1%
20	Indiana	7,153	1.7%
21	Arkansas	5,539	1.4%
22	Wisconsin	5,346	1.3%
23	Massachusetts	5,009	1.2%
24	Kentucky	3,552	0.9%
25	Connecticut	3,421	0.8%
26	Oklahoma	3,243	0.8%
27	Minnesota	3,022	0.7%
28	Washington	2,075	0.5%
29	Arizona	2,036	0.5%
30	Nevada	2,025	0.5%
31	Delaware	2,018	0.5%
32	Kansas	1,891	0.5%
33	Colorado	1,534	0.4%
34	Nebraska	1,031	0.3%
35	Iowa	958	0.2%
36	Rhode Island	814	0.2%
37	Oregon	654	0.2%
38	West Virginia	539	0.1%
39	New Mexico	326	0.1%
40	Alaska	186	0.0%
41	Utah	182	0.0%
42	Hawaii	138	0.0%
43	New Hampshire	103	0.0%
44	Maine	64	0.0%
45	South Dakota	56	0.0%
46	Idaho	43	0.0%
47	North Dakota	32	0.0%
48	Vermont	29	0.0%
49	Wyoming	28	0.0%
50	Montana	27	0.0%
	District of Columbia	3,792	0.9%

Source: Morgan Quitno Press using data from U.S. Dept. of Health and Human Services, Nat'l Center for Health Statistics "National Vital Statistics Reports" (Vol. 53, No. 9, November 23, 2004)
*Preliminary data by state of residence. By race of mother.

Births to Unmarried Black Women
As a Percent of All Births to Black Women in 2003
National Percent = 68.2% of Live Births*

<u>ALPHA ORDER</u>

RANK	STATE	PERCENT
20	Alabama	69.3
45	Alaska	45.8
32	Arizona	62.1
6	Arkansas	75.8
33	California	62.0
41	Colorado	52.2
25	Connecticut	66.0
18	Delaware	70.0
22	Florida	66.9
26	Georgia	65.5
50	Hawaii	26.6
47	Idaho	39.8
3	Illinois	76.3
4	Indiana	76.2
10	Iowa	74.4
21	Kansas	68.4
14	Kentucky	73.1
5	Louisiana	76.0
48	Maine	34.8
35	Maryland	58.5
36	Massachusetts	58.2
12	Michigan	73.7
37	Minnesota	56.2
8	Mississippi	74.7
2	Missouri	77.0
38	Montana	52.9
17	Nebraska	70.3
19	Nevada	69.7
46	New Hampshire	42.2
29	New Jersey	63.5
34	New Mexico	61.2
23	New York	66.5
24	North Carolina	66.3
49	North Dakota	29.4
7	Ohio	75.4
16	Oklahoma	71.0
28	Oregon	63.9
11	Pennsylvania	74.2
27	Rhode Island	64.6
15	South Carolina	72.5
44	South Dakota	45.9
13	Tennessee	73.4
30	Texas	62.6
43	Utah	47.4
39	Vermont	52.8
31	Virginia	62.3
42	Washington	51.5
8	West Virginia	74.7
1	Wisconsin	82.3
39	Wyoming	52.8

<u>RANK ORDER</u>

RANK	STATE	PERCENT
1	Wisconsin	82.3
2	Missouri	77.0
3	Illinois	76.3
4	Indiana	76.2
5	Louisiana	76.0
6	Arkansas	75.8
7	Ohio	75.4
8	Mississippi	74.7
8	West Virginia	74.7
10	Iowa	74.4
11	Pennsylvania	74.2
12	Michigan	73.7
13	Tennessee	73.4
14	Kentucky	73.1
15	South Carolina	72.5
16	Oklahoma	71.0
17	Nebraska	70.3
18	Delaware	70.0
19	Nevada	69.7
20	Alabama	69.3
21	Kansas	68.4
22	Florida	66.9
23	New York	66.5
24	North Carolina	66.3
25	Connecticut	66.0
26	Georgia	65.5
27	Rhode Island	64.6
28	Oregon	63.9
29	New Jersey	63.5
30	Texas	62.6
31	Virginia	62.3
32	Arizona	62.1
33	California	62.0
34	New Mexico	61.2
35	Maryland	58.5
36	Massachusetts	58.2
37	Minnesota	56.2
38	Montana	52.9
39	Vermont	52.8
39	Wyoming	52.8
41	Colorado	52.2
42	Washington	51.5
43	Utah	47.4
44	South Dakota	45.9
45	Alaska	45.8
46	New Hampshire	42.2
47	Idaho	39.8
48	Maine	34.8
49	North Dakota	29.4
50	Hawaii	26.6
	District of Columbia	72.6

Source: U.S. Department of Health and Human Services, National Center for Health Statistics
"National Vital Statistics Reports" (Vol. 53, No. 9, November 23, 2004)
Preliminary data by state of residence. By race of mother.

Births to Unmarried Hispanic Women in 2003

National Total = 410,515 Live Births*

ALPHA ORDER

RANK	STATE	BIRTHS	% of USA
39	Alabama	706	0.2%
42	Alaska	314	0.1%
5	Arizona	21,053	5.1%
33	Arkansas	1,369	0.3%
1	California	116,151	28.3%
8	Colorado	8,837	2.2%
16	Connecticut	4,687	1.1%
38	Delaware	806	0.2%
4	Florida	22,494	5.5%
9	Georgia	8,165	2.0%
34	Hawaii	1,134	0.3%
36	Idaho	1,073	0.3%
6	Illinois	18,779	4.6%
19	Indiana	3,382	0.8%
35	Iowa	1,076	0.3%
26	Kansas	2,444	0.6%
37	Kentucky	850	0.2%
40	Louisiana	576	0.1%
48	Maine	55	0.0%
21	Maryland	2,909	0.7%
13	Massachusetts	6,131	1.5%
20	Michigan	3,365	0.8%
25	Minnesota	2,473	0.6%
43	Mississippi	215	0.1%
29	Missouri	1,583	0.4%
46	Montana	162	0.0%
31	Nebraska	1,504	0.4%
15	Nevada	5,627	1.4%
44	New Hampshire	209	0.1%
7	New Jersey	14,100	3.4%
10	New Mexico	8,126	2.0%
3	New York	33,425	8.1%
11	North Carolina	7,994	1.9%
47	North Dakota	56	0.0%
22	Ohio	2,766	0.7%
27	Oklahoma	2,426	0.6%
18	Oregon	3,646	0.9%
12	Pennsylvania	6,181	1.5%
32	Rhode Island	1,425	0.3%
30	South Carolina	1,542	0.4%
45	South Dakota	166	0.0%
28	Tennessee	2,339	0.6%
2	Texas	71,746	17.5%
23	Utah	2,730	0.7%
NA	Vermont**	NA	NA
17	Virginia	4,415	1.1%
14	Washington	5,642	1.4%
49	West Virginia	33	0.0%
24	Wisconsin	2,542	0.6%
41	Wyoming	333	0.1%

RANK ORDER

RANK	STATE	BIRTHS	% of USA
1	California	116,151	28.3%
2	Texas	71,746	17.5%
3	New York	33,425	8.1%
4	Florida	22,494	5.5%
5	Arizona	21,053	5.1%
6	Illinois	18,779	4.6%
7	New Jersey	14,100	3.4%
8	Colorado	8,837	2.2%
9	Georgia	8,165	2.0%
10	New Mexico	8,126	2.0%
11	North Carolina	7,994	1.9%
12	Pennsylvania	6,181	1.5%
13	Massachusetts	6,131	1.5%
14	Washington	5,642	1.4%
15	Nevada	5,627	1.4%
16	Connecticut	4,687	1.1%
17	Virginia	4,415	1.1%
18	Oregon	3,646	0.9%
19	Indiana	3,382	0.8%
20	Michigan	3,365	0.8%
21	Maryland	2,909	0.7%
22	Ohio	2,766	0.7%
23	Utah	2,730	0.7%
24	Wisconsin	2,542	0.6%
25	Minnesota	2,473	0.6%
26	Kansas	2,444	0.6%
27	Oklahoma	2,426	0.6%
28	Tennessee	2,339	0.6%
29	Missouri	1,583	0.4%
30	South Carolina	1,542	0.4%
31	Nebraska	1,504	0.4%
32	Rhode Island	1,425	0.3%
33	Arkansas	1,369	0.3%
34	Hawaii	1,134	0.3%
35	Iowa	1,076	0.3%
36	Idaho	1,073	0.3%
37	Kentucky	850	0.2%
38	Delaware	806	0.2%
39	Alabama	706	0.2%
40	Louisiana	576	0.1%
41	Wyoming	333	0.1%
42	Alaska	314	0.1%
43	Mississippi	215	0.1%
44	New Hampshire	209	0.1%
45	South Dakota	166	0.0%
46	Montana	162	0.0%
47	North Dakota	56	0.0%
48	Maine	55	0.0%
49	West Virginia	33	0.0%
NA	Vermont**	NA	NA
	District of Columbia	560	0.1%

Source: Morgan Quitno Press using data from U.S. Dept. of Health and Human Services, Nat'l Center for Health Statistics
"National Vital Statistics Reports" (Vol. 53, No. 9, November 23, 2004)
*Preliminary data by state of residence. Hispanic can be of any race.
**Not available. Fewer than 20 births to unmarried Hispanic women.

Births to Unmarried Hispanic Women
As a Percent of All Births to Hispanic Women in 2003
National Percent = 45.0% of Live Births*

ALPHA ORDER

RANK	STATE	PERCENT
49	Alabama	24.3
40	Alaska	40.5
9	Arizona	52.9
37	Arkansas	41.4
29	California	43.2
38	Colorado	41.3
2	Connecticut	62.1
4	Delaware	58.9
39	Florida	41.0
23	Georgia	44.7
27	Hawaii	43.3
44	Idaho	36.5
24	Illinois	44.2
12	Indiana	50.0
33	Iowa	42.7
22	Kansas	44.9
27	Kentucky	43.3
45	Louisiana	34.2
48	Maine	32.9
18	Maryland	46.2
1	Massachusetts	62.5
25	Michigan	43.9
11	Minnesota	50.1
17	Mississippi	46.6
21	Missouri	45.5
34	Montana	42.6
26	Nebraska	43.6
19	Nevada	46.1
41	New Hampshire	39.7
8	New Jersey	53.2
7	New Mexico	54.7
3	New York	60.4
14	North Carolina	49.7
46	North Dakota	33.3
10	Ohio	50.8
32	Oklahoma	42.9
29	Oregon	43.2
4	Pennsylvania	58.9
6	Rhode Island	56.7
31	South Carolina	43.0
15	South Dakota	48.8
16	Tennessee	47.4
42	Texas	38.8
43	Utah	38.6
NA	Vermont**	NA
35	Virginia	42.5
36	Washington	42.4
46	West Virginia	33.3
20	Wisconsin	45.9
12	Wyoming	50.0

RANK ORDER

RANK	STATE	PERCENT
1	Massachusetts	62.5
2	Connecticut	62.1
3	New York	60.4
4	Delaware	58.9
4	Pennsylvania	58.9
6	Rhode Island	56.7
7	New Mexico	54.7
8	New Jersey	53.2
9	Arizona	52.9
10	Ohio	50.8
11	Minnesota	50.1
12	Indiana	50.0
12	Wyoming	50.0
14	North Carolina	49.7
15	South Dakota	48.8
16	Tennessee	47.4
17	Mississippi	46.6
18	Maryland	46.2
19	Nevada	46.1
20	Wisconsin	45.9
21	Missouri	45.5
22	Kansas	44.9
23	Georgia	44.7
24	Illinois	44.2
25	Michigan	43.9
26	Nebraska	43.6
27	Hawaii	43.3
27	Kentucky	43.3
29	California	43.2
29	Oregon	43.2
31	South Carolina	43.0
32	Oklahoma	42.9
33	Iowa	42.7
34	Montana	42.6
35	Virginia	42.5
36	Washington	42.4
37	Arkansas	41.4
38	Colorado	41.3
39	Florida	41.0
40	Alaska	40.5
41	New Hampshire	39.7
42	Texas	38.8
43	Utah	38.6
44	Idaho	36.5
45	Louisiana	34.2
46	North Dakota	33.3
46	West Virginia	33.3
48	Maine	32.9
49	Alabama	24.3
NA	Vermont**	NA

| | District of Columbia | 58.7 |

Source: U.S. Department of Health and Human Services, National Center for Health Statistics
    "National Vital Statistics Reports" (Vol. 53, No. 9, November 23, 2004)
Preliminary data by state of residence. Hispanic can be of any race.
**Not available. Fewer than 20 births to unmarried Hispanic women.*

Pregnancy Rate in 2001

National Rate = 67.9 Births and Abortions per 1,000 Women 15-49 Years Old*

ALPHA ORDER

RANK	STATE	RATE
21	Alabama	64.7
NA	Alaska**	NA
9	Arizona	72.4
23	Arkansas	64.6
NA	California**	NA
33	Colorado	60.7
23	Connecticut	64.6
5	Delaware	75.2
6	Florida	75.1
8	Georgia	74.2
43	Hawaii	55.4
25	Idaho	64.3
10	Illinois	71.6
29	Indiana	63.3
36	Iowa	59.9
7	Kansas	75.0
41	Kentucky	55.9
19	Louisiana	65.2
45	Maine	50.2
34	Maryland	60.6
28	Massachusetts	63.4
30	Michigan	63.0
27	Minnesota	63.6
31	Mississippi	62.1
39	Missouri	58.1
38	Montana	58.9
15	Nebraska	66.7
2	Nevada	79.5
NA	New Hampshire**	NA
13	New Jersey	69.2
12	New Mexico	69.6
4	New York	76.6
11	North Carolina	70.5
42	North Dakota	55.7
18	Ohio	65.3
26	Oklahoma	64.1
14	Oregon	67.5
37	Pennsylvania	59.3
17	Rhode Island	65.4
35	South Carolina	60.1
32	South Dakota	60.8
21	Tennessee	64.7
3	Texas	79.3
1	Utah	85.1
46	Vermont	49.7
20	Virginia	65.0
16	Washington	66.4
44	West Virginia	51.5
40	Wisconsin	58.0
47	Wyoming	48.8

RANK ORDER

RANK	STATE	RATE
1	Utah	85.1
2	Nevada	79.5
3	Texas	79.3
4	New York	76.6
5	Delaware	75.2
6	Florida	75.1
7	Kansas	75.0
8	Georgia	74.2
9	Arizona	72.4
10	Illinois	71.6
11	North Carolina	70.5
12	New Mexico	69.6
13	New Jersey	69.2
14	Oregon	67.5
15	Nebraska	66.7
16	Washington	66.4
17	Rhode Island	65.4
18	Ohio	65.3
19	Louisiana	65.2
20	Virginia	65.0
21	Alabama	64.7
21	Tennessee	64.7
23	Arkansas	64.6
23	Connecticut	64.6
25	Idaho	64.3
26	Oklahoma	64.1
27	Minnesota	63.6
28	Massachusetts	63.4
29	Indiana	63.3
30	Michigan	63.0
31	Mississippi	62.1
32	South Dakota	60.8
33	Colorado	60.7
34	Maryland	60.6
35	South Carolina	60.1
36	Iowa	59.9
37	Pennsylvania	59.3
38	Montana	58.9
39	Missouri	58.1
40	Wisconsin	58.0
41	Kentucky	55.9
42	North Dakota	55.7
43	Hawaii	55.4
44	West Virginia	51.5
45	Maine	50.2
46	Vermont	49.7
47	Wyoming	48.8
NA	Alaska**	NA
NA	California**	NA
NA	New Hampshire**	NA

District of Columbia 77.9

Source: Morgan Quitno Press using data from US Dept of Health & Human Serv's, Centers for Disease Control-Prevention "Abortion Surveillance-United States, 2001" (Morbidity and Mortality Weekly Report, Vol. 53, No. SS-9, 11/26/04)
The sum of live births and legal induced abortions per 1,000 women aged 15-49 years old. Births by state of residence, abortions by state of occurrence. Miscarriages are not included in these rates. National rate includes only states reporting abortions and births.
***Not available.*

Pregnancy Rate for 15 to 19 Year Old Women in 2001

National Rate = 62.0 Births and Abortions per 1,000 Women 15-19 Years Old*

ALPHA ORDER

RANK	STATE	RATE
11	Alabama	71.8
NA	Alaska**	NA
8	Arizona	72.9
7	Arkansas	74.1
NA	California**	NA
26	Colorado	54.1
27	Connecticut	53.4
6	Delaware	74.2
NA	Florida**	NA
4	Georgia	78.0
18	Hawaii	64.2
37	Idaho	44.1
16	Illinois	66.4
25	Indiana	55.8
39	Iowa	44.0
15	Kansas	67.6
24	Kentucky	56.1
12	Louisiana	69.2
43	Maine	39.3
33	Maryland	49.6
41	Massachusetts	43.7
29	Michigan	52.7
42	Minnesota	41.7
10	Mississippi	72.6
30	Missouri	52.6
32	Montana	51.0
34	Nebraska	49.2
1	Nevada	84.0
NA	New Hampshire**	NA
31	New Jersey	51.4
3	New Mexico	78.4
14	New York	68.4
5	North Carolina	74.3
45	North Dakota	38.7
22	Ohio	59.2
13	Oklahoma	68.6
20	Oregon	62.4
35	Pennsylvania	48.7
19	Rhode Island	63.3
17	South Carolina	65.7
36	South Dakota	44.5
9	Tennessee	72.8
2	Texas	80.2
39	Utah	44.0
46	Vermont	38.5
23	Virginia	56.4
21	Washington	59.6
28	West Virginia	53.3
37	Wisconsin	44.1
44	Wyoming	39.1

RANK ORDER

RANK	STATE	RATE
1	Nevada	84.0
2	Texas	80.2
3	New Mexico	78.4
4	Georgia	78.0
5	North Carolina	74.3
6	Delaware	74.2
7	Arkansas	74.1
8	Arizona	72.9
9	Tennessee	72.8
10	Mississippi	72.6
11	Alabama	71.8
12	Louisiana	69.2
13	Oklahoma	68.6
14	New York	68.4
15	Kansas	67.6
16	Illinois	66.4
17	South Carolina	65.7
18	Hawaii	64.2
19	Rhode Island	63.3
20	Oregon	62.4
21	Washington	59.6
22	Ohio	59.2
23	Virginia	56.4
24	Kentucky	56.1
25	Indiana	55.8
26	Colorado	54.1
27	Connecticut	53.4
28	West Virginia	53.3
29	Michigan	52.7
30	Missouri	52.6
31	New Jersey	51.4
32	Montana	51.0
33	Maryland	49.6
34	Nebraska	49.2
35	Pennsylvania	48.7
36	South Dakota	44.5
37	Idaho	44.1
37	Wisconsin	44.1
39	Iowa	44.0
39	Utah	44.0
41	Massachusetts	43.7
42	Minnesota	41.7
43	Maine	39.3
44	Wyoming	39.1
45	North Dakota	38.7
46	Vermont	38.5
NA	Alaska**	NA
NA	California**	NA
NA	Florida**	NA
NA	New Hampshire**	NA

District of Columbia   136.1

Source: Morgan Quitno Press using data from US Dept of Health & Human Serv's, Centers for Disease Control-Prevention
"Abortion Surveillance-United States, 2001" (Morbidity and Mortality Weekly Report, Vol. 53, No. SS-9, 11/26/04)
*The sum of live births and legal induced abortions per 1,000 women aged 15-19 years old. Births by state of
residence, abortions by state of occurrence. Miscarriages are not included in these rates. National rate includes
only states reporting abortions and births.
**Not available.

29

Percent Change in Pregnancy Rate for 15 to 19 Year Old Women: 1997 to 2001

National Percent Change = 13.0% Decrease*

ALPHA ORDER			RANK ORDER		
RANK	STATE	PERCENT CHANGE	RANK	STATE	PERCENT CHANGE
28	Alabama	(13.6)	1	North Dakota	(4.7)
NA	Alaska**	NA	2	South Dakota	(6.5)
24	Arizona	(12.9)	3	Idaho	(6.6)
27	Arkansas	(13.5)	4	New Jersey	(7.1)
NA	California**	NA	5	Nevada	(7.2)
31	Colorado	(14.5)	6	Nebraska	(7.7)
39	Connecticut	(19.2)	6	New Mexico	(7.7)
43	Delaware	(31.2)	8	Hawaii	(7.9)
NA	Florida**	NA	9	Kansas	(8.4)
34	Georgia	(15.2)	10	West Virginia	(9.2)
8	Hawaii	(7.9)	11	Wisconsin	(9.3)
3	Idaho	(6.6)	12	Maryland	(9.8)
NA	Illinois**	NA	12	Utah	(9.8)
35	Indiana	(15.6)	14	Montana	(10.1)
NA	Iowa**	NA	15	Mississippi	(10.5)
9	Kansas	(8.4)	15	Pennsylvania	(10.5)
39	Kentucky	(19.2)	17	Minnesota	(11.5)
18	Louisiana	(11.6)	18	Louisiana	(11.6)
32	Maine	(14.9)	19	Michigan	(11.9)
12	Maryland	(9.8)	20	Wyoming	(12.1)
42	Massachusetts	(23.2)	21	South Carolina	(12.4)
19	Michigan	(11.9)	21	Tennessee	(12.4)
17	Minnesota	(11.5)	21	Texas	(12.4)
15	Mississippi	(10.5)	24	Arizona	(12.9)
26	Missouri	(13.3)	25	North Carolina	(13.2)
14	Montana	(10.1)	26	Missouri	(13.3)
6	Nebraska	(7.7)	27	Arkansas	(13.5)
5	Nevada	(7.2)	28	Alabama	(13.6)
NA	New Hampshire**	NA	29	Ohio	(13.8)
4	New Jersey	(7.1)	30	Virginia	(14.2)
6	New Mexico	(7.7)	31	Colorado	(14.5)
37	New York	(17.5)	32	Maine	(14.9)
25	North Carolina	(13.2)	33	Washington	(15.0)
1	North Dakota	(4.7)	34	Georgia	(15.2)
29	Ohio	(13.8)	35	Indiana	(15.6)
NA	Oklahoma**	NA	36	Oregon	(16.5)
36	Oregon	(16.5)	37	New York	(17.5)
15	Pennsylvania	(10.5)	38	Rhode Island	(17.7)
38	Rhode Island	(17.7)	39	Connecticut	(19.2)
21	South Carolina	(12.4)	39	Kentucky	(19.2)
2	South Dakota	(6.5)	41	Vermont	(21.1)
21	Tennessee	(12.4)	42	Massachusetts	(23.2)
21	Texas	(12.4)	43	Delaware	(31.2)
12	Utah	(9.8)	NA	Alaska**	NA
41	Vermont	(21.1)	NA	California**	NA
30	Virginia	(14.2)	NA	Florida**	NA
33	Washington	(15.0)	NA	Illinois**	NA
10	West Virginia	(9.2)	NA	Iowa**	NA
11	Wisconsin	(9.3)	NA	New Hampshire**	NA
20	Wyoming	(12.1)	NA	Oklahoma**	NA

District of Columbia (35.8)

Source: Morgan Quitno Press using data from US Dept of Health & Human Serv's, Centers for Disease Control-Prevention "Abortion Surveillance-United States, 2001" (Morbidity and Mortality Weekly Report, Vol. 53, No. SS-9, 11/26/04)
*The sum of live births and legal induced abortions per 1,000 women aged 15-19 years old. Births by state of residence, abortions by state of occurrence. Miscarriages are not included in these rates. National rate includes only states reporting abortions and births.
**Not available.

Births to Teenage Mothers in 2003

National Total = 421,379 Live Births*

ALPHA ORDER

RANK	STATE	BIRTHS	% of USA
17	Alabama	8,287	2.0%
45	Alaska	1,073	0.3%
11	Arizona	11,740	2.8%
27	Arkansas	5,762	1.4%
2	California	50,313	11.9%
24	Colorado	6,798	1.6%
36	Connecticut	2,871	0.7%
41	Delaware	1,217	0.3%
3	Florida	23,139	5.5%
6	Georgia	16,185	3.8%
40	Hawaii	1,522	0.4%
39	Idaho	2,093	0.5%
5	Illinois	17,711	4.2%
14	Indiana	9,526	2.3%
35	Iowa	3,322	0.8%
32	Kansas	4,107	1.0%
21	Kentucky	6,910	1.6%
13	Louisiana	9,729	2.3%
43	Maine	1,137	0.3%
25	Maryland	6,438	1.5%
29	Massachusetts	4,735	1.1%
10	Michigan	12,439	3.0%
28	Minnesota	4,981	1.2%
22	Mississippi	6,863	1.6%
16	Missouri	8,787	2.1%
42	Montana	1,210	0.3%
38	Nebraska	2,333	0.6%
33	Nevada	3,802	0.9%
47	New Hampshire	820	0.2%
19	New Jersey	7,209	1.7%
30	New Mexico	4,594	1.1%
4	New York	17,793	4.2%
8	North Carolina	13,487	3.2%
49	North Dakota	630	0.1%
7	Ohio	15,958	3.8%
20	Oklahoma	7,017	1.7%
31	Oregon	4,184	1.0%
9	Pennsylvania	12,659	3.0%
44	Rhode Island	1,082	0.3%
18	South Carolina	7,403	1.8%
46	South Dakota	1,037	0.2%
12	Tennessee	10,415	2.5%
1	Texas	52,611	12.5%
34	Utah	3,341	0.8%
50	Vermont	422	0.1%
15	Virginia	9,009	2.1%
23	Washington	6,840	1.6%
37	West Virginia	2,572	0.6%
26	Wisconsin	6,305	1.5%
48	Wyoming	812	0.2%

RANK ORDER

RANK	STATE	BIRTHS	% of USA
1	Texas	52,611	12.5%
2	California	50,313	11.9%
3	Florida	23,139	5.5%
4	New York	17,793	4.2%
5	Illinois	17,711	4.2%
6	Georgia	16,185	3.8%
7	Ohio	15,958	3.8%
8	North Carolina	13,487	3.2%
9	Pennsylvania	12,659	3.0%
10	Michigan	12,439	3.0%
11	Arizona	11,740	2.8%
12	Tennessee	10,415	2.5%
13	Louisiana	9,729	2.3%
14	Indiana	9,526	2.3%
15	Virginia	9,009	2.1%
16	Missouri	8,787	2.1%
17	Alabama	8,287	2.0%
18	South Carolina	7,403	1.8%
19	New Jersey	7,209	1.7%
20	Oklahoma	7,017	1.7%
21	Kentucky	6,910	1.6%
22	Mississippi	6,863	1.6%
23	Washington	6,840	1.6%
24	Colorado	6,798	1.6%
25	Maryland	6,438	1.5%
26	Wisconsin	6,305	1.5%
27	Arkansas	5,762	1.4%
28	Minnesota	4,981	1.2%
29	Massachusetts	4,735	1.1%
30	New Mexico	4,594	1.1%
31	Oregon	4,184	1.0%
32	Kansas	4,107	1.0%
33	Nevada	3,802	0.9%
34	Utah	3,341	0.8%
35	Iowa	3,322	0.8%
36	Connecticut	2,871	0.7%
37	West Virginia	2,572	0.6%
38	Nebraska	2,333	0.6%
39	Idaho	2,093	0.5%
40	Hawaii	1,522	0.4%
41	Delaware	1,217	0.3%
42	Montana	1,210	0.3%
43	Maine	1,137	0.3%
44	Rhode Island	1,082	0.3%
45	Alaska	1,073	0.3%
46	South Dakota	1,037	0.2%
47	New Hampshire	820	0.2%
48	Wyoming	812	0.2%
49	North Dakota	630	0.1%
50	Vermont	422	0.1%
	District of Columbia	867	0.2%

Source: Morgan Quitno Press using data from U.S. Dept. of Health and Human Services, Nat'l Center for Health Statistics
  "National Vital Statistics Reports" (Vol. 53, No. 9, November 23, 2004)
*Live births to women 15 to 19 years old by state of residence.

Teenage Birth Rate in 2003

National Rate = 46.1 Live Births per 1,000 Women 15 to 19 Years Old*

ALPHA ORDER

RANK	STATE	RATE
13	Alabama	55.8
32	Alaska	38.6
4	Arizona	67.0
5	Arkansas	66.3
25	California	42.9
18	Colorado	48.4
47	Connecticut	26.8
15	Delaware	51.5
21	Florida	44.9
8	Georgia	62.2
28	Hawaii	41.4
26	Idaho	42.8
22	Illinois	44.6
19	Indiana	48.3
33	Iowa	38.3
20	Kansas	47.6
14	Kentucky	55.1
6	Louisiana	63.9
46	Maine	27.9
36	Maryland	37.5
48	Massachusetts	25.8
38	Michigan	37.2
43	Minnesota	29.9
1	Mississippi	70.5
17	Missouri	48.8
33	Montana	38.3
27	Nebraska	42.4
11	Nevada	56.5
50	New Hampshire	20.2
45	New Jersey	29.1
2	New Mexico	70.1
42	New York	31.8
11	North Carolina	56.5
44	North Dakota	29.8
24	Ohio	43.9
7	Oklahoma	62.5
31	Oregon	39.2
40	Pennsylvania	34.9
35	Rhode Island	38.0
10	South Carolina	57.3
29	South Dakota	40.3
9	Tennessee	58.4
3	Texas	69.4
37	Utah	37.3
49	Vermont	21.9
30	Virginia	39.7
41	Washington	33.5
16	West Virginia	50.5
39	Wisconsin	36.3
23	Wyoming	44.0

RANK ORDER

RANK	STATE	RATE
1	Mississippi	70.5
2	New Mexico	70.1
3	Texas	69.4
4	Arizona	67.0
5	Arkansas	66.3
6	Louisiana	63.9
7	Oklahoma	62.5
8	Georgia	62.2
9	Tennessee	58.4
10	South Carolina	57.3
11	Nevada	56.5
11	North Carolina	56.5
13	Alabama	55.8
14	Kentucky	55.1
15	Delaware	51.5
16	West Virginia	50.5
17	Missouri	48.8
18	Colorado	48.4
19	Indiana	48.3
20	Kansas	47.6
21	Florida	44.9
22	Illinois	44.6
23	Wyoming	44.0
24	Ohio	43.9
25	California	42.9
26	Idaho	42.8
27	Nebraska	42.4
28	Hawaii	41.4
29	South Dakota	40.3
30	Virginia	39.7
31	Oregon	39.2
32	Alaska	38.6
33	Iowa	38.3
33	Montana	38.3
35	Rhode Island	38.0
36	Maryland	37.5
37	Utah	37.3
38	Michigan	37.2
39	Wisconsin	36.3
40	Pennsylvania	34.9
41	Washington	33.5
42	New York	31.8
43	Minnesota	29.9
44	North Dakota	29.8
45	New Jersey	29.1
46	Maine	27.9
47	Connecticut	26.8
48	Massachusetts	25.8
49	Vermont	21.9
50	New Hampshire	20.2

| | District of Columbia | 102.7 |

Source: Morgan Quitno Press using data from U.S. Dept. of Health and Human Services, Nat'l Center for Health Statistics "National Vital Statistics Reports" (Vol. 53, No. 9, November 23, 2004)

*By state of residence.

Births to Teenage Mothers as a Percent of Births in 2003

National Percent = 10.3% of Live Births*

ALPHA ORDER

RANK	STATE	PERCENT
5	Alabama	13.9
21	Alaska	10.6
10	Arizona	12.9
3	Arkansas	15.1
30	California	9.3
25	Colorado	9.8
45	Connecticut	6.7
20	Delaware	10.8
19	Florida	10.9
14	Georgia	11.9
39	Hawaii	8.4
27	Idaho	9.6
26	Illinois	9.7
18	Indiana	11.0
36	Iowa	8.7
24	Kansas	10.4
11	Kentucky	12.5
4	Louisiana	14.9
40	Maine	8.2
37	Maryland	8.6
49	Massachusetts	5.9
28	Michigan	9.5
43	Minnesota	7.1
2	Mississippi	16.2
15	Missouri	11.4
21	Montana	10.6
32	Nebraska	9.0
17	Nevada	11.3
50	New Hampshire	5.7
48	New Jersey	6.2
1	New Mexico	16.5
44	New York	7.0
15	North Carolina	11.4
42	North Dakota	7.9
23	Ohio	10.5
5	Oklahoma	13.9
31	Oregon	9.1
32	Pennsylvania	9.0
40	Rhode Island	8.2
8	South Carolina	13.3
29	South Dakota	9.4
9	Tennessee	13.2
7	Texas	13.8
45	Utah	6.7
47	Vermont	6.4
35	Virginia	8.9
38	Washington	8.5
12	West Virginia	12.3
32	Wisconsin	9.0
13	Wyoming	12.1

RANK ORDER

RANK	STATE	PERCENT
1	New Mexico	16.5
2	Mississippi	16.2
3	Arkansas	15.1
4	Louisiana	14.9
5	Alabama	13.9
5	Oklahoma	13.9
7	Texas	13.8
8	South Carolina	13.3
9	Tennessee	13.2
10	Arizona	12.9
11	Kentucky	12.5
12	West Virginia	12.3
13	Wyoming	12.1
14	Georgia	11.9
15	Missouri	11.4
15	North Carolina	11.4
17	Nevada	11.3
18	Indiana	11.0
19	Florida	10.9
20	Delaware	10.8
21	Alaska	10.6
21	Montana	10.6
23	Ohio	10.5
24	Kansas	10.4
25	Colorado	9.8
26	Illinois	9.7
27	Idaho	9.6
28	Michigan	9.5
29	South Dakota	9.4
30	California	9.3
31	Oregon	9.1
32	Nebraska	9.0
32	Pennsylvania	9.0
32	Wisconsin	9.0
35	Virginia	8.9
36	Iowa	8.7
37	Maryland	8.6
38	Washington	8.5
39	Hawaii	8.4
40	Maine	8.2
40	Rhode Island	8.2
42	North Dakota	7.9
43	Minnesota	7.1
44	New York	7.0
45	Connecticut	6.7
45	Utah	6.7
47	Vermont	6.4
48	New Jersey	6.2
49	Massachusetts	5.9
50	New Hampshire	5.7
	District of Columbia	11.4

Source: U.S. Department of Health and Human Services, National Center for Health Statistics
    "National Vital Statistics Reports" (Vol. 53, No. 9, November 23, 2004)
*Live births to women 15 to 19 years old by state of residence.

Percent Change in Teenage Birth Rate: 1999 to 2003

National Percent Change = 7.1% Decrease*

ALPHA ORDER

RANK	STATE	PERCENT CHANGE
38	Alabama	(11.1)
35	Alaska	(7.7)
23	Arizona	(3.7)
20	Arkansas	(2.6)
45	California	(15.4)
13	Colorado	0.0
50	Connecticut	(19.5)
27	Delaware	(5.2)
48	Florida	(16.1)
24	Georgia	(4.5)
28	Hawaii	(5.5)
18	Idaho	(2.1)
42	Illinois	(12.7)
30	Indiana	(6.4)
6	Iowa	7.0
12	Kansas	0.4
19	Kentucky	(2.3)
10	Louisiana	1.8
30	Maine	(6.4)
41	Maryland	(12.0)
37	Massachusetts	(10.1)
36	Michigan	(8.1)
14	Minnesota	(0.3)
21	Mississippi	(2.8)
17	Missouri	(1.6)
2	Montana	9.1
1	Nebraska	14.6
40	Nevada	(11.9)
47	New Hampshire	(15.8)
39	New Jersey	(11.3)
8	New Mexico	4.0
43	New York	(14.1)
26	North Carolina	(5.0)
4	North Dakota	7.6
25	Ohio	(4.6)
9	Oklahoma	3.3
46	Oregon	(15.7)
22	Pennsylvania	(3.6)
15	Rhode Island	(0.5)
29	South Carolina	(5.8)
5	South Dakota	7.2
32	Tennessee	(6.9)
16	Texas	(1.0)
34	Utah	(7.2)
44	Vermont	(14.8)
33	Virginia	(7.0)
49	Washington	(16.5)
7	West Virginia	5.4
11	Wisconsin	1.7
3	Wyoming	8.9

RANK ORDER

RANK	STATE	PERCENT CHANGE
1	Nebraska	14.6
2	Montana	9.1
3	Wyoming	8.9
4	North Dakota	7.6
5	South Dakota	7.2
6	Iowa	7.0
7	West Virginia	5.4
8	New Mexico	4.0
9	Oklahoma	3.3
10	Louisiana	1.8
11	Wisconsin	1.7
12	Kansas	0.4
13	Colorado	0.0
14	Minnesota	(0.3)
15	Rhode Island	(0.5)
16	Texas	(1.0)
17	Missouri	(1.6)
18	Idaho	(2.1)
19	Kentucky	(2.3)
20	Arkansas	(2.6)
21	Mississippi	(2.8)
22	Pennsylvania	(3.6)
23	Arizona	(3.7)
24	Georgia	(4.5)
25	Ohio	(4.6)
26	North Carolina	(5.0)
27	Delaware	(5.2)
28	Hawaii	(5.5)
29	South Carolina	(5.8)
30	Indiana	(6.4)
30	Maine	(6.4)
32	Tennessee	(6.9)
33	Virginia	(7.0)
34	Utah	(7.2)
35	Alaska	(7.7)
36	Michigan	(8.1)
37	Massachusetts	(10.1)
38	Alabama	(11.1)
39	New Jersey	(11.3)
40	Nevada	(11.9)
41	Maryland	(12.0)
42	Illinois	(12.7)
43	New York	(14.1)
44	Vermont	(14.8)
45	California	(15.4)
46	Oregon	(15.7)
47	New Hampshire	(15.8)
48	Florida	(16.1)
49	Washington	(16.5)
50	Connecticut	(19.5)

District of Columbia   23.0

Source: Morgan Quitno Press using data from U.S. Dept. of Health and Human Services, Nat'l Center for Health Statistics "National Vital Statistics Reports" (Vol. 53, No. 9, November 23, 2004 and Vol. 49, No. 1, April 17, 2001)
*By state of residence. Births to women aged 15 to 19 years old.

Births to White Teenage Mothers in 2003

National Total = 303,409 Live Births*

ALPHA ORDER

RANK	STATE	BIRTHS	% of USA
20	Alabama	4,623	1.5%
47	Alaska	519	0.2%
7	Arizona	9,871	3.3%
23	Arkansas	4,026	1.3%
2	California	42,927	14.1%
15	Colorado	6,129	2.0%
37	Connecticut	2,122	0.7%
45	Delaware	711	0.2%
3	Florida	14,857	4.9%
8	Georgia	8,897	2.9%
50	Hawaii	319	0.1%
38	Idaho	1,992	0.7%
6	Illinois	11,093	3.7%
12	Indiana	7,569	2.5%
33	Iowa	2,962	1.0%
29	Kansas	3,502	1.2%
16	Kentucky	5,935	2.0%
24	Louisiana	4,008	1.3%
40	Maine	1,096	0.4%
35	Maryland	2,884	1.0%
28	Massachusetts	3,633	1.2%
10	Michigan	8,140	2.7%
30	Minnesota	3,450	1.1%
34	Mississippi	2,900	1.0%
14	Missouri	6,381	2.1%
41	Montana	865	0.3%
39	Nebraska	1,871	0.6%
32	Nevada	3,046	1.0%
43	New Hampshire	805	0.3%
21	New Jersey	4,434	1.5%
25	New Mexico	3,845	1.3%
4	New York	11,596	3.8%
11	North Carolina	8,035	2.6%
48	North Dakota	441	0.1%
5	Ohio	11,293	3.7%
19	Oklahoma	4,947	1.6%
26	Oregon	3,785	1.2%
9	Pennsylvania	8,325	2.7%
42	Rhode Island	829	0.3%
27	South Carolina	3,735	1.2%
46	South Dakota	597	0.2%
13	Tennessee	7,074	2.3%
1	Texas	44,496	14.7%
31	Utah	3,077	1.0%
49	Vermont	417	0.1%
18	Virginia	5,105	1.7%
17	Washington	5,525	1.8%
36	West Virginia	2,441	0.8%
22	Wisconsin	4,218	1.4%
44	Wyoming	731	0.2%

RANK ORDER

RANK	STATE	BIRTHS	% of USA
1	Texas	44,496	14.7%
2	California	42,927	14.1%
3	Florida	14,857	4.9%
4	New York	11,596	3.8%
5	Ohio	11,293	3.7%
6	Illinois	11,093	3.7%
7	Arizona	9,871	3.3%
8	Georgia	8,897	2.9%
9	Pennsylvania	8,325	2.7%
10	Michigan	8,140	2.7%
11	North Carolina	8,035	2.6%
12	Indiana	7,569	2.5%
13	Tennessee	7,074	2.3%
14	Missouri	6,381	2.1%
15	Colorado	6,129	2.0%
16	Kentucky	5,935	2.0%
17	Washington	5,525	1.8%
18	Virginia	5,105	1.7%
19	Oklahoma	4,947	1.6%
20	Alabama	4,623	1.5%
21	New Jersey	4,434	1.5%
22	Wisconsin	4,218	1.4%
23	Arkansas	4,026	1.3%
24	Louisiana	4,008	1.3%
25	New Mexico	3,845	1.3%
26	Oregon	3,785	1.2%
27	South Carolina	3,735	1.2%
28	Massachusetts	3,633	1.2%
29	Kansas	3,502	1.2%
30	Minnesota	3,450	1.1%
31	Utah	3,077	1.0%
32	Nevada	3,046	1.0%
33	Iowa	2,962	1.0%
34	Mississippi	2,900	1.0%
35	Maryland	2,884	1.0%
36	West Virginia	2,441	0.8%
37	Connecticut	2,122	0.7%
38	Idaho	1,992	0.7%
39	Nebraska	1,871	0.6%
40	Maine	1,096	0.4%
41	Montana	865	0.3%
42	Rhode Island	829	0.3%
43	New Hampshire	805	0.3%
44	Wyoming	731	0.2%
45	Delaware	711	0.2%
46	South Dakota	597	0.2%
47	Alaska	519	0.2%
48	North Dakota	441	0.1%
49	Vermont	417	0.1%
50	Hawaii	319	0.1%
	District of Columbia	40	0.0%

Source: Morgan Quitno Press using data from U.S. Dept. of Health and Human Services, Nat'l Center for Health Statistics
"National Vital Statistics Reports" (Vol. 53, No. 9, November 23, 2004)
*Live births to women 15 to 19 years old by state of residence.

White Teenage Birth Rate in 2003

National Rate = 38.5 Births per 1,000 White Teenage Women*

ALPHA ORDER

RANK	STATE	RATE
11	Alabama	46.1
36	Alaska	27.0
3	Arizona	60.9
4	Arkansas	55.5
13	California	44.4
14	Colorado	44.2
43	Connecticut	22.2
24	Delaware	36.0
23	Florida	37.2
9	Georgia	48.2
50	Hawaii	17.8
21	Idaho	39.1
28	Illinois	33.2
18	Indiana	39.6
30	Iowa	30.2
19	Kansas	39.2
8	Kentucky	48.7
17	Louisiana	41.1
38	Maine	24.8
39	Maryland	24.3
46	Massachusetts	20.9
33	Michigan	28.4
44	Minnesota	21.0
5	Mississippi	51.4
22	Missouri	37.8
34	Montana	28.0
29	Nebraska	31.8
6	Nevada	51.3
49	New Hampshire	18.3
44	New Jersey	21.0
2	New Mexico	64.2
37	New York	25.9
16	North Carolina	43.3
47	North Dakota	20.6
27	Ohio	33.7
7	Oklahoma	51.0
25	Oregon	34.4
41	Pennsylvania	23.7
35	Rhode Island	27.7
15	South Carolina	43.6
42	South Dakota	23.4
10	Tennessee	48.1
1	Texas	65.9
26	Utah	34.2
48	Vermont	19.4
32	Virginia	29.2
31	Washington	29.7
12	West Virginia	45.2
40	Wisconsin	24.0
19	Wyoming	39.2

RANK ORDER

RANK	STATE	RATE
1	Texas	65.9
2	New Mexico	64.2
3	Arizona	60.9
4	Arkansas	55.5
5	Mississippi	51.4
6	Nevada	51.3
7	Oklahoma	51.0
8	Kentucky	48.7
9	Georgia	48.2
10	Tennessee	48.1
11	Alabama	46.1
12	West Virginia	45.2
13	California	44.4
14	Colorado	44.2
15	South Carolina	43.6
16	North Carolina	43.3
17	Louisiana	41.1
18	Indiana	39.6
19	Kansas	39.2
19	Wyoming	39.2
21	Idaho	39.1
22	Missouri	37.8
23	Florida	37.2
24	Delaware	36.0
25	Oregon	34.4
26	Utah	34.2
27	Ohio	33.7
28	Illinois	33.2
29	Nebraska	31.8
30	Iowa	30.2
31	Washington	29.7
32	Virginia	29.2
33	Michigan	28.4
34	Montana	28.0
35	Rhode Island	27.7
36	Alaska	27.0
37	New York	25.9
38	Maine	24.8
39	Maryland	24.3
40	Wisconsin	24.0
41	Pennsylvania	23.7
42	South Dakota	23.4
43	Connecticut	22.2
44	Minnesota	21.0
44	New Jersey	21.0
46	Massachusetts	20.9
47	North Dakota	20.6
48	Vermont	19.4
49	New Hampshire	18.3
50	Hawaii	17.8

District of Columbia 6.6

Source: Morgan Quitno Press using data from U.S. Dept. of Health and Human Services, Nat'l Center for Health Statistics
"National Vital Statistics Reports" (Vol. 53, No. 9, November 23, 2004)
*Live births to women age 15 to 19 years old by state of residence. Rates calculated using Census 2003 estimates
for females ages 15 to 19 years old in the category of "White Alone or in Combination."

Births to White Teenage Mothers as a Percent of White Births in 2003

National Percent = 9.4% of White Live Births*

ALPHA ORDER

RANK	STATE	PERCENT
11	Alabama	11.3
31	Alaska	8.0
4	Arizona	12.5
3	Arkansas	13.4
19	California	9.8
20	Colorado	9.7
46	Connecticut	6.0
25	Delaware	9.0
22	Florida	9.4
15	Georgia	10.1
40	Hawaii	6.6
21	Idaho	9.5
34	Illinois	7.8
16	Indiana	10.0
28	Iowa	8.3
16	Kansas	10.0
8	Kentucky	12.0
13	Louisiana	10.7
30	Maine	8.2
44	Maryland	6.3
49	Massachusetts	5.5
33	Michigan	7.9
48	Minnesota	5.8
6	Mississippi	12.3
16	Missouri	10.0
27	Montana	8.8
31	Nebraska	8.0
12	Nevada	11.0
47	New Hampshire	5.9
50	New Jersey	5.2
1	New Mexico	16.5
44	New York	6.3
23	North Carolina	9.3
43	North Dakota	6.4
25	Ohio	9.0
4	Oklahoma	12.5
24	Oregon	9.1
36	Pennsylvania	7.3
35	Rhode Island	7.4
14	South Carolina	10.3
39	South Dakota	6.7
9	Tennessee	11.6
2	Texas	13.7
41	Utah	6.5
41	Vermont	6.5
37	Virginia	7.1
28	Washington	8.3
7	West Virginia	12.2
38	Wisconsin	7.0
9	Wyoming	11.6

RANK ORDER

RANK	STATE	PERCENT
1	New Mexico	16.5
2	Texas	13.7
3	Arkansas	13.4
4	Arizona	12.5
4	Oklahoma	12.5
6	Mississippi	12.3
7	West Virginia	12.2
8	Kentucky	12.0
9	Tennessee	11.6
9	Wyoming	11.6
11	Alabama	11.3
12	Nevada	11.0
13	Louisiana	10.7
14	South Carolina	10.3
15	Georgia	10.1
16	Indiana	10.0
16	Kansas	10.0
16	Missouri	10.0
19	California	9.8
20	Colorado	9.7
21	Idaho	9.5
22	Florida	9.4
23	North Carolina	9.3
24	Oregon	9.1
25	Delaware	9.0
25	Ohio	9.0
27	Montana	8.8
28	Iowa	8.3
28	Washington	8.3
30	Maine	8.2
31	Alaska	8.0
31	Nebraska	8.0
33	Michigan	7.9
34	Illinois	7.8
35	Rhode Island	7.4
36	Pennsylvania	7.3
37	Virginia	7.1
38	Wisconsin	7.0
39	South Dakota	6.7
40	Hawaii	6.6
41	Utah	6.5
41	Vermont	6.5
43	North Dakota	6.4
44	Maryland	6.3
44	New York	6.3
46	Connecticut	6.0
47	New Hampshire	5.9
48	Minnesota	5.8
49	Massachusetts	5.5
50	New Jersey	5.2
	District of Columbia	1.9

Source: U.S. Department of Health and Human Services, National Center for Health Statistics
   "National Vital Statistics Reports" (Vol. 53, No. 9, November 23, 2004)
*Live births to women 15 to 19 years old by state of residence.

Births to Black Teenage Mothers in 2003

National Total = 103,699 Live Births*

ALPHA ORDER

RANK	STATE	BIRTHS	% of USA
14	Alabama	3,610	3.5%
41	Alaska	57	0.1%
28	Arizona	587	0.6%
21	Arkansas	1,644	1.6%
9	California	4,542	4.4%
33	Colorado	470	0.5%
27	Connecticut	721	0.7%
31	Delaware	505	0.5%
1	Florida	7,907	7.6%
3	Georgia	7,062	6.8%
42	Hawaii	37	0.0%
NA	Idaho**	NA	NA
4	Illinois	6,447	6.2%
20	Indiana	1,868	1.8%
35	Iowa	288	0.3%
30	Kansas	520	0.5%
24	Kentucky	913	0.9%
6	Louisiana	5,661	5.5%
NA	Maine**	NA	NA
16	Maryland	3,444	3.3%
25	Massachusetts	878	0.8%
11	Michigan	4,041	3.9%
26	Minnesota	731	0.7%
12	Mississippi	3,912	3.8%
19	Missouri	2,244	2.2%
NA	Montana**	NA	NA
34	Nebraska	305	0.3%
31	Nevada	505	0.5%
NA	New Hampshire**	NA	NA
18	New Jersey	2,676	2.6%
39	New Mexico	95	0.1%
5	New York	5,772	5.6%
7	North Carolina	4,918	4.7%
NA	North Dakota**	NA	NA
8	Ohio	4,566	4.4%
23	Oklahoma	932	0.9%
37	Oregon	148	0.1%
10	Pennsylvania	4,096	3.9%
36	Rhode Island	170	0.2%
15	South Carolina	3,577	3.4%
43	South Dakota	21	0.0%
17	Tennessee	3,218	3.1%
2	Texas	7,562	7.3%
40	Utah	60	0.1%
NA	Vermont**	NA	NA
13	Virginia	3,730	3.6%
29	Washington	524	0.5%
38	West Virginia	138	0.1%
22	Wisconsin	1,585	1.5%
NA	Wyoming**	NA	NA

RANK ORDER

RANK	STATE	BIRTHS	% of USA
1	Florida	7,907	7.6%
2	Texas	7,562	7.3%
3	Georgia	7,062	6.8%
4	Illinois	6,447	6.2%
5	New York	5,772	5.6%
6	Louisiana	5,661	5.5%
7	North Carolina	4,918	4.7%
8	Ohio	4,566	4.4%
9	California	4,542	4.4%
10	Pennsylvania	4,096	3.9%
11	Michigan	4,041	3.9%
12	Mississippi	3,912	3.8%
13	Virginia	3,730	3.6%
14	Alabama	3,610	3.5%
15	South Carolina	3,577	3.4%
16	Maryland	3,444	3.3%
17	Tennessee	3,218	3.1%
18	New Jersey	2,676	2.6%
19	Missouri	2,244	2.2%
20	Indiana	1,868	1.8%
21	Arkansas	1,644	1.6%
22	Wisconsin	1,585	1.5%
23	Oklahoma	932	0.9%
24	Kentucky	913	0.9%
25	Massachusetts	878	0.8%
26	Minnesota	731	0.7%
27	Connecticut	721	0.7%
28	Arizona	587	0.6%
29	Washington	524	0.5%
30	Kansas	520	0.5%
31	Delaware	505	0.5%
31	Nevada	505	0.5%
33	Colorado	470	0.5%
34	Nebraska	305	0.3%
35	Iowa	288	0.3%
36	Rhode Island	170	0.2%
37	Oregon	148	0.1%
38	West Virginia	138	0.1%
39	New Mexico	95	0.1%
40	Utah	60	0.1%
41	Alaska	57	0.1%
42	Hawaii	37	0.0%
43	South Dakota	21	0.0%
NA	Idaho**	NA	NA
NA	Maine**	NA	NA
NA	Montana**	NA	NA
NA	New Hampshire**	NA	NA
NA	North Dakota**	NA	NA
NA	Vermont**	NA	NA
NA	Wyoming**	NA	NA
	District of Columbia	815	0.8%

Source: Morgan Quitno Press using data from U.S. Dept. of Health and Human Services, Nat'l Center for Health Statistics
    "National Vital Statistics Reports" (Vol. 53, No. 9, November 23, 2004)
*Live births to women 15 to 19 years old by state of residence.
**Not available. Fewer than 20 births to black teenage women.

Black Teenage Birth Rate in 2003

National Rate = 64.3 Births per 1,000 Black Teenage Women*

RANK	STATE	RATE	RANK	STATE	RATE
16	Alabama	68.8	1	Wisconsin	97.8
41	Alaska	40.0	2	Iowa	85.6
25	Arizona	65.1	3	Nebraska	82.5
7	Arkansas	79.5	4	Indiana	81.9
40	California	40.7	5	Louisiana	81.3
31	Colorado	53.3	6	Mississippi	80.9
34	Connecticut	46.2	7	Arkansas	79.5
11	Delaware	75.8	8	Ohio	79.0
26	Florida	63.2	9	Illinois	78.2
20	Georgia	67.0	10	Tennessee	77.8
43	Hawaii	21.3	11	Delaware	75.8
NA	Idaho**	NA	12	Missouri	75.7
9	Illinois	78.2	13	Pennsylvania	74.3
4	Indiana	81.9	14	Nevada	73.7
2	Iowa	85.6	15	Minnesota	71.4
21	Kansas	66.7	16	Alabama	68.8
18	Kentucky	68.5	17	Oklahoma	68.7
5	Louisiana	81.3	18	Kentucky	68.5
NA	Maine**	NA	19	Texas	67.7
29	Maryland	55.1	20	Georgia	67.0
35	Massachusetts	45.6	21	Kansas	66.7
23	Michigan	66.5	21	South Carolina	66.7
15	Minnesota	71.4	23	Michigan	66.5
6	Mississippi	80.9	24	North Carolina	65.5
12	Missouri	75.7	25	Arizona	65.1
NA	Montana**	NA	26	Florida	63.2
3	Nebraska	82.5	27	Virginia	60.4
14	Nevada	73.7	28	Rhode Island	55.7
NA	New Hampshire**	NA	29	Maryland	55.1
33	New Jersey	50.8	30	South Dakota	54.5
37	New Mexico	41.7	31	Colorado	53.3
38	New York	41.3	32	West Virginia	52.9
24	North Carolina	65.5	33	New Jersey	50.8
NA	North Dakota**	NA	34	Connecticut	46.2
8	Ohio	79.0	35	Massachusetts	45.6
17	Oklahoma	68.7	36	Washington	45.0
39	Oregon	41.0	37	New Mexico	41.7
13	Pennsylvania	74.3	38	New York	41.3
28	Rhode Island	55.7	39	Oregon	41.0
21	South Carolina	66.7	40	California	40.7
30	South Dakota	54.5	41	Alaska	40.0
10	Tennessee	77.8	42	Utah	38.5
19	Texas	67.7	43	Hawaii	21.3
42	Utah	38.5	NA	Idaho**	NA
NA	Vermont**	NA	NA	Maine**	NA
27	Virginia	60.4	NA	Montana**	NA
36	Washington	45.0	NA	New Hampshire**	NA
32	West Virginia	52.9	NA	North Dakota**	NA
1	Wisconsin	97.8	NA	Vermont**	NA
NA	Wyoming**	NA	NA	Wyoming**	NA
				District of Columbia	110.3

Source: Morgan Quitno Press using data from U.S. Dept. of Health and Human Services, Nat'l Center for Health Statistics
   "National Vital Statistics Reports" (Vol. 53, No. 9, November 23, 2004)
*Live births to women age 15 to 19 years old by state of residence. Rates calculated using Census 2003 estimates
for females ages 15 to 19 years old in the category of "Black Alone or in Combination."
**Insufficient number of births for a reliable figure.

Births to Black Teenage Mothers as a Percent of Black Births in 2003

National Percent = 17.3% of Black Live Births*

ALPHA ORDER

RANK	STATE	PERCENT
9	Alabama	20.1
33	Alaska	14.1
20	Arizona	17.9
2	Arkansas	22.5
34	California	13.9
30	Colorado	16.0
34	Connecticut	13.9
24	Delaware	17.5
27	Florida	16.7
29	Georgia	16.4
43	Hawaii	7.1
NA	Idaho**	NA
7	Illinois	20.4
11	Indiana	19.9
3	Iowa	22.4
17	Kansas	18.8
17	Kentucky	18.8
4	Louisiana	21.5
NA	Maine**	NA
34	Maryland	13.9
42	Massachusetts	10.2
20	Michigan	17.9
37	Minnesota	13.6
5	Mississippi	21.3
9	Missouri	20.1
NA	Montana**	NA
6	Nebraska	20.8
25	Nevada	17.4
NA	New Hampshire**	NA
39	New Jersey	13.3
23	New Mexico	17.8
41	New York	12.0
19	North Carolina	18.1
NA	North Dakota**	NA
12	Ohio	19.8
7	Oklahoma	20.4
32	Oregon	14.5
15	Pennsylvania	19.2
38	Rhode Island	13.5
14	South Carolina	19.5
26	South Dakota	17.2
12	Tennessee	19.8
20	Texas	17.9
31	Utah	15.6
NA	Vermont**	NA
28	Virginia	16.5
40	Washington	13.0
16	West Virginia	19.1
1	Wisconsin	24.4
NA	Wyoming**	NA

RANK ORDER

RANK	STATE	PERCENT
1	Wisconsin	24.4
2	Arkansas	22.5
3	Iowa	22.4
4	Louisiana	21.5
5	Mississippi	21.3
6	Nebraska	20.8
7	Illinois	20.4
7	Oklahoma	20.4
9	Alabama	20.1
9	Missouri	20.1
11	Indiana	19.9
12	Ohio	19.8
12	Tennessee	19.8
14	South Carolina	19.5
15	Pennsylvania	19.2
16	West Virginia	19.1
17	Kansas	18.8
17	Kentucky	18.8
19	North Carolina	18.1
20	Arizona	17.9
20	Michigan	17.9
20	Texas	17.9
23	New Mexico	17.8
24	Delaware	17.5
25	Nevada	17.4
26	South Dakota	17.2
27	Florida	16.7
28	Virginia	16.5
29	Georgia	16.4
30	Colorado	16.0
31	Utah	15.6
32	Oregon	14.5
33	Alaska	14.1
34	California	13.9
34	Connecticut	13.9
34	Maryland	13.9
37	Minnesota	13.6
38	Rhode Island	13.5
39	New Jersey	13.3
40	Washington	13.0
41	New York	12.0
42	Massachusetts	10.2
43	Hawaii	7.1
NA	Idaho**	NA
NA	Maine**	NA
NA	Montana**	NA
NA	New Hampshire**	NA
NA	North Dakota**	NA
NA	Vermont**	NA
NA	Wyoming**	NA

District of Columbia 15.6

Source: U.S. Department of Health and Human Services, National Center for Health Statistics
    "National Vital Statistics Reports" (Vol. 53, No. 9, November 23, 2004)
Live births to women 15 to 19 years old by state of residence.
**Not available. Fewer than 20 births to black teenage women.*

Births to Young Teenagers: 2000 to 2002

National Total = 23,615 Live Births*

ALPHA ORDER

RANK	STATE	BIRTHS	% of USA
15	Alabama	556	2.4%
43	Alaska	45	0.2%
13	Arizona	625	2.6%
22	Arkansas	346	1.5%
2	California	2,448	10.4%
24	Colorado	336	1.4%
32	Connecticut	178	0.8%
37	Delaware	85	0.4%
3	Florida	1,458	6.2%
4	Georgia	1,118	4.7%
41	Hawaii	59	0.2%
42	Idaho	53	0.2%
5	Illinois	1,050	4.4%
20	Indiana	391	1.7%
35	Iowa	111	0.5%
34	Kansas	157	0.7%
25	Kentucky	332	1.4%
10	Louisiana	743	3.1%
46	Maine	20	0.1%
18	Maryland	475	2.0%
29	Massachusetts	241	1.0%
11	Michigan	659	2.8%
30	Minnesota	230	1.0%
12	Mississippi	626	2.7%
21	Missouri	379	1.6%
45	Montana	26	0.1%
38	Nebraska	83	0.4%
33	Nevada	175	0.7%
49	New Hampshire	12	0.1%
19	New Jersey	421	1.8%
28	New Mexico	246	1.0%
6	New York	972	4.1%
7	North Carolina	906	3.8%
48	North Dakota	14	0.1%
8	Ohio	848	3.6%
23	Oklahoma	338	1.4%
31	Oregon	183	0.8%
9	Pennsylvania	792	3.4%
40	Rhode Island	68	0.3%
16	South Carolina	537	2.3%
44	South Dakota	44	0.2%
14	Tennessee	624	2.6%
1	Texas	3,204	13.6%
36	Utah	102	0.4%
50	Vermont	7	0.0%
17	Virginia	506	2.1%
26	Washington	308	1.3%
39	West Virginia	82	0.3%
27	Wisconsin	287	1.2%
46	Wyoming	20	0.1%

RANK ORDER

RANK	STATE	BIRTHS	% of USA
1	Texas	3,204	13.6%
2	California	2,448	10.4%
3	Florida	1,458	6.2%
4	Georgia	1,118	4.7%
5	Illinois	1,050	4.4%
6	New York	972	4.1%
7	North Carolina	906	3.8%
8	Ohio	848	3.6%
9	Pennsylvania	792	3.4%
10	Louisiana	743	3.1%
11	Michigan	659	2.8%
12	Mississippi	626	2.7%
13	Arizona	625	2.6%
14	Tennessee	624	2.6%
15	Alabama	556	2.4%
16	South Carolina	537	2.3%
17	Virginia	506	2.1%
18	Maryland	475	2.0%
19	New Jersey	421	1.8%
20	Indiana	391	1.7%
21	Missouri	379	1.6%
22	Arkansas	346	1.5%
23	Oklahoma	338	1.4%
24	Colorado	336	1.4%
25	Kentucky	332	1.4%
26	Washington	308	1.3%
27	Wisconsin	287	1.2%
28	New Mexico	246	1.0%
29	Massachusetts	241	1.0%
30	Minnesota	230	1.0%
31	Oregon	183	0.8%
32	Connecticut	178	0.8%
33	Nevada	175	0.7%
34	Kansas	157	0.7%
35	Iowa	111	0.5%
36	Utah	102	0.4%
37	Delaware	85	0.4%
38	Nebraska	83	0.4%
39	West Virginia	82	0.3%
40	Rhode Island	68	0.3%
41	Hawaii	59	0.2%
42	Idaho	53	0.2%
43	Alaska	45	0.2%
44	South Dakota	44	0.2%
45	Montana	26	0.1%
46	Maine	20	0.1%
46	Wyoming	20	0.1%
48	North Dakota	14	0.1%
49	New Hampshire	12	0.1%
50	Vermont	7	0.0%
	District of Columbia	89	0.4%

Source: U.S. Department of Health and Human Services, National Center for Health Statistics
   "National Vital Statistics Reports" (Vol. 53, No. 7, November 15, 2004)
*Births to 10 to 14 years old during the three years of 2000 to 2002 by state of residence.

Young Teen Birthrate: 2000 to 2002

National Rate = 0.8 Live Births per 1,000 10 to 14 Year Old Females*

<table>
<tr><td colspan="3">ALPHA ORDER</td><td colspan="3">RANK ORDER</td></tr>
<tr><td>RANK</td><td>STATE</td><td>RATE</td><td>RANK</td><td>STATE</td><td>RATE</td></tr>
<tr><td>5</td><td>Alabama</td><td>1.2</td><td>1</td><td>Mississippi</td><td>2.0</td></tr>
<tr><td>28</td><td>Alaska</td><td>0.5</td><td>2</td><td>Louisiana</td><td>1.5</td></tr>
<tr><td>8</td><td>Arizona</td><td>1.1</td><td>3</td><td>South Carolina</td><td>1.3</td></tr>
<tr><td>5</td><td>Arkansas</td><td>1.2</td><td>3</td><td>Texas</td><td>1.3</td></tr>
<tr><td>23</td><td>California</td><td>0.6</td><td>5</td><td>Alabama</td><td>1.2</td></tr>
<tr><td>19</td><td>Colorado</td><td>0.7</td><td>5</td><td>Arkansas</td><td>1.2</td></tr>
<tr><td>28</td><td>Connecticut</td><td>0.5</td><td>5</td><td>Georgia</td><td>1.2</td></tr>
<tr><td>8</td><td>Delaware</td><td>1.1</td><td>8</td><td>Arizona</td><td>1.1</td></tr>
<tr><td>13</td><td>Florida</td><td>0.9</td><td>8</td><td>Delaware</td><td>1.1</td></tr>
<tr><td>5</td><td>Georgia</td><td>1.2</td><td>8</td><td>New Mexico</td><td>1.1</td></tr>
<tr><td>28</td><td>Hawaii</td><td>0.5</td><td>8</td><td>North Carolina</td><td>1.1</td></tr>
<tr><td>45</td><td>Idaho</td><td>0.3</td><td>8</td><td>Tennessee</td><td>1.1</td></tr>
<tr><td>15</td><td>Illinois</td><td>0.8</td><td>13</td><td>Florida</td><td>0.9</td></tr>
<tr><td>23</td><td>Indiana</td><td>0.6</td><td>13</td><td>Oklahoma</td><td>0.9</td></tr>
<tr><td>39</td><td>Iowa</td><td>0.4</td><td>15</td><td>Illinois</td><td>0.8</td></tr>
<tr><td>28</td><td>Kansas</td><td>0.5</td><td>15</td><td>Kentucky</td><td>0.8</td></tr>
<tr><td>15</td><td>Kentucky</td><td>0.8</td><td>15</td><td>Maryland</td><td>0.8</td></tr>
<tr><td>2</td><td>Louisiana</td><td>1.5</td><td>15</td><td>Nevada</td><td>0.8</td></tr>
<tr><td>47</td><td>Maine</td><td>0.2</td><td>19</td><td>Colorado</td><td>0.7</td></tr>
<tr><td>15</td><td>Maryland</td><td>0.8</td><td>19</td><td>Ohio</td><td>0.7</td></tr>
<tr><td>39</td><td>Massachusetts</td><td>0.4</td><td>19</td><td>Rhode Island</td><td>0.7</td></tr>
<tr><td>23</td><td>Michigan</td><td>0.6</td><td>19</td><td>Virginia</td><td>0.7</td></tr>
<tr><td>39</td><td>Minnesota</td><td>0.4</td><td>23</td><td>California</td><td>0.6</td></tr>
<tr><td>1</td><td>Mississippi</td><td>2.0</td><td>23</td><td>Indiana</td><td>0.6</td></tr>
<tr><td>23</td><td>Missouri</td><td>0.6</td><td>23</td><td>Michigan</td><td>0.6</td></tr>
<tr><td>45</td><td>Montana</td><td>0.3</td><td>23</td><td>Missouri</td><td>0.6</td></tr>
<tr><td>39</td><td>Nebraska</td><td>0.4</td><td>23</td><td>Pennsylvania</td><td>0.6</td></tr>
<tr><td>15</td><td>Nevada</td><td>0.8</td><td>28</td><td>Alaska</td><td>0.5</td></tr>
<tr><td>NA</td><td>New Hampshire**</td><td>NA</td><td>28</td><td>Connecticut</td><td>0.5</td></tr>
<tr><td>28</td><td>New Jersey</td><td>0.5</td><td>28</td><td>Hawaii</td><td>0.5</td></tr>
<tr><td>8</td><td>New Mexico</td><td>1.1</td><td>28</td><td>Kansas</td><td>0.5</td></tr>
<tr><td>28</td><td>New York</td><td>0.5</td><td>28</td><td>New Jersey</td><td>0.5</td></tr>
<tr><td>8</td><td>North Carolina</td><td>1.1</td><td>28</td><td>New York</td><td>0.5</td></tr>
<tr><td>NA</td><td>North Dakota**</td><td>NA</td><td>28</td><td>Oregon</td><td>0.5</td></tr>
<tr><td>19</td><td>Ohio</td><td>0.7</td><td>28</td><td>South Dakota</td><td>0.5</td></tr>
<tr><td>13</td><td>Oklahoma</td><td>0.9</td><td>28</td><td>Washington</td><td>0.5</td></tr>
<tr><td>28</td><td>Oregon</td><td>0.5</td><td>28</td><td>West Virginia</td><td>0.5</td></tr>
<tr><td>23</td><td>Pennsylvania</td><td>0.6</td><td>28</td><td>Wisconsin</td><td>0.5</td></tr>
<tr><td>19</td><td>Rhode Island</td><td>0.7</td><td>39</td><td>Iowa</td><td>0.4</td></tr>
<tr><td>3</td><td>South Carolina</td><td>1.3</td><td>39</td><td>Massachusetts</td><td>0.4</td></tr>
<tr><td>28</td><td>South Dakota</td><td>0.5</td><td>39</td><td>Minnesota</td><td>0.4</td></tr>
<tr><td>8</td><td>Tennessee</td><td>1.1</td><td>39</td><td>Nebraska</td><td>0.4</td></tr>
<tr><td>3</td><td>Texas</td><td>1.3</td><td>39</td><td>Utah</td><td>0.4</td></tr>
<tr><td>39</td><td>Utah</td><td>0.4</td><td>39</td><td>Wyoming</td><td>0.4</td></tr>
<tr><td>NA</td><td>Vermont**</td><td>NA</td><td>45</td><td>Idaho</td><td>0.3</td></tr>
<tr><td>19</td><td>Virginia</td><td>0.7</td><td>45</td><td>Montana</td><td>0.3</td></tr>
<tr><td>28</td><td>Washington</td><td>0.5</td><td>47</td><td>Maine</td><td>0.2</td></tr>
<tr><td>28</td><td>West Virginia</td><td>0.5</td><td>NA</td><td>New Hampshire**</td><td>NA</td></tr>
<tr><td>28</td><td>Wisconsin</td><td>0.5</td><td>NA</td><td>North Dakota**</td><td>NA</td></tr>
<tr><td>39</td><td>Wyoming</td><td>0.4</td><td>NA</td><td>Vermont**</td><td>NA</td></tr>
<tr><td></td><td></td><td></td><td></td><td>District of Columbia</td><td>2.0</td></tr>
</table>

Source: U.S. Department of Health and Human Services, National Center for Health Statistics
   "National Vital Statistics Reports" (Vol. 53, No. 7, November 15, 2004)
*Births to 10 to 14 years old during the three years of 2000 to 2002 by state of residence.
**Insufficient data for a reliable rate.

Births to Women 35 to 54 Years Old in 2002

National Total = 555,202 Live Births*

ALPHA ORDER

RANK ORDER

RANK	STATE	BIRTHS	% of USA		RANK	STATE	BIRTHS	% of USA
27	Alabama	5,052	0.9%		1	California	87,615	15.8%
45	Alaska	1,352	0.2%		2	New York	48,802	8.8%
18	Arizona	9,673	1.7%		3	Texas	39,097	7.0%
38	Arkansas	2,744	0.5%		4	Florida	29,372	5.3%
1	California	87,615	15.8%		5	Illinois	26,258	4.7%
17	Colorado	9,709	1.7%		6	New Jersey	24,261	4.4%
20	Connecticut	9,169	1.7%		7	Pennsylvania	22,143	4.0%
44	Delaware	1,499	0.3%		8	Massachusetts	18,383	3.3%
4	Florida	29,372	5.3%		9	Ohio	17,784	3.2%
12	Georgia	15,735	2.8%		10	Michigan	16,755	3.0%
36	Hawaii	2,880	0.5%		11	Virginia	15,747	2.8%
41	Idaho	2,034	0.4%		12	Georgia	15,735	2.8%
5	Illinois	26,258	4.7%		13	Maryland	13,539	2.4%
21	Indiana	8,712	1.6%		14	North Carolina	13,311	2.4%
31	Iowa	4,073	0.7%		15	Washington	11,650	2.1%
30	Kansas	4,293	0.8%		16	Minnesota	10,281	1.9%
28	Kentucky	4,841	0.9%		17	Colorado	9,709	1.7%
24	Louisiana	5,775	1.0%		18	Arizona	9,673	1.7%
42	Maine	1,887	0.3%		19	Wisconsin	9,297	1.7%
13	Maryland	13,539	2.4%		20	Connecticut	9,169	1.7%
8	Massachusetts	18,383	3.3%		21	Indiana	8,712	1.6%
10	Michigan	16,755	3.0%		22	Missouri	8,289	1.5%
16	Minnesota	10,281	1.9%		23	Tennessee	7,411	1.3%
34	Mississippi	3,024	0.5%		24	Louisiana	5,775	1.0%
22	Missouri	8,289	1.5%		25	Oregon	5,774	1.0%
46	Montana	1,264	0.2%		26	South Carolina	5,750	1.0%
35	Nebraska	2,949	0.5%		27	Alabama	5,052	0.9%
32	Nevada	4,058	0.7%		28	Kentucky	4,841	0.9%
39	New Hampshire	2,675	0.5%		29	Utah	4,304	0.8%
6	New Jersey	24,261	4.4%		30	Kansas	4,293	0.8%
37	New Mexico	2,858	0.5%		31	Iowa	4,073	0.7%
2	New York	48,802	8.8%		32	Nevada	4,058	0.7%
14	North Carolina	13,311	2.4%		33	Oklahoma	4,034	0.7%
49	North Dakota	878	0.2%		34	Mississippi	3,024	0.5%
9	Ohio	17,784	3.2%		35	Nebraska	2,949	0.5%
33	Oklahoma	4,034	0.7%		36	Hawaii	2,880	0.5%
25	Oregon	5,774	1.0%		37	New Mexico	2,858	0.5%
7	Pennsylvania	22,143	4.0%		38	Arkansas	2,744	0.5%
40	Rhode Island	2,264	0.4%		39	New Hampshire	2,675	0.5%
26	South Carolina	5,750	1.0%		40	Rhode Island	2,264	0.4%
48	South Dakota	1,107	0.2%		41	Idaho	2,034	0.4%
23	Tennessee	7,411	1.3%		42	Maine	1,887	0.3%
3	Texas	39,097	7.0%		43	West Virginia	1,712	0.3%
29	Utah	4,304	0.8%		44	Delaware	1,499	0.3%
47	Vermont	1,109	0.2%		45	Alaska	1,352	0.2%
11	Virginia	15,747	2.8%		46	Montana	1,264	0.2%
15	Washington	11,650	2.1%		47	Vermont	1,109	0.2%
43	West Virginia	1,712	0.3%		48	South Dakota	1,107	0.2%
19	Wisconsin	9,297	1.7%		49	North Dakota	878	0.2%
50	Wyoming	600	0.1%		50	Wyoming	600	0.1%
						District of Columbia	1,419	0.3%

Source: Morgan Quitno Press using data from U.S. Dept of Health & Human Services, National Center for Health Statistics
   (unpublished data)
*By state of residence.

Births to Women 35 to 54 Years Old as a Percent of All Births in 2002

National Percent = 13.8% of Live Births*

ALPHA ORDER

RANK	STATE	PERCENT
46	Alabama	8.6
19	Alaska	13.6
31	Arizona	11.0
49	Arkansas	7.3
9	California	16.6
17	Colorado	14.2
2	Connecticut	21.8
21	Delaware	13.5
16	Florida	14.3
26	Georgia	11.8
10	Hawaii	16.5
40	Idaho	9.7
15	Illinois	14.5
39	Indiana	10.2
34	Iowa	10.8
33	Kansas	10.9
43	Kentucky	8.9
43	Louisiana	8.9
18	Maine	13.9
5	Maryland	18.5
1	Massachusetts	22.8
22	Michigan	12.9
13	Minnesota	15.1
49	Mississippi	7.3
31	Missouri	11.0
28	Montana	11.4
27	Nebraska	11.6
24	Nevada	12.5
5	New Hampshire	18.5
3	New Jersey	21.1
37	New Mexico	10.3
4	New York	19.4
29	North Carolina	11.3
29	North Dakota	11.3
25	Ohio	12.0
48	Oklahoma	8.0
23	Oregon	12.8
12	Pennsylvania	15.5
7	Rhode Island	17.6
35	South Carolina	10.5
37	South Dakota	10.3
41	Tennessee	9.6
35	Texas	10.5
45	Utah	8.8
8	Vermont	17.4
11	Virginia	15.8
14	Washington	14.7
47	West Virginia	8.3
19	Wisconsin	13.6
42	Wyoming	9.2

RANK ORDER

RANK	STATE	PERCENT
1	Massachusetts	22.8
2	Connecticut	21.8
3	New Jersey	21.1
4	New York	19.4
5	Maryland	18.5
5	New Hampshire	18.5
7	Rhode Island	17.6
8	Vermont	17.4
9	California	16.6
10	Hawaii	16.5
11	Virginia	15.8
12	Pennsylvania	15.5
13	Minnesota	15.1
14	Washington	14.7
15	Illinois	14.5
16	Florida	14.3
17	Colorado	14.2
18	Maine	13.9
19	Alaska	13.6
19	Wisconsin	13.6
21	Delaware	13.5
22	Michigan	12.9
23	Oregon	12.8
24	Nevada	12.5
25	Ohio	12.0
26	Georgia	11.8
27	Nebraska	11.6
28	Montana	11.4
29	North Carolina	11.3
29	North Dakota	11.3
31	Arizona	11.0
31	Missouri	11.0
33	Kansas	10.9
34	Iowa	10.8
35	South Carolina	10.5
35	Texas	10.5
37	New Mexico	10.3
37	South Dakota	10.3
39	Indiana	10.2
40	Idaho	9.7
41	Tennessee	9.6
42	Wyoming	9.2
43	Kentucky	8.9
43	Louisiana	8.9
45	Utah	8.8
46	Alabama	8.6
47	West Virginia	8.3
48	Oklahoma	8.0
49	Arkansas	7.3
49	Mississippi	7.3
	District of Columbia	18.9

Source: Morgan Quitno Press using data from U.S. Dept of Health & Human Services, National Center for Health Statistics
(unpublished data)
*By state of residence.

Births by Vaginal Delivery in 2003

National Total = 2,961,930 Live Births*

ALPHA ORDER

RANK	STATE	BIRTHS	% of USA
24	Alabama	41,973	1.4%
47	Alaska	7,966	0.3%
13	Arizona	70,802	2.4%
34	Arkansas	26,902	0.9%
1	California	390,057	13.2%
20	Colorado	53,964	1.8%
30	Connecticut	31,193	1.1%
46	Delaware	7,997	0.3%
4	Florida	146,902	5.0%
8	Georgia	98,881	3.3%
40	Hawaii	14,129	0.5%
38	Idaho	17,180	0.6%
5	Illinois	135,664	4.6%
14	Indiana	64,430	2.2%
33	Iowa	28,484	1.0%
31	Kansas	29,027	1.0%
27	Kentucky	38,641	1.3%
23	Louisiana	44,599	1.5%
42	Maine	10,216	0.3%
22	Maryland	53,522	1.8%
16	Massachusetts	56,737	1.9%
9	Michigan	96,370	3.3%
21	Minnesota	53,810	1.8%
32	Mississippi	28,679	1.0%
18	Missouri	56,036	1.9%
44	Montana	8,710	0.3%
37	Nebraska	18,743	0.6%
35	Nevada	24,358	0.8%
41	New Hampshire	10,579	0.4%
11	New Jersey	77,784	2.6%
36	New Mexico	22,192	0.7%
3	New York	181,998	6.1%
10	North Carolina	85,892	2.9%
48	North Dakota	6,037	0.2%
6	Ohio	113,835	3.8%
28	Oklahoma	35,642	1.2%
29	Oregon	34,527	1.2%
7	Pennsylvania	101,416	3.4%
43	Rhode Island	9,459	0.3%
26	South Carolina	39,128	1.3%
45	South Dakota	8,232	0.3%
17	Tennessee	56,335	1.9%
2	Texas	266,105	9.0%
25	Utah	40,295	1.4%
50	Vermont	5,101	0.2%
12	Virginia	72,579	2.5%
15	Washington	58,424	2.0%
39	West Virginia	14,301	0.5%
19	Wisconsin	54,711	1.8%
49	Wyoming	5,111	0.2%

RANK ORDER

RANK	STATE	BIRTHS	% of USA
1	California	390,057	13.2%
2	Texas	266,105	9.0%
3	New York	181,998	6.1%
4	Florida	146,902	5.0%
5	Illinois	135,664	4.6%
6	Ohio	113,835	3.8%
7	Pennsylvania	101,416	3.4%
8	Georgia	98,881	3.3%
9	Michigan	96,370	3.3%
10	North Carolina	85,892	2.9%
11	New Jersey	77,784	2.6%
12	Virginia	72,579	2.5%
13	Arizona	70,802	2.4%
14	Indiana	64,430	2.2%
15	Washington	58,424	2.0%
16	Massachusetts	56,737	1.9%
17	Tennessee	56,335	1.9%
18	Missouri	56,036	1.9%
19	Wisconsin	54,711	1.8%
20	Colorado	53,964	1.8%
21	Minnesota	53,810	1.8%
22	Maryland	53,522	1.8%
23	Louisiana	44,599	1.5%
24	Alabama	41,973	1.4%
25	Utah	40,295	1.4%
26	South Carolina	39,128	1.3%
27	Kentucky	38,641	1.3%
28	Oklahoma	35,642	1.2%
29	Oregon	34,527	1.2%
30	Connecticut	31,193	1.1%
31	Kansas	29,027	1.0%
32	Mississippi	28,679	1.0%
33	Iowa	28,484	1.0%
34	Arkansas	26,902	0.9%
35	Nevada	24,358	0.8%
36	New Mexico	22,192	0.7%
37	Nebraska	18,743	0.6%
38	Idaho	17,180	0.6%
39	West Virginia	14,301	0.5%
40	Hawaii	14,129	0.5%
41	New Hampshire	10,579	0.4%
42	Maine	10,216	0.3%
43	Rhode Island	9,459	0.3%
44	Montana	8,710	0.3%
45	South Dakota	8,232	0.3%
46	Delaware	7,997	0.3%
47	Alaska	7,966	0.3%
48	North Dakota	6,037	0.2%
49	Wyoming	5,111	0.2%
50	Vermont	5,101	0.2%
	District of Columbia	5,522	0.2%

Source: Morgan Quitno Press using data from U.S. Dept. of Health and Human Services, Nat'l Center for Health Statistics
   "National Vital Statistics Reports" (Vol. 53, No. 9, November 23, 2004)
*By state of residence.

Percent of Births by Vaginal Delivery in 2003

National Percent = 72.4% of Live Births*

ALPHA ORDER

RANK	STATE	PERCENT
42	Alabama	70.4
4	Alaska	78.7
7	Arizona	77.8
41	Arkansas	70.5
31	California	72.1
7	Colorado	77.8
24	Connecticut	72.8
38	Delaware	71.0
46	Florida	69.2
25	Georgia	72.7
6	Hawaii	78.0
3	Idaho	78.8
19	Illinois	74.3
18	Indiana	74.4
16	Iowa	74.6
22	Kansas	73.5
44	Kentucky	69.9
48	Louisiana	68.3
20	Maine	73.7
36	Maryland	71.5
39	Massachusetts	70.7
21	Michigan	73.6
10	Minnesota	76.7
49	Mississippi	67.7
25	Missouri	72.7
11	Montana	76.3
30	Nebraska	72.3
29	Nevada	72.4
22	New Hampshire	73.5
50	New Jersey	66.9
2	New Mexico	79.7
35	New York	71.6
27	North Carolina	72.6
13	North Dakota	75.7
15	Ohio	74.9
40	Oklahoma	70.6
14	Oregon	75.1
31	Pennsylvania	72.1
33	Rhode Island	71.7
43	South Carolina	70.3
16	South Dakota	74.6
37	Tennessee	71.4
45	Texas	69.8
1	Utah	80.8
9	Vermont	77.4
33	Virginia	71.7
27	Washington	72.6
47	West Virginia	68.4
5	Wisconsin	78.1
12	Wyoming	76.2

RANK ORDER

RANK	STATE	PERCENT
1	Utah	80.8
2	New Mexico	79.7
3	Idaho	78.8
4	Alaska	78.7
5	Wisconsin	78.1
6	Hawaii	78.0
7	Arizona	77.8
7	Colorado	77.8
9	Vermont	77.4
10	Minnesota	76.7
11	Montana	76.3
12	Wyoming	76.2
13	North Dakota	75.7
14	Oregon	75.1
15	Ohio	74.9
16	Iowa	74.6
16	South Dakota	74.6
18	Indiana	74.4
19	Illinois	74.3
20	Maine	73.7
21	Michigan	73.6
22	Kansas	73.5
22	New Hampshire	73.5
24	Connecticut	72.8
25	Georgia	72.7
25	Missouri	72.7
27	North Carolina	72.6
27	Washington	72.6
29	Nevada	72.4
30	Nebraska	72.3
31	California	72.1
31	Pennsylvania	72.1
33	Rhode Island	71.7
33	Virginia	71.7
35	New York	71.6
36	Maryland	71.5
37	Tennessee	71.4
38	Delaware	71.0
39	Massachusetts	70.7
40	Oklahoma	70.6
41	Arkansas	70.5
42	Alabama	70.4
43	South Carolina	70.3
44	Kentucky	69.9
45	Texas	69.8
46	Florida	69.2
47	West Virginia	68.4
48	Louisiana	68.3
49	Mississippi	67.7
50	New Jersey	66.9

District of Columbia 72.6

Source: Morgan Quitno Press using data from U.S. Dept. of Health and Human Services, Nat'l Center for Health Statistics
"National Vital Statistics Reports" (Vol. 53, No. 9, November 23, 2004)
*By state of residence.

Births by Cesarean Delivery in 2003

National Total = 1,129,133 Live Cesarean Births*

ALPHA ORDER

RANK	STATE	BIRTHS	% of USA
21	Alabama	17,648	1.6%
47	Alaska	2,156	0.2%
20	Arizona	20,203	1.8%
31	Arkansas	11,257	1.0%
1	California	150,938	13.4%
25	Colorado	15,399	1.4%
29	Connecticut	11,655	1.0%
44	Delaware	3,267	0.3%
4	Florida	65,384	5.8%
9	Georgia	37,131	3.3%
40	Hawaii	3,985	0.4%
39	Idaho	4,622	0.4%
5	Illinois	46,926	4.2%
15	Indiana	22,170	2.0%
33	Iowa	9,698	0.9%
32	Kansas	10,466	0.9%
22	Kentucky	16,640	1.5%
19	Louisiana	20,699	1.8%
43	Maine	3,645	0.3%
17	Maryland	21,334	1.9%
13	Massachusetts	23,513	2.1%
10	Michigan	34,567	3.1%
24	Minnesota	16,347	1.4%
28	Mississippi	13,683	1.2%
18	Missouri	21,043	1.9%
46	Montana	2,706	0.2%
36	Nebraska	7,181	0.6%
35	Nevada	9,286	0.8%
41	New Hampshire	3,814	0.3%
7	New Jersey	38,485	3.4%
38	New Mexico	5,653	0.5%
3	New York	72,189	6.4%
11	North Carolina	32,416	2.9%
48	North Dakota	1,938	0.2%
8	Ohio	38,148	3.4%
27	Oklahoma	14,842	1.3%
30	Oregon	11,448	1.0%
6	Pennsylvania	39,244	3.5%
42	Rhode Island	3,733	0.3%
23	South Carolina	16,530	1.5%
45	South Dakota	2,803	0.2%
14	Tennessee	22,566	2.0%
2	Texas	115,134	10.2%
34	Utah	9,575	0.8%
50	Vermont	1,490	0.1%
12	Virginia	28,647	2.5%
16	Washington	22,050	2.0%
37	West Virginia	6,607	0.6%
26	Wisconsin	15,342	1.4%
49	Wyoming	1,597	0.1%

RANK ORDER

RANK	STATE	BIRTHS	% of USA
1	California	150,938	13.4%
2	Texas	115,134	10.2%
3	New York	72,189	6.4%
4	Florida	65,384	5.8%
5	Illinois	46,926	4.2%
6	Pennsylvania	39,244	3.5%
7	New Jersey	38,485	3.4%
8	Ohio	38,148	3.4%
9	Georgia	37,131	3.3%
10	Michigan	34,567	3.1%
11	North Carolina	32,416	2.9%
12	Virginia	28,647	2.5%
13	Massachusetts	23,513	2.1%
14	Tennessee	22,566	2.0%
15	Indiana	22,170	2.0%
16	Washington	22,050	2.0%
17	Maryland	21,334	1.9%
18	Missouri	21,043	1.9%
19	Louisiana	20,699	1.8%
20	Arizona	20,203	1.8%
21	Alabama	17,648	1.6%
22	Kentucky	16,640	1.5%
23	South Carolina	16,530	1.5%
24	Minnesota	16,347	1.4%
25	Colorado	15,399	1.4%
26	Wisconsin	15,342	1.4%
27	Oklahoma	14,842	1.3%
28	Mississippi	13,683	1.2%
29	Connecticut	11,655	1.0%
30	Oregon	11,448	1.0%
31	Arkansas	11,257	1.0%
32	Kansas	10,466	0.9%
33	Iowa	9,698	0.9%
34	Utah	9,575	0.8%
35	Nevada	9,286	0.8%
36	Nebraska	7,181	0.6%
37	West Virginia	6,607	0.6%
38	New Mexico	5,653	0.5%
39	Idaho	4,622	0.4%
40	Hawaii	3,985	0.4%
41	New Hampshire	3,814	0.3%
42	Rhode Island	3,733	0.3%
43	Maine	3,645	0.3%
44	Delaware	3,267	0.3%
45	South Dakota	2,803	0.2%
46	Montana	2,706	0.2%
47	Alaska	2,156	0.2%
48	North Dakota	1,938	0.2%
49	Wyoming	1,597	0.1%
50	Vermont	1,490	0.1%
	District of Columbia	2,084	0.2%

Source: Morgan Quitno Press using data from U.S. Dept. of Health and Human Services, Nat'l Center for Health Statistics
  "National Vital Statistics Reports" (Vol. 53, No. 9, November 23, 2004)
*By state of residence.

Percent of Births by Cesarean Delivery in 2003

National Percent = 27.6% of Live Births*

ALPHA ORDER				RANK ORDER

RANK	STATE	PERCENT	RANK	STATE	PERCENT
9	Alabama	29.6	1	New Jersey	33.1
47	Alaska	21.3	2	Mississippi	32.3
43	Arizona	22.2	3	Louisiana	31.7
10	Arkansas	29.5	4	West Virginia	31.6
19	California	27.9	5	Florida	30.8
43	Colorado	22.2	6	Texas	30.2
27	Connecticut	27.2	7	Kentucky	30.1
13	Delaware	29.0	8	South Carolina	29.7
5	Florida	30.8	9	Alabama	29.6
25	Georgia	27.3	10	Arkansas	29.5
45	Hawaii	22.0	11	Oklahoma	29.4
48	Idaho	21.2	12	Massachusetts	29.3
32	Illinois	25.7	13	Delaware	29.0
33	Indiana	25.6	14	Tennessee	28.6
34	Iowa	25.4	15	Maryland	28.5
28	Kansas	26.5	16	New York	28.4
7	Kentucky	30.1	17	Rhode Island	28.3
3	Louisiana	31.7	17	Virginia	28.3
31	Maine	26.3	19	California	27.9
15	Maryland	28.5	19	Pennsylvania	27.9
12	Massachusetts	29.3	21	Nebraska	27.7
30	Michigan	26.4	22	Nevada	27.6
41	Minnesota	23.3	23	North Carolina	27.4
2	Mississippi	32.3	23	Washington	27.4
25	Missouri	27.3	25	Georgia	27.3
40	Montana	23.7	25	Missouri	27.3
21	Nebraska	27.7	27	Connecticut	27.2
22	Nevada	27.6	28	Kansas	26.5
28	New Hampshire	26.5	28	New Hampshire	26.5
1	New Jersey	33.1	30	Michigan	26.4
49	New Mexico	20.3	31	Maine	26.3
16	New York	28.4	32	Illinois	25.7
23	North Carolina	27.4	33	Indiana	25.6
38	North Dakota	24.3	34	Iowa	25.4
36	Ohio	25.1	34	South Dakota	25.4
11	Oklahoma	29.4	36	Ohio	25.1
37	Oregon	24.9	37	Oregon	24.9
19	Pennsylvania	27.9	38	North Dakota	24.3
17	Rhode Island	28.3	39	Wyoming	23.8
8	South Carolina	29.7	40	Montana	23.7
34	South Dakota	25.4	41	Minnesota	23.3
14	Tennessee	28.6	42	Vermont	22.6
6	Texas	30.2	43	Arizona	22.2
50	Utah	19.2	43	Colorado	22.2
42	Vermont	22.6	45	Hawaii	22.0
17	Virginia	28.3	46	Wisconsin	21.9
23	Washington	27.4	47	Alaska	21.3
4	West Virginia	31.6	48	Idaho	21.2
46	Wisconsin	21.9	49	New Mexico	20.3
39	Wyoming	23.8	50	Utah	19.2
				District of Columbia	27.4

Source: U.S. Department of Health and Human Services, National Center for Health Statistics
   "National Vital Statistics Reports" (Vol. 53, No. 9, November 23, 2004)
*By state of residence.

Percent Change in Rate of Cesarean Births: 1999 to 2003

National Percent Change = 25.5% Increase*

ALPHA ORDER				RANK ORDER		
RANK	STATE	PERCENT CHANGE		RANK	STATE	PERCENT CHANGE
45	Alabama	19.4		1	Hawaii	59.4
3	Alaska	43.9		2	Washington	45.0
31	Arizona	24.7		3	Alaska	43.9
49	Arkansas	16.1		4	Rhode Island	38.0
35	California	22.9		5	Vermont	37.8
16	Colorado	28.3		6	Oregon	35.3
11	Connecticut	29.5		7	Pennsylvania	33.5
22	Delaware	26.1		8	New Hampshire	33.2
12	Florida	29.4		9	Massachusetts	30.8
26	Georgia	25.8		10	Virginia	30.4
1	Hawaii	59.4		11	Connecticut	29.5
38	Idaho	22.5		12	Florida	29.4
17	Illinois	27.9		12	Ohio	29.4
30	Indiana	24.9		14	Kentucky	29.2
18	Iowa	27.6		15	Wisconsin	28.8
29	Kansas	25.0		16	Colorado	28.3
14	Kentucky	29.2		17	Illinois	27.9
47	Louisiana	18.3		18	Iowa	27.6
39	Maine	22.3		19	West Virginia	27.4
36	Maryland	22.8		20	Texas	26.9
9	Massachusetts	30.8		21	Nevada	26.6
28	Michigan	25.7		22	Delaware	26.1
34	Minnesota	23.3		22	Montana	26.1
47	Mississippi	18.3		24	Nebraska	25.9
26	Missouri	25.8		24	New Jersey	25.9
22	Montana	26.1		26	Georgia	25.8
24	Nebraska	25.9		26	Missouri	25.8
21	Nevada	26.6		28	Michigan	25.7
8	New Hampshire	33.2		29	Kansas	25.0
24	New Jersey	25.9		30	Indiana	24.9
33	New Mexico	23.8		31	Arizona	24.7
43	New York	20.3		32	North Dakota	24.6
42	North Carolina	20.7		33	New Mexico	23.8
32	North Dakota	24.6		34	Minnesota	23.3
12	Ohio	29.4		35	California	22.9
40	Oklahoma	22.0		36	Maryland	22.8
6	Oregon	35.3		37	South Carolina	22.7
7	Pennsylvania	33.5		38	Idaho	22.5
4	Rhode Island	38.0		39	Maine	22.3
37	South Carolina	22.7		40	Oklahoma	22.0
50	South Dakota	13.9		41	Wyoming	21.4
46	Tennessee	19.2		42	North Carolina	20.7
20	Texas	26.9		43	New York	20.3
44	Utah	20.0		44	Utah	20.0
5	Vermont	37.8		45	Alabama	19.4
10	Virginia	30.4		46	Tennessee	19.2
2	Washington	45.0		47	Louisiana	18.3
19	West Virginia	27.4		47	Mississippi	18.3
15	Wisconsin	28.8		49	Arkansas	16.1
41	Wyoming	21.4		50	South Dakota	13.9
					District of Columbia	23.4

Source: Morgan Quitno Press using data from U.S. Dept. of Health and Human Services, Nat'l Center for Health Statistics "National Vital Statistics Reports" (Vol. 53, No. 9, November 23, 2004 and Vol. 49, No. 1, April 17, 2001)
By state of residence.

Percent of Vaginal Births After a Cesarean (VBAC) in 2002

National Percent = 12.6% of Live Births to Women Who Have Had a Cesarean*

ALPHA ORDER

RANK	STATE	PERCENT
42	Alabama	9.4
4	Alaska	20.8
36	Arizona	11.4
33	Arkansas	11.9
47	California	8.0
6	Colorado	18.6
25	Connecticut	13.3
29	Delaware	12.8
46	Florida	8.3
38	Georgia	11.1
15	Hawaii	16.7
11	Idaho	17.4
12	Illinois	17.1
31	Indiana	12.2
32	Iowa	12.0
34	Kansas	11.7
42	Kentucky	9.4
50	Louisiana	6.4
39	Maine	10.4
13	Maryland	17.0
22	Massachusetts	14.9
27	Michigan	13.0
18	Minnesota	16.4
49	Mississippi	6.9
24	Missouri	14.1
20	Montana	16.1
40	Nebraska	9.8
37	Nevada	11.3
21	New Hampshire	15.7
14	New Jersey	16.8
3	New Mexico	21.5
9	New York	18.2
26	North Carolina	13.2
15	North Dakota	16.7
5	Ohio	18.9
45	Oklahoma	8.4
19	Oregon	16.3
7	Pennsylvania	18.4
27	Rhode Island	13.0
41	South Carolina	9.5
15	South Dakota	16.7
35	Tennessee	11.6
47	Texas	8.0
2	Utah	24.1
1	Vermont	25.6
30	Virginia	12.6
23	Washington	14.6
44	West Virginia	9.3
8	Wisconsin	18.3
10	Wyoming	18.0

RANK ORDER

RANK	STATE	PERCENT
1	Vermont	25.6
2	Utah	24.1
3	New Mexico	21.5
4	Alaska	20.8
5	Ohio	18.9
6	Colorado	18.6
7	Pennsylvania	18.4
8	Wisconsin	18.3
9	New York	18.2
10	Wyoming	18.0
11	Idaho	17.4
12	Illinois	17.1
13	Maryland	17.0
14	New Jersey	16.8
15	Hawaii	16.7
15	North Dakota	16.7
15	South Dakota	16.7
18	Minnesota	16.4
19	Oregon	16.3
20	Montana	16.1
21	New Hampshire	15.7
22	Massachusetts	14.9
23	Washington	14.6
24	Missouri	14.1
25	Connecticut	13.3
26	North Carolina	13.2
27	Michigan	13.0
27	Rhode Island	13.0
29	Delaware	12.8
30	Virginia	12.6
31	Indiana	12.2
32	Iowa	12.0
33	Arkansas	11.9
34	Kansas	11.7
35	Tennessee	11.6
36	Arizona	11.4
37	Nevada	11.3
38	Georgia	11.1
39	Maine	10.4
40	Nebraska	9.8
41	South Carolina	9.5
42	Alabama	9.4
42	Kentucky	9.4
44	West Virginia	9.3
45	Oklahoma	8.4
46	Florida	8.3
47	California	8.0
47	Texas	8.0
49	Mississippi	6.9
50	Louisiana	6.4
	District of Columbia	8.4

Source: U.S. Department of Health and Human Services, National Center for Health Statistics
    "National Vital Statistics Reports" (Vol. 52, No. 10, December 17, 2003)
*Vaginal births after a cesarean delivery as a percent of all births to women with a previous cesarean delivery
giving birth in 2002.

Assisted Reproductive Technology Procedures in 2001

National Total = 105,479 Procedures*

ALPHA ORDER

RANK	STATE	PROCEDURES	% of USA
32	Alabama	558	0.5%
49	Alaska	82	0.1%
20	Arizona	1,484	1.4%
38	Arkansas	419	0.4%
1	California	13,124	12.4%
19	Colorado	1,666	1.6%
14	Connecticut	2,115	2.0%
36	Delaware	440	0.4%
7	Florida	4,539	4.3%
13	Georgia	2,453	2.3%
39	Hawaii	402	0.4%
48	Idaho	97	0.1%
4	Illinois	7,933	7.5%
17	Indiana	1,792	1.7%
22	Iowa	842	0.8%
24	Kansas	795	0.8%
27	Kentucky	770	0.7%
31	Louisiana	700	0.7%
46	Maine	126	0.1%
8	Maryland	4,082	3.9%
3	Massachusetts	8,151	7.7%
10	Michigan	3,286	3.1%
15	Minnesota	2,092	2.0%
40	Mississippi	313	0.3%
21	Missouri	1,454	1.4%
47	Montana	116	0.1%
25	Nebraska	786	0.7%
35	Nevada	465	0.4%
33	New Hampshire	554	0.5%
5	New Jersey	6,011	5.7%
42	New Mexico	190	0.2%
2	New York	12,379	11.7%
18	North Carolina	1,775	1.7%
44	North Dakota	154	0.1%
12	Ohio	2,996	2.8%
34	Oklahoma	548	0.5%
28	Oregon	760	0.7%
9	Pennsylvania	3,941	3.7%
29	Rhode Island	723	0.7%
26	South Carolina	774	0.7%
45	South Dakota	130	0.1%
23	Tennessee	839	0.8%
6	Texas	5,568	5.3%
37	Utah	436	0.4%
43	Vermont	167	0.2%
11	Virginia	3,080	2.9%
16	Washington	1,994	1.9%
41	West Virginia	223	0.2%
30	Wisconsin	709	0.7%
50	Wyoming	47	0.0%

RANK ORDER

RANK	STATE	PROCEDURES	% of USA
1	California	13,124	12.4%
2	New York	12,379	11.7%
3	Massachusetts	8,151	7.7%
4	Illinois	7,933	7.5%
5	New Jersey	6,011	5.7%
6	Texas	5,568	5.3%
7	Florida	4,539	4.3%
8	Maryland	4,082	3.9%
9	Pennsylvania	3,941	3.7%
10	Michigan	3,286	3.1%
11	Virginia	3,080	2.9%
12	Ohio	2,996	2.8%
13	Georgia	2,453	2.3%
14	Connecticut	2,115	2.0%
15	Minnesota	2,092	2.0%
16	Washington	1,994	1.9%
17	Indiana	1,792	1.7%
18	North Carolina	1,775	1.7%
19	Colorado	1,666	1.6%
20	Arizona	1,484	1.4%
21	Missouri	1,454	1.4%
22	Iowa	842	0.8%
23	Tennessee	839	0.8%
24	Kansas	795	0.8%
25	Nebraska	786	0.7%
26	South Carolina	774	0.7%
27	Kentucky	770	0.7%
28	Oregon	760	0.7%
29	Rhode Island	723	0.7%
30	Wisconsin	709	0.7%
31	Louisiana	700	0.7%
32	Alabama	558	0.5%
33	New Hampshire	554	0.5%
34	Oklahoma	548	0.5%
35	Nevada	465	0.4%
36	Delaware	440	0.4%
37	Utah	436	0.4%
38	Arkansas	419	0.4%
39	Hawaii	402	0.4%
40	Mississippi	313	0.3%
41	West Virginia	223	0.2%
42	New Mexico	190	0.2%
43	Vermont	167	0.2%
44	North Dakota	154	0.1%
45	South Dakota	130	0.1%
46	Maine	126	0.1%
47	Montana	116	0.1%
48	Idaho	97	0.1%
49	Alaska	82	0.1%
50	Wyoming	47	0.0%
	District of Columbia	399	0.4%

Source: U.S. Department of Health and Human Services, Centers for Disease Control and Prevention
"Assisted Reproductive Technology, 2001" (Morbidity and Mortality Weekly Report, Vol. 53, No. SS-01, 04/30/04)
*By patient's residence. Does not include 2,089 procedures for patients with residences outside the U.S. Assisted reproductive technology (ART) includes treatments in which both eggs and sperm are handled in the laboratory. In 2001, 76% of ART treatments were freshly fertilized embryos using the patient's eggs, 14% were thawed embryos using the patient's eggs, 8% were freshly fertilized embryos from donor eggs and 3% were thawed embryos from donor eggs.

Infants Born from Assisted Reproductive Technology Procedures in 2001

National Total = 39,963 Live Births*

ALPHA ORDER

RANK	STATE	BIRTHS	% of USA
31	Alabama	242	0.6%
49	Alaska	29	0.1%
21	Arizona	578	1.4%
36	Arkansas	191	0.5%
1	California	4,943	12.4%
15	Colorado	883	2.2%
16	Connecticut	791	2.0%
37	Delaware	155	0.4%
7	Florida	1,832	4.6%
14	Georgia	918	2.3%
39	Hawaii	133	0.3%
47	Idaho	47	0.1%
4	Illinois	2,551	6.4%
19	Indiana	614	1.5%
22	Iowa	433	1.1%
26	Kansas	318	0.8%
27	Kentucky	282	0.7%
34	Louisiana	214	0.5%
46	Maine	52	0.1%
8	Maryland	1,449	3.6%
3	Massachusetts	2,915	7.3%
11	Michigan	1,198	3.0%
13	Minnesota	929	2.3%
40	Mississippi	102	0.3%
20	Missouri	596	1.5%
45	Montana	62	0.2%
30	Nebraska	263	0.7%
35	Nevada	192	0.5%
32	New Hampshire	230	0.6%
5	New Jersey	2,470	6.2%
41	New Mexico	91	0.2%
2	New York	4,498	11.3%
17	North Carolina	752	1.9%
44	North Dakota	63	0.2%
10	Ohio	1,216	3.0%
28	Oklahoma	275	0.7%
25	Oregon	341	0.9%
9	Pennsylvania	1,287	3.2%
29	Rhode Island	269	0.7%
24	South Carolina	350	0.9%
48	South Dakota	36	0.1%
23	Tennessee	392	1.0%
6	Texas	2,265	5.7%
37	Utah	155	0.4%
43	Vermont	66	0.2%
12	Virginia	1,141	2.9%
18	Washington	723	1.8%
42	West Virginia	76	0.2%
33	Wisconsin	217	0.5%
50	Wyoming	18	0.0%

RANK ORDER

RANK	STATE	BIRTHS	% of USA
1	California	4,943	12.4%
2	New York	4,498	11.3%
3	Massachusetts	2,915	7.3%
4	Illinois	2,551	6.4%
5	New Jersey	2,470	6.2%
6	Texas	2,265	5.7%
7	Florida	1,832	4.6%
8	Maryland	1,449	3.6%
9	Pennsylvania	1,287	3.2%
10	Ohio	1,216	3.0%
11	Michigan	1,198	3.0%
12	Virginia	1,141	2.9%
13	Minnesota	929	2.3%
14	Georgia	918	2.3%
15	Colorado	883	2.2%
16	Connecticut	791	2.0%
17	North Carolina	752	1.9%
18	Washington	723	1.8%
19	Indiana	614	1.5%
20	Missouri	596	1.5%
21	Arizona	578	1.4%
22	Iowa	433	1.1%
23	Tennessee	392	1.0%
24	South Carolina	350	0.9%
25	Oregon	341	0.9%
26	Kansas	318	0.8%
27	Kentucky	282	0.7%
28	Oklahoma	275	0.7%
29	Rhode Island	269	0.7%
30	Nebraska	263	0.7%
31	Alabama	242	0.6%
32	New Hampshire	230	0.6%
33	Wisconsin	217	0.5%
34	Louisiana	214	0.5%
35	Nevada	192	0.5%
36	Arkansas	191	0.5%
37	Delaware	155	0.4%
37	Utah	155	0.4%
39	Hawaii	133	0.3%
40	Mississippi	102	0.3%
41	New Mexico	91	0.2%
42	West Virginia	76	0.2%
43	Vermont	66	0.2%
44	North Dakota	63	0.2%
45	Montana	62	0.2%
46	Maine	52	0.1%
47	Idaho	47	0.1%
48	South Dakota	36	0.1%
49	Alaska	29	0.1%
50	Wyoming	18	0.0%
	District of Columbia	120	0.3%

Source: U.S. Department of Health and Human Services, Centers for Disease Control and Prevention
"Assisted Reproductive Technology, 2001" (Morbidity and Mortality Weekly Report, Vol. 53, No. SS-01, 04/30/04)
*By patient's residence. Does not include 714 births to patients with residences outside the U.S. Assisted reproductive technology (ART) includes treatments in which both eggs and sperm are handled in the laboratory. In 2001, 76% of ART treatments were freshly fertilized embryos using the patient's eggs, 14% were thawed embryos using the patient's eggs, 8% were freshly fertilized embryos from donor eggs and 3% were thawed embryos from donor eggs.

Percent of Assisted Reproductive Technology Procedures that Resulted in Live Births in 2001
National Percent = 27.3%*

<table>
<tr><td colspan="3">ALPHA ORDER</td><td colspan="3">RANK ORDER</td></tr>
<tr><td>RANK</td><td>STATE</td><td>PERCENT</td><td>RANK</td><td>STATE</td><td>PERCENT</td></tr>
<tr><td>19</td><td>Alabama</td><td>29.0</td><td>1</td><td>Iowa</td><td>36.1</td></tr>
<tr><td>32</td><td>Alaska</td><td>26.8</td><td>2</td><td>Colorado</td><td>35.9</td></tr>
<tr><td>25</td><td>Arizona</td><td>28.4</td><td>3</td><td>Oklahoma</td><td>35.8</td></tr>
<tr><td>10</td><td>Arkansas</td><td>32.7</td><td>4</td><td>Idaho</td><td>35.1</td></tr>
<tr><td>29</td><td>California</td><td>27.1</td><td>5</td><td>New Mexico</td><td>34.2</td></tr>
<tr><td>2</td><td>Colorado</td><td>35.9</td><td>6</td><td>Maine</td><td>34.1</td></tr>
<tr><td>27</td><td>Connecticut</td><td>27.6</td><td>7</td><td>Montana</td><td>33.6</td></tr>
<tr><td>39</td><td>Delaware</td><td>25.5</td><td>8</td><td>Minnesota</td><td>32.9</td></tr>
<tr><td>20</td><td>Florida</td><td>28.9</td><td>9</td><td>South Carolina</td><td>32.8</td></tr>
<tr><td>28</td><td>Georgia</td><td>27.2</td><td>10</td><td>Arkansas</td><td>32.7</td></tr>
<tr><td>47</td><td>Hawaii</td><td>23.6</td><td>11</td><td>Oregon</td><td>32.1</td></tr>
<tr><td>4</td><td>Idaho</td><td>35.1</td><td>12</td><td>Tennessee</td><td>31.6</td></tr>
<tr><td>44</td><td>Illinois</td><td>23.8</td><td>13</td><td>New Hampshire</td><td>31.2</td></tr>
<tr><td>43</td><td>Indiana</td><td>24.2</td><td>14</td><td>North Dakota</td><td>29.9</td></tr>
<tr><td>1</td><td>Iowa</td><td>36.1</td><td>15</td><td>Wyoming</td><td>29.8</td></tr>
<tr><td>16</td><td>Kansas</td><td>29.4</td><td>16</td><td>Kansas</td><td>29.4</td></tr>
<tr><td>38</td><td>Kentucky</td><td>25.8</td><td>17</td><td>New Jersey</td><td>29.3</td></tr>
<tr><td>50</td><td>Louisiana</td><td>20.7</td><td>18</td><td>North Carolina</td><td>29.1</td></tr>
<tr><td>6</td><td>Maine</td><td>34.1</td><td>19</td><td>Alabama</td><td>29.0</td></tr>
<tr><td>39</td><td>Maryland</td><td>25.5</td><td>20</td><td>Florida</td><td>28.9</td></tr>
<tr><td>30</td><td>Massachusetts</td><td>26.9</td><td>21</td><td>Missouri</td><td>28.7</td></tr>
<tr><td>33</td><td>Michigan</td><td>26.7</td><td>21</td><td>Ohio</td><td>28.7</td></tr>
<tr><td>8</td><td>Minnesota</td><td>32.9</td><td>21</td><td>Vermont</td><td>28.7</td></tr>
<tr><td>42</td><td>Mississippi</td><td>24.9</td><td>24</td><td>Texas</td><td>28.6</td></tr>
<tr><td>21</td><td>Missouri</td><td>28.7</td><td>25</td><td>Arizona</td><td>28.4</td></tr>
<tr><td>7</td><td>Montana</td><td>33.6</td><td>25</td><td>Nevada</td><td>28.4</td></tr>
<tr><td>46</td><td>Nebraska</td><td>23.7</td><td>27</td><td>Connecticut</td><td>27.6</td></tr>
<tr><td>25</td><td>Nevada</td><td>28.4</td><td>28</td><td>Georgia</td><td>27.2</td></tr>
<tr><td>13</td><td>New Hampshire</td><td>31.2</td><td>29</td><td>California</td><td>27.1</td></tr>
<tr><td>17</td><td>New Jersey</td><td>29.3</td><td>30</td><td>Massachusetts</td><td>26.9</td></tr>
<tr><td>5</td><td>New Mexico</td><td>34.2</td><td>30</td><td>Virginia</td><td>26.9</td></tr>
<tr><td>34</td><td>New York</td><td>26.5</td><td>32</td><td>Alaska</td><td>26.8</td></tr>
<tr><td>18</td><td>North Carolina</td><td>29.1</td><td>33</td><td>Michigan</td><td>26.7</td></tr>
<tr><td>14</td><td>North Dakota</td><td>29.9</td><td>34</td><td>New York</td><td>26.5</td></tr>
<tr><td>21</td><td>Ohio</td><td>28.7</td><td>34</td><td>Washington</td><td>26.5</td></tr>
<tr><td>3</td><td>Oklahoma</td><td>35.8</td><td>34</td><td>West Virginia</td><td>26.5</td></tr>
<tr><td>11</td><td>Oregon</td><td>32.1</td><td>37</td><td>Utah</td><td>26.4</td></tr>
<tr><td>44</td><td>Pennsylvania</td><td>23.8</td><td>38</td><td>Kentucky</td><td>25.8</td></tr>
<tr><td>41</td><td>Rhode Island</td><td>25.0</td><td>39</td><td>Delaware</td><td>25.5</td></tr>
<tr><td>9</td><td>South Carolina</td><td>32.8</td><td>39</td><td>Maryland</td><td>25.5</td></tr>
<tr><td>49</td><td>South Dakota</td><td>20.8</td><td>41</td><td>Rhode Island</td><td>25.0</td></tr>
<tr><td>12</td><td>Tennessee</td><td>31.6</td><td>42</td><td>Mississippi</td><td>24.9</td></tr>
<tr><td>24</td><td>Texas</td><td>28.6</td><td>43</td><td>Indiana</td><td>24.2</td></tr>
<tr><td>37</td><td>Utah</td><td>26.4</td><td>44</td><td>Illinois</td><td>23.8</td></tr>
<tr><td>21</td><td>Vermont</td><td>28.7</td><td>44</td><td>Pennsylvania</td><td>23.8</td></tr>
<tr><td>30</td><td>Virginia</td><td>26.9</td><td>46</td><td>Nebraska</td><td>23.7</td></tr>
<tr><td>34</td><td>Washington</td><td>26.5</td><td>47</td><td>Hawaii</td><td>23.6</td></tr>
<tr><td>34</td><td>West Virginia</td><td>26.5</td><td>48</td><td>Wisconsin</td><td>21.7</td></tr>
<tr><td>48</td><td>Wisconsin</td><td>21.7</td><td>49</td><td>South Dakota</td><td>20.8</td></tr>
<tr><td>15</td><td>Wyoming</td><td>29.8</td><td>50</td><td>Louisiana</td><td>20.7</td></tr>
<tr><td></td><td></td><td></td><td></td><td>District of Columbia</td><td>22.6</td></tr>
</table>

Source: U.S. Department of Health and Human Services, Centers for Disease Control and Prevention
"Assisted Reproductive Technology, 2001" (Morbidity and Mortality Weekly Report, Vol. 53, No. SS-01, 04/30/04)
*By patient's residence. Assisted reproductive technology (ART) includes treatments in which both eggs and sperm are handled in the laboratory. In 2001, 76% of ART treatments were freshly fertilized embryos using the patient's eggs, 14% were thawed embryos using the patient's eggs, 8% were freshly fertilized embryos from donor eggs and 3% were thawed embryos from donor eggs.

Percent of Total Live Births Resulting from
Assisted Reproductive Technology Procedures in 2001
National Percent = 1.0% of Live Births*

RANK	STATE	PERCENT
39	Alabama	0.4
42	Alaska	0.3
27	Arizona	0.7
35	Arkansas	0.5
16	California	0.9
11	Colorado	1.3
5	Connecticut	1.9
8	Delaware	1.4
16	Florida	0.9
27	Georgia	0.7
21	Hawaii	0.8
49	Idaho	0.2
8	Illinois	1.4
27	Indiana	0.7
12	Iowa	1.2
21	Kansas	0.8
35	Kentucky	0.5
42	Louisiana	0.3
39	Maine	0.4
4	Maryland	2.0
1	Massachusetts	3.6
16	Michigan	0.9
8	Minnesota	1.4
49	Mississippi	0.2
21	Missouri	0.8
30	Montana	0.6
14	Nebraska	1.1
30	Nevada	0.6
7	New Hampshire	1.6
2	New Jersey	2.1
42	New Mexico	0.3
6	New York	1.8
30	North Carolina	0.6
21	North Dakota	0.8
21	Ohio	0.8
35	Oklahoma	0.5
21	Oregon	0.8
16	Pennsylvania	0.9
2	Rhode Island	2.1
30	South Carolina	0.6
42	South Dakota	0.3
35	Tennessee	0.5
30	Texas	0.6
42	Utah	0.3
15	Vermont	1.0
12	Virginia	1.2
16	Washington	0.9
39	West Virginia	0.4
42	Wisconsin	0.3
42	Wyoming	0.3

RANK	STATE	PERCENT
1	Massachusetts	3.6
2	New Jersey	2.1
2	Rhode Island	2.1
4	Maryland	2.0
5	Connecticut	1.9
6	New York	1.8
7	New Hampshire	1.6
8	Delaware	1.4
8	Illinois	1.4
8	Minnesota	1.4
11	Colorado	1.3
12	Iowa	1.2
12	Virginia	1.2
14	Nebraska	1.1
15	Vermont	1.0
16	California	0.9
16	Florida	0.9
16	Michigan	0.9
16	Pennsylvania	0.9
16	Washington	0.9
21	Hawaii	0.8
21	Kansas	0.8
21	Missouri	0.8
21	North Dakota	0.8
21	Ohio	0.8
21	Oregon	0.8
27	Arizona	0.7
27	Georgia	0.7
27	Indiana	0.7
30	Montana	0.6
30	Nevada	0.6
30	North Carolina	0.6
30	South Carolina	0.6
30	Texas	0.6
35	Arkansas	0.5
35	Kentucky	0.5
35	Oklahoma	0.5
35	Tennessee	0.5
39	Alabama	0.4
39	Maine	0.4
39	West Virginia	0.4
42	Alaska	0.3
42	Louisiana	0.3
42	New Mexico	0.3
42	South Dakota	0.3
42	Utah	0.3
42	Wisconsin	0.3
42	Wyoming	0.3
49	Idaho	0.2
49	Mississippi	0.2

District of Columbia 1.6

Source: Morgan Quitno Press using data from US Dept of Health & Human Serv's, Centers for Disease Control-Prevention "Assisted Reproductive Technology, 2001" (Morbidity and Mortality Weekly Report, Vol. 53, No. SS-01, 04/30/04) "National Vital Statistics Reports" (Vol. 51, No. 2, December 18, 2002)
By patient's residence. Does not include births or procedures to patients with residences outside the U.S. Assisted reproductive technology (ART) includes treatments in which both eggs and sperm are handled in the laboratory (i.e. in vitro fertilization and related procedures).

Percent of Infants Born in Multiple-Birth Deliveries as a Percent of All Infants Born Through Assisted Reproductive Technology Procedures in 2001
National Percent = 53.4% of Births*

ALPHA ORDER

RANK	STATE	PERCENT
5	Alabama	60.7
44	Alaska	48.3
38	Arizona	50.7
20	Arkansas	54.5
25	California	54.1
2	Colorado	61.4
37	Connecticut	50.9
28	Delaware	52.9
22	Florida	54.3
32	Georgia	52.1
17	Hawaii	54.9
15	Idaho	55.3
40	Illinois	50.1
19	Indiana	54.7
9	Iowa	57.0
42	Kansas	49.4
22	Kentucky	54.3
8	Louisiana	58.4
49	Maine	32.7
24	Maryland	54.2
45	Massachusetts	48.0
36	Michigan	51.0
39	Minnesota	50.3
47	Mississippi	47.1
11	Missouri	56.7
1	Montana	69.4
28	Nebraska	52.9
6	Nevada	59.4
46	New Hampshire	47.4
16	New Jersey	55.0
13	New Mexico	56.0
31	New York	52.3
7	North Carolina	58.8
30	North Dakota	52.4
12	Ohio	56.5
17	Oklahoma	54.9
13	Oregon	56.0
33	Pennsylvania	51.9
3	Rhode Island	61.3
35	South Carolina	51.1
41	South Dakota	50.0
4	Tennessee	61.2
10	Texas	56.8
43	Utah	48.4
20	Vermont	54.5
27	Virginia	53.1
34	Washington	51.2
48	West Virginia	44.7
26	Wisconsin	53.5
NA	Wyoming**	NA

RANK ORDER

RANK	STATE	PERCENT
1	Montana	69.4
2	Colorado	61.4
3	Rhode Island	61.3
4	Tennessee	61.2
5	Alabama	60.7
6	Nevada	59.4
7	North Carolina	58.8
8	Louisiana	58.4
9	Iowa	57.0
10	Texas	56.8
11	Missouri	56.7
12	Ohio	56.5
13	New Mexico	56.0
13	Oregon	56.0
15	Idaho	55.3
16	New Jersey	55.0
17	Hawaii	54.9
17	Oklahoma	54.9
19	Indiana	54.7
20	Arkansas	54.5
20	Vermont	54.5
22	Florida	54.3
22	Kentucky	54.3
24	Maryland	54.2
25	California	54.1
26	Wisconsin	53.5
27	Virginia	53.1
28	Delaware	52.9
28	Nebraska	52.9
30	North Dakota	52.4
31	New York	52.3
32	Georgia	52.1
33	Pennsylvania	51.9
34	Washington	51.2
35	South Carolina	51.1
36	Michigan	51.0
37	Connecticut	50.9
38	Arizona	50.7
39	Minnesota	50.3
40	Illinois	50.1
41	South Dakota	50.0
42	Kansas	49.4
43	Utah	48.4
44	Alaska	48.3
45	Massachusetts	48.0
46	New Hampshire	47.4
47	Mississippi	47.1
48	West Virginia	44.7
49	Maine	32.7
NA	Wyoming**	NA
	District of Columbia	48.3

Source: U.S. Department of Health and Human Services, Centers for Disease Control and Prevention
   "Assisted Reproductive Technology, 2001" (Morbidity and Mortality Weekly Report, Vol. 53, No. SS-01, 04/30/04)
By patient's residence. Includes births and procedures to patients with residences outside the U.S. Assisted reproductive technology (ART) includes treatments in which both eggs and sperm are handled in the laboratory (i.e. in vitro fertilization and related procedures).
**Not available.*

Percent of Mothers Beginning Prenatal Care in First Trimester in 2003

National Percent = 84.1% of Mothers*

ALPHA ORDER

RANK	STATE	PERCENT
28	Alabama	83.9
36	Alaska	81.3
47	Arizona	76.6
36	Arkansas	81.3
11	California	87.3
42	Colorado	79.3
6	Connecticut	88.6
25	Delaware	84.3
17	Florida	85.8
27	Georgia	84.0
32	Hawaii	82.5
35	Idaho	81.4
19	Illinois	85.4
34	Indiana	81.6
5	Iowa	88.9
8	Kansas	87.7
13	Kentucky	87.1
26	Louisiana	84.1
10	Maine	87.5
29	Maryland	83.7
4	Massachusetts	90.0
16	Michigan	86.2
14	Minnesota	86.5
21	Mississippi	85.2
7	Missouri	88.4
23	Montana	84.5
30	Nebraska	83.4
48	Nevada	75.7
1	New Hampshire	92.8
41	New Jersey	80.2
50	New Mexico	68.8
33	New York	82.4
23	North Carolina	84.5
11	North Dakota	87.3
8	Ohio	87.7
44	Oklahoma	77.5
38	Oregon	81.1
44	Pennsylvania	77.5
2	Rhode Island	91.2
44	South Carolina	77.5
43	South Dakota	78.4
30	Tennessee	83.4
39	Texas	80.9
40	Utah	80.3
3	Vermont	90.6
20	Virginia	85.3
49	Washington	75.6
18	West Virginia	85.7
22	Wisconsin	84.9
15	Wyoming	86.4

RANK ORDER

RANK	STATE	PERCENT
1	New Hampshire	92.8
2	Rhode Island	91.2
3	Vermont	90.6
4	Massachusetts	90.0
5	Iowa	88.9
6	Connecticut	88.6
7	Missouri	88.4
8	Kansas	87.7
8	Ohio	87.7
10	Maine	87.5
11	California	87.3
11	North Dakota	87.3
13	Kentucky	87.1
14	Minnesota	86.5
15	Wyoming	86.4
16	Michigan	86.2
17	Florida	85.8
18	West Virginia	85.7
19	Illinois	85.4
20	Virginia	85.3
21	Mississippi	85.2
22	Wisconsin	84.9
23	Montana	84.5
23	North Carolina	84.5
25	Delaware	84.3
26	Louisiana	84.1
27	Georgia	84.0
28	Alabama	83.9
29	Maryland	83.7
30	Nebraska	83.4
30	Tennessee	83.4
32	Hawaii	82.5
33	New York	82.4
34	Indiana	81.6
35	Idaho	81.4
36	Alaska	81.3
36	Arkansas	81.3
38	Oregon	81.1
39	Texas	80.9
40	Utah	80.3
41	New Jersey	80.2
42	Colorado	79.3
43	South Dakota	78.4
44	Oklahoma	77.5
44	Pennsylvania	77.5
44	South Carolina	77.5
47	Arizona	76.6
48	Nevada	75.7
49	Washington	75.6
50	New Mexico	68.8
	District of Columbia	76.1

Source: U.S. Department of Health and Human Services, National Center for Health Statistics
    "National Vital Statistics Reports" (Vol. 53, No. 9, November 23, 2004)
*Final data by state of residence.

Percent of White Mothers Beginning Prenatal Care in First Trimester in 2003

National Percent = 85.7% of White Mothers*

ALPHA ORDER				RANK ORDER		
RANK	STATE	PERCENT		RANK	STATE	PERCENT
21	Alabama	87.4		1	New Hampshire	93.0
31	Alaska	85.8		2	Rhode Island	92.5
47	Arizona	76.9		3	Massachusetts	91.4
36	Arkansas	83.2		4	Mississippi	90.8
21	California	87.4		5	Vermont	90.7
45	Colorado	79.8		6	Louisiana	90.0
7	Connecticut	89.8		7	Connecticut	89.8
27	Delaware	86.2		8	Missouri	89.7
15	Florida	88.1		9	North Dakota	89.6
27	Georgia	86.2		10	Iowa	89.5
32	Hawaii	85.7		11	Ohio	89.3
39	Idaho	81.6		12	Michigan	89.0
19	Illinois	87.8		13	Minnesota	88.9
37	Indiana	83.1		14	Kansas	88.5
10	Iowa	89.5		15	Florida	88.1
14	Kansas	88.5		15	Maryland	88.1
20	Kentucky	87.7		17	Maine	87.9
6	Louisiana	90.0		17	Virginia	87.9
17	Maine	87.9		19	Illinois	87.8
15	Maryland	88.1		20	Kentucky	87.7
3	Massachusetts	91.4		21	Alabama	87.4
12	Michigan	89.0		21	California	87.4
13	Minnesota	88.9		23	Wyoming	87.1
4	Mississippi	90.8		24	Montana	87.0
8	Missouri	89.7		25	North Carolina	86.9
24	Montana	87.0		25	Wisconsin	86.9
34	Nebraska	84.4		27	Delaware	86.2
49	Nevada	75.8		27	Georgia	86.2
1	New Hampshire	93.0		27	Tennessee	86.2
35	New Jersey	83.4		27	West Virginia	86.2
50	New Mexico	70.2		31	Alaska	85.8
33	New York	85.2		32	Hawaii	85.7
25	North Carolina	86.9		33	New York	85.2
9	North Dakota	89.6		34	Nebraska	84.4
11	Ohio	89.3		35	New Jersey	83.4
46	Oklahoma	79.3		36	Arkansas	83.2
40	Oregon	81.4		37	Indiana	83.1
44	Pennsylvania	80.2		38	South Dakota	82.8
2	Rhode Island	92.5		39	Idaho	81.6
42	South Carolina	81.1		40	Oregon	81.4
38	South Dakota	82.8		41	Utah	81.2
27	Tennessee	86.2		42	South Carolina	81.1
42	Texas	81.1		42	Texas	81.1
41	Utah	81.2		44	Pennsylvania	80.2
5	Vermont	90.7		45	Colorado	79.8
17	Virginia	87.9		46	Oklahoma	79.3
48	Washington	76.5		47	Arizona	76.9
27	West Virginia	86.2		48	Washington	76.5
25	Wisconsin	86.9		49	Nevada	75.8
23	Wyoming	87.1		50	New Mexico	70.2
					District of Columbia	86.4

Source: U.S. Department of Health and Human Services, National Center for Health Statistics
"National Vital Statistics Reports" (Vol. 53, No. 9, November 23, 2004)
*Final data by state of residence.

Percent of Black Mothers Beginning Prenatal Care in First Trimester in 2003

National Percent = 76.0% of Black Mothers*

ALPHA ORDER

RANK	STATE	PERCENT
26	Alabama	75.7
7	Alaska	84.6
25	Arizona	76.0
33	Arkansas	73.5
8	California	84.1
40	Colorado	70.9
11	Connecticut	81.0
17	Delaware	78.7
20	Florida	77.9
15	Georgia	79.1
2	Hawaii	88.7
3	Idaho	88.2
30	Illinois	74.2
44	Indiana	69.3
22	Iowa	76.9
14	Kansas	80.1
13	Kentucky	80.9
27	Louisiana	75.5
29	Maine	74.5
28	Maryland	75.1
10	Massachusetts	81.5
37	Michigan	72.8
39	Minnesota	72.4
19	Mississippi	78.0
11	Missouri	81.0
4	Montana	86.3
38	Nebraska	72.7
41	Nevada	70.7
5	New Hampshire	85.2
48	New Jersey	64.4
46	New Mexico	68.8
35	New York	73.1
24	North Carolina	76.8
5	North Dakota	85.2
16	Ohio	78.8
45	Oklahoma	69.2
18	Oregon	78.2
50	Pennsylvania	60.4
9	Rhode Island	83.3
42	South Carolina	70.5
47	South Dakota	64.8
36	Tennessee	73.0
21	Texas	77.0
49	Utah	63.5
31	Vermont	74.0
22	Virginia	76.9
43	Washington	69.8
33	West Virginia	73.5
32	Wisconsin	73.7
1	Wyoming	96.2

RANK ORDER

RANK	STATE	PERCENT
1	Wyoming	96.2
2	Hawaii	88.7
3	Idaho	88.2
4	Montana	86.3
5	New Hampshire	85.2
5	North Dakota	85.2
7	Alaska	84.6
8	California	84.1
9	Rhode Island	83.3
10	Massachusetts	81.5
11	Connecticut	81.0
11	Missouri	81.0
13	Kentucky	80.9
14	Kansas	80.1
15	Georgia	79.1
16	Ohio	78.8
17	Delaware	78.7
18	Oregon	78.2
19	Mississippi	78.0
20	Florida	77.9
21	Texas	77.0
22	Iowa	76.9
22	Virginia	76.9
24	North Carolina	76.8
25	Arizona	76.0
26	Alabama	75.7
27	Louisiana	75.5
28	Maryland	75.1
29	Maine	74.5
30	Illinois	74.2
31	Vermont	74.0
32	Wisconsin	73.7
33	Arkansas	73.5
33	West Virginia	73.5
35	New York	73.1
36	Tennessee	73.0
37	Michigan	72.8
38	Nebraska	72.7
39	Minnesota	72.4
40	Colorado	70.9
41	Nevada	70.7
42	South Carolina	70.5
43	Washington	69.8
44	Indiana	69.3
45	Oklahoma	69.2
46	New Mexico	68.8
47	South Dakota	64.8
48	New Jersey	64.4
49	Utah	63.5
50	Pennsylvania	60.4
	District of Columbia	70.9

Source: U.S. Department of Health and Human Services, National Center for Health Statistics
   "National Vital Statistics Reports" (Vol. 53, No. 9, November 23, 2004)
*Final data by state of residence.

Percent of Hispanic Mothers Beginning Prenatal Care in First Trimester in 2003

National Percent = 77.4% of Hispanic Mothers*

ALPHA ORDER				RANK ORDER		
RANK	STATE	PERCENT		RANK	STATE	PERCENT
50	Alabama	52.0		1	Rhode Island	87.3
11	Alaska	80.6		2	California	85.2
39	Arizona	66.7		3	New Hampshire	84.3
26	Arkansas	71.5		4	Florida	84.2
2	California	85.2		5	Massachusetts	83.9
38	Colorado	67.0		6	Louisiana	83.2
17	Connecticut	78.2		7	Vermont	83.0
25	Delaware	71.9		8	Missouri	81.0
4	Florida	84.2		9	Hawaii	80.8
35	Georgia	69.1		9	Maine	80.8
9	Hawaii	80.8		11	Alaska	80.6
37	Idaho	68.2		11	Montana	80.6
14	Illinois	80.0		13	Wyoming	80.2
41	Indiana	66.0		14	Illinois	80.0
23	Iowa	74.9		15	North Dakota	79.5
20	Kansas	77.2		16	Ohio	79.0
24	Kentucky	74.0		17	Connecticut	78.2
6	Louisiana	83.2		18	Michigan	77.7
9	Maine	80.8		19	Mississippi	77.6
33	Maryland	69.5		20	Kansas	77.2
5	Massachusetts	83.9		21	New York	76.2
18	Michigan	77.7		22	Texas	75.5
28	Minnesota	71.0		23	Iowa	74.9
19	Mississippi	77.6		24	Kentucky	74.0
8	Missouri	81.0		25	Delaware	71.9
11	Montana	80.6		26	Arkansas	71.5
31	Nebraska	69.8		27	Virginia	71.2
45	Nevada	64.1		28	Minnesota	71.0
3	New Hampshire	84.3		29	Wisconsin	70.7
36	New Jersey	68.6		30	Oregon	69.9
40	New Mexico	66.2		31	Nebraska	69.8
21	New York	76.2		32	North Carolina	69.6
32	North Carolina	69.6		33	Maryland	69.5
15	North Dakota	79.5		34	West Virginia	69.4
16	Ohio	79.0		35	Georgia	69.1
43	Oklahoma	65.0		36	New Jersey	68.6
30	Oregon	69.9		37	Idaho	68.2
48	Pennsylvania	62.1		38	Colorado	67.0
1	Rhode Island	87.3		39	Arizona	66.7
49	South Carolina	57.1		40	New Mexico	66.2
46	South Dakota	64.0		41	Indiana	66.0
47	Tennessee	63.7		42	Utah	65.1
22	Texas	75.5		43	Oklahoma	65.0
42	Utah	65.1		44	Washington	64.4
7	Vermont	83.0		45	Nevada	64.1
27	Virginia	71.2		46	South Dakota	64.0
44	Washington	64.4		47	Tennessee	63.7
34	West Virginia	69.4		48	Pennsylvania	62.1
29	Wisconsin	70.7		49	South Carolina	57.1
13	Wyoming	80.2		50	Alabama	52.0
					District of Columbia	69.3

Source: U.S. Department of Health and Human Services, National Center for Health Statistics
"National Vital Statistics Reports" (Vol. 53, No. 9, November 23, 2004)
*Final data by state of residence. Persons of Hispanic origin may be of any race.

Percent of Mothers Receiving Late or No Prenatal Care in 2002

National Percent = 3.6% of Mothers*

ALPHA ORDER			RANK ORDER		
RANK	STATE	PERCENT	RANK	STATE	PERCENT
15	Alabama	3.8	1	New Mexico	7.9
11	Alaska	4.6	2	Nevada	7.1
3	Arizona	6.6	3	Arizona	6.6
6	Arkansas	4.9	4	Oklahoma	5.4
40	California	2.6	5	Texas	5.0
12	Colorado	4.5	6	Arkansas	4.9
45	Connecticut	2.0	6	New Jersey	4.9
19	Delaware	3.5	6	Utah	4.9
31	Florida	2.9	9	New York	4.7
25	Georgia	3.4	9	South Carolina	4.7
19	Hawaii	3.5	11	Alaska	4.6
25	Idaho	3.4	12	Colorado	4.5
31	Illinois	2.9	13	South Dakota	4.4
19	Indiana	3.5	14	Tennessee	3.9
43	Iowa	2.2	15	Alabama	3.8
36	Kansas	2.8	15	Oregon	3.8
41	Kentucky	2.5	17	Louisiana	3.6
17	Louisiana	3.6	17	Maryland	3.6
48	Maine	1.6	19	Delaware	3.5
17	Maryland	3.6	19	Hawaii	3.5
45	Massachusetts	2.0	19	Indiana	3.5
19	Michigan	3.5	19	Michigan	3.5
42	Minnesota	2.3	19	Pennsylvania	3.5
28	Mississippi	3.1	19	Virginia	3.5
38	Missouri	2.7	25	Georgia	3.4
36	Montana	2.8	25	Idaho	3.4
28	Nebraska	3.1	27	Wisconsin	3.2
2	Nevada	7.1	28	Mississippi	3.1
50	New Hampshire	1.4	28	Nebraska	3.1
6	New Jersey	4.9	28	Washington	3.1
1	New Mexico	7.9	31	Florida	2.9
9	New York	4.7	31	Illinois	2.9
31	North Carolina	2.9	31	North Carolina	2.9
38	North Dakota	2.7	31	Ohio	2.9
31	Ohio	2.9	31	Wyoming	2.9
4	Oklahoma	5.4	36	Kansas	2.8
15	Oregon	3.8	36	Montana	2.8
19	Pennsylvania	3.5	38	Missouri	2.7
49	Rhode Island	1.5	38	North Dakota	2.7
9	South Carolina	4.7	40	California	2.6
13	South Dakota	4.4	41	Kentucky	2.5
14	Tennessee	3.9	42	Minnesota	2.3
5	Texas	5.0	43	Iowa	2.2
6	Utah	4.9	43	West Virginia	2.2
47	Vermont	1.7	45	Connecticut	2.0
19	Virginia	3.5	45	Massachusetts	2.0
28	Washington	3.1	47	Vermont	1.7
43	West Virginia	2.2	48	Maine	1.6
27	Wisconsin	3.2	49	Rhode Island	1.5
31	Wyoming	2.9	50	New Hampshire	1.4
				District of Columbia	7.4

*Source: U.S. Department of Health and Human Services, National Center for Health Statistics
"National Vital Statistics Reports" (Vol. 52, No. 10, December 17, 2003)
Final data by state of residence. "Late" means care begun in third trimester.

Percent of White Mothers Receiving Late or No Prenatal Care in 2002

National Percent = 3.1% of White Mothers*

ALPHA ORDER

RANK	STATE	PERCENT
16	Alabama	2.9
9	Alaska	3.8
3	Arizona	6.5
8	Arkansas	4.2
25	California	2.6
7	Colorado	4.4
42	Connecticut	1.8
16	Delaware	2.9
31	Florida	2.3
16	Georgia	2.9
28	Hawaii	2.5
14	Idaho	3.3
36	Illinois	2.1
15	Indiana	3.0
39	Iowa	2.0
28	Kansas	2.5
31	Kentucky	2.3
44	Louisiana	1.7
46	Maine	1.6
31	Maryland	2.3
48	Massachusetts	1.5
28	Michigan	2.5
44	Minnesota	1.7
42	Mississippi	1.8
36	Missouri	2.1
40	Montana	1.9
21	Nebraska	2.8
2	Nevada	7.0
49	New Hampshire	1.4
10	New Jersey	3.7
1	New Mexico	7.4
10	New York	3.7
35	North Carolina	2.2
40	North Dakota	1.9
31	Ohio	2.3
5	Oklahoma	4.9
10	Oregon	3.7
21	Pennsylvania	2.8
50	Rhode Island	1.2
13	South Carolina	3.4
23	South Dakota	2.7
16	Tennessee	2.9
4	Texas	5.0
6	Utah	4.5
46	Vermont	1.6
23	Virginia	2.7
16	Washington	2.9
36	West Virginia	2.1
25	Wisconsin	2.6
25	Wyoming	2.6

RANK ORDER

RANK	STATE	PERCENT
1	New Mexico	7.4
2	Nevada	7.0
3	Arizona	6.5
4	Texas	5.0
5	Oklahoma	4.9
6	Utah	4.5
7	Colorado	4.4
8	Arkansas	4.2
9	Alaska	3.8
10	New Jersey	3.7
10	New York	3.7
10	Oregon	3.7
13	South Carolina	3.4
14	Idaho	3.3
15	Indiana	3.0
16	Alabama	2.9
16	Delaware	2.9
16	Georgia	2.9
16	Tennessee	2.9
16	Washington	2.9
21	Nebraska	2.8
21	Pennsylvania	2.8
23	South Dakota	2.7
23	Virginia	2.7
25	California	2.6
25	Wisconsin	2.6
25	Wyoming	2.6
28	Hawaii	2.5
28	Kansas	2.5
28	Michigan	2.5
31	Florida	2.3
31	Kentucky	2.3
31	Maryland	2.3
31	Ohio	2.3
35	North Carolina	2.2
36	Illinois	2.1
36	Missouri	2.1
36	West Virginia	2.1
39	Iowa	2.0
40	Montana	1.9
40	North Dakota	1.9
42	Connecticut	1.8
42	Mississippi	1.8
44	Louisiana	1.7
44	Minnesota	1.7
46	Maine	1.6
46	Vermont	1.6
48	Massachusetts	1.5
49	New Hampshire	1.4
50	Rhode Island	1.2
	District of Columbia	3.7

Source: U.S. Department of Health and Human Services, National Center for Health Statistics
    "National Vital Statistics Reports" (Vol. 52, No. 10, December 17, 2003)
*Final data by state of residence. "Late" means care begun in third trimester.

Percent of Black Mothers Receiving Late or No Prenatal Care in 2002

National Percent = 6.2% of Black Mothers*

ALPHA ORDER

RANK	STATE	PERCENT
23	Alabama	5.7
NA	Alaska**	NA
26	Arizona	5.5
8	Arkansas	7.5
39	California	3.4
11	Colorado	7.3
38	Connecticut	3.5
23	Delaware	5.7
31	Florida	4.9
34	Georgia	4.5
NA	Hawaii**	NA
NA	Idaho**	NA
15	Illinois	6.7
13	Indiana	7.1
26	Iowa	5.5
30	Kansas	5.0
36	Kentucky	4.4
19	Louisiana	6.1
NA	Maine**	NA
16	Maryland	6.2
28	Massachusetts	5.1
5	Michigan	7.9
16	Minnesota	6.2
32	Mississippi	4.6
25	Missouri	5.6
NA	Montana**	NA
20	Nebraska	6.0
3	Nevada	8.6
NA	New Hampshire**	NA
2	New Jersey	11.0
5	New Mexico	7.9
4	New York	8.4
28	North Carolina	5.1
NA	North Dakota**	NA
16	Ohio	6.2
8	Oklahoma	7.5
34	Oregon	4.5
7	Pennsylvania	7.8
39	Rhode Island	3.4
13	South Carolina	7.1
NA	South Dakota**	NA
8	Tennessee	7.5
22	Texas	5.8
1	Utah	14.2
NA	Vermont**	NA
21	Virginia	5.9
32	Washington	4.6
36	West Virginia	4.4
11	Wisconsin	7.3
NA	Wyoming**	NA

RANK ORDER

RANK	STATE	PERCENT
1	Utah	14.2
2	New Jersey	11.0
3	Nevada	8.6
4	New York	8.4
5	Michigan	7.9
5	New Mexico	7.9
7	Pennsylvania	7.8
8	Arkansas	7.5
8	Oklahoma	7.5
8	Tennessee	7.5
11	Colorado	7.3
11	Wisconsin	7.3
13	Indiana	7.1
13	South Carolina	7.1
15	Illinois	6.7
16	Maryland	6.2
16	Minnesota	6.2
16	Ohio	6.2
19	Louisiana	6.1
20	Nebraska	6.0
21	Virginia	5.9
22	Texas	5.8
23	Alabama	5.7
23	Delaware	5.7
25	Missouri	5.6
26	Arizona	5.5
26	Iowa	5.5
28	Massachusetts	5.1
28	North Carolina	5.1
30	Kansas	5.0
31	Florida	4.9
32	Mississippi	4.6
32	Washington	4.6
34	Georgia	4.5
34	Oregon	4.5
36	Kentucky	4.4
36	West Virginia	4.4
38	Connecticut	3.5
39	California	3.4
39	Rhode Island	3.4
NA	Alaska**	NA
NA	Hawaii**	NA
NA	Idaho**	NA
NA	Maine**	NA
NA	Montana**	NA
NA	New Hampshire**	NA
NA	North Dakota**	NA
NA	South Dakota**	NA
NA	Vermont**	NA
NA	Wyoming**	NA
	District of Columbia	10.0

Source: U.S. Department of Health and Human Services, National Center for Health Statistics
"National Vital Statistics Reports" (Vol. 52, No. 10, December 17, 2003)
*Final data by state of residence. "Late" means care begun in third trimester.
**Insufficient data.

Percent of Hispanic Mothers Receiving Late or No Prenatal Care in 2002

National Percent = 5.5% of Hispanic Mothers*

ALPHA ORDER

RANK	STATE	PERCENT
1	Alabama	19.0
24	Alaska	5.9
5	Arizona	10.4
8	Arkansas	9.4
42	California	3.1
11	Colorado	7.9
36	Connecticut	3.8
24	Delaware	5.9
40	Florida	3.3
14	Georgia	7.1
41	Hawaii	3.2
21	Idaho	6.4
37	Illinois	3.5
11	Indiana	7.9
30	Iowa	5.6
17	Kansas	6.6
17	Kentucky	6.6
39	Louisiana	3.4
NA	Maine**	NA
24	Maryland	5.9
43	Massachusetts	3.0
35	Michigan	4.7
28	Minnesota	5.8
17	Mississippi	6.6
34	Missouri	4.8
NA	Montana**	NA
16	Nebraska	6.8
3	Nevada	11.1
NA	New Hampshire**	NA
14	New Jersey	7.1
9	New Mexico	8.8
24	New York	5.9
23	North Carolina	6.1
NA	North Dakota**	NA
33	Ohio	5.1
10	Oklahoma	8.3
31	Oregon	5.5
29	Pennsylvania	5.7
44	Rhode Island	2.1
5	South Carolina	10.4
4	South Dakota	10.8
2	Tennessee	12.2
17	Texas	6.6
7	Utah	9.5
NA	Vermont**	NA
13	Virginia	7.5
32	Washington	5.2
NA	West Virginia**	NA
22	Wisconsin	6.3
37	Wyoming	3.5

RANK ORDER

RANK	STATE	PERCENT
1	Alabama	19.0
2	Tennessee	12.2
3	Nevada	11.1
4	South Dakota	10.8
5	Arizona	10.4
5	South Carolina	10.4
7	Utah	9.5
8	Arkansas	9.4
9	New Mexico	8.8
10	Oklahoma	8.3
11	Colorado	7.9
11	Indiana	7.9
13	Virginia	7.5
14	Georgia	7.1
14	New Jersey	7.1
16	Nebraska	6.8
17	Kansas	6.6
17	Kentucky	6.6
17	Mississippi	6.6
17	Texas	6.6
21	Idaho	6.4
22	Wisconsin	6.3
23	North Carolina	6.1
24	Alaska	5.9
24	Delaware	5.9
24	Maryland	5.9
24	New York	5.9
28	Minnesota	5.8
29	Pennsylvania	5.7
30	Iowa	5.6
31	Oregon	5.5
32	Washington	5.2
33	Ohio	5.1
34	Missouri	4.8
35	Michigan	4.7
36	Connecticut	3.8
37	Illinois	3.5
37	Wyoming	3.5
39	Louisiana	3.4
40	Florida	3.3
41	Hawaii	3.2
42	California	3.1
43	Massachusetts	3.0
44	Rhode Island	2.1
NA	Maine**	NA
NA	Montana**	NA
NA	New Hampshire**	NA
NA	North Dakota**	NA
NA	Vermont**	NA
NA	West Virginia**	NA

District of Columbia	7.9

*Source: U.S. Department of Health and Human Services, National Center for Health Statistics
"National Vital Statistics Reports" (Vol. 52, No. 10, December 17, 2003)*
Final data by state of residence. "Late" means care begun in third trimester.
**Insufficient data.*

Reported Legal Abortions in 2001

Reporting States' Total = 853,485 Abortions*

RANK	STATE	ABORTIONS	% of USA
18	Alabama	13,382	1.6%
NA	Alaska**	NA	NA
25	Arizona	8,302	1.0%
29	Arkansas	5,924	0.7%
NA	California**	NA	NA
34	Colorado	4,633	0.5%
19	Connecticut	13,265	1.6%
33	Delaware	4,869	0.6%
2	Florida	85,589	10.0%
8	Georgia	33,248	3.9%
35	Hawaii	3,999	0.5%
46	Idaho	738	0.1%
4	Illinois	46,546	5.5%
21	Indiana	11,875	1.4%
30	Iowa	5,722	0.7%
20	Kansas	12,284	1.4%
37	Kentucky	3,764	0.4%
22	Louisiana	10,932	1.3%
40	Maine	2,515	0.3%
17	Maryland	13,502	1.6%
11	Massachusetts	26,293	3.1%
10	Michigan	28,220	3.3%
15	Minnesota	14,832	1.7%
39	Mississippi	3,566	0.4%
26	Missouri	7,797	0.9%
41	Montana	2,350	0.3%
36	Nebraska	3,982	0.5%
24	Nevada	10,110	1.2%
NA	New Hampshire**	NA	NA
7	New Jersey	33,606	3.9%
32	New Mexico	5,166	0.6%
1	New York	127,102	14.9%
9	North Carolina	30,419	3.6%
44	North Dakota	1,216	0.1%
5	Ohio	37,464	4.4%
27	Oklahoma	7,038	0.8%
16	Oregon	14,272	1.7%
6	Pennsylvania	36,820	4.3%
31	Rhode Island	5,455	0.6%
28	South Carolina	7,014	0.8%
45	South Dakota	895	0.1%
14	Tennessee	17,405	2.0%
3	Texas	77,409	9.1%
38	Utah	3,594	0.4%
43	Vermont	1,519	0.2%
13	Virginia	24,586	2.9%
12	Washington	25,620	3.0%
42	West Virginia	2,332	0.3%
23	Wisconsin	10,925	1.3%
47	Wyoming	4	0.0%

RANK	STATE	ABORTIONS	% of USA
1	New York	127,102	14.9%
2	Florida	85,589	10.0%
3	Texas	77,409	9.1%
4	Illinois	46,546	5.5%
5	Ohio	37,464	4.4%
6	Pennsylvania	36,820	4.3%
7	New Jersey	33,606	3.9%
8	Georgia	33,248	3.9%
9	North Carolina	30,419	3.6%
10	Michigan	28,220	3.3%
11	Massachusetts	26,293	3.1%
12	Washington	25,620	3.0%
13	Virginia	24,586	2.9%
14	Tennessee	17,405	2.0%
15	Minnesota	14,832	1.7%
16	Oregon	14,272	1.7%
17	Maryland	13,502	1.6%
18	Alabama	13,382	1.6%
19	Connecticut	13,265	1.6%
20	Kansas	12,284	1.4%
21	Indiana	11,875	1.4%
22	Louisiana	10,932	1.3%
23	Wisconsin	10,925	1.3%
24	Nevada	10,110	1.2%
25	Arizona	8,302	1.0%
26	Missouri	7,797	0.9%
27	Oklahoma	7,038	0.8%
28	South Carolina	7,014	0.8%
29	Arkansas	5,924	0.7%
30	Iowa	5,722	0.7%
31	Rhode Island	5,455	0.6%
32	New Mexico	5,166	0.6%
33	Delaware	4,869	0.6%
34	Colorado	4,633	0.5%
35	Hawaii	3,999	0.5%
36	Nebraska	3,982	0.5%
37	Kentucky	3,764	0.4%
38	Utah	3,594	0.4%
39	Mississippi	3,566	0.4%
40	Maine	2,515	0.3%
41	Montana	2,350	0.3%
42	West Virginia	2,332	0.3%
43	Vermont	1,519	0.2%
44	North Dakota	1,216	0.1%
45	South Dakota	895	0.1%
46	Idaho	738	0.1%
47	Wyoming	4	0.0%
NA	Alaska**	NA	NA
NA	California**	NA	NA
NA	New Hampshire**	NA	NA
	District of Columbia	5,385	0.6%

Source: U.S. Department of Health and Human Services, Centers for Disease Control and Prevention
"Abortion Surveillance-United States, 2001" (Morbidity and Mortality Weekly Report, Vol. 53, No. SS-9, 11/26/04)
*By state of occurrence. Total is for reporting states only.
**Not reported.

Percent Change in Reported Legal Abortions: 1997 to 2001

National Percent Change = 5.9% Decrease*

ALPHA ORDER

RANK	STATE	PERCENT CHANGE
10	Alabama	2.4
NA	Alaska**	NA
43	Arizona	(26.3)
9	Arkansas	2.5
NA	California**	NA
46	Colorado	(49.5)
19	Connecticut	(3.9)
24	Delaware	(5.2)
7	Florida	4.8
26	Georgia	(6.9)
33	Hawaii	(11.5)
34	Idaho	(15.9)
28	Illinois	(7.2)
32	Indiana	(10.1)
44	Iowa	(42.9)
5	Kansas	9.2
45	Kentucky	(46.5)
26	Louisiana	(6.9)
14	Maine	(1.2)
2	Maryland	36.8
29	Massachusetts	(7.7)
21	Michigan	(4.4)
8	Minnesota	4.2
38	Mississippi	(17.5)
41	Missouri	(23.6)
35	Montana	(16.3)
40	Nebraska	(22.4)
1	Nevada	46.8
NA	New Hampshire**	NA
3	New Jersey	9.6
20	New Mexico	(4.0)
31	New York	(9.8)
17	North Carolina	(3.4)
12	North Dakota	(0.8)
15	Ohio	(2.0)
4	Oklahoma	9.5
18	Oregon	(3.8)
12	Pennsylvania	(0.8)
11	Rhode Island	(0.4)
42	South Carolina	(23.9)
16	South Dakota	(2.6)
22	Tennessee	(4.8)
30	Texas	(8.6)
6	Utah	5.5
39	Vermont	(22.3)
25	Virginia	(5.8)
23	Washington	(4.9)
36	West Virginia	(17.0)
37	Wisconsin	(17.3)
47	Wyoming	(97.9)

RANK ORDER

RANK	STATE	PERCENT CHANGE
1	Nevada	46.8
2	Maryland	36.8
3	New Jersey	9.6
4	Oklahoma	9.5
5	Kansas	9.2
6	Utah	5.5
7	Florida	4.8
8	Minnesota	4.2
9	Arkansas	2.5
10	Alabama	2.4
11	Rhode Island	(0.4)
12	North Dakota	(0.8)
12	Pennsylvania	(0.8)
14	Maine	(1.2)
15	Ohio	(2.0)
16	South Dakota	(2.6)
17	North Carolina	(3.4)
18	Oregon	(3.8)
19	Connecticut	(3.9)
20	New Mexico	(4.0)
21	Michigan	(4.4)
22	Tennessee	(4.8)
23	Washington	(4.9)
24	Delaware	(5.2)
25	Virginia	(5.8)
26	Georgia	(6.9)
26	Louisiana	(6.9)
28	Illinois	(7.2)
29	Massachusetts	(7.7)
30	Texas	(8.6)
31	New York	(9.8)
32	Indiana	(10.1)
33	Hawaii	(11.5)
34	Idaho	(15.9)
35	Montana	(16.3)
36	West Virginia	(17.0)
37	Wisconsin	(17.3)
38	Mississippi	(17.5)
39	Vermont	(22.3)
40	Nebraska	(22.4)
41	Missouri	(23.6)
42	South Carolina	(23.9)
43	Arizona	(26.3)
44	Iowa	(42.9)
45	Kentucky	(46.5)
46	Colorado	(49.5)
47	Wyoming	(97.9)
NA	Alaska**	NA
NA	California**	NA
NA	New Hampshire**	NA

District of Columbia   (38.6)

Source: Morgan Quitno Press using data from US Dept of Health & Human Serv's, Centers for Disease Control-Prevention
"Abortion Surveillance-United States, 2001" (Morbidity and Mortality Weekly Report, Vol. 53, No. SS-9, 11/26/04)
"Abortion Surveillance-United States, 1997" (Morbidity and Mortality Weekly Report, Vol. 49, No. SS-11, 12/08/00)
*By state of occurrence. Percent change is only for states reporting in both years.
**Not reported.

Reported Legal Abortions per 1,000 Live Births in 2001

Reporting States' Ratio = 246 Abortions per 1,000 Live Births*

RANK	STATE	RATIO		RANK	STATE	RATIO
21	Alabama	221		1	New York	500
NA	Alaska**	NA		2	Delaware	453
40	Arizona	97		3	Rhode Island	429
30	Arkansas	160		4	Florida	416
NA	California**	NA		5	Massachusetts	324
44	Colorado	69		6	Nevada	322
10	Connecticut	311		6	Washington	322
2	Delaware	453		8	Kansas	316
4	Florida	416		9	Oregon	315
15	Georgia	249		10	Connecticut	311
19	Hawaii	234		11	New Jersey	290
46	Idaho	36		12	North Carolina	257
14	Illinois	253		12	Pennsylvania	257
36	Indiana	137		14	Illinois	253
34	Iowa	152		15	Georgia	249
8	Kansas	316		15	Virginia	249
44	Kentucky	69		17	Ohio	247
29	Louisiana	167		18	Vermont	239
28	Maine	183		19	Hawaii	234
27	Maryland	184		20	Tennessee	222
5	Massachusetts	324		21	Alabama	221
24	Michigan	212		22	Minnesota	220
22	Minnesota	220		23	Montana	214
42	Mississippi	84		24	Michigan	212
39	Missouri	103		24	Texas	212
23	Montana	214		26	New Mexico	190
30	Nebraska	160		27	Maryland	184
6	Nevada	322		28	Maine	183
NA	New Hampshire**	NA		29	Louisiana	167
11	New Jersey	290		30	Arkansas	160
26	New Mexico	190		30	Nebraska	160
1	New York	500		32	North Dakota	159
12	North Carolina	257		33	Wisconsin	158
32	North Dakota	159		34	Iowa	152
17	Ohio	247		35	Oklahoma	140
35	Oklahoma	140		36	Indiana	137
9	Oregon	315		37	South Carolina	126
12	Pennsylvania	257		38	West Virginia	114
3	Rhode Island	429		39	Missouri	103
37	South Carolina	126		40	Arizona	97
41	South Dakota	85		41	South Dakota	85
20	Tennessee	222		42	Mississippi	84
24	Texas	212		43	Utah	75
43	Utah	75		44	Colorado	69
18	Vermont	239		44	Kentucky	69
15	Virginia	249		46	Idaho	36
6	Washington	322		NA	Alaska**	NA
38	West Virginia	114		NA	California**	NA
33	Wisconsin	158		NA	New Hampshire**	NA
NA	Wyoming**	NA		NA	Wyoming**	NA

	District of Columbia	706

Source: U.S. Department of Health and Human Services, Centers for Disease Control and Prevention
    "Abortion Surveillance-United States, 2001" (Morbidity and Mortality Weekly Report, Vol. 53, No. SS-9, 11/26/04)
By state of occurrence. National figure is for reporting states only.
**Not reported.*

Reported Legal Abortions per 1,000 Women Ages 15 to 44 in 2001

Reporting States' Rate = 16 Abortions per 1,000 Women Ages 15 to 44*

ALPHA ORDER

RANK	STATE	RATE
19	Alabama	14
NA	Alaska**	NA
37	Arizona	8
27	Arkansas	11
NA	California**	NA
44	Colorado	5
9	Connecticut	19
2	Delaware	28
3	Florida	26
12	Georgia	17
15	Hawaii	16
46	Idaho	3
12	Illinois	17
32	Indiana	9
32	Iowa	9
6	Kansas	21
45	Kentucky	4
27	Louisiana	11
32	Maine	9
27	Maryland	11
11	Massachusetts	18
23	Michigan	13
19	Minnesota	14
40	Mississippi	6
40	Missouri	6
23	Montana	13
27	Nebraska	11
4	Nevada	23
NA	New Hampshire**	NA
9	New Jersey	19
23	New Mexico	13
1	New York	30
12	North Carolina	17
32	North Dakota	9
17	Ohio	15
31	Oklahoma	10
7	Oregon	20
19	Pennsylvania	14
4	Rhode Island	23
37	South Carolina	8
40	South Dakota	6
19	Tennessee	14
15	Texas	16
39	Utah	7
26	Vermont	12
17	Virginia	15
7	Washington	20
40	West Virginia	6
32	Wisconsin	9
NA	Wyoming**	NA

RANK ORDER

RANK	STATE	RATE
1	New York	30
2	Delaware	28
3	Florida	26
4	Nevada	23
4	Rhode Island	23
6	Kansas	21
7	Oregon	20
7	Washington	20
9	Connecticut	19
9	New Jersey	19
11	Massachusetts	18
12	Georgia	17
12	Illinois	17
12	North Carolina	17
15	Hawaii	16
15	Texas	16
17	Ohio	15
17	Virginia	15
19	Alabama	14
19	Minnesota	14
19	Pennsylvania	14
19	Tennessee	14
23	Michigan	13
23	Montana	13
23	New Mexico	13
26	Vermont	12
27	Arkansas	11
27	Louisiana	11
27	Maryland	11
27	Nebraska	11
31	Oklahoma	10
32	Indiana	9
32	Iowa	9
32	Maine	9
32	North Dakota	9
32	Wisconsin	9
37	Arizona	8
37	South Carolina	8
39	Utah	7
40	Mississippi	6
40	Missouri	6
40	South Dakota	6
40	West Virginia	6
44	Colorado	5
45	Kentucky	4
46	Idaho	3
NA	Alaska**	NA
NA	California**	NA
NA	New Hampshire**	NA
NA	Wyoming**	NA

District of Columbia   37

Source: U.S. Department of Health and Human Services, Centers for Disease Control and Prevention
    "Abortion Surveillance-United States, 2001" (Morbidity and Mortality Weekly Report, Vol. 53, No. SS-9, 11/26/04)
*By state of occurrence. National figure is for reporting states only.
**Not reported.

Percent of Legal Abortions Obtained by Out-Of-State Residents in 2001

Reporting States' Percent = 8.7% of Abortions*

ALPHA ORDER

RANK ORDER

RANK	STATE	PERCENT	RANK	STATE	PERCENT
6	Alabama	18.1	1	Kansas	48.9
NA	Alaska**	NA	2	North Dakota	38.3
41	Arizona	0.9	3	Delaware	28.3
8	Arkansas	15.9	4	Rhode Island	24.8
NA	California**	NA	5	Tennessee	19.2
7	Colorado	16.7	6	Alabama	18.1
38	Connecticut	3.3	7	Colorado	16.7
3	Delaware	28.3	8	Arkansas	15.9
NA	Florida**	NA	9	Nebraska	15.8
17	Georgia	10.5	10	South Dakota	15.2
42	Hawaii	0.3	11	Kentucky	14.8
37	Idaho	3.5	12	Vermont	14.2
18	Illinois	9.8	13	North Carolina	13.8
33	Indiana	4.2	14	Oregon	12.6
NA	Iowa**	NA	15	Montana	12.2
1	Kansas	48.9	16	West Virginia	10.9
11	Kentucky	14.8	17	Georgia	10.5
NA	Louisiana**	NA	18	Illinois	9.8
39	Maine	2.9	19	Minnesota	9.3
26	Maryland	5.9	20	Missouri	9.1
23	Massachusetts	6.3	21	Ohio	8.7
36	Michigan	3.6	22	Nevada	7.3
19	Minnesota	9.3	23	Massachusetts	6.3
31	Mississippi	4.3	24	Utah	6.2
20	Missouri	9.1	25	Virginia	6.1
15	Montana	12.2	26	Maryland	5.9
9	Nebraska	15.8	27	South Carolina	5.3
22	Nevada	7.3	28	Pennsylvania	4.9
NA	New Hampshire**	NA	28	Washington	4.9
35	New Jersey	3.7	30	New Mexico	4.5
30	New Mexico	4.5	31	Mississippi	4.3
NA	New York**	NA	31	Oklahoma	4.3
13	North Carolina	13.8	33	Indiana	4.2
2	North Dakota	38.3	34	Texas	3.9
21	Ohio	8.7	35	New Jersey	3.7
31	Oklahoma	4.3	36	Michigan	3.6
14	Oregon	12.6	37	Idaho	3.5
28	Pennsylvania	4.9	38	Connecticut	3.3
4	Rhode Island	24.8	39	Maine	2.9
27	South Carolina	5.3	40	Wisconsin	2.0
10	South Dakota	15.2	41	Arizona	0.9
5	Tennessee	19.2	42	Hawaii	0.3
34	Texas	3.9	43	Wyoming	0.0
24	Utah	6.2	NA	Alaska**	NA
12	Vermont	14.2	NA	California**	NA
25	Virginia	6.1	NA	Florida**	NA
28	Washington	4.9	NA	Iowa**	NA
16	West Virginia	10.9	NA	Louisiana**	NA
40	Wisconsin	2.0	NA	New Hampshire**	NA
43	Wyoming	0.0	NA	New York**	NA

	District of Columbia	56.0

Source: U.S. Department of Health and Human Services, Centers for Disease Control and Prevention
   "Abortion Surveillance-United States, 2001" (Morbidity and Mortality Weekly Report, Vol. 53, No. SS-9, 11/26/04)
*By state of occurrence. National figure is for reporting states only.
**Not reported.

Percent of Reported Legal Abortions Obtained by White Women in 2001

Reporting States' Percent = 54.1% of Abortions*

ALPHA ORDER

RANK	STATE	PERCENT
30	Alabama	46.6
NA	Alaska**	NA
NA	Arizona**	NA
21	Arkansas	59.7
NA	California**	NA
12	Colorado	79.5
NA	Connecticut**	NA
25	Delaware	54.7
NA	Florida**	NA
33	Georgia	41.0
38	Hawaii	26.1
3	Idaho	92.0
NA	Illinois**	NA
20	Indiana	62.9
11	Iowa	80.4
14	Kansas	72.4
16	Kentucky	71.0
34	Louisiana	35.9
4	Maine	90.7
35	Maryland	30.3
24	Massachusetts	54.9
NA	Michigan**	NA
19	Minnesota	65.1
37	Mississippi	26.9
23	Missouri	57.5
6	Montana	85.2
NA	Nebraska**	NA
NA	Nevada**	NA
NA	New Hampshire**	NA
36	New Jersey	30.1
8	New Mexico	84.0
32	New York**	42.2
31	North Carolina	44.1
7	North Dakota	85.1
22	Ohio	58.8
18	Oklahoma	66.7
9	Oregon	83.7
26	Pennsylvania	54.2
NA	Rhode Island**	NA
27	South Carolina	53.8
10	South Dakota	82.0
28	Tennessee	53.3
14	Texas	72.4
13	Utah	76.6
2	Vermont	94.6
29	Virginia	50.1
NA	Washington**	NA
5	West Virginia	87.3
17	Wisconsin	68.0
1	Wyoming	100.0

RANK ORDER

RANK	STATE	PERCENT
1	Wyoming	100.0
2	Vermont	94.6
3	Idaho	92.0
4	Maine	90.7
5	West Virginia	87.3
6	Montana	85.2
7	North Dakota	85.1
8	New Mexico	84.0
9	Oregon	83.7
10	South Dakota	82.0
11	Iowa	80.4
12	Colorado	79.5
13	Utah	76.6
14	Kansas	72.4
14	Texas	72.4
16	Kentucky	71.0
17	Wisconsin	68.0
18	Oklahoma	66.7
19	Minnesota	65.1
20	Indiana	62.9
21	Arkansas	59.7
22	Ohio	58.8
23	Missouri	57.5
24	Massachusetts	54.9
25	Delaware	54.7
26	Pennsylvania	54.2
27	South Carolina	53.8
28	Tennessee	53.3
29	Virginia	50.1
30	Alabama	46.6
31	North Carolina	44.1
32	New York**	42.2
33	Georgia	41.0
34	Louisiana	35.9
35	Maryland	30.3
36	New Jersey	30.1
37	Mississippi	26.9
38	Hawaii	26.1
NA	Alaska**	NA
NA	Arizona**	NA
NA	California**	NA
NA	Connecticut**	NA
NA	Florida**	NA
NA	Illinois**	NA
NA	Michigan**	NA
NA	Nebraska**	NA
NA	Nevada**	NA
NA	New Hampshire**	NA
NA	Rhode Island**	NA
NA	Washington**	NA

District of Columbia 8.9

Source: U.S. Department of Health and Human Services, Centers for Disease Control and Prevention
"Abortion Surveillance-United States, 2001" (Morbidity and Mortality Weekly Report, Vol. 53, No. SS-9, 11/26/04)
*By state of occurrence. Includes those of Hispanic ethnicity. National percent is for reporting states only.
**Not reported. New York's number is for New York City only.

Percent of Reported Legal Abortions Obtained by Black Women in 2001

Reporting States' Percent = 35.7% of Abortions*

RANK	STATE	PERCENT
5	Alabama	51.0
NA	Alaska**	NA
NA	Arizona**	NA
16	Arkansas	34.3
NA	California**	NA
28	Colorado	4.8
NA	Connecticut**	NA
11	Delaware	42.1
NA	Florida**	NA
3	Georgia	54.6
29	Hawaii	3.3
35	Idaho	1.8
NA	Illinois**	NA
17	Indiana	27.4
26	Iowa	7.8
19	Kansas	22.0
20	Kentucky	21.8
4	Louisiana	52.5
33	Maine	2.1
2	Maryland	60.3
23	Massachusetts	18.1
NA	Michigan**	NA
22	Minnesota	19.0
1	Mississippi	72.2
13	Missouri	37.9
37	Montana	0.3
NA	Nebraska**	NA
NA	Nevada**	NA
NA	New Hampshire**	NA
7	New Jersey	45.2
30	New Mexico	3.1
6	New York**	49.2
9	North Carolina	43.3
36	North Dakota	1.2
15	Ohio	35.1
24	Oklahoma	17.7
27	Oregon	5.8
12	Pennsylvania	42.0
NA	Rhode Island**	NA
8	South Carolina	43.4
32	South Dakota	2.3
10	Tennessee	43.1
21	Texas	20.6
31	Utah	2.4
34	Vermont	2.0
13	Virginia	37.9
NA	Washington**	NA
25	West Virginia	10.4
18	Wisconsin	24.7
38	Wyoming	0.0

RANK	STATE	PERCENT
1	Mississippi	72.2
2	Maryland	60.3
3	Georgia	54.6
4	Louisiana	52.5
5	Alabama	51.0
6	New York**	49.2
7	New Jersey	45.2
8	South Carolina	43.4
9	North Carolina	43.3
10	Tennessee	43.1
11	Delaware	42.1
12	Pennsylvania	42.0
13	Missouri	37.9
13	Virginia	37.9
15	Ohio	35.1
16	Arkansas	34.3
17	Indiana	27.4
18	Wisconsin	24.7
19	Kansas	22.0
20	Kentucky	21.8
21	Texas	20.6
22	Minnesota	19.0
23	Massachusetts	18.1
24	Oklahoma	17.7
25	West Virginia	10.4
26	Iowa	7.8
27	Oregon	5.8
28	Colorado	4.8
29	Hawaii	3.3
30	New Mexico	3.1
31	Utah	2.4
32	South Dakota	2.3
33	Maine	2.1
34	Vermont	2.0
35	Idaho	1.8
36	North Dakota	1.2
37	Montana	0.3
38	Wyoming	0.0
NA	Alaska**	NA
NA	Arizona**	NA
NA	California**	NA
NA	Connecticut**	NA
NA	Florida**	NA
NA	Illinois**	NA
NA	Michigan**	NA
NA	Nebraska**	NA
NA	Nevada**	NA
NA	New Hampshire**	NA
NA	Rhode Island**	NA
NA	Washington**	NA
	District of Columbia	75.2

Source: U.S. Department of Health and Human Services, Centers for Disease Control and Prevention
    "Abortion Surveillance-United States, 2001" (Morbidity and Mortality Weekly Report, Vol. 53, No. SS-9, 11/26/04)
*By state of occurrence. National percent is for reporting states only.
**Not reported. New York's number is for New York City only.

Percent of Reported Legal Abortions Obtained by Hispanic Women in 2001

Reporting States' Percent = 16.7%*

ALPHA ORDER

RANK	STATE	PERCENT
24	Alabama	2.6
NA	Alaska**	NA
NA	Arizona**	NA
26	Arkansas	1.7
NA	California**	NA
6	Colorado	15.9
NA	Connecticut**	NA
12	Delaware	6.8
NA	Florida**	NA
16	Georgia	5.0
18	Hawaii	4.6
8	Idaho	12.5
NA	Illinois**	NA
13	Indiana	5.5
NA	Iowa**	NA
11	Kansas	7.1
31	Kentucky	0.0
NA	Louisiana**	NA
28	Maine	1.1
NA	Maryland**	NA
NA	Massachusetts**	NA
NA	Michigan**	NA
14	Minnesota	5.3
30	Mississippi	0.6
25	Missouri	2.1
NA	Montana**	NA
NA	Nebraska**	NA
NA	Nevada**	NA
NA	New Hampshire**	NA
5	New Jersey	21.9
2	New Mexico	48.7
4	New York**	25.6
NA	North Carolina**	NA
22	North Dakota	2.8
23	Ohio	2.7
14	Oklahoma	5.3
9	Oregon	10.0
16	Pennsylvania	5.0
NA	Rhode Island**	NA
21	South Carolina	3.0
19	South Dakota	4.5
20	Tennessee	3.3
3	Texas	37.5
7	Utah	15.2
27	Vermont	1.4
NA	Virginia**	NA
NA	Washington**	NA
29	West Virginia	0.7
10	Wisconsin	7.8
1	Wyoming	50.0

RANK ORDER

RANK	STATE	PERCENT
1	Wyoming	50.0
2	New Mexico	48.7
3	Texas	37.5
4	New York**	25.6
5	New Jersey	21.9
6	Colorado	15.9
7	Utah	15.2
8	Idaho	12.5
9	Oregon	10.0
10	Wisconsin	7.8
11	Kansas	7.1
12	Delaware	6.8
13	Indiana	5.5
14	Minnesota	5.3
14	Oklahoma	5.3
16	Georgia	5.0
16	Pennsylvania	5.0
18	Hawaii	4.6
19	South Dakota	4.5
20	Tennessee	3.3
21	South Carolina	3.0
22	North Dakota	2.8
23	Ohio	2.7
24	Alabama	2.6
25	Missouri	2.1
26	Arkansas	1.7
27	Vermont	1.4
28	Maine	1.1
29	West Virginia	0.7
30	Mississippi	0.6
31	Kentucky	0.0
NA	Alaska**	NA
NA	Arizona**	NA
NA	California**	NA
NA	Connecticut**	NA
NA	Florida**	NA
NA	Illinois**	NA
NA	Iowa**	NA
NA	Louisiana**	NA
NA	Maryland**	NA
NA	Massachusetts**	NA
NA	Michigan**	NA
NA	Montana**	NA
NA	Nebraska**	NA
NA	Nevada**	NA
NA	New Hampshire**	NA
NA	North Carolina**	NA
NA	Rhode Island**	NA
NA	Virginia**	NA
NA	Washington**	NA
	District of Columbia**	NA

Source: U.S. Department of Health and Human Services, Centers for Disease Control and Prevention
    "Abortion Surveillance-United States, 2001" (Morbidity and Mortality Weekly Report, Vol. 53, No. SS-9, 11/26/04)
*By state of occurrence. National percent is for reporting states only. Hispanic can be of any race.
**Not reported. New York's number is for New York City only.

Percent of Reported Legal Abortions Obtained by Married Women in 2001

Reporting States' Percent = 17.8% of Abortions*

ALPHA ORDER

RANK	STATE	PERCENT
39	Alabama	13.2
NA	Alaska**	NA
NA	Arizona**	NA
34	Arkansas	15.0
NA	California**	NA
4	Colorado	23.3
NA	Connecticut**	NA
32	Delaware	15.7
NA	Florida**	NA
18	Georgia	18.2
12	Hawaii	19.9
5	Idaho	22.8
28	Illinois	16.7
37	Indiana	14.1
9	Iowa	21.1
18	Kansas	18.2
26	Kentucky	17.0
NA	Louisiana**	NA
NA	Maine**	NA
38	Maryland	13.4
14	Massachusetts	18.7
35	Michigan	14.7
12	Minnesota	19.9
36	Mississippi	14.2
10	Missouri	20.8
16	Montana	18.4
NA	Nebraska**	NA
3	Nevada	23.9
NA	New Hampshire**	NA
27	New Jersey	16.9
33	New Mexico	15.6
31	New York**	15.8
11	North Carolina	20.5
22	North Dakota	17.4
24	Ohio	17.2
15	Oklahoma	18.5
7	Oregon	22.3
29	Pennsylvania	16.1
NA	Rhode Island**	NA
30	South Carolina	16.0
6	South Dakota	22.5
18	Tennessee	18.2
8	Texas	21.4
2	Utah	24.7
18	Vermont	18.2
17	Virginia	18.3
NA	Washington**	NA
25	West Virginia	17.1
22	Wisconsin	17.4
1	Wyoming	50.0

RANK ORDER

RANK	STATE	PERCENT
1	Wyoming	50.0
2	Utah	24.7
3	Nevada	23.9
4	Colorado	23.3
5	Idaho	22.8
6	South Dakota	22.5
7	Oregon	22.3
8	Texas	21.4
9	Iowa	21.1
10	Missouri	20.8
11	North Carolina	20.5
12	Hawaii	19.9
12	Minnesota	19.9
14	Massachusetts	18.7
15	Oklahoma	18.5
16	Montana	18.4
17	Virginia	18.3
18	Georgia	18.2
18	Kansas	18.2
18	Tennessee	18.2
18	Vermont	18.2
22	North Dakota	17.4
22	Wisconsin	17.4
24	Ohio	17.2
25	West Virginia	17.1
26	Kentucky	17.0
27	New Jersey	16.9
28	Illinois	16.7
29	Pennsylvania	16.1
30	South Carolina	16.0
31	New York**	15.8
32	Delaware	15.7
33	New Mexico	15.6
34	Arkansas	15.0
35	Michigan	14.7
36	Mississippi	14.2
37	Indiana	14.1
38	Maryland	13.4
39	Alabama	13.2
NA	Alaska**	NA
NA	Arizona**	NA
NA	California**	NA
NA	Connecticut**	NA
NA	Florida**	NA
NA	Louisiana**	NA
NA	Maine**	NA
NA	Nebraska**	NA
NA	New Hampshire**	NA
NA	Rhode Island**	NA
NA	Washington**	NA
	District of Columbia**	NA

Source: U.S. Department of Health and Human Services, Centers for Disease Control and Prevention
   "Abortion Surveillance-United States, 2001" (Morbidity and Mortality Weekly Report, Vol. 53, No. SS-9, 11/26/04)
By state of occurrence. National percent is for reporting states only.
**Not reported. New York's number is for New York City only.*

Percent of Reported Legal Abortions Obtained by Unmarried Women in 2001

Reporting States' Percent = 79.0% of Abortions*

<table>
<tr><td colspan="3">ALPHA ORDER</td><td colspan="3">RANK ORDER</td></tr>
<tr><td>RANK</td><td>STATE</td><td>PERCENT</td><td>RANK</td><td>STATE</td><td>PERCENT</td></tr>
<tr><td>10</td><td>Alabama</td><td>82.4</td><td>1</td><td>Mississippi</td><td>85.5</td></tr>
<tr><td>NA</td><td>Alaska**</td><td>NA</td><td>2</td><td>Delaware</td><td>84.3</td></tr>
<tr><td>NA</td><td>Arizona**</td><td>NA</td><td>3</td><td>Michigan</td><td>84.2</td></tr>
<tr><td>6</td><td>Arkansas</td><td>83.4</td><td>4</td><td>South Carolina</td><td>84.0</td></tr>
<tr><td>NA</td><td>California**</td><td>NA</td><td>5</td><td>Pennsylvania</td><td>83.8</td></tr>
<tr><td>30</td><td>Colorado</td><td>76.0</td><td>6</td><td>Arkansas</td><td>83.4</td></tr>
<tr><td>NA</td><td>Connecticut**</td><td>NA</td><td>7</td><td>Kentucky</td><td>83.0</td></tr>
<tr><td>2</td><td>Delaware</td><td>84.3</td><td>7</td><td>New Mexico</td><td>83.0</td></tr>
<tr><td>NA</td><td>Florida**</td><td>NA</td><td>9</td><td>New Jersey</td><td>82.9</td></tr>
<tr><td>19</td><td>Georgia</td><td>80.3</td><td>10</td><td>Alabama</td><td>82.4</td></tr>
<tr><td>20</td><td>Hawaii</td><td>79.9</td><td>10</td><td>North Dakota</td><td>82.4</td></tr>
<tr><td>25</td><td>Idaho</td><td>77.1</td><td>12</td><td>Wisconsin</td><td>82.3</td></tr>
<tr><td>17</td><td>Illinois</td><td>81.0</td><td>13</td><td>Kansas</td><td>81.6</td></tr>
<tr><td>33</td><td>Indiana</td><td>73.5</td><td>13</td><td>New York**</td><td>81.6</td></tr>
<tr><td>22</td><td>Iowa</td><td>78.2</td><td>13</td><td>Tennessee</td><td>81.6</td></tr>
<tr><td>13</td><td>Kansas</td><td>81.6</td><td>16</td><td>Ohio</td><td>81.4</td></tr>
<tr><td>7</td><td>Kentucky</td><td>83.0</td><td>17</td><td>Illinois</td><td>81.0</td></tr>
<tr><td>NA</td><td>Louisiana**</td><td>NA</td><td>18</td><td>West Virginia</td><td>80.7</td></tr>
<tr><td>NA</td><td>Maine**</td><td>NA</td><td>19</td><td>Georgia</td><td>80.3</td></tr>
<tr><td>27</td><td>Maryland</td><td>76.8</td><td>20</td><td>Hawaii</td><td>79.9</td></tr>
<tr><td>32</td><td>Massachusetts</td><td>73.7</td><td>21</td><td>Vermont</td><td>78.7</td></tr>
<tr><td>3</td><td>Michigan</td><td>84.2</td><td>22</td><td>Iowa</td><td>78.2</td></tr>
<tr><td>24</td><td>Minnesota</td><td>77.4</td><td>23</td><td>Missouri</td><td>78.0</td></tr>
<tr><td>1</td><td>Mississippi</td><td>85.5</td><td>24</td><td>Minnesota</td><td>77.4</td></tr>
<tr><td>23</td><td>Missouri</td><td>78.0</td><td>25</td><td>Idaho</td><td>77.1</td></tr>
<tr><td>36</td><td>Montana</td><td>72.3</td><td>25</td><td>South Dakota</td><td>77.1</td></tr>
<tr><td>NA</td><td>Nebraska**</td><td>NA</td><td>27</td><td>Maryland</td><td>76.8</td></tr>
<tr><td>34</td><td>Nevada</td><td>73.1</td><td>28</td><td>Oregon</td><td>76.3</td></tr>
<tr><td>NA</td><td>New Hampshire**</td><td>NA</td><td>29</td><td>Texas</td><td>76.1</td></tr>
<tr><td>9</td><td>New Jersey</td><td>82.9</td><td>30</td><td>Colorado</td><td>76.0</td></tr>
<tr><td>7</td><td>New Mexico</td><td>83.0</td><td>31</td><td>Virginia</td><td>74.1</td></tr>
<tr><td>13</td><td>New York**</td><td>81.6</td><td>32</td><td>Massachusetts</td><td>73.7</td></tr>
<tr><td>38</td><td>North Carolina</td><td>66.5</td><td>33</td><td>Indiana</td><td>73.5</td></tr>
<tr><td>10</td><td>North Dakota</td><td>82.4</td><td>34</td><td>Nevada</td><td>73.1</td></tr>
<tr><td>16</td><td>Ohio</td><td>81.4</td><td>35</td><td>Oklahoma</td><td>72.6</td></tr>
<tr><td>35</td><td>Oklahoma</td><td>72.6</td><td>36</td><td>Montana</td><td>72.3</td></tr>
<tr><td>28</td><td>Oregon</td><td>76.3</td><td>37</td><td>Utah</td><td>69.9</td></tr>
<tr><td>5</td><td>Pennsylvania</td><td>83.8</td><td>38</td><td>North Carolina</td><td>66.5</td></tr>
<tr><td>NA</td><td>Rhode Island**</td><td>NA</td><td>39</td><td>Wyoming</td><td>50.0</td></tr>
<tr><td>4</td><td>South Carolina</td><td>84.0</td><td>NA</td><td>Alaska**</td><td>NA</td></tr>
<tr><td>25</td><td>South Dakota</td><td>77.1</td><td>NA</td><td>Arizona**</td><td>NA</td></tr>
<tr><td>13</td><td>Tennessee</td><td>81.6</td><td>NA</td><td>California**</td><td>NA</td></tr>
<tr><td>29</td><td>Texas</td><td>76.1</td><td>NA</td><td>Connecticut**</td><td>NA</td></tr>
<tr><td>37</td><td>Utah</td><td>69.9</td><td>NA</td><td>Florida**</td><td>NA</td></tr>
<tr><td>21</td><td>Vermont</td><td>78.7</td><td>NA</td><td>Louisiana**</td><td>NA</td></tr>
<tr><td>31</td><td>Virginia</td><td>74.1</td><td>NA</td><td>Maine**</td><td>NA</td></tr>
<tr><td>NA</td><td>Washington**</td><td>NA</td><td>NA</td><td>Nebraska**</td><td>NA</td></tr>
<tr><td>18</td><td>West Virginia</td><td>80.7</td><td>NA</td><td>New Hampshire**</td><td>NA</td></tr>
<tr><td>12</td><td>Wisconsin</td><td>82.3</td><td>NA</td><td>Rhode Island**</td><td>NA</td></tr>
<tr><td>39</td><td>Wyoming</td><td>50.0</td><td>NA</td><td>Washington**</td><td>NA</td></tr>
<tr><td></td><td></td><td></td><td></td><td>District of Columbia**</td><td>NA</td></tr>
</table>

Source: U.S. Department of Health and Human Services, Centers for Disease Control and Prevention
   "Abortion Surveillance-United States, 2001" (Morbidity and Mortality Weekly Report, Vol. 53, No. SS-9, 11/26/04)
*By state of occurrence. National percent is for reporting states only.
**Not reported. New York's number is for New York City only.

Reported Legal Abortions Obtained by Teenagers in 2001

Reporting States' Total = 126,518 Abortions Obtained by Teenagers*

ALPHA ORDER

RANK	STATE	ABORTIONS	% of USA
16	Alabama	2,511	2.0%
NA	Alaska**	NA	NA
22	Arizona	1,535	1.2%
26	Arkansas	1,184	0.9%
NA	California**	NA	NA
29	Colorado	1,006	0.8%
13	Connecticut	2,806	2.2%
33	Delaware	748	0.6%
NA	Florida**	NA	NA
6	Georgia	5,481	4.3%
31	Hawaii	907	0.7%
43	Idaho	172	0.1%
NA	Illinois**	NA	NA
19	Indiana	2,038	1.6%
27	Iowa	1,160	0.9%
17	Kansas	2,431	1.9%
35	Kentucky	641	0.5%
20	Louisiana	1,953	1.5%
37	Maine	552	0.4%
NA	Maryland**	NA	NA
11	Massachusetts	3,813	3.0%
7	Michigan	5,184	4.1%
15	Minnesota	2,513	2.0%
34	Mississippi	671	0.5%
25	Missouri	1,295	1.0%
38	Montana	539	0.4%
32	Nebraska	827	0.7%
21	Nevada	1,848	1.5%
NA	New Hampshire**	NA	NA
5	New Jersey	6,220	4.9%
28	New Mexico	1,118	0.9%
1	New York	23,285	18.4%
8	North Carolina	5,182	4.1%
41	North Dakota	289	0.2%
3	Ohio	6,771	5.4%
24	Oklahoma	1,366	1.1%
14	Oregon	2,686	2.1%
4	Pennsylvania	6,748	5.3%
30	Rhode Island	969	0.8%
23	South Carolina	1,385	1.1%
42	South Dakota	194	0.2%
12	Tennessee	3,125	2.5%
2	Texas	11,483	9.1%
36	Utah	611	0.5%
40	Vermont	329	0.3%
10	Virginia	4,104	3.2%
9	Washington	5,181	4.1%
39	West Virginia	462	0.4%
18	Wisconsin	2,041	1.6%
44	Wyoming	1	0.0%

RANK ORDER

RANK	STATE	ABORTIONS	% of USA
1	New York	23,285	18.4%
2	Texas	11,483	9.1%
3	Ohio	6,771	5.4%
4	Pennsylvania	6,748	5.3%
5	New Jersey	6,220	4.9%
6	Georgia	5,481	4.3%
7	Michigan	5,184	4.1%
8	North Carolina	5,182	4.1%
9	Washington	5,181	4.1%
10	Virginia	4,104	3.2%
11	Massachusetts	3,813	3.0%
12	Tennessee	3,125	2.5%
13	Connecticut	2,806	2.2%
14	Oregon	2,686	2.1%
15	Minnesota	2,513	2.0%
16	Alabama	2,511	2.0%
17	Kansas	2,431	1.9%
18	Wisconsin	2,041	1.6%
19	Indiana	2,038	1.6%
20	Louisiana	1,953	1.5%
21	Nevada	1,848	1.5%
22	Arizona	1,535	1.2%
23	South Carolina	1,385	1.1%
24	Oklahoma	1,366	1.1%
25	Missouri	1,295	1.0%
26	Arkansas	1,184	0.9%
27	Iowa	1,160	0.9%
28	New Mexico	1,118	0.9%
29	Colorado	1,006	0.8%
30	Rhode Island	969	0.8%
31	Hawaii	907	0.7%
32	Nebraska	827	0.7%
33	Delaware	748	0.6%
34	Mississippi	671	0.5%
35	Kentucky	641	0.5%
36	Utah	611	0.5%
37	Maine	552	0.4%
38	Montana	539	0.4%
39	West Virginia	462	0.4%
40	Vermont	329	0.3%
41	North Dakota	289	0.2%
42	South Dakota	194	0.2%
43	Idaho	172	0.1%
44	Wyoming	1	0.0%
NA	Alaska**	NA	NA
NA	California**	NA	NA
NA	Florida**	NA	NA
NA	Illinois**	NA	NA
NA	Maryland**	NA	NA
NA	New Hampshire**	NA	NA
	District of Columbia	1,153	0.9%

Source: U.S. Department of Health and Human Services, Centers for Disease Control and Prevention
     "Abortion Surveillance-United States, 2001" (Morbidity and Mortality Weekly Report, Vol. 53, No. SS-9, 11/26/04)
*Nineteen years old and younger by state of occurrence. National total is for reporting states only.
**Not reported.

Percent of Reported Legal Abortions Obtained by Teenagers in 2001

Reporting States' Percent = 18.0% of Abortions*

<table>
<tr><td colspan="3">ALPHA ORDER</td><td colspan="3">RANK ORDER</td></tr>
<tr><td>RANK</td><td>STATE</td><td>PERCENT</td><td>RANK</td><td>STATE</td><td>PERCENT</td></tr>
<tr><td>24</td><td>Alabama</td><td>18.8</td><td>1</td><td>Wyoming</td><td>25.0</td></tr>
<tr><td>NA</td><td>Alaska**</td><td>NA</td><td>2</td><td>North Dakota</td><td>23.7</td></tr>
<tr><td>26</td><td>Arizona</td><td>18.5</td><td>3</td><td>Idaho</td><td>23.3</td></tr>
<tr><td>16</td><td>Arkansas</td><td>20.0</td><td>4</td><td>Montana</td><td>23.0</td></tr>
<tr><td>NA</td><td>California**</td><td>NA</td><td>5</td><td>Hawaii</td><td>22.7</td></tr>
<tr><td>7</td><td>Colorado</td><td>21.7</td><td>6</td><td>Maine</td><td>21.9</td></tr>
<tr><td>12</td><td>Connecticut</td><td>21.1</td><td>7</td><td>Colorado</td><td>21.7</td></tr>
<tr><td>11</td><td>Delaware</td><td>21.4</td><td>7</td><td>New Mexico</td><td>21.7</td></tr>
<tr><td>NA</td><td>Florida**</td><td>NA</td><td>7</td><td>Vermont</td><td>21.7</td></tr>
<tr><td>44</td><td>Georgia</td><td>16.5</td><td>10</td><td>South Dakota</td><td>21.6</td></tr>
<tr><td>5</td><td>Hawaii</td><td>22.7</td><td>11</td><td>Delaware</td><td>21.4</td></tr>
<tr><td>3</td><td>Idaho</td><td>23.3</td><td>12</td><td>Connecticut</td><td>21.1</td></tr>
<tr><td>19</td><td>Illinois</td><td>19.7</td><td>13</td><td>Nebraska</td><td>20.8</td></tr>
<tr><td>37</td><td>Indiana</td><td>17.2</td><td>14</td><td>Iowa</td><td>20.3</td></tr>
<tr><td>14</td><td>Iowa</td><td>20.3</td><td>15</td><td>Washington</td><td>20.2</td></tr>
<tr><td>17</td><td>Kansas</td><td>19.8</td><td>16</td><td>Arkansas</td><td>20.0</td></tr>
<tr><td>38</td><td>Kentucky</td><td>17.0</td><td>17</td><td>Kansas</td><td>19.8</td></tr>
<tr><td>34</td><td>Louisiana</td><td>17.9</td><td>17</td><td>West Virginia</td><td>19.8</td></tr>
<tr><td>6</td><td>Maine</td><td>21.9</td><td>19</td><td>Illinois</td><td>19.7</td></tr>
<tr><td>34</td><td>Maryland</td><td>17.9</td><td>19</td><td>South Carolina</td><td>19.7</td></tr>
<tr><td>46</td><td>Massachusetts</td><td>14.5</td><td>21</td><td>Oklahoma</td><td>19.4</td></tr>
<tr><td>29</td><td>Michigan</td><td>18.3</td><td>22</td><td>Wisconsin</td><td>19.1</td></tr>
<tr><td>41</td><td>Minnesota</td><td>16.9</td><td>23</td><td>Mississippi</td><td>18.9</td></tr>
<tr><td>23</td><td>Mississippi</td><td>18.9</td><td>24</td><td>Alabama</td><td>18.8</td></tr>
<tr><td>43</td><td>Missouri</td><td>16.6</td><td>24</td><td>Oregon</td><td>18.8</td></tr>
<tr><td>4</td><td>Montana</td><td>23.0</td><td>26</td><td>Arizona</td><td>18.5</td></tr>
<tr><td>13</td><td>Nebraska</td><td>20.8</td><td>26</td><td>New Jersey</td><td>18.5</td></tr>
<tr><td>29</td><td>Nevada</td><td>18.3</td><td>28</td><td>Pennsylvania</td><td>18.4</td></tr>
<tr><td>NA</td><td>New Hampshire**</td><td>NA</td><td>29</td><td>Michigan</td><td>18.3</td></tr>
<tr><td>26</td><td>New Jersey</td><td>18.5</td><td>29</td><td>Nevada</td><td>18.3</td></tr>
<tr><td>7</td><td>New Mexico</td><td>21.7</td><td>29</td><td>New York</td><td>18.3</td></tr>
<tr><td>29</td><td>New York</td><td>18.3</td><td>32</td><td>Ohio</td><td>18.1</td></tr>
<tr><td>38</td><td>North Carolina</td><td>17.0</td><td>33</td><td>Tennessee</td><td>18.0</td></tr>
<tr><td>2</td><td>North Dakota</td><td>23.7</td><td>34</td><td>Louisiana</td><td>17.9</td></tr>
<tr><td>32</td><td>Ohio</td><td>18.1</td><td>34</td><td>Maryland</td><td>17.9</td></tr>
<tr><td>21</td><td>Oklahoma</td><td>19.4</td><td>36</td><td>Rhode Island</td><td>17.8</td></tr>
<tr><td>24</td><td>Oregon</td><td>18.8</td><td>37</td><td>Indiana</td><td>17.2</td></tr>
<tr><td>28</td><td>Pennsylvania</td><td>18.4</td><td>38</td><td>Kentucky</td><td>17.0</td></tr>
<tr><td>36</td><td>Rhode Island</td><td>17.8</td><td>38</td><td>North Carolina</td><td>17.0</td></tr>
<tr><td>19</td><td>South Carolina</td><td>19.7</td><td>38</td><td>Utah</td><td>17.0</td></tr>
<tr><td>10</td><td>South Dakota</td><td>21.6</td><td>41</td><td>Minnesota</td><td>16.9</td></tr>
<tr><td>33</td><td>Tennessee</td><td>18.0</td><td>42</td><td>Virginia</td><td>16.7</td></tr>
<tr><td>45</td><td>Texas</td><td>14.8</td><td>43</td><td>Missouri</td><td>16.6</td></tr>
<tr><td>38</td><td>Utah</td><td>17.0</td><td>44</td><td>Georgia</td><td>16.5</td></tr>
<tr><td>7</td><td>Vermont</td><td>21.7</td><td>45</td><td>Texas</td><td>14.8</td></tr>
<tr><td>42</td><td>Virginia</td><td>16.7</td><td>46</td><td>Massachusetts</td><td>14.5</td></tr>
<tr><td>15</td><td>Washington</td><td>20.2</td><td>NA</td><td>Alaska**</td><td>NA</td></tr>
<tr><td>17</td><td>West Virginia</td><td>19.8</td><td>NA</td><td>California**</td><td>NA</td></tr>
<tr><td>22</td><td>Wisconsin</td><td>19.1</td><td>NA</td><td>Florida**</td><td>NA</td></tr>
<tr><td>1</td><td>Wyoming</td><td>25.0</td><td>NA</td><td>New Hampshire**</td><td>NA</td></tr>
<tr><td></td><td></td><td></td><td></td><td>District of Columbia</td><td>21.5</td></tr>
</table>

Source: U.S. Department of Health and Human Services, Centers for Disease Control and Prevention
    "Abortion Surveillance-United States, 2001" (Morbidity and Mortality Weekly Report, Vol. 53, No. SS-9, 11/26/04)
*Nineteen years old and younger by state of occurrence. National total is for reporting states only.
**Not reported.

Reported Legal Abortions Obtained by Teenagers 17 Years and Younger in 2001

Reporting States' Total = 47,947 Abortions*

ALPHA ORDER

RANK	STATE	ABORTIONS	% of USA
16	Alabama	917	1.9%
NA	Alaska**	NA	NA
23	Arizona	588	1.2%
26	Arkansas	457	1.0%
NA	California**	NA	NA
29	Colorado	409	0.9%
12	Connecticut	1,171	2.4%
31	Delaware	348	0.7%
NA	Florida**	NA	NA
6	Georgia	2,077	4.3%
30	Hawaii	378	0.8%
43	Idaho	58	0.1%
NA	Illinois**	NA	NA
20	Indiana	708	1.5%
27	Iowa	424	0.9%
15	Kansas	970	2.0%
34	Kentucky	246	0.5%
19	Louisiana	752	1.6%
36	Maine	220	0.5%
NA	Maryland**	NA	NA
11	Massachusetts	1,202	2.5%
8	Michigan	1,938	4.0%
17	Minnesota	838	1.7%
35	Mississippi	240	0.5%
28	Missouri	420	0.9%
37	Montana	209	0.4%
32	Nebraska	301	0.6%
21	Nevada	705	1.5%
NA	New Hampshire**	NA	NA
3	New Jersey	2,617	5.5%
25	New Mexico	472	1.0%
1	New York	9,781	20.4%
9	North Carolina	1,867	3.9%
41	North Dakota	108	0.2%
4	Ohio	2,537	5.3%
24	Oklahoma	515	1.1%
14	Oregon	974	2.0%
5	Pennsylvania	2,328	4.9%
33	Rhode Island	282	0.6%
22	South Carolina	615	1.3%
42	South Dakota	74	0.2%
13	Tennessee	1,145	2.4%
2	Texas	3,713	7.7%
38	Utah	185	0.4%
40	Vermont	149	0.3%
10	Virginia	1,465	3.1%
7	Washington	2,066	4.3%
39	West Virginia	175	0.4%
18	Wisconsin	797	1.7%
44	Wyoming	0	0.0%

RANK ORDER

RANK	STATE	ABORTIONS	% of USA
1	New York	9,781	20.4%
2	Texas	3,713	7.7%
3	New Jersey	2,617	5.5%
4	Ohio	2,537	5.3%
5	Pennsylvania	2,328	4.9%
6	Georgia	2,077	4.3%
7	Washington	2,066	4.3%
8	Michigan	1,938	4.0%
9	North Carolina	1,867	3.9%
10	Virginia	1,465	3.1%
11	Massachusetts	1,202	2.5%
12	Connecticut	1,171	2.4%
13	Tennessee	1,145	2.4%
14	Oregon	974	2.0%
15	Kansas	970	2.0%
16	Alabama	917	1.9%
17	Minnesota	838	1.7%
18	Wisconsin	797	1.7%
19	Louisiana	752	1.6%
20	Indiana	708	1.5%
21	Nevada	705	1.5%
22	South Carolina	615	1.3%
23	Arizona	588	1.2%
24	Oklahoma	515	1.1%
25	New Mexico	472	1.0%
26	Arkansas	457	1.0%
27	Iowa	424	0.9%
28	Missouri	420	0.9%
29	Colorado	409	0.9%
30	Hawaii	378	0.8%
31	Delaware	348	0.7%
32	Nebraska	301	0.6%
33	Rhode Island	282	0.6%
34	Kentucky	246	0.5%
35	Mississippi	240	0.5%
36	Maine	220	0.5%
37	Montana	209	0.4%
38	Utah	185	0.4%
39	West Virginia	175	0.4%
40	Vermont	149	0.3%
41	North Dakota	108	0.2%
42	South Dakota	74	0.2%
43	Idaho	58	0.1%
44	Wyoming	0	0.0%
NA	Alaska**	NA	NA
NA	California**	NA	NA
NA	Florida**	NA	NA
NA	Illinois**	NA	NA
NA	Maryland**	NA	NA
NA	New Hampshire**	NA	NA

District of Columbia   506   1.1%

Source: U.S. Department of Health and Human Services, Centers for Disease Control and Prevention
    "Abortion Surveillance-United States, 2001" (Morbidity and Mortality Weekly Report, Vol. 53, No. SS-9, 11/26/04)
*By state of occurrence. National total is for reporting states only.
**Not reported.

Percent of Reported Legal Abortions Obtained
By Teenagers 17 Years and Younger in 2001
Reporting States' Percent = 6.8% of Abortions*

ALPHA ORDER

RANK	STATE	PERCENT
25	Alabama	6.9
NA	Alaska**	NA
23	Arizona	7.1
16	Arkansas	7.7
NA	California**	NA
7	Colorado	8.8
7	Connecticut	8.8
1	Delaware	10.0
NA	Florida**	NA
34	Georgia	6.2
3	Hawaii	9.5
13	Idaho	7.9
NA	Illinois**	NA
36	Indiana	6.0
20	Iowa	7.4
13	Kansas	7.9
32	Kentucky	6.5
25	Louisiana	6.9
10	Maine	8.7
NA	Maryland**	NA
43	Massachusetts	4.6
25	Michigan	6.9
38	Minnesota	5.6
30	Mississippi	6.7
39	Missouri	5.4
5	Montana	8.9
18	Nebraska	7.6
24	Nevada	7.0
NA	New Hampshire**	NA
15	New Jersey	7.8
4	New Mexico	9.1
16	New York	7.7
35	North Carolina	6.1
5	North Dakota	8.9
28	Ohio	6.8
22	Oklahoma	7.3
28	Oregon	6.8
33	Pennsylvania	6.3
40	Rhode Island	5.2
7	South Carolina	8.8
11	South Dakota	8.3
31	Tennessee	6.6
42	Texas	4.8
41	Utah	5.1
2	Vermont	9.8
36	Virginia	6.0
12	Washington	8.1
19	West Virginia	7.5
20	Wisconsin	7.4
44	Wyoming	0.0

RANK ORDER

RANK	STATE	PERCENT
1	Delaware	10.0
2	Vermont	9.8
3	Hawaii	9.5
4	New Mexico	9.1
5	Montana	8.9
5	North Dakota	8.9
7	Colorado	8.8
7	Connecticut	8.8
7	South Carolina	8.8
10	Maine	8.7
11	South Dakota	8.3
12	Washington	8.1
13	Idaho	7.9
13	Kansas	7.9
15	New Jersey	7.8
16	Arkansas	7.7
16	New York	7.7
18	Nebraska	7.6
19	West Virginia	7.5
20	Iowa	7.4
20	Wisconsin	7.4
22	Oklahoma	7.3
23	Arizona	7.1
24	Nevada	7.0
25	Alabama	6.9
25	Louisiana	6.9
25	Michigan	6.9
28	Ohio	6.8
28	Oregon	6.8
30	Mississippi	6.7
31	Tennessee	6.6
32	Kentucky	6.5
33	Pennsylvania	6.3
34	Georgia	6.2
35	North Carolina	6.1
36	Indiana	6.0
36	Virginia	6.0
38	Minnesota	5.6
39	Missouri	5.4
40	Rhode Island	5.2
41	Utah	5.1
42	Texas	4.8
43	Massachusetts	4.6
44	Wyoming	0.0
NA	Alaska**	NA
NA	California**	NA
NA	Florida**	NA
NA	Illinois**	NA
NA	Maryland**	NA
NA	New Hampshire**	NA

District of Columbia   9.4

Source: Morgan Quitno Press using data from US Dept of Health & Human Serv's, Centers for Disease Control-Prevention
    "Abortion Surveillance-United States, 2001" (Morbidity and Mortality Weekly Report, Vol. 53, No. SS-9, 11/26/04)
*By state of occurrence. National percent is for reporting states only.
**Not reported.

Percent of Teenage Abortions Obtained
By Teenagers 17 Years and Younger in 2001
Reporting States' Percent = 37.9% of Teenage Abortions*

ALPHA ORDER

RANK	STATE	PERCENT
29	Alabama	36.5
NA	Alaska**	NA
18	Arizona	38.3
15	Arkansas	38.6
NA	California**	NA
9	Colorado	40.7
7	Connecticut	41.7
1	Delaware	46.5
NA	Florida**	NA
21	Georgia	37.9
7	Hawaii	41.7
37	Idaho	33.7
NA	Illinois**	NA
35	Indiana	34.7
27	Iowa	36.6
10	Kansas	39.9
17	Kentucky	38.4
16	Louisiana	38.5
10	Maine	39.9
NA	Maryland**	NA
41	Massachusetts	31.5
25	Michigan	37.4
38	Minnesota	33.3
33	Mississippi	35.8
39	Missouri	32.4
14	Montana	38.8
30	Nebraska	36.4
19	Nevada	38.1
NA	New Hampshire**	NA
5	New Jersey	42.1
4	New Mexico	42.2
6	New York	42.0
32	North Carolina	36.0
25	North Dakota	37.4
24	Ohio	37.5
23	Oklahoma	37.7
31	Oregon	36.3
36	Pennsylvania	34.5
43	Rhode Island	29.1
3	South Carolina	44.4
19	South Dakota	38.1
27	Tennessee	36.6
40	Texas	32.3
42	Utah	30.3
2	Vermont	45.3
34	Virginia	35.7
10	Washington	39.9
21	West Virginia	37.9
13	Wisconsin	39.0
44	Wyoming	0.0

RANK ORDER

RANK	STATE	PERCENT
1	Delaware	46.5
2	Vermont	45.3
3	South Carolina	44.4
4	New Mexico	42.2
5	New Jersey	42.1
6	New York	42.0
7	Connecticut	41.7
7	Hawaii	41.7
9	Colorado	40.7
10	Kansas	39.9
10	Maine	39.9
10	Washington	39.9
13	Wisconsin	39.0
14	Montana	38.8
15	Arkansas	38.6
16	Louisiana	38.5
17	Kentucky	38.4
18	Arizona	38.3
19	Nevada	38.1
19	South Dakota	38.1
21	Georgia	37.9
21	West Virginia	37.9
23	Oklahoma	37.7
24	Ohio	37.5
25	Michigan	37.4
25	North Dakota	37.4
27	Iowa	36.6
27	Tennessee	36.6
29	Alabama	36.5
30	Nebraska	36.4
31	Oregon	36.3
32	North Carolina	36.0
33	Mississippi	35.8
34	Virginia	35.7
35	Indiana	34.7
36	Pennsylvania	34.5
37	Idaho	33.7
38	Minnesota	33.3
39	Missouri	32.4
40	Texas	32.3
41	Massachusetts	31.5
42	Utah	30.3
43	Rhode Island	29.1
44	Wyoming	0.0
NA	Alaska**	NA
NA	California**	NA
NA	Florida**	NA
NA	Illinois**	NA
NA	Maryland**	NA
NA	New Hampshire**	NA

District of Columbia 43.9

Source: U.S. Department of Health and Human Services, Centers for Disease Control and Prevention
"Abortion Surveillance-United States, 2001" (Morbidity and Mortality Weekly Report, Vol. 53, No. SS-9, 11/26/04)
*By state of occurrence. National percent is for reporting states only.
**Not reported.

Reported Legal Abortions Performed at 12 Weeks or Less of Gestation in 2001

Reporting States' Total = 532,922 Abortions*

ALPHA ORDER

RANK ORDER

RANK	STATE	ABORTIONS	% of USA
13	Alabama	11,818	2.2%
NA	Alaska**	NA	NA
21	Arizona	7,205	1.4%
26	Arkansas	4,862	0.9%
NA	California**	NA	NA
28	Colorado	3,921	0.7%
15	Connecticut	10,772	2.0%
33	Delaware	3,083	0.6%
NA	Florida**	NA	NA
5	Georgia	28,789	5.4%
29	Hawaii	3,301	0.6%
40	Idaho	715	0.1%
NA	Illinois**	NA	NA
14	Indiana	11,284	2.1%
24	Iowa	5,307	1.0%
16	Kansas	10,360	1.9%
30	Kentucky	3,234	0.6%
19	Louisiana	8,680	1.6%
34	Maine	2,450	0.5%
NA	Maryland**	NA	NA
NA	Massachusetts**	NA	NA
7	Michigan	24,955	4.7%
11	Minnesota	13,243	2.5%
32	Mississippi	3,098	0.6%
20	Missouri	7,216	1.4%
35	Montana	1,996	0.4%
NA	Nebraska**	NA	NA
18	Nevada	8,970	1.7%
NA	New Hampshire**	NA	NA
6	New Jersey	26,815	5.0%
27	New Mexico	4,385	0.8%
1	New York**	79,015	14.8%
NA	North Carolina**	NA	NA
38	North Dakota	1,084	0.2%
4	Ohio	31,782	6.0%
23	Oklahoma	6,344	1.2%
12	Oregon	12,444	2.3%
3	Pennsylvania	32,235	6.0%
25	Rhode Island	4,959	0.9%
22	South Carolina	6,616	1.2%
39	South Dakota	856	0.2%
10	Tennessee	16,652	3.1%
2	Texas	68,198	12.8%
31	Utah	3,125	0.6%
37	Vermont	1,434	0.3%
8	Virginia	23,636	4.4%
9	Washington	22,414	4.2%
36	West Virginia	1,995	0.4%
17	Wisconsin	9,228	1.7%
41	Wyoming	4	0.0%

RANK	STATE	ABORTIONS	% of USA
1	New York**	79,015	14.8%
2	Texas	68,198	12.8%
3	Pennsylvania	32,235	6.0%
4	Ohio	31,782	6.0%
5	Georgia	28,789	5.4%
6	New Jersey	26,815	5.0%
7	Michigan	24,955	4.7%
8	Virginia	23,636	4.4%
9	Washington	22,414	4.2%
10	Tennessee	16,652	3.1%
11	Minnesota	13,243	2.5%
12	Oregon	12,444	2.3%
13	Alabama	11,818	2.2%
14	Indiana	11,284	2.1%
15	Connecticut	10,772	2.0%
16	Kansas	10,360	1.9%
17	Wisconsin	9,228	1.7%
18	Nevada	8,970	1.7%
19	Louisiana	8,680	1.6%
20	Missouri	7,216	1.4%
21	Arizona	7,205	1.4%
22	South Carolina	6,616	1.2%
23	Oklahoma	6,344	1.2%
24	Iowa	5,307	1.0%
25	Rhode Island	4,959	0.9%
26	Arkansas	4,862	0.9%
27	New Mexico	4,385	0.8%
28	Colorado	3,921	0.7%
29	Hawaii	3,301	0.6%
30	Kentucky	3,234	0.6%
31	Utah	3,125	0.6%
32	Mississippi	3,098	0.6%
33	Delaware	3,083	0.6%
34	Maine	2,450	0.5%
35	Montana	1,996	0.4%
36	West Virginia	1,995	0.4%
37	Vermont	1,434	0.3%
38	North Dakota	1,084	0.2%
39	South Dakota	856	0.2%
40	Idaho	715	0.1%
41	Wyoming	4	0.0%
NA	Alaska**	NA	NA
NA	California**	NA	NA
NA	Florida**	NA	NA
NA	Illinois**	NA	NA
NA	Maryland**	NA	NA
NA	Massachusetts**	NA	NA
NA	Nebraska**	NA	NA
NA	New Hampshire**	NA	NA
NA	North Carolina**	NA	NA

District of Columbia		4,442	0.8%

Source: Morgan Quitno Press using data from US Dept of Health & Human Serv's, Centers for Disease Control-Prevention
    "Abortion Surveillance-United States, 2001" (Morbidity and Mortality Weekly Report, Vol. 53, No. SS-9, 11/26/04)
*By state of occurrence. National total is for reporting states only.
**Not reported. New York's number is for New York City only.

Percent of Reported Legal Abortions Performed At 12 Weeks or Less of Gestation in 2001
Reporting States' Percent = 87.3% of Abortions*

ALPHA ORDER				RANK ORDER		
RANK	STATE	PERCENT		RANK	STATE	PERCENT
19	Alabama	88.3		1	Wyoming	100.0
NA	Alaska**	NA		2	Maine	97.4
26	Arizona	86.8		3	Idaho	96.9
38	Arkansas	82.1		4	Virginia	96.1
NA	California**	NA		5	Tennessee	95.7
35	Colorado	84.6		6	South Dakota	95.6
39	Connecticut	81.2		7	Indiana	95.0
17	Delaware	88.4		8	Vermont	94.4
NA	Florida**	NA		9	South Carolina	94.3
27	Georgia	86.6		10	Iowa	92.7
37	Hawaii	82.5		11	Missouri	92.5
3	Idaho	96.9		12	Rhode Island	90.9
NA	Illinois**	NA		13	Oklahoma	90.1
7	Indiana	95.0		14	Minnesota	89.3
10	Iowa	92.7		15	North Dakota	89.1
36	Kansas	84.3		16	Nevada	88.7
30	Kentucky	85.9		17	Delaware	88.4
41	Louisiana	79.4		17	Michigan	88.4
2	Maine	97.4		19	Alabama	88.3
NA	Maryland**	NA		20	Texas	88.1
NA	Massachusetts**	NA		21	Pennsylvania	87.5
17	Michigan	88.4		21	Washington	87.5
14	Minnesota	89.3		23	Oregon	87.2
25	Mississippi	86.9		24	Utah	87.0
11	Missouri	92.5		25	Mississippi	86.9
32	Montana	84.9		26	Arizona	86.8
NA	Nebraska**	NA		27	Georgia	86.6
16	Nevada	88.7		28	Wisconsin	86.2
NA	New Hampshire**	NA		29	New York**	86.1
40	New Jersey	79.8		30	Kentucky	85.9
32	New Mexico	84.9		31	West Virginia	85.5
29	New York**	86.1		32	Montana	84.9
NA	North Carolina**	NA		32	New Mexico	84.9
15	North Dakota	89.1		34	Ohio	84.8
34	Ohio	84.8		35	Colorado	84.6
13	Oklahoma	90.1		36	Kansas	84.3
23	Oregon	87.2		37	Hawaii	82.5
21	Pennsylvania	87.5		38	Arkansas	82.1
12	Rhode Island	90.9		39	Connecticut	81.2
9	South Carolina	94.3		40	New Jersey	79.8
6	South Dakota	95.6		41	Louisiana	79.4
5	Tennessee	95.7		NA	Alaska**	NA
20	Texas	88.1		NA	California**	NA
24	Utah	87.0		NA	Florida**	NA
8	Vermont	94.4		NA	Illinois**	NA
4	Virginia	96.1		NA	Maryland**	NA
21	Washington	87.5		NA	Massachusetts**	NA
31	West Virginia	85.5		NA	Nebraska**	NA
28	Wisconsin	86.2		NA	New Hampshire**	NA
1	Wyoming	100.0		NA	North Carolina**	NA
				District of Columbia		82.5

Source: Morgan Quitno Press using data from US Dept of Health & Human Serv's, Centers for Disease Control-Prevention "Abortion Surveillance-United States, 2001" (Morbidity and Mortality Weekly Report, Vol. 53, No. SS-9, 11/26/04)
By state of occurrence. National percent is for reporting states only.
**Not reported. New York's number is for New York City only.*

Reported Legal Abortions Performed At or After 21 Weeks of Gestation in 2001

Reporting States' Total = 8,654 Abortions*

ALPHA ORDER

RANK	STATE	ABORTIONS	% of USA
18	Alabama	52	0.6%
NA	Alaska**	NA	NA
27	Arizona	11	0.1%
31	Arkansas	6	0.1%
NA	California**	NA	NA
13	Colorado	159	1.8%
21	Connecticut	25	0.3%
29	Delaware	8	0.1%
NA	Florida**	NA	NA
2	Georgia	778	9.0%
16	Hawaii	64	0.7%
34	Idaho	3	0.0%
NA	Illinois**	NA	NA
36	Indiana	2	0.0%
37	Iowa	1	0.0%
5	Kansas	689	8.0%
17	Kentucky	62	0.7%
9	Louisiana	340	3.9%
34	Maine	3	0.0%
NA	Maryland**	NA	NA
NA	Massachusetts**	NA	NA
11	Michigan	202	2.3%
14	Minnesota	131	1.5%
29	Mississippi	8	0.1%
24	Missouri	17	0.2%
22	Montana	22	0.3%
NA	Nebraska**	NA	NA
19	Nevada	50	0.6%
NA	New Hampshire**	NA	NA
3	New Jersey	760	8.8%
20	New Mexico	44	0.5%
1	New York**	2,155	24.9%
NA	North Carolina**	NA	NA
38	North Dakota	0	0.0%
6	Ohio	683	7.9%
26	Oklahoma	15	0.2%
10	Oregon	296	3.4%
7	Pennsylvania	505	5.8%
27	Rhode Island	11	0.1%
22	South Carolina	22	0.3%
32	South Dakota	5	0.1%
24	Tennessee	17	0.2%
4	Texas	746	8.6%
38	Utah	0	0.0%
38	Vermont	0	0.0%
15	Virginia	67	0.8%
8	Washington	504	5.8%
33	West Virginia	4	0.0%
12	Wisconsin	187	2.2%
38	Wyoming	0	0.0%

RANK ORDER

RANK	STATE	ABORTIONS	% of USA
1	New York**	2,155	24.9%
2	Georgia	778	9.0%
3	New Jersey	760	8.8%
4	Texas	746	8.6%
5	Kansas	689	8.0%
6	Ohio	683	7.9%
7	Pennsylvania	505	5.8%
8	Washington	504	5.8%
9	Louisiana	340	3.9%
10	Oregon	296	3.4%
11	Michigan	202	2.3%
12	Wisconsin	187	2.2%
13	Colorado	159	1.8%
14	Minnesota	131	1.5%
15	Virginia	67	0.8%
16	Hawaii	64	0.7%
17	Kentucky	62	0.7%
18	Alabama	52	0.6%
19	Nevada	50	0.6%
20	New Mexico	44	0.5%
21	Connecticut	25	0.3%
22	Montana	22	0.3%
22	South Carolina	22	0.3%
24	Missouri	17	0.2%
24	Tennessee	17	0.2%
26	Oklahoma	15	0.2%
27	Arizona	11	0.1%
27	Rhode Island	11	0.1%
29	Delaware	8	0.1%
29	Mississippi	8	0.1%
31	Arkansas	6	0.1%
32	South Dakota	5	0.1%
33	West Virginia	4	0.0%
34	Idaho	3	0.0%
34	Maine	3	0.0%
36	Indiana	2	0.0%
37	Iowa	1	0.0%
38	North Dakota	0	0.0%
38	Utah	0	0.0%
38	Vermont	0	0.0%
38	Wyoming	0	0.0%
NA	Alaska**	NA	NA
NA	California**	NA	NA
NA	Florida**	NA	NA
NA	Illinois**	NA	NA
NA	Maryland**	NA	NA
NA	Massachusetts**	NA	NA
NA	Nebraska**	NA	NA
NA	New Hampshire**	NA	NA
NA	North Carolina**	NA	NA

District of Columbia   0   0.0%

Source: Morgan Quitno Press using data from US Dept of Health & Human Serv's, Centers for Disease Control-Prevention "Abortion Surveillance-United States, 2001" (Morbidity and Mortality Weekly Report, Vol. 53, No. SS-9, 11/26/04)
*By state of occurrence. National total is for reporting states only.
**Not reported. New York's number is for New York City only.

Percent of Reported Legal Abortions Performed At or After
21 Weeks of Gestation in 2001
Reporting States' Percent = 1.4% of Abortions*

ALPHA ORDER

RANK ORDER

RANK	STATE	PERCENT	RANK	STATE	PERCENT
21	Alabama	0.4	1	Kansas	5.6
NA	Alaska**	NA	2	Colorado	3.4
32	Arizona	0.1	3	Louisiana	3.1
32	Arkansas	0.1	4	Georgia	2.3
NA	California**	NA	4	New Jersey	2.3
2	Colorado	3.4	4	New York**	2.3
25	Connecticut	0.2	7	Oregon	2.1
25	Delaware	0.2	8	Washington	2.0
NA	Florida**	NA	9	Ohio	1.8
4	Georgia	2.3	10	Wisconsin	1.7
11	Hawaii	1.6	11	Hawaii	1.6
21	Idaho	0.4	11	Kentucky	1.6
NA	Illinois**	NA	13	Pennsylvania	1.4
36	Indiana	0.0	14	Texas	1.0
36	Iowa	0.0	15	Minnesota	0.9
1	Kansas	5.6	15	Montana	0.9
11	Kentucky	1.6	15	New Mexico	0.9
3	Louisiana	3.1	18	Michigan	0.7
32	Maine	0.1	19	South Dakota	0.6
NA	Maryland**	NA	20	Nevada	0.5
NA	Massachusetts**	NA	21	Alabama	0.4
18	Michigan	0.7	21	Idaho	0.4
15	Minnesota	0.9	23	South Carolina	0.3
25	Mississippi	0.2	23	Virginia	0.3
25	Missouri	0.2	25	Connecticut	0.2
15	Montana	0.9	25	Delaware	0.2
NA	Nebraska**	NA	25	Mississippi	0.2
20	Nevada	0.5	25	Missouri	0.2
NA	New Hampshire**	NA	25	Oklahoma	0.2
4	New Jersey	2.3	25	Rhode Island	0.2
15	New Mexico	0.9	25	West Virginia	0.2
4	New York**	2.3	32	Arizona	0.1
NA	North Carolina**	NA	32	Arkansas	0.1
36	North Dakota	0.0	32	Maine	0.1
9	Ohio	1.8	32	Tennessee	0.1
25	Oklahoma	0.2	36	Indiana	0.0
7	Oregon	2.1	36	Iowa	0.0
13	Pennsylvania	1.4	36	North Dakota	0.0
25	Rhode Island	0.2	36	Utah	0.0
23	South Carolina	0.3	36	Vermont	0.0
19	South Dakota	0.6	36	Wyoming	0.0
32	Tennessee	0.1	NA	Alaska**	NA
14	Texas	1.0	NA	California**	NA
36	Utah	0.0	NA	Florida**	NA
36	Vermont	0.0	NA	Illinois**	NA
23	Virginia	0.3	NA	Maryland**	NA
8	Washington	2.0	NA	Massachusetts**	NA
25	West Virginia	0.2	NA	Nebraska**	NA
10	Wisconsin	1.7	NA	New Hampshire**	NA
36	Wyoming	0.0	NA	North Carolina**	NA

District of Columbia   0.0

Source: Morgan Quitno Press using data from US Dept of Health & Human Serv's, Centers for Disease Control-Prevention
    "Abortion Surveillance-United States, 2001" (Morbidity and Mortality Weekly Report, Vol. 53, No. SS-9, 11/26/04)
*By state of occurrence. National percent is for reporting states only.
**Not reported. New York's number is for New York City only.

II. DEATHS

II. DEATHS (Continued)

Deaths in 2002

National Total = 2,443,387 Deaths*

ALPHA ORDER

RANK	STATE	DEATHS	% of USA
18	Alabama	46,069	1.9%
50	Alaska	3,030	0.1%
21	Arizona	42,816	1.8%
31	Arkansas	28,513	1.2%
1	California	234,565	9.6%
29	Colorado	29,210	1.2%
28	Connecticut	30,122	1.2%
46	Delaware	6,861	0.3%
2	Florida	167,814	6.9%
11	Georgia	65,449	2.7%
43	Hawaii	8,801	0.4%
41	Idaho	9,923	0.4%
7	Illinois	106,667	4.4%
16	Indiana	55,396	2.3%
32	Iowa	27,978	1.1%
33	Kansas	25,021	1.0%
23	Kentucky	40,697	1.7%
22	Louisiana	41,984	1.7%
39	Maine	12,694	0.5%
20	Maryland	43,970	1.8%
13	Massachusetts	56,928	2.3%
8	Michigan	87,795	3.6%
24	Minnesota	38,510	1.6%
30	Mississippi	28,853	1.2%
15	Missouri	55,940	2.3%
44	Montana	8,506	0.3%
36	Nebraska	15,738	0.6%
35	Nevada	16,927	0.7%
42	New Hampshire	9,853	0.4%
9	New Jersey	74,009	3.0%
37	New Mexico	14,344	0.6%
3	New York	158,118	6.5%
10	North Carolina	72,027	2.9%
47	North Dakota	5,892	0.2%
6	Ohio	109,766	4.5%
26	Oklahoma	35,502	1.5%
27	Oregon	31,119	1.3%
5	Pennsylvania	130,223	5.3%
40	Rhode Island	10,246	0.4%
25	South Carolina	37,736	1.5%
45	South Dakota	6,898	0.3%
14	Tennessee	56,606	2.3%
4	Texas	155,524	6.4%
38	Utah	13,116	0.5%
48	Vermont	5,075	0.2%
12	Virginia	57,196	2.3%
19	Washington	45,338	1.9%
34	West Virginia	21,016	0.9%
17	Wisconsin	46,981	1.9%
49	Wyoming	4,174	0.2%

RANK ORDER

RANK	STATE	DEATHS	% of USA
1	California	234,565	9.6%
2	Florida	167,814	6.9%
3	New York	158,118	6.5%
4	Texas	155,524	6.4%
5	Pennsylvania	130,223	5.3%
6	Ohio	109,766	4.5%
7	Illinois	106,667	4.4%
8	Michigan	87,795	3.6%
9	New Jersey	74,009	3.0%
10	North Carolina	72,027	2.9%
11	Georgia	65,449	2.7%
12	Virginia	57,196	2.3%
13	Massachusetts	56,928	2.3%
14	Tennessee	56,606	2.3%
15	Missouri	55,940	2.3%
16	Indiana	55,396	2.3%
17	Wisconsin	46,981	1.9%
18	Alabama	46,069	1.9%
19	Washington	45,338	1.9%
20	Maryland	43,970	1.8%
21	Arizona	42,816	1.8%
22	Louisiana	41,984	1.7%
23	Kentucky	40,697	1.7%
24	Minnesota	38,510	1.6%
25	South Carolina	37,736	1.5%
26	Oklahoma	35,502	1.5%
27	Oregon	31,119	1.3%
28	Connecticut	30,122	1.2%
29	Colorado	29,210	1.2%
30	Mississippi	28,853	1.2%
31	Arkansas	28,513	1.2%
32	Iowa	27,978	1.1%
33	Kansas	25,021	1.0%
34	West Virginia	21,016	0.9%
35	Nevada	16,927	0.7%
36	Nebraska	15,738	0.6%
37	New Mexico	14,344	0.6%
38	Utah	13,116	0.5%
39	Maine	12,694	0.5%
40	Rhode Island	10,246	0.4%
41	Idaho	9,923	0.4%
42	New Hampshire	9,853	0.4%
43	Hawaii	8,801	0.4%
44	Montana	8,506	0.3%
45	South Dakota	6,898	0.3%
46	Delaware	6,861	0.3%
47	North Dakota	5,892	0.2%
48	Vermont	5,075	0.2%
49	Wyoming	4,174	0.2%
50	Alaska	3,030	0.1%
	District of Columbia	5,851	0.2%

Source: U.S. Department of Health and Human Services, National Center for Health Statistics
  "National Vital Statistics Reports" (Vol. 53, No. 5, October 12, 2004)
Final data by state of residence.

Age-Adjusted Death Rate in 2002

National Rate = 845.3 Deaths per 100,000 Population*

<u>ALPHA ORDER</u>

RANK	STATE	RATE
3	Alabama	998.1
37	Alaska	789.1
33	Arizona	795.7
8	Arkansas	964.4
47	California	757.8
36	Colorado	790.2
46	Connecticut	762.4
26	Delaware	838.2
38	Florida	786.4
9	Georgia	949.1
50	Hawaii	660.6
34	Idaho	793.0
22	Illinois	856.0
15	Indiana	899.6
44	Iowa	774.5
25	Kansas	843.5
4	Kentucky	993.9
2	Louisiana	1,000.5
24	Maine	846.5
19	Maryland	864.1
35	Massachusetts	791.9
16	Michigan	876.2
49	Minnesota	747.5
1	Mississippi	1,036.3
11	Missouri	916.7
23	Montana	849.7
29	Nebraska	814.8
12	Nevada	916.5
42	New Hampshire	781.7
31	New Jersey	808.7
28	New Mexico	815.0
40	New York	783.3
14	North Carolina	906.1
48	North Dakota	749.8
13	Ohio	908.2
7	Oklahoma	973.2
27	Oregon	834.2
20	Pennsylvania	862.1
30	Rhode Island	809.5
10	South Carolina	946.9
45	South Dakota	771.2
6	Tennessee	981.5
17	Texas	870.0
41	Utah	782.0
43	Vermont	775.0
21	Virginia	856.6
39	Washington	785.3
5	West Virginia	991.7
32	Wisconsin	799.8
18	Wyoming	864.3

<u>RANK ORDER</u>

RANK	STATE	RATE
1	Mississippi	1,036.3
2	Louisiana	1,000.5
3	Alabama	998.1
4	Kentucky	993.9
5	West Virginia	991.7
6	Tennessee	981.5
7	Oklahoma	973.2
8	Arkansas	964.4
9	Georgia	949.1
10	South Carolina	946.9
11	Missouri	916.7
12	Nevada	916.5
13	Ohio	908.2
14	North Carolina	906.1
15	Indiana	899.6
16	Michigan	876.2
17	Texas	870.0
18	Wyoming	864.3
19	Maryland	864.1
20	Pennsylvania	862.1
21	Virginia	856.6
22	Illinois	856.0
23	Montana	849.7
24	Maine	846.5
25	Kansas	843.5
26	Delaware	838.2
27	Oregon	834.2
28	New Mexico	815.0
29	Nebraska	814.8
30	Rhode Island	809.5
31	New Jersey	808.7
32	Wisconsin	799.8
33	Arizona	795.7
34	Idaho	793.0
35	Massachusetts	791.9
36	Colorado	790.2
37	Alaska	789.1
38	Florida	786.4
39	Washington	785.3
40	New York	783.3
41	Utah	782.0
42	New Hampshire	781.7
43	Vermont	775.0
44	Iowa	774.5
45	South Dakota	771.2
46	Connecticut	762.4
47	California	757.8
48	North Dakota	749.8
49	Minnesota	747.5
50	Hawaii	660.6

	District of Columbia	1,021.4

Source: U.S. Department of Health and Human Services, National Center for Health Statistics
"National Vital Statistics Reports" (Vol. 53, No. 5, October 12, 2004)
Final data by state of residence. Age-adjusted rates eliminate the distorting effects of the aging of the population. Rates based on the year 2000 standard population.

Death Rate in 2002

National Rate = 847.3 Deaths per 100,000 Population*

ALPHA ORDER

RANK	STATE	RATE
4	Alabama	1,026.8
50	Alaska	470.7
36	Arizona	784.7
3	Arkansas	1,052.1
47	California	668.0
48	Colorado	648.2
26	Connecticut	870.5
30	Delaware	849.8
7	Florida	1,004.1
42	Georgia	764.6
46	Hawaii	707.0
44	Idaho	739.9
31	Illinois	846.5
22	Indiana	899.4
14	Iowa	952.7
18	Kansas	921.3
8	Kentucky	994.3
15	Louisiana	936.6
10	Maine	980.6
35	Maryland	805.6
23	Massachusetts	885.7
25	Michigan	873.5
41	Minnesota	767.2
6	Mississippi	1,004.7
9	Missouri	986.1
16	Montana	935.3
20	Nebraska	910.1
38	Nevada	778.8
40	New Hampshire	772.8
29	New Jersey	861.5
39	New Mexico	773.2
33	New York	825.4
27	North Carolina	865.7
17	North Dakota	929.2
12	Ohio	961.1
5	Oklahoma	1,016.2
24	Oregon	883.7
2	Pennsylvania	1,055.7
13	Rhode Island	957.8
19	South Carolina	918.8
21	South Dakota	906.4
11	Tennessee	976.4
45	Texas	714.1
49	Utah	566.3
34	Vermont	823.1
37	Virginia	784.2
43	Washington	747.0
1	West Virginia	1,166.3
28	Wisconsin	863.4
32	Wyoming	837.0

RANK ORDER

RANK	STATE	RATE
1	West Virginia	1,166.3
2	Pennsylvania	1,055.7
3	Arkansas	1,052.1
4	Alabama	1,026.8
5	Oklahoma	1,016.2
6	Mississippi	1,004.7
7	Florida	1,004.1
8	Kentucky	994.3
9	Missouri	986.1
10	Maine	980.6
11	Tennessee	976.4
12	Ohio	961.1
13	Rhode Island	957.8
14	Iowa	952.7
15	Louisiana	936.6
16	Montana	935.3
17	North Dakota	929.2
18	Kansas	921.3
19	South Carolina	918.8
20	Nebraska	910.1
21	South Dakota	906.4
22	Indiana	899.4
23	Massachusetts	885.7
24	Oregon	883.7
25	Michigan	873.5
26	Connecticut	870.5
27	North Carolina	865.7
28	Wisconsin	863.4
29	New Jersey	861.5
30	Delaware	849.8
31	Illinois	846.5
32	Wyoming	837.0
33	New York	825.4
34	Vermont	823.1
35	Maryland	805.6
36	Arizona	784.7
37	Virginia	784.2
38	Nevada	778.8
39	New Mexico	773.2
40	New Hampshire	772.8
41	Minnesota	767.2
42	Georgia	764.6
43	Washington	747.0
44	Idaho	739.9
45	Texas	714.1
46	Hawaii	707.0
47	California	668.0
48	Colorado	648.2
49	Utah	566.3
50	Alaska	470.7

| | District of Columbia | 1,024.9 |

Source: U.S. Department of Health and Human Services, National Center for Health Statistics
"National Vital Statistics Reports" (Vol. 53, No. 5, October 12, 2004)
Final data by state of residence. Not age-adjusted.

Percent Change in Death Rate: 1993 to 2002

National Percent Change = 3.7% Decrease*

ALPHA ORDER

RANK	STATE	PERCENT CHANGE
7	Alabama	4.0
1	Alaska	18.1
48	Arizona	(7.1)
36	Arkansas	(3.8)
45	California	(6.1)
29	Colorado	(2.7)
23	Connecticut	(1.7)
33	Delaware	(3.5)
45	Florida	(6.1)
44	Georgia	(5.9)
3	Hawaii	12.4
32	Idaho	(3.0)
49	Illinois	(7.7)
24	Indiana	(1.9)
37	Iowa	(3.9)
21	Kansas	(1.2)
11	Kentucky	2.3
13	Louisiana	1.5
7	Maine	4.0
20	Maryland	(1.1)
39	Massachusetts	(4.2)
19	Michigan	0.1
43	Minnesota	(4.8)
17	Mississippi	0.5
37	Missouri	(3.9)
5	Montana	5.3
28	Nebraska	(2.3)
34	Nevada	(3.7)
24	New Hampshire	(1.9)
47	New Jersey	(6.9)
4	New Mexico	6.5
50	New York	(12.5)
34	North Carolina	(3.7)
12	North Dakota	1.6
10	Ohio	3.5
14	Oklahoma	1.3
30	Oregon	(2.8)
18	Pennsylvania	0.4
27	Rhode Island	(2.2)
6	South Carolina	4.3
40	South Dakota	(4.3)
15	Tennessee	1.0
41	Texas	(4.4)
16	Utah	0.6
41	Vermont	(4.4)
22	Virginia	(1.5)
31	Washington	(2.9)
9	West Virginia	3.9
26	Wisconsin	(2.1)
2	Wyoming	12.7

RANK ORDER

RANK	STATE	PERCENT CHANGE
1	Alaska	18.1
2	Wyoming	12.7
3	Hawaii	12.4
4	New Mexico	6.5
5	Montana	5.3
6	South Carolina	4.3
7	Alabama	4.0
7	Maine	4.0
9	West Virginia	3.9
10	Ohio	3.5
11	Kentucky	2.3
12	North Dakota	1.6
13	Louisiana	1.5
14	Oklahoma	1.3
15	Tennessee	1.0
16	Utah	0.6
17	Mississippi	0.5
18	Pennsylvania	0.4
19	Michigan	0.1
20	Maryland	(1.1)
21	Kansas	(1.2)
22	Virginia	(1.5)
23	Connecticut	(1.7)
24	Indiana	(1.9)
24	New Hampshire	(1.9)
26	Wisconsin	(2.1)
27	Rhode Island	(2.2)
28	Nebraska	(2.3)
29	Colorado	(2.7)
30	Oregon	(2.8)
31	Washington	(2.9)
32	Idaho	(3.0)
33	Delaware	(3.5)
34	Nevada	(3.7)
34	North Carolina	(3.7)
36	Arkansas	(3.8)
37	Iowa	(3.9)
37	Missouri	(3.9)
39	Massachusetts	(4.2)
40	South Dakota	(4.3)
41	Texas	(4.4)
41	Vermont	(4.4)
43	Minnesota	(4.8)
44	Georgia	(5.9)
45	California	(6.1)
45	Florida	(6.1)
47	New Jersey	(6.9)
48	Arizona	(7.1)
49	Illinois	(7.7)
50	New York	(12.5)

District of Columbia   (17.5)

Source: Morgan Quitno Press using data from US Dept of Health & Human Services, National Center for Health Statistics
  "National Vital Statistics Reports" (Vol. 53, No. 5, October 12, 2004)
  "Monthly Vital Statistics Report" (Vol. 44, No. 7(S), February 29, 1996)
*Final data by state of residence. Not age-adjusted.

Infant Deaths in 2002

National Total = 28,034 Infant Deaths*

ALPHA ORDER

RANK	STATE	DEATHS	% of USA
19	Alabama	539	1.9%
47	Alaska	55	0.2%
17	Arizona	559	2.0%
29	Arkansas	312	1.1%
1	California	2,889	10.3%
24	Colorado	415	1.5%
31	Connecticut	274	1.0%
41	Delaware	96	0.3%
3	Florida	1,548	5.5%
6	Georgia	1,192	4.3%
40	Hawaii	127	0.5%
39	Idaho	128	0.5%
5	Illinois	1,339	4.8%
14	Indiana	657	2.3%
34	Iowa	199	0.7%
30	Kansas	281	1.0%
27	Kentucky	392	1.4%
13	Louisiana	665	2.4%
46	Maine	59	0.2%
18	Maryland	551	2.0%
26	Massachusetts	395	1.4%
9	Michigan	1,057	3.8%
28	Minnesota	364	1.3%
23	Mississippi	428	1.5%
16	Missouri	637	2.3%
43	Montana	83	0.3%
37	Nebraska	178	0.6%
35	Nevada	197	0.7%
44	New Hampshire	72	0.3%
15	New Jersey	655	2.3%
38	New Mexico	174	0.6%
4	New York	1,519	5.4%
10	North Carolina	959	3.4%
48	North Dakota	49	0.2%
7	Ohio	1,180	4.2%
25	Oklahoma	410	1.5%
33	Oregon	260	0.9%
8	Pennsylvania	1,091	3.9%
42	Rhode Island	90	0.3%
20	South Carolina	507	1.8%
45	South Dakota	70	0.2%
12	Tennessee	727	2.6%
2	Texas	2,368	8.4%
32	Utah	273	1.0%
50	Vermont	28	0.1%
11	Virginia	741	2.6%
22	Washington	456	1.6%
36	West Virginia	188	0.7%
21	Wisconsin	472	1.7%
49	Wyoming	44	0.2%

RANK ORDER

RANK	STATE	DEATHS	% of USA
1	California	2,889	10.3%
2	Texas	2,368	8.4%
3	Florida	1,548	5.5%
4	New York	1,519	5.4%
5	Illinois	1,339	4.8%
6	Georgia	1,192	4.3%
7	Ohio	1,180	4.2%
8	Pennsylvania	1,091	3.9%
9	Michigan	1,057	3.8%
10	North Carolina	959	3.4%
11	Virginia	741	2.6%
12	Tennessee	727	2.6%
13	Louisiana	665	2.4%
14	Indiana	657	2.3%
15	New Jersey	655	2.3%
16	Missouri	637	2.3%
17	Arizona	559	2.0%
18	Maryland	551	2.0%
19	Alabama	539	1.9%
20	South Carolina	507	1.8%
21	Wisconsin	472	1.7%
22	Washington	456	1.6%
23	Mississippi	428	1.5%
24	Colorado	415	1.5%
25	Oklahoma	410	1.5%
26	Massachusetts	395	1.4%
27	Kentucky	392	1.4%
28	Minnesota	364	1.3%
29	Arkansas	312	1.1%
30	Kansas	281	1.0%
31	Connecticut	274	1.0%
32	Utah	273	1.0%
33	Oregon	260	0.9%
34	Iowa	199	0.7%
35	Nevada	197	0.7%
36	West Virginia	188	0.7%
37	Nebraska	178	0.6%
38	New Mexico	174	0.6%
39	Idaho	128	0.5%
40	Hawaii	127	0.5%
41	Delaware	96	0.3%
42	Rhode Island	90	0.3%
43	Montana	83	0.3%
44	New Hampshire	72	0.3%
45	South Dakota	70	0.2%
46	Maine	59	0.2%
47	Alaska	55	0.2%
48	North Dakota	49	0.2%
49	Wyoming	44	0.2%
50	Vermont	28	0.1%
	District of Columbia	85	0.3%

Source: U.S. Department of Health and Human Services, National Center for Health Statistics
"National Vital Statistics Reports" (Vol. 53, No. 5, October 12, 2004)
*Final data. Deaths under 1 year old by state of residence.

Infant Mortality Rate in 2002

National Rate = 7.0 Infant Deaths per 1,000 Live Births*

ALPHA ORDER

RANK ORDER

RANK	STATE	RATE		RANK	STATE	RATE
5	Alabama	9.1		1	Louisiana	10.3
43	Alaska	5.5		1	Mississippi	10.3
31	Arizona	6.4		3	Tennessee	9.4
10	Arkansas	8.3		4	South Carolina	9.3
43	California	5.5		5	Alabama	9.1
35	Colorado	6.1		5	West Virginia	9.1
29	Connecticut	6.5		7	Georgia	8.9
8	Delaware	8.7		8	Delaware	8.7
17	Florida	7.5		9	Missouri	8.5
7	Georgia	8.9		10	Arkansas	8.3
22	Hawaii	7.3		11	North Carolina	8.2
35	Idaho	6.1		12	Michigan	8.1
20	Illinois	7.4		12	Oklahoma	8.1
15	Indiana	7.7		14	Ohio	7.9
46	Iowa	5.3		15	Indiana	7.7
24	Kansas	7.1		16	Pennsylvania	7.6
23	Kentucky	7.2		17	Florida	7.5
1	Louisiana	10.3		17	Maryland	7.5
49	Maine	4.4		17	Montana	7.5
17	Maryland	7.5		20	Illinois	7.4
48	Massachusetts	4.9		20	Virginia	7.4
12	Michigan	8.1		22	Hawaii	7.3
45	Minnesota	5.4		23	Kentucky	7.2
1	Mississippi	10.3		24	Kansas	7.1
9	Missouri	8.5		25	Nebraska	7.0
17	Montana	7.5		25	Rhode Island	7.0
25	Nebraska	7.0		27	Wisconsin	6.9
37	Nevada	6.0		28	Wyoming	6.7
47	New Hampshire	5.0		29	Connecticut	6.5
41	New Jersey	5.7		29	South Dakota	6.5
33	New Mexico	6.3		31	Arizona	6.4
37	New York	6.0		31	Texas	6.4
11	North Carolina	8.2		33	New Mexico	6.3
33	North Dakota	6.3		33	North Dakota	6.3
14	Ohio	7.9		35	Colorado	6.1
12	Oklahoma	8.1		35	Idaho	6.1
39	Oregon	5.8		37	Nevada	6.0
16	Pennsylvania	7.6		37	New York	6.0
25	Rhode Island	7.0		39	Oregon	5.8
4	South Carolina	9.3		39	Washington	5.8
29	South Dakota	6.5		41	New Jersey	5.7
3	Tennessee	9.4		42	Utah	5.6
31	Texas	6.4		43	Alaska	5.5
42	Utah	5.6		43	California	5.5
49	Vermont	4.4		45	Minnesota	5.4
20	Virginia	7.4		46	Iowa	5.3
39	Washington	5.8		47	New Hampshire	5.0
5	West Virginia	9.1		48	Massachusetts	4.9
27	Wisconsin	6.9		49	Maine	4.4
28	Wyoming	6.7		49	Vermont	4.4
					District of Columbia	11.3

Source: U.S. Department of Health and Human Services, National Center for Health Statistics
   "National Vital Statistics Reports" (Vol. 53, No. 5, October 12, 2004)
Final data. Deaths under 1 year old by state of residence.

Percent Change in Infant Mortality Rate: 1993 to 2002

National Percent Change = 16.7% Decrease*

ALPHA ORDER

RANK	STATE	PERCENT CHANGE
18	Alabama	(11.7)
48	Alaska	(32.9)
29	Arizona	(15.8)
31	Arkansas	(17.0)
32	California	(19.1)
38	Colorado	(22.8)
12	Connecticut	(8.5)
6	Delaware	(1.1)
21	Florida	(12.8)
23	Georgia	(14.4)
2	Hawaii	1.4
28	Idaho	(15.3)
43	Illinois	(25.3)
30	Indiana	(16.3)
40	Iowa	(23.2)
33	Kansas	(19.3)
19	Kentucky	(12.2)
8	Louisiana	(4.6)
50	Maine	(35.3)
41	Maryland	(23.5)
36	Massachusetts	(21.0)
24	Michigan	(14.7)
44	Minnesota	(28.0)
14	Mississippi	(10.4)
4	Missouri	1.2
2	Montana	1.4
39	Nebraska	(23.1)
14	Nevada	(10.4)
16	New Hampshire	(10.7)
46	New Jersey	(31.3)
42	New Mexico	(25.0)
45	New York	(28.6)
37	North Carolina	(21.9)
35	North Dakota	(20.3)
22	Ohio	(14.1)
11	Oklahoma	(8.0)
34	Oregon	(19.4)
17	Pennsylvania	(11.6)
7	Rhode Island	(4.1)
10	South Carolina	(7.9)
47	South Dakota	(31.6)
5	Tennessee	0.0
24	Texas	(14.7)
9	Utah	(6.7)
49	Vermont	(34.3)
26	Virginia	(14.9)
13	Washington	(9.4)
1	West Virginia	5.8
20	Wisconsin	(12.7)
27	Wyoming	(15.2)

RANK ORDER

RANK	STATE	PERCENT CHANGE
1	West Virginia	5.8
2	Hawaii	1.4
2	Montana	1.4
4	Missouri	1.2
5	Tennessee	0.0
6	Delaware	(1.1)
7	Rhode Island	(4.1)
8	Louisiana	(4.6)
9	Utah	(6.7)
10	South Carolina	(7.9)
11	Oklahoma	(8.0)
12	Connecticut	(8.5)
13	Washington	(9.4)
14	Mississippi	(10.4)
14	Nevada	(10.4)
16	New Hampshire	(10.7)
17	Pennsylvania	(11.6)
18	Alabama	(11.7)
19	Kentucky	(12.2)
20	Wisconsin	(12.7)
21	Florida	(12.8)
22	Ohio	(14.1)
23	Georgia	(14.4)
24	Michigan	(14.7)
24	Texas	(14.7)
26	Virginia	(14.9)
27	Wyoming	(15.2)
28	Idaho	(15.3)
29	Arizona	(15.8)
30	Indiana	(16.3)
31	Arkansas	(17.0)
32	California	(19.1)
33	Kansas	(19.3)
34	Oregon	(19.4)
35	North Dakota	(20.3)
36	Massachusetts	(21.0)
37	North Carolina	(21.9)
38	Colorado	(22.8)
39	Nebraska	(23.1)
40	Iowa	(23.2)
41	Maryland	(23.5)
42	New Mexico	(25.0)
43	Illinois	(25.3)
44	Minnesota	(28.0)
45	New York	(28.6)
46	New Jersey	(31.3)
47	South Dakota	(31.6)
48	Alaska	(32.9)
49	Vermont	(34.3)
50	Maine	(35.3)

District of Columbia — (35.1)

Source: Morgan Quitno Press using data from US Dept of Health & Human Services, National Center for Health Statistics
   "National Vital Statistics Reports" (Vol. 53, No. 5, October 12, 2004)
   "Monthly Vital Statistics Report" (Vol. 44, No. 7(S), February 29, 1996)
*Final data by state of residence. Infant deaths are those occurring under 1 year, exclusive of fetal deaths.

White Infant Deaths in 2002

National Total = 18,369 Deaths*

ALPHA ORDER

RANK	STATE	DEATHS	% of USA
23	Alabama	283	1.5%
49	Alaska	27	0.1%
12	Arizona	475	2.6%
31	Arkansas	201	1.1%
1	California	2,212	12.0%
18	Colorado	342	1.9%
32	Connecticut	191	1.0%
43	Delaware	58	0.3%
4	Florida	893	4.9%
9	Georgia	569	3.1%
50	Hawaii	18	0.1%
39	Idaho	123	0.7%
5	Illinois	780	4.2%
11	Indiana	503	2.7%
33	Iowa	179	1.0%
29	Kansas	228	1.2%
20	Kentucky	318	1.7%
26	Louisiana	253	1.4%
44	Maine	56	0.3%
27	Maryland	240	1.3%
21	Massachusetts	302	1.6%
8	Michigan	619	3.4%
22	Minnesota	290	1.6%
35	Mississippi	155	0.8%
13	Missouri	443	2.4%
42	Montana	68	0.4%
36	Nebraska	141	0.8%
37	Nevada	138	0.8%
40	New Hampshire	72	0.4%
16	New Jersey	382	2.1%
38	New Mexico	132	0.7%
3	New York	977	5.3%
10	North Carolina	505	2.7%
47	North Dakota	38	0.2%
7	Ohio	761	4.1%
24	Oklahoma	279	1.5%
28	Oregon	229	1.2%
6	Pennsylvania	772	4.2%
41	Rhode Island	71	0.4%
30	South Carolina	213	1.2%
45	South Dakota	42	0.2%
14	Tennessee	419	2.3%
2	Texas	1,773	9.7%
25	Utah	255	1.4%
48	Vermont	28	0.2%
15	Virginia	394	2.1%
17	Washington	366	2.0%
34	West Virginia	169	0.9%
19	Wisconsin	329	1.8%
45	Wyoming	42	0.2%

RANK ORDER

RANK	STATE	DEATHS	% of USA
1	California	2,212	12.0%
2	Texas	1,773	9.7%
3	New York	977	5.3%
4	Florida	893	4.9%
5	Illinois	780	4.2%
6	Pennsylvania	772	4.2%
7	Ohio	761	4.1%
8	Michigan	619	3.4%
9	Georgia	569	3.1%
10	North Carolina	505	2.7%
11	Indiana	503	2.7%
12	Arizona	475	2.6%
13	Missouri	443	2.4%
14	Tennessee	419	2.3%
15	Virginia	394	2.1%
16	New Jersey	382	2.1%
17	Washington	366	2.0%
18	Colorado	342	1.9%
19	Wisconsin	329	1.8%
20	Kentucky	318	1.7%
21	Massachusetts	302	1.6%
22	Minnesota	290	1.6%
23	Alabama	283	1.5%
24	Oklahoma	279	1.5%
25	Utah	255	1.4%
26	Louisiana	253	1.4%
27	Maryland	240	1.3%
28	Oregon	229	1.2%
29	Kansas	228	1.2%
30	South Carolina	213	1.2%
31	Arkansas	201	1.1%
32	Connecticut	191	1.0%
33	Iowa	179	1.0%
34	West Virginia	169	0.9%
35	Mississippi	155	0.8%
36	Nebraska	141	0.8%
37	Nevada	138	0.8%
38	New Mexico	132	0.7%
39	Idaho	123	0.7%
40	New Hampshire	72	0.4%
41	Rhode Island	71	0.4%
42	Montana	68	0.4%
43	Delaware	58	0.3%
44	Maine	56	0.3%
45	South Dakota	42	0.2%
45	Wyoming	42	0.2%
47	North Dakota	38	0.2%
48	Vermont	28	0.2%
49	Alaska	27	0.1%
50	Hawaii	18	0.1%
	District of Columbia	16	0.1%

Source: U.S. Department of Health and Human Services, National Center for Health Statistics
    "National Vital Statistics Reports" (Vol. 53, No. 5, October 12, 2004)
*Final data. Deaths of infants under 1 year old, exclusive of fetal deaths. Based on race of the mother.

White Infant Mortality Rate in 2002

National Rate = 5.8 White Infant Deaths per 1,000 White Live Births*

ALPHA ORDER

RANK	STATE	RATE
3	Alabama	7.1
49	Alaska	4.2
18	Arizona	6.2
8	Arkansas	6.9
40	California	5.2
32	Colorado	5.5
32	Connecticut	5.5
2	Delaware	7.3
25	Florida	5.8
13	Georgia	6.6
NA	Hawaii**	NA
20	Idaho	6.1
27	Illinois	5.6
11	Indiana	6.8
41	Iowa	5.1
16	Kansas	6.5
13	Kentucky	6.6
8	Louisiana	6.9
48	Maine	4.3
38	Maryland	5.3
45	Massachusetts	4.5
22	Michigan	6.0
43	Minnesota	5.0
8	Mississippi	6.9
3	Missouri	7.1
3	Montana	7.1
20	Nebraska	6.1
41	Nevada	5.1
38	New Hampshire	5.3
45	New Jersey	4.5
26	New Mexico	5.7
37	New York	5.4
24	North Carolina	5.9
27	North Dakota	5.6
18	Ohio	6.2
3	Oklahoma	7.1
27	Oregon	5.6
13	Pennsylvania	6.6
17	Rhode Island	6.4
22	South Carolina	6.0
44	South Dakota	4.9
7	Tennessee	7.0
27	Texas	5.6
32	Utah	5.5
45	Vermont	4.5
32	Virginia	5.5
32	Washington	5.5
1	West Virginia	8.5
27	Wisconsin	5.6
11	Wyoming	6.8

RANK ORDER

RANK	STATE	RATE
1	West Virginia	8.5
2	Delaware	7.3
3	Alabama	7.1
3	Missouri	7.1
3	Montana	7.1
3	Oklahoma	7.1
7	Tennessee	7.0
8	Arkansas	6.9
8	Louisiana	6.9
8	Mississippi	6.9
11	Indiana	6.8
11	Wyoming	6.8
13	Georgia	6.6
13	Kentucky	6.6
13	Pennsylvania	6.6
16	Kansas	6.5
17	Rhode Island	6.4
18	Arizona	6.2
18	Ohio	6.2
20	Idaho	6.1
20	Nebraska	6.1
22	Michigan	6.0
22	South Carolina	6.0
24	North Carolina	5.9
25	Florida	5.8
26	New Mexico	5.7
27	Illinois	5.6
27	North Dakota	5.6
27	Oregon	5.6
27	Texas	5.6
27	Wisconsin	5.6
32	Colorado	5.5
32	Connecticut	5.5
32	Utah	5.5
32	Virginia	5.5
32	Washington	5.5
37	New York	5.4
38	Maryland	5.3
38	New Hampshire	5.3
40	California	5.2
41	Iowa	5.1
41	Nevada	5.1
43	Minnesota	5.0
44	South Dakota	4.9
45	Massachusetts	4.5
45	New Jersey	4.5
45	Vermont	4.5
48	Maine	4.3
49	Alaska	4.2
NA	Hawaii**	NA
	District of Columbia**	NA

*Source: U.S. Department of Health and Human Services, National Center for Health Statistics
    "National Vital Statistics Reports" (Vol. 53, No. 5, October 12, 2004)*
Final data. Deaths of infants under 1 year old, exclusive of fetal deaths. Based on race of the mother.
***Not available, fewer than 20 white infant deaths.*

Percent Change in White Infant Mortality Rate: 1993 to 2002

National Percent Change = 14.7% Decrease*

ALPHA ORDER

RANK	STATE	PERCENT CHANGE
14	Alabama	(10.1)
47	Alaska	(33.3)
14	Arizona	(10.1)
40	Arkansas	(24.2)
27	California	(17.5)
41	Colorado	(25.7)
7	Connecticut	(5.2)
1	Delaware	28.1
17	Florida	(12.1)
10	Georgia	(8.3)
NA	Hawaii**	NA
18	Idaho	(12.9)
36	Illinois	(21.1)
24	Indiana	(15.0)
35	Iowa	(20.3)
20	Kansas	(13.3)
19	Kentucky	(13.2)
8	Louisiana	(6.8)
49	Maine	(37.7)
26	Maryland	(15.9)
36	Massachusetts	(21.1)
25	Michigan	(15.5)
45	Minnesota	(29.6)
29	Mississippi	(17.9)
5	Missouri	0.0
4	Montana	2.9
43	Nebraska	(26.5)
28	Nevada	(17.7)
9	New Hampshire	(7.0)
42	New Jersey	(26.2)
38	New Mexico	(21.9)
31	New York	(18.2)
39	North Carolina	(23.4)
44	North Dakota	(29.1)
32	Ohio	(18.4)
23	Oklahoma	(14.5)
33	Oregon	(20.0)
5	Pennsylvania	0.0
13	Rhode Island	(9.9)
16	South Carolina	(10.4)
48	South Dakota	(35.5)
3	Tennessee	4.5
21	Texas	(13.8)
10	Utah	(8.3)
46	Vermont	(32.8)
29	Virginia	(17.9)
10	Washington	(8.3)
2	West Virginia	4.9
33	Wisconsin	(20.0)
22	Wyoming	(13.9)

RANK ORDER

RANK	STATE	PERCENT CHANGE
1	Delaware	28.1
2	West Virginia	4.9
3	Tennessee	4.5
4	Montana	2.9
5	Missouri	0.0
5	Pennsylvania	0.0
7	Connecticut	(5.2)
8	Louisiana	(6.8)
9	New Hampshire	(7.0)
10	Georgia	(8.3)
10	Utah	(8.3)
10	Washington	(8.3)
13	Rhode Island	(9.9)
14	Alabama	(10.1)
14	Arizona	(10.1)
16	South Carolina	(10.4)
17	Florida	(12.1)
18	Idaho	(12.9)
19	Kentucky	(13.2)
20	Kansas	(13.3)
21	Texas	(13.8)
22	Wyoming	(13.9)
23	Oklahoma	(14.5)
24	Indiana	(15.0)
25	Michigan	(15.5)
26	Maryland	(15.9)
27	California	(17.5)
28	Nevada	(17.7)
29	Mississippi	(17.9)
29	Virginia	(17.9)
31	New York	(18.2)
32	Ohio	(18.4)
33	Oregon	(20.0)
33	Wisconsin	(20.0)
35	Iowa	(20.3)
36	Illinois	(21.1)
36	Massachusetts	(21.1)
38	New Mexico	(21.9)
39	North Carolina	(23.4)
40	Arkansas	(24.2)
41	Colorado	(25.7)
42	New Jersey	(26.2)
43	Nebraska	(26.5)
44	North Dakota	(29.1)
45	Minnesota	(29.6)
46	Vermont	(32.8)
47	Alaska	(33.3)
48	South Dakota	(35.5)
49	Maine	(37.7)
NA	Hawaii**	NA

District of Columbia**   NA

Source: Morgan Quitno Press using data from US Dept of Health & Human Services, National Center for Health Statistics
   "National Vital Statistics Reports" (Vol. 53, No. 5, October 12, 2004)
   "Monthly Vital Statistics Report" (Vol. 44, No. 7(S), February 29, 1996)
*Final data. Deaths of infants under 1 year old, exclusive of fetal deaths. Based on race of the mother.
**Not available, fewer than 20 white infant deaths.

Black Infant Deaths in 2002

National Total = 8,524 Deaths*

ALPHA ORDER

RANK	STATE	DEATHS	% of USA
17	Alabama	255	3.0%
41	Alaska	6	0.1%
32	Arizona	36	0.4%
22	Arkansas	103	1.2%
7	California	420	4.9%
27	Colorado	62	0.7%
25	Connecticut	74	0.9%
33	Delaware	35	0.4%
1	Florida	629	7.4%
2	Georgia	588	6.9%
40	Hawaii	7	0.1%
46	Idaho	1	0.0%
4	Illinois	519	6.1%
20	Indiana	143	1.7%
36	Iowa	17	0.2%
30	Kansas	44	0.5%
26	Kentucky	70	0.8%
9	Louisiana	401	4.7%
46	Maine	1	0.0%
14	Maryland	298	3.5%
24	Massachusetts	76	0.9%
8	Michigan	416	4.9%
28	Minnesota	50	0.6%
16	Mississippi	269	3.2%
19	Missouri	189	2.2%
43	Montana	3	0.0%
34	Nebraska	30	0.4%
29	Nevada	48	0.6%
48	New Hampshire	0	0.0%
17	New Jersey	255	3.0%
39	New Mexico	11	0.1%
5	New York	493	5.8%
6	North Carolina	430	5.0%
45	North Dakota	2	0.0%
10	Ohio	400	4.7%
23	Oklahoma	81	1.0%
38	Oregon	13	0.2%
12	Pennsylvania	305	3.6%
37	Rhode Island	15	0.2%
15	South Carolina	287	3.4%
43	South Dakota	3	0.0%
13	Tennessee	299	3.5%
3	Texas	561	6.6%
41	Utah	6	0.1%
48	Vermont	0	0.0%
11	Virginia	323	3.8%
31	Washington	43	0.5%
35	West Virginia	19	0.2%
21	Wisconsin	121	1.4%
48	Wyoming	0	0.0%

RANK ORDER

RANK	STATE	DEATHS	% of USA
1	Florida	629	7.4%
2	Georgia	588	6.9%
3	Texas	561	6.6%
4	Illinois	519	6.1%
5	New York	493	5.8%
6	North Carolina	430	5.0%
7	California	420	4.9%
8	Michigan	416	4.9%
9	Louisiana	401	4.7%
10	Ohio	400	4.7%
11	Virginia	323	3.8%
12	Pennsylvania	305	3.6%
13	Tennessee	299	3.5%
14	Maryland	298	3.5%
15	South Carolina	287	3.4%
16	Mississippi	269	3.2%
17	Alabama	255	3.0%
17	New Jersey	255	3.0%
19	Missouri	189	2.2%
20	Indiana	143	1.7%
21	Wisconsin	121	1.4%
22	Arkansas	103	1.2%
23	Oklahoma	81	1.0%
24	Massachusetts	76	0.9%
25	Connecticut	74	0.9%
26	Kentucky	70	0.8%
27	Colorado	62	0.7%
28	Minnesota	50	0.6%
29	Nevada	48	0.6%
30	Kansas	44	0.5%
31	Washington	43	0.5%
32	Arizona	36	0.4%
33	Delaware	35	0.4%
34	Nebraska	30	0.4%
35	West Virginia	19	0.2%
36	Iowa	17	0.2%
37	Rhode Island	15	0.2%
38	Oregon	13	0.2%
39	New Mexico	11	0.1%
40	Hawaii	7	0.1%
41	Alaska	6	0.1%
41	Utah	6	0.1%
43	Montana	3	0.0%
43	South Dakota	3	0.0%
45	North Dakota	2	0.0%
46	Idaho	1	0.0%
46	Maine	1	0.0%
48	New Hampshire	0	0.0%
48	Vermont	0	0.0%
48	Wyoming	0	0.0%
	District of Columbia	67	0.8%

Source: U.S. Department of Health and Human Services, National Center for Health Statistics
"National Vital Statistics Reports" (Vol. 53, No. 5, October 12, 2004)
*Final data. Deaths of infants under 1 year old, exclusive of fetal deaths. Based on race of the mother.

Black Infant Mortality Rate in 2002

National Rate = 14.4 Black Infant Deaths per 1,000 Black Live Births*

ALPHA ORDER

RANK	STATE	RATE
21	Alabama	13.9
NA	Alaska**	NA
26	Arizona	13.0
21	Arkansas	13.9
27	California	12.9
1	Colorado	21.1
19	Connecticut	14.2
27	Delaware	12.9
24	Florida	13.6
23	Georgia	13.7
NA	Hawaii**	NA
NA	Idaho**	NA
10	Illinois	16.3
13	Indiana	15.3
NA	Iowa**	NA
14	Kansas	15.2
19	Kentucky	14.2
16	Louisiana	15.0
NA	Maine**	NA
31	Maryland	12.3
34	Massachusetts	9.1
4	Michigan	18.5
32	Minnesota	10.3
17	Mississippi	14.8
9	Missouri	17.1
NA	Montana**	NA
2	Nebraska	20.8
5	Nevada	18.4
NA	New Hampshire**	NA
29	New Jersey	12.8
NA	New Mexico**	NA
33	New York	9.9
12	North Carolina	15.6
NA	North Dakota**	NA
7	Ohio	17.7
8	Oklahoma	17.2
NA	Oregon**	NA
15	Pennsylvania	15.1
NA	Rhode Island**	NA
11	South Carolina	15.8
NA	South Dakota**	NA
6	Tennessee	18.3
25	Texas	13.5
NA	Utah**	NA
NA	Vermont**	NA
18	Virginia	14.6
30	Washington	12.7
NA	West Virginia**	NA
3	Wisconsin	18.9
NA	Wyoming**	NA

RANK ORDER

RANK	STATE	RATE
1	Colorado	21.1
2	Nebraska	20.8
3	Wisconsin	18.9
4	Michigan	18.5
5	Nevada	18.4
6	Tennessee	18.3
7	Ohio	17.7
8	Oklahoma	17.2
9	Missouri	17.1
10	Illinois	16.3
11	South Carolina	15.8
12	North Carolina	15.6
13	Indiana	15.3
14	Kansas	15.2
15	Pennsylvania	15.1
16	Louisiana	15.0
17	Mississippi	14.8
18	Virginia	14.6
19	Connecticut	14.2
19	Kentucky	14.2
21	Alabama	13.9
21	Arkansas	13.9
23	Georgia	13.7
24	Florida	13.6
25	Texas	13.5
26	Arizona	13.0
27	California	12.9
27	Delaware	12.9
29	New Jersey	12.8
30	Washington	12.7
31	Maryland	12.3
32	Minnesota	10.3
33	New York	9.9
34	Massachusetts	9.1
NA	Alaska**	NA
NA	Hawaii**	NA
NA	Idaho**	NA
NA	Iowa**	NA
NA	Maine**	NA
NA	Montana**	NA
NA	New Hampshire**	NA
NA	New Mexico**	NA
NA	North Dakota**	NA
NA	Oregon**	NA
NA	Rhode Island**	NA
NA	South Dakota**	NA
NA	Utah**	NA
NA	Vermont**	NA
NA	West Virginia**	NA
NA	Wyoming**	NA

District of Columbia   14.5

Source: U.S. Department of Health and Human Services, National Center for Health Statistics
"National Vital Statistics Reports" (Vol. 53, No. 5, October 12, 2004)
*Final data. Deaths of infants under 1 year old, exclusive of fetal deaths. Based on race of the mother.
**Not available, fewer than 20 black infant deaths.

Percent Change in Black Infant Mortality Rate: 1993 to 2002

National Percent Change = 12.7% Decrease*

ALPHA ORDER

RANK	STATE	PERCENT CHANGE
16	Alabama	(7.9)
NA	Alaska**	NA
34	Arizona	(41.2)
6	Arkansas	3.7
23	California	(17.3)
2	Colorado	24.1
18	Connecticut	(9.0)
31	Delaware	(35.2)
19	Florida	(11.1)
20	Georgia	(16.0)
NA	Hawaii**	NA
NA	Idaho**	NA
22	Illinois	(16.8)
21	Indiana	(16.4)
NA	Iowa**	NA
32	Kansas	(35.3)
10	Kentucky	(0.7)
14	Louisiana	(3.8)
NA	Maine**	NA
30	Maryland	(30.1)
24	Massachusetts	(20.2)
12	Michigan	(1.6)
28	Minnesota	(27.0)
8	Mississippi	0.7
4	Missouri	15.5
NA	Montana**	NA
25	Nebraska	(20.6)
1	Nevada	31.4
NA	New Hampshire**	NA
27	New Jersey	(26.9)
NA	New Mexico**	NA
33	New York	(35.7)
17	North Carolina	(8.8)
NA	North Dakota**	NA
11	Ohio	(1.1)
5	Oklahoma	4.9
NA	Oregon**	NA
26	Pennsylvania	(23.4)
NA	Rhode Island**	NA
9	South Carolina	0.6
NA	South Dakota**	NA
7	Tennessee	2.2
15	Texas	(7.5)
NA	Utah**	NA
NA	Vermont**	NA
13	Virginia	(2.0)
29	Washington	(28.7)
NA	West Virginia**	NA
3	Wisconsin	18.1
NA	Wyoming**	NA

RANK ORDER

RANK	STATE	PERCENT CHANGE
1	Nevada	31.4
2	Colorado	24.1
3	Wisconsin	18.1
4	Missouri	15.5
5	Oklahoma	4.9
6	Arkansas	3.7
7	Tennessee	2.2
8	Mississippi	0.7
9	South Carolina	0.6
10	Kentucky	(0.7)
11	Ohio	(1.1)
12	Michigan	(1.6)
13	Virginia	(2.0)
14	Louisiana	(3.8)
15	Texas	(7.5)
16	Alabama	(7.9)
17	North Carolina	(8.8)
18	Connecticut	(9.0)
19	Florida	(11.1)
20	Georgia	(16.0)
21	Indiana	(16.4)
22	Illinois	(16.8)
23	California	(17.3)
24	Massachusetts	(20.2)
25	Nebraska	(20.6)
26	Pennsylvania	(23.4)
27	New Jersey	(26.9)
28	Minnesota	(27.0)
29	Washington	(28.7)
30	Maryland	(30.1)
31	Delaware	(35.2)
32	Kansas	(35.3)
33	New York	(35.7)
34	Arizona	(41.2)
NA	Alaska**	NA
NA	Hawaii**	NA
NA	Idaho**	NA
NA	Iowa**	NA
NA	Maine**	NA
NA	Montana**	NA
NA	New Hampshire**	NA
NA	New Mexico**	NA
NA	North Dakota**	NA
NA	Oregon**	NA
NA	Rhode Island**	NA
NA	South Dakota**	NA
NA	Utah**	NA
NA	Vermont**	NA
NA	West Virginia**	NA
NA	Wyoming**	NA

District of Columbia   (29.6)

Source: Morgan Quitno Press using data from US Dept of Health & Human Services, National Center for Health Statistics
"National Vital Statistics Reports" (Vol. 53, No. 5, October 12, 2004)
"Monthly Vital Statistics Report" (Vol. 44, No. 7(S), February 29, 1996)
*Final data. Deaths of infants under 1 year old, exclusive of fetal deaths. Based on race of the mother.
**Not available, fewer than 20 black infant deaths.

Neonatal Deaths in 2002

National Total = 18,747 Deaths*

ALPHA ORDER

RANK ORDER

RANK	STATE	DEATHS	% of USA	RANK	STATE	DEATHS	% of USA
20	Alabama	345	1.8%	1	California	1,934	10.3%
49	Alaska	20	0.1%	2	Texas	1,451	7.7%
18	Arizona	361	1.9%	3	New York	1,074	5.7%
30	Arkansas	191	1.0%	4	Florida	1,032	5.5%
1	California	1,934	10.3%	5	Illinois	911	4.9%
25	Colorado	275	1.5%	6	Ohio	800	4.3%
29	Connecticut	198	1.1%	6	Pennsylvania	800	4.3%
41	Delaware	78	0.4%	8	Georgia	792	4.2%
4	Florida	1,032	5.5%	9	Michigan	720	3.8%
8	Georgia	792	4.2%	10	North Carolina	659	3.5%
40	Hawaii	83	0.4%	11	Virginia	513	2.7%
39	Idaho	84	0.4%	12	New Jersey	471	2.5%
5	Illinois	911	4.9%	13	Tennessee	456	2.4%
14	Indiana	448	2.4%	14	Indiana	448	2.4%
34	Iowa	134	0.7%	15	Louisiana	429	2.3%
30	Kansas	191	1.0%	16	Missouri	417	2.2%
28	Kentucky	228	1.2%	17	Maryland	394	2.1%
15	Louisiana	429	2.3%	18	Arizona	361	1.9%
45	Maine	43	0.2%	19	South Carolina	346	1.8%
17	Maryland	394	2.1%	20	Alabama	345	1.8%
22	Massachusetts	298	1.6%	21	Wisconsin	330	1.8%
9	Michigan	720	3.8%	22	Massachusetts	298	1.6%
27	Minnesota	240	1.3%	23	Washington	291	1.6%
24	Mississippi	281	1.5%	24	Mississippi	281	1.5%
16	Missouri	417	2.2%	25	Colorado	275	1.5%
43	Montana	54	0.3%	26	Oklahoma	257	1.4%
36	Nebraska	121	0.6%	27	Minnesota	240	1.3%
35	Nevada	126	0.7%	28	Kentucky	228	1.2%
44	New Hampshire	51	0.3%	29	Connecticut	198	1.1%
12	New Jersey	471	2.5%	30	Arkansas	191	1.0%
37	New Mexico	120	0.6%	30	Kansas	191	1.0%
3	New York	1,074	5.7%	32	Utah	186	1.0%
10	North Carolina	659	3.5%	33	Oregon	172	0.9%
47	North Dakota	32	0.2%	34	Iowa	134	0.7%
6	Ohio	800	4.3%	35	Nevada	126	0.7%
26	Oklahoma	257	1.4%	36	Nebraska	121	0.6%
33	Oregon	172	0.9%	37	New Mexico	120	0.6%
6	Pennsylvania	800	4.3%	38	West Virginia	109	0.6%
42	Rhode Island	62	0.3%	39	Idaho	84	0.4%
19	South Carolina	346	1.8%	40	Hawaii	83	0.4%
46	South Dakota	38	0.2%	41	Delaware	78	0.4%
13	Tennessee	456	2.4%	42	Rhode Island	62	0.3%
2	Texas	1,451	7.7%	43	Montana	54	0.3%
32	Utah	186	1.0%	44	New Hampshire	51	0.3%
50	Vermont	19	0.1%	45	Maine	43	0.2%
11	Virginia	513	2.7%	46	South Dakota	38	0.2%
23	Washington	291	1.6%	47	North Dakota	32	0.2%
38	West Virginia	109	0.6%	48	Wyoming	25	0.1%
21	Wisconsin	330	1.8%	49	Alaska	20	0.1%
48	Wyoming	25	0.1%	50	Vermont	19	0.1%
					District of Columbia	57	0.3%

Source: U.S. Department of Health and Human Services, National Center for Health Statistics
"National Vital Statistics Reports" (Vol. 53, No. 5, October 12, 2004)
*Final data. Deaths of infants under 28 days, exclusive of fetal deaths.

Neonatal Death Rate in 2002

National Rate = 4.7 Deaths per 1,000 Live Births*

ALPHA ORDER

RANK	STATE	RATE
5	Alabama	5.9
49	Alaska	2.0
31	Arizona	4.1
16	Arkansas	5.1
41	California	3.7
34	Colorado	4.0
26	Connecticut	4.7
1	Delaware	7.0
19	Florida	5.0
5	Georgia	5.9
26	Hawaii	4.7
34	Idaho	4.0
19	Illinois	5.0
14	Indiana	5.3
44	Iowa	3.6
22	Kansas	4.8
30	Kentucky	4.2
3	Louisiana	6.6
48	Maine	3.2
12	Maryland	5.4
41	Massachusetts	3.7
10	Michigan	5.5
46	Minnesota	3.5
2	Mississippi	6.8
10	Missouri	5.5
21	Montana	4.9
22	Nebraska	4.8
36	Nevada	3.9
46	New Hampshire	3.5
31	New Jersey	4.1
28	New Mexico	4.3
28	New York	4.3
8	North Carolina	5.6
31	North Dakota	4.1
12	Ohio	5.4
16	Oklahoma	5.1
38	Oregon	3.8
8	Pennsylvania	5.6
22	Rhode Island	4.8
4	South Carolina	6.3
44	South Dakota	3.6
5	Tennessee	5.9
36	Texas	3.9
38	Utah	3.8
NA	Vermont**	NA
16	Virginia	5.1
41	Washington	3.7
14	West Virginia	5.3
22	Wisconsin	4.8
38	Wyoming	3.8

RANK ORDER

RANK	STATE	RATE
1	Delaware	7.0
2	Mississippi	6.8
3	Louisiana	6.6
4	South Carolina	6.3
5	Alabama	5.9
5	Georgia	5.9
5	Tennessee	5.9
8	North Carolina	5.6
8	Pennsylvania	5.6
10	Michigan	5.5
10	Missouri	5.5
12	Maryland	5.4
12	Ohio	5.4
14	Indiana	5.3
14	West Virginia	5.3
16	Arkansas	5.1
16	Oklahoma	5.1
16	Virginia	5.1
19	Florida	5.0
19	Illinois	5.0
21	Montana	4.9
22	Kansas	4.8
22	Nebraska	4.8
22	Rhode Island	4.8
22	Wisconsin	4.8
26	Connecticut	4.7
26	Hawaii	4.7
28	New Mexico	4.3
28	New York	4.3
30	Kentucky	4.2
31	Arizona	4.1
31	New Jersey	4.1
31	North Dakota	4.1
34	Colorado	4.0
34	Idaho	4.0
36	Nevada	3.9
36	Texas	3.9
38	Oregon	3.8
38	Utah	3.8
38	Wyoming	3.8
41	California	3.7
41	Massachusetts	3.7
41	Washington	3.7
44	Iowa	3.6
44	South Dakota	3.6
46	Minnesota	3.5
46	New Hampshire	3.5
48	Maine	3.2
49	Alaska	2.0
NA	Vermont**	NA

District of Columbia   7.6

Source: U.S. Department of Health and Human Services, National Center for Health Statistics
    "National Vital Statistics Reports" (Vol. 53, No. 5, October 12, 2004)
*Final data. Deaths of infants under 28 days, exclusive of fetal deaths.
**Not available. Fewer than 20 neonatal deaths.

White Neonatal Deaths in 2002

National Total = 12,354 Deaths*

RANK	STATE	DEATHS	% of USA
23	Alabama	182	1.5%
50	Alaska	11	0.1%
12	Arizona	318	2.6%
32	Arkansas	123	1.0%
1	California	1,505	12.2%
20	Colorado	227	1.8%
30	Connecticut	144	1.2%
41	Delaware	48	0.4%
4	Florida	596	4.8%
9	Georgia	360	2.9%
49	Hawaii	12	0.1%
39	Idaho	82	0.7%
6	Illinois	557	4.5%
10	Indiana	347	2.8%
32	Iowa	123	1.0%
29	Kansas	155	1.3%
22	Kentucky	193	1.6%
27	Louisiana	162	1.3%
44	Maine	41	0.3%
24	Maryland	178	1.4%
17	Massachusetts	234	1.9%
8	Michigan	430	3.5%
21	Minnesota	205	1.7%
35	Mississippi	99	0.8%
13	Missouri	292	2.4%
43	Montana	45	0.4%
36	Nebraska	96	0.8%
38	Nevada	90	0.7%
40	New Hampshire	51	0.4%
14	New Jersey	273	2.2%
37	New Mexico	92	0.7%
3	New York	709	5.7%
11	North Carolina	326	2.6%
45	North Dakota	25	0.2%
7	Ohio	512	4.1%
26	Oklahoma	172	1.4%
28	Oregon	158	1.3%
5	Pennsylvania	581	4.7%
41	Rhode Island	48	0.4%
31	South Carolina	138	1.1%
45	South Dakota	25	0.2%
16	Tennessee	250	2.0%
2	Texas	1,082	8.8%
25	Utah	176	1.4%
48	Vermont	19	0.2%
15	Virginia	260	2.1%
19	Washington	230	1.9%
34	West Virginia	100	0.8%
17	Wisconsin	234	1.9%
47	Wyoming	24	0.2%

RANK	STATE	DEATHS	% of USA
1	California	1,505	12.2%
2	Texas	1,082	8.8%
3	New York	709	5.7%
4	Florida	596	4.8%
5	Pennsylvania	581	4.7%
6	Illinois	557	4.5%
7	Ohio	512	4.1%
8	Michigan	430	3.5%
9	Georgia	360	2.9%
10	Indiana	347	2.8%
11	North Carolina	326	2.6%
12	Arizona	318	2.6%
13	Missouri	292	2.4%
14	New Jersey	273	2.2%
15	Virginia	260	2.1%
16	Tennessee	250	2.0%
17	Massachusetts	234	1.9%
17	Wisconsin	234	1.9%
19	Washington	230	1.9%
20	Colorado	227	1.8%
21	Minnesota	205	1.7%
22	Kentucky	193	1.6%
23	Alabama	182	1.5%
24	Maryland	178	1.4%
25	Utah	176	1.4%
26	Oklahoma	172	1.4%
27	Louisiana	162	1.3%
28	Oregon	158	1.3%
29	Kansas	155	1.3%
30	Connecticut	144	1.2%
31	South Carolina	138	1.1%
32	Arkansas	123	1.0%
32	Iowa	123	1.0%
34	West Virginia	100	0.8%
35	Mississippi	99	0.8%
36	Nebraska	96	0.8%
37	New Mexico	92	0.7%
38	Nevada	90	0.7%
39	Idaho	82	0.7%
40	New Hampshire	51	0.4%
41	Delaware	48	0.4%
41	Rhode Island	48	0.4%
43	Montana	45	0.4%
44	Maine	41	0.3%
45	North Dakota	25	0.2%
45	South Dakota	25	0.2%
47	Wyoming	24	0.2%
48	Vermont	19	0.2%
49	Hawaii	12	0.1%
50	Alaska	11	0.1%
	District of Columbia	14	0.1%

Source: U.S. Department of Health and Human Services, National Center for Health Statistics
"National Vital Statistics Reports" (Vol. 53, No. 5, October 12, 2004)
*Final data. Deaths of infants under 28 days, exclusive of fetal deaths. Based on race of the mother.

White Neonatal Death Rate in 2002

National Rate = 3.9 White Neonatal Deaths per 1,000 White Live Births*

ALPHA ORDER

RANK	STATE	RATE
7	Alabama	4.6
NA	Alaska**	NA
20	Arizona	4.1
13	Arkansas	4.2
38	California	3.5
36	Colorado	3.6
13	Connecticut	4.2
1	Delaware	6.1
26	Florida	3.9
13	Georgia	4.2
NA	Hawaii**	NA
20	Idaho	4.1
22	Illinois	4.0
4	Indiana	4.7
38	Iowa	3.5
8	Kansas	4.4
22	Kentucky	4.0
8	Louisiana	4.4
46	Maine	3.1
26	Maryland	3.9
38	Massachusetts	3.5
13	Michigan	4.2
38	Minnesota	3.5
8	Mississippi	4.4
4	Missouri	4.7
4	Montana	4.7
13	Nebraska	4.2
44	Nevada	3.3
34	New Hampshire	3.7
45	New Jersey	3.2
22	New Mexico	4.0
26	New York	3.9
31	North Carolina	3.8
34	North Dakota	3.7
13	Ohio	4.2
8	Oklahoma	4.4
31	Oregon	3.8
3	Pennsylvania	4.9
12	Rhode Island	4.3
26	South Carolina	3.9
47	South Dakota	2.9
13	Tennessee	4.2
43	Texas	3.4
31	Utah	3.8
NA	Vermont**	NA
36	Virginia	3.6
38	Washington	3.5
2	West Virginia	5.0
22	Wisconsin	4.0
26	Wyoming	3.9

RANK ORDER

RANK	STATE	RATE
1	Delaware	6.1
2	West Virginia	5.0
3	Pennsylvania	4.9
4	Indiana	4.7
4	Missouri	4.7
4	Montana	4.7
7	Alabama	4.6
8	Kansas	4.4
8	Louisiana	4.4
8	Mississippi	4.4
8	Oklahoma	4.4
12	Rhode Island	4.3
13	Arkansas	4.2
13	Connecticut	4.2
13	Georgia	4.2
13	Michigan	4.2
13	Nebraska	4.2
13	Ohio	4.2
13	Tennessee	4.2
20	Arizona	4.1
20	Idaho	4.1
22	Illinois	4.0
22	Kentucky	4.0
22	New Mexico	4.0
22	Wisconsin	4.0
26	Florida	3.9
26	Maryland	3.9
26	New York	3.9
26	South Carolina	3.9
26	Wyoming	3.9
31	North Carolina	3.8
31	Oregon	3.8
31	Utah	3.8
34	New Hampshire	3.7
34	North Dakota	3.7
36	Colorado	3.6
36	Virginia	3.6
38	California	3.5
38	Iowa	3.5
38	Massachusetts	3.5
38	Minnesota	3.5
38	Washington	3.5
43	Texas	3.4
44	Nevada	3.3
45	New Jersey	3.2
46	Maine	3.1
47	South Dakota	2.9
NA	Alaska**	NA
NA	Hawaii**	NA
NA	Vermont**	NA
	District of Columbia**	NA

Source: U.S. Department of Health and Human Services, National Center for Health Statistics
   "National Vital Statistics Reports" (Vol. 53, No. 5, October 12, 2004)
*Final data. Deaths of infants under 28 days, exclusive of fetal deaths. Based on race of the mother.
**Not available. Fewer than 20 white neonatal deaths.

Black Neonatal Deaths in 2002

National Total = 5,646 Deaths*

ALPHA ORDER

RANK ORDER

RANK	STATE	DEATHS	% of USA		RANK	STATE	DEATHS	% of USA
18	Alabama	163	2.9%		1	Florida	419	7.4%
45	Alaska	1	0.0%		2	Georgia	404	7.2%
34	Arizona	16	0.3%		3	Texas	347	6.1%
22	Arkansas	62	1.1%		4	New York	334	5.9%
9	California	260	4.6%		5	Illinois	324	5.7%
26	Colorado	40	0.7%		6	North Carolina	318	5.6%
25	Connecticut	47	0.8%		7	Michigan	272	4.8%
30	Delaware	28	0.5%		7	Ohio	272	4.8%
1	Florida	419	7.4%		9	California	260	4.6%
2	Georgia	404	7.2%		10	Louisiana	259	4.6%
39	Hawaii	5	0.1%		11	Virginia	239	4.2%
46	Idaho	0	0.0%		12	Maryland	206	3.6%
5	Illinois	324	5.7%		12	Pennsylvania	206	3.6%
20	Indiana	90	1.6%		14	South Carolina	203	3.6%
36	Iowa	9	0.2%		14	Tennessee	203	3.6%
29	Kansas	29	0.5%		16	New Jersey	184	3.3%
27	Kentucky	33	0.6%		17	Mississippi	178	3.2%
10	Louisiana	259	4.6%		18	Alabama	163	2.9%
46	Maine	0	0.0%		19	Missouri	121	2.1%
12	Maryland	206	3.6%		20	Indiana	90	1.6%
24	Massachusetts	51	0.9%		21	Wisconsin	83	1.5%
7	Michigan	272	4.8%		22	Arkansas	62	1.1%
32	Minnesota	24	0.4%		23	Oklahoma	52	0.9%
17	Mississippi	178	3.2%		24	Massachusetts	51	0.9%
19	Missouri	121	2.1%		25	Connecticut	47	0.8%
42	Montana	2	0.0%		26	Colorado	40	0.7%
33	Nebraska	22	0.4%		27	Kentucky	33	0.6%
30	Nevada	28	0.5%		28	Washington	30	0.5%
46	New Hampshire	0	0.0%		29	Kansas	29	0.5%
16	New Jersey	184	3.3%		30	Delaware	28	0.5%
38	New Mexico	7	0.1%		30	Nevada	28	0.5%
4	New York	334	5.9%		32	Minnesota	24	0.4%
6	North Carolina	318	5.6%		33	Nebraska	22	0.4%
42	North Dakota	2	0.0%		34	Arizona	16	0.3%
7	Ohio	272	4.8%		35	Rhode Island	11	0.2%
23	Oklahoma	52	0.9%		36	Iowa	9	0.2%
39	Oregon	5	0.1%		36	West Virginia	9	0.2%
12	Pennsylvania	206	3.6%		38	New Mexico	7	0.1%
35	Rhode Island	11	0.2%		39	Hawaii	5	0.1%
14	South Carolina	203	3.6%		39	Oregon	5	0.1%
42	South Dakota	2	0.0%		41	Utah	3	0.1%
14	Tennessee	203	3.6%		42	Montana	2	0.0%
3	Texas	347	6.1%		42	North Dakota	2	0.0%
41	Utah	3	0.1%		42	South Dakota	2	0.0%
46	Vermont	0	0.0%		45	Alaska	1	0.0%
11	Virginia	239	4.2%		46	Idaho	0	0.0%
28	Washington	30	0.5%		46	Maine	0	0.0%
36	West Virginia	9	0.2%		46	New Hampshire	0	0.0%
21	Wisconsin	83	1.5%		46	Vermont	0	0.0%
46	Wyoming	0	0.0%		46	Wyoming	0	0.0%
						District of Columbia	43	0.8%

Source: U.S. Department of Health and Human Services, National Center for Health Statistics
    "National Vital Statistics Reports" (Vol. 53, No. 5, October 12, 2004)
*Final data. Deaths of infants under 28 days, exclusive of fetal deaths. Based on race of the mother.

Black Neonatal Death Rate in 2002

National Rate = 9.5 Black Neonatal Deaths per 1,000 Black Live Births*

ALPHA ORDER			RANK ORDER		
RANK	STATE	RATE	RANK	STATE	RATE
24	Alabama	8.9	1	Nebraska	15.3
NA	Alaska**	NA	2	Colorado	13.6
NA	Arizona**	NA	3	Wisconsin	12.9
27	Arkansas	8.3	4	Tennessee	12.5
29	California	8.0	5	Michigan	12.1
2	Colorado	13.6	5	Ohio	12.1
23	Connecticut	9.0	7	North Carolina	11.5
13	Delaware	10.3	8	South Carolina	11.2
22	Florida	9.1	9	Oklahoma	11.1
20	Georgia	9.4	10	Missouri	11.0
NA	Hawaii**	NA	11	Virginia	10.8
NA	Idaho**	NA	12	Nevada	10.7
14	Illinois	10.2	13	Delaware	10.3
19	Indiana	9.6	14	Illinois	10.2
NA	Iowa**	NA	14	Pennsylvania	10.2
16	Kansas	10.0	16	Kansas	10.0
30	Kentucky	6.7	17	Mississippi	9.8
18	Louisiana	9.7	18	Louisiana	9.7
NA	Maine**	NA	19	Indiana	9.6
26	Maryland	8.5	20	Georgia	9.4
32	Massachusetts	6.1	21	New Jersey	9.2
5	Michigan	12.1	22	Florida	9.1
33	Minnesota	4.9	23	Connecticut	9.0
17	Mississippi	9.8	24	Alabama	8.9
10	Missouri	11.0	25	Washington	8.8
NA	Montana**	NA	26	Maryland	8.5
1	Nebraska	15.3	27	Arkansas	8.3
12	Nevada	10.7	27	Texas	8.3
NA	New Hampshire**	NA	29	California	8.0
21	New Jersey	9.2	30	Kentucky	6.7
NA	New Mexico**	NA	30	New York	6.7
30	New York	6.7	32	Massachusetts	6.1
7	North Carolina	11.5	33	Minnesota	4.9
NA	North Dakota**	NA	NA	Alaska**	NA
5	Ohio	12.1	NA	Arizona**	NA
9	Oklahoma	11.1	NA	Hawaii**	NA
NA	Oregon**	NA	NA	Idaho**	NA
14	Pennsylvania	10.2	NA	Iowa**	NA
NA	Rhode Island**	NA	NA	Maine**	NA
8	South Carolina	11.2	NA	Montana**	NA
NA	South Dakota**	NA	NA	New Hampshire**	NA
4	Tennessee	12.5	NA	New Mexico**	NA
27	Texas	8.3	NA	North Dakota**	NA
NA	Utah**	NA	NA	Oregon**	NA
NA	Vermont**	NA	NA	Rhode Island**	NA
11	Virginia	10.8	NA	South Dakota**	NA
25	Washington	8.8	NA	Utah**	NA
NA	West Virginia**	NA	NA	Vermont**	NA
3	Wisconsin	12.9	NA	West Virginia**	NA
NA	Wyoming**	NA	NA	Wyoming**	NA
				District of Columbia	9.3

Source: U.S. Department of Health and Human Services, National Center for Health Statistics
     "National Vital Statistics Reports" (Vol. 53, No. 5, October 12, 2004)
*Final data. Deaths of infants under 28 days, exclusive of fetal deaths. Based on race of the mother.
**Not available. Fewer than 20 black neonatal deaths.

Deaths by AIDS in 2002

National Total = 14,095 Deaths*

ALPHA ORDER

RANK	STATE	DEATHS	% of USA
18	Alabama	190	1.3%
42	Alaska	16	0.1%
21	Arizona	165	1.2%
29	Arkansas	81	0.6%
3	California	1,435	10.2%
25	Colorado	105	0.7%
19	Connecticut	186	1.3%
32	Delaware	70	0.5%
2	Florida	1,719	12.2%
6	Georgia	708	5.0%
37	Hawaii	26	0.2%
45	Idaho	11	0.1%
9	Illinois	490	3.5%
24	Indiana	118	0.8%
36	Iowa	29	0.2%
34	Kansas	37	0.3%
26	Kentucky	98	0.7%
11	Louisiana	364	2.6%
44	Maine	12	0.1%
7	Maryland	610	4.3%
17	Massachusetts	232	1.6%
16	Michigan	240	1.7%
33	Minnesota	53	0.4%
20	Mississippi	185	1.3%
22	Missouri	123	0.9%
46	Montana	8	0.1%
39	Nebraska	21	0.1%
31	Nevada	76	0.5%
43	New Hampshire	13	0.1%
5	New Jersey	762	5.4%
35	New Mexico	35	0.2%
1	New York	1,980	14.0%
10	North Carolina	486	3.4%
50	North Dakota	1	0.0%
15	Ohio	241	1.7%
27	Oklahoma	91	0.6%
27	Oregon	91	0.6%
8	Pennsylvania	497	3.5%
38	Rhode Island	23	0.2%
13	South Carolina	301	2.1%
48	South Dakota	5	0.0%
12	Tennessee	347	2.5%
4	Texas	1,075	7.6%
41	Utah	19	0.1%
46	Vermont	8	0.1%
14	Virginia	261	1.9%
23	Washington	119	0.8%
40	West Virginia	20	0.1%
30	Wisconsin	77	0.5%
49	Wyoming	2	0.0%

RANK ORDER

RANK	STATE	DEATHS	% of USA
1	New York	1,980	14.0%
2	Florida	1,719	12.2%
3	California	1,435	10.2%
4	Texas	1,075	7.6%
5	New Jersey	762	5.4%
6	Georgia	708	5.0%
7	Maryland	610	4.3%
8	Pennsylvania	497	3.5%
9	Illinois	490	3.5%
10	North Carolina	486	3.4%
11	Louisiana	364	2.6%
12	Tennessee	347	2.5%
13	South Carolina	301	2.1%
14	Virginia	261	1.9%
15	Ohio	241	1.7%
16	Michigan	240	1.7%
17	Massachusetts	232	1.6%
18	Alabama	190	1.3%
19	Connecticut	186	1.3%
20	Mississippi	185	1.3%
21	Arizona	165	1.2%
22	Missouri	123	0.9%
23	Washington	119	0.8%
24	Indiana	118	0.8%
25	Colorado	105	0.7%
26	Kentucky	98	0.7%
27	Oklahoma	91	0.6%
27	Oregon	91	0.6%
29	Arkansas	81	0.6%
30	Wisconsin	77	0.5%
31	Nevada	76	0.5%
32	Delaware	70	0.5%
33	Minnesota	53	0.4%
34	Kansas	37	0.3%
35	New Mexico	35	0.2%
36	Iowa	29	0.2%
37	Hawaii	26	0.2%
38	Rhode Island	23	0.2%
39	Nebraska	21	0.1%
40	West Virginia	20	0.1%
41	Utah	19	0.1%
42	Alaska	16	0.1%
43	New Hampshire	13	0.1%
44	Maine	12	0.1%
45	Idaho	11	0.1%
46	Montana	8	0.1%
46	Vermont	8	0.1%
48	South Dakota	5	0.0%
49	Wyoming	2	0.0%
50	North Dakota	1	0.0%
	District of Columbia	233	1.7%

Source: U.S. Department of Health and Human Services, National Center for Health Statistics
   "National Vital Statistics Reports" (Vol. 53, No. 5, October 12, 2004)
*AIDS is Acquired Immunodeficiency Syndrome. It is a specific group of diseases or conditions which are indicative
of severe immunosuppression related to infection with the Human Immunodeficiency Virus (HIV).

Death Rate by AIDS in 2002

National Rate = 4.9 Deaths per 100,000 Population*

ALPHA ORDER

RANK	STATE	RATE
14	Alabama	4.2
NA	Alaska**	NA
21	Arizona	3.0
21	Arkansas	3.0
15	California	4.1
27	Colorado	2.3
12	Connecticut	5.4
5	Delaware	8.7
2	Florida	10.3
6	Georgia	8.3
30	Hawaii	2.1
NA	Idaho**	NA
17	Illinois	3.9
33	Indiana	1.9
40	Iowa	1.0
35	Kansas	1.4
25	Kentucky	2.4
7	Louisiana	8.1
NA	Maine**	NA
1	Maryland	11.2
18	Massachusetts	3.6
25	Michigan	2.4
38	Minnesota	1.1
9	Mississippi	6.4
28	Missouri	2.2
NA	Montana**	NA
37	Nebraska	1.2
20	Nevada	3.5
NA	New Hampshire**	NA
4	New Jersey	8.9
33	New Mexico	1.9
2	New York	10.3
11	North Carolina	5.8
NA	North Dakota**	NA
30	Ohio	2.1
23	Oklahoma	2.6
23	Oregon	2.6
16	Pennsylvania	4.0
28	Rhode Island	2.2
8	South Carolina	7.3
NA	South Dakota**	NA
10	Tennessee	6.0
13	Texas	4.9
NA	Utah**	NA
NA	Vermont**	NA
18	Virginia	3.6
32	Washington	2.0
38	West Virginia	1.1
35	Wisconsin	1.4
NA	Wyoming**	NA

RANK ORDER

RANK	STATE	RATE
1	Maryland	11.2
2	Florida	10.3
2	New York	10.3
4	New Jersey	8.9
5	Delaware	8.7
6	Georgia	8.3
7	Louisiana	8.1
8	South Carolina	7.3
9	Mississippi	6.4
10	Tennessee	6.0
11	North Carolina	5.8
12	Connecticut	5.4
13	Texas	4.9
14	Alabama	4.2
15	California	4.1
16	Pennsylvania	4.0
17	Illinois	3.9
18	Massachusetts	3.6
18	Virginia	3.6
20	Nevada	3.5
21	Arizona	3.0
21	Arkansas	3.0
23	Oklahoma	2.6
23	Oregon	2.6
25	Kentucky	2.4
25	Michigan	2.4
27	Colorado	2.3
28	Missouri	2.2
28	Rhode Island	2.2
30	Hawaii	2.1
30	Ohio	2.1
32	Washington	2.0
33	Indiana	1.9
33	New Mexico	1.9
35	Kansas	1.4
35	Wisconsin	1.4
37	Nebraska	1.2
38	Minnesota	1.1
38	West Virginia	1.1
40	Iowa	1.0
NA	Alaska**	NA
NA	Idaho**	NA
NA	Maine**	NA
NA	Montana**	NA
NA	New Hampshire**	NA
NA	North Dakota**	NA
NA	South Dakota**	NA
NA	Utah**	NA
NA	Vermont**	NA
NA	Wyoming**	NA

District of Columbia   40.8

Source: U.S. Department of Health and Human Services, National Center for Health Statistics
"National Vital Statistics Reports" (Vol. 53, No. 5, October 12, 2004)
*AIDS is Acquired Immunodeficiency Syndrome. It is a specific group of diseases or conditions which are indicative of severe immunosuppression related to infection with the Human Immunodeficiency Virus (HIV). Not age-adjusted.
**Insufficient data to determine a reliable rate.

Age-Adjusted Death Rate by AIDS in 2002

National Rate = 4.9 Deaths per 100,000 Population*

ALPHA ORDER

RANK	STATE	RATE
14	Alabama	4.3
NA	Alaska**	NA
21	Arizona	3.3
22	Arkansas	3.2
15	California	4.2
26	Colorado	2.3
12	Connecticut	5.2
4	Delaware	8.5
2	Florida	10.4
7	Georgia	8.2
30	Hawaii	2.1
NA	Idaho**	NA
17	Illinois	3.9
32	Indiana	2.0
39	Iowa	1.0
35	Kansas	1.4
26	Kentucky	2.3
6	Louisiana	8.4
NA	Maine**	NA
1	Maryland	10.7
18	Massachusetts	3.5
25	Michigan	2.4
39	Minnesota	1.0
9	Mississippi	6.8
28	Missouri	2.2
NA	Montana**	NA
37	Nebraska	1.3
18	Nevada	3.5
NA	New Hampshire**	NA
4	New Jersey	8.5
32	New Mexico	2.0
3	New York	10.2
11	North Carolina	5.8
NA	North Dakota**	NA
28	Ohio	2.2
23	Oklahoma	2.7
24	Oregon	2.6
16	Pennsylvania	4.0
30	Rhode Island	2.1
8	South Carolina	7.4
NA	South Dakota**	NA
10	Tennessee	5.9
13	Texas	5.1
NA	Utah**	NA
NA	Vermont**	NA
18	Virginia	3.5
34	Washington	1.9
38	West Virginia	1.1
35	Wisconsin	1.4
NA	Wyoming**	NA

RANK ORDER

RANK	STATE	RATE
1	Maryland	10.7
2	Florida	10.4
3	New York	10.2
4	Delaware	8.5
4	New Jersey	8.5
6	Louisiana	8.4
7	Georgia	8.2
8	South Carolina	7.4
9	Mississippi	6.8
10	Tennessee	5.9
11	North Carolina	5.8
12	Connecticut	5.2
13	Texas	5.1
14	Alabama	4.3
15	California	4.2
16	Pennsylvania	4.0
17	Illinois	3.9
18	Massachusetts	3.5
18	Nevada	3.5
18	Virginia	3.5
21	Arizona	3.3
22	Arkansas	3.2
23	Oklahoma	2.7
24	Oregon	2.6
25	Michigan	2.4
26	Colorado	2.3
26	Kentucky	2.3
28	Missouri	2.2
28	Ohio	2.2
30	Hawaii	2.1
30	Rhode Island	2.1
32	Indiana	2.0
32	New Mexico	2.0
34	Washington	1.9
35	Kansas	1.4
35	Wisconsin	1.4
37	Nebraska	1.3
38	West Virginia	1.1
39	Iowa	1.0
39	Minnesota	1.0
NA	Alaska**	NA
NA	Idaho**	NA
NA	Maine**	NA
NA	Montana**	NA
NA	New Hampshire**	NA
NA	North Dakota**	NA
NA	South Dakota**	NA
NA	Utah**	NA
NA	Vermont**	NA
NA	Wyoming**	NA

District of Columbia   40.8

Source: U.S. Department of Health and Human Services, National Center for Health Statistics
  "National Vital Statistics Reports" (Vol. 53, No. 5, October 12, 2004)
*AIDS is Acquired Immunodeficiency Syndrome. It is a specific group of diseases or conditions which are indicative of severe immunosuppression related to infection with the Human Immunodeficiency Virus (HIV). Age-adjusted rates based on the year 2000 standard population.
**Insufficient data to determine a reliable rate.

Estimated Deaths by Cancer in 2005

National Estimated Total = 570,280 Deaths

ALPHA ORDER

RANK	STATE	DEATHS	% of USA
20	Alabama	10,100	1.8%
50	Alaska	800	0.1%
21	Arizona	9,920	1.7%
32	Arkansas	6,210	1.1%
1	California	56,090	9.8%
29	Colorado	6,680	1.2%
28	Connecticut	7,030	1.2%
46	Delaware	1,580	0.3%
2	Florida	39,960	7.0%
11	Georgia	14,810	2.6%
44	Hawaii	1,990	0.3%
42	Idaho	2,280	0.4%
6	Illinois	24,810	4.4%
14	Indiana	13,250	2.3%
30	Iowa	6,610	1.2%
33	Kansas	5,370	0.9%
23	Kentucky	9,560	1.7%
22	Louisiana	9,670	1.7%
38	Maine	3,220	0.6%
19	Maryland	10,570	1.9%
13	Massachusetts	13,720	2.4%
8	Michigan	20,860	3.7%
24	Minnesota	9,510	1.7%
31	Mississippi	6,220	1.1%
16	Missouri	12,550	2.2%
43	Montana	2,040	0.4%
36	Nebraska	3,460	0.6%
35	Nevada	4,620	0.8%
40	New Hampshire	2,620	0.5%
9	New Jersey	17,860	3.1%
37	New Mexico	3,230	0.6%
3	New York	36,160	6.3%
10	North Carolina	16,830	3.0%
47	North Dakota	1,280	0.2%
7	Ohio	24,790	4.3%
26	Oklahoma	7,670	1.3%
27	Oregon	7,360	1.3%
5	Pennsylvania	29,840	5.2%
41	Rhode Island	2,440	0.4%
25	South Carolina	9,080	1.6%
45	South Dakota	1,620	0.3%
15	Tennessee	12,910	2.3%
4	Texas	36,090	6.3%
39	Utah	2,650	0.5%
48	Vermont	1,260	0.2%
12	Virginia	13,990	2.5%
17	Washington	11,360	2.0%
34	West Virginia	4,650	0.8%
18	Wisconsin	10,940	1.9%
49	Wyoming	990	0.2%

RANK ORDER

RANK	STATE	DEATHS	% of USA
1	California	56,090	9.8%
2	Florida	39,960	7.0%
3	New York	36,160	6.3%
4	Texas	36,090	6.3%
5	Pennsylvania	29,840	5.2%
6	Illinois	24,810	4.4%
7	Ohio	24,790	4.3%
8	Michigan	20,860	3.7%
9	New Jersey	17,860	3.1%
10	North Carolina	16,830	3.0%
11	Georgia	14,810	2.6%
12	Virginia	13,990	2.5%
13	Massachusetts	13,720	2.4%
14	Indiana	13,250	2.3%
15	Tennessee	12,910	2.3%
16	Missouri	12,550	2.2%
17	Washington	11,360	2.0%
18	Wisconsin	10,940	1.9%
19	Maryland	10,570	1.9%
20	Alabama	10,100	1.8%
21	Arizona	9,920	1.7%
22	Louisiana	9,670	1.7%
23	Kentucky	9,560	1.7%
24	Minnesota	9,510	1.7%
25	South Carolina	9,080	1.6%
26	Oklahoma	7,670	1.3%
27	Oregon	7,360	1.3%
28	Connecticut	7,030	1.2%
29	Colorado	6,680	1.2%
30	Iowa	6,610	1.2%
31	Mississippi	6,220	1.1%
32	Arkansas	6,210	1.1%
33	Kansas	5,370	0.9%
34	West Virginia	4,650	0.8%
35	Nevada	4,620	0.8%
36	Nebraska	3,460	0.6%
37	New Mexico	3,230	0.6%
38	Maine	3,220	0.6%
39	Utah	2,650	0.5%
40	New Hampshire	2,620	0.5%
41	Rhode Island	2,440	0.4%
42	Idaho	2,280	0.4%
43	Montana	2,040	0.4%
44	Hawaii	1,990	0.3%
45	South Dakota	1,620	0.3%
46	Delaware	1,580	0.3%
47	North Dakota	1,280	0.2%
48	Vermont	1,260	0.2%
49	Wyoming	990	0.2%
50	Alaska	800	0.1%
	District of Columbia	1,170	0.2%

Source: American Cancer Society
"Cancer Facts & Figures 2005" (Copyright 2005, American Cancer Society)

Estimated Death Rate by Cancer in 2005

National Estimated Rate = 194.2 Deaths per 100,000 Population*

ALPHA ORDER

RANK	STATE	RATE
9	Alabama	222.9
49	Alaska	122.1
41	Arizona	172.7
7	Arkansas	225.6
47	California	156.3
48	Colorado	145.2
27	Connecticut	200.7
35	Delaware	190.3
5	Florida	229.7
43	Georgia	167.7
46	Hawaii	157.6
44	Idaho	163.6
34	Illinois	195.1
19	Indiana	212.4
8	Iowa	223.7
32	Kansas	196.3
4	Kentucky	230.6
17	Louisiana	214.1
2	Maine	244.4
36	Maryland	190.2
18	Massachusetts	213.8
21	Michigan	206.3
39	Minnesota	186.4
16	Mississippi	214.3
12	Missouri	218.1
10	Montana	220.1
29	Nebraska	198.0
30	Nevada	197.9
26	New Hampshire	201.6
22	New Jersey	205.3
42	New Mexico	169.7
37	New York	188.1
31	North Carolina	197.0
25	North Dakota	201.8
14	Ohio	216.3
13	Oklahoma	217.7
23	Oregon	204.8
3	Pennsylvania	240.5
6	Rhode Island	225.8
14	South Carolina	216.3
20	South Dakota	210.1
11	Tennessee	218.8
45	Texas	160.5
50	Utah	110.9
24	Vermont	202.8
38	Virginia	187.5
40	Washington	183.1
1	West Virginia	256.1
28	Wisconsin	198.6
33	Wyoming	195.4

RANK ORDER

RANK	STATE	RATE
1	West Virginia	256.1
2	Maine	244.4
3	Pennsylvania	240.5
4	Kentucky	230.6
5	Florida	229.7
6	Rhode Island	225.8
7	Arkansas	225.6
8	Iowa	223.7
9	Alabama	222.9
10	Montana	220.1
11	Tennessee	218.8
12	Missouri	218.1
13	Oklahoma	217.7
14	Ohio	216.3
14	South Carolina	216.3
16	Mississippi	214.3
17	Louisiana	214.1
18	Massachusetts	213.8
19	Indiana	212.4
20	South Dakota	210.1
21	Michigan	206.3
22	New Jersey	205.3
23	Oregon	204.8
24	Vermont	202.8
25	North Dakota	201.8
26	New Hampshire	201.6
27	Connecticut	200.7
28	Wisconsin	198.6
29	Nebraska	198.0
30	Nevada	197.9
31	North Carolina	197.0
32	Kansas	196.3
33	Wyoming	195.4
34	Illinois	195.1
35	Delaware	190.3
36	Maryland	190.2
37	New York	188.1
38	Virginia	187.5
39	Minnesota	186.4
40	Washington	183.1
41	Arizona	172.7
42	New Mexico	169.7
43	Georgia	167.7
44	Idaho	163.6
45	Texas	160.5
46	Hawaii	157.6
47	California	156.3
48	Colorado	145.2
49	Alaska	122.1
50	Utah	110.9
	District of Columbia	211.4

Source: Morgan Quitno Press using data from American Cancer Society
        "Cancer Facts & Figures 2005" (Copyright 2005, American Cancer Society)
*Rates calculated using 2004 Census resident population estimates. Not age-adjusted.

Age-Adjusted Death Rate by Cancer for Males in 2001

National Rate = 251.1 Deaths per 100,000 Male Population*

ALPHA ORDER

RANK	STATE	RATE
4	Alabama	290.4
38	Alaska	235.5
46	Arizona	212.3
8	Arkansas	277.3
44	California	221.3
47	Colorado	210.9
39	Connecticut	234.7
14	Delaware	265.5
37	Florida	236.2
11	Georgia	272.5
49	Hawaii	195.7
45	Idaho	220.0
19	Illinois	263.5
9	Indiana	274.2
32	Iowa	241.2
34	Kansas	239.2
3	Kentucky	298.9
2	Louisiana	303.8
17	Maine	264.7
15	Maryland	265.3
22	Massachusetts	258.3
24	Michigan	255.7
40	Minnesota	234.2
1	Mississippi	306.7
20	Missouri	262.4
30	Montana	244.4
43	Nebraska	231.6
28	Nevada	249.5
23	New Hampshire	256.7
25	New Jersey	255.2
48	New Mexico	209.0
35	New York	238.3
10	North Carolina	272.7
41	North Dakota	234.0
12	Ohio	269.3
16	Oklahoma	265.2
33	Oregon	240.9
21	Pennsylvania	260.9
18	Rhode Island	264.4
7	South Carolina	281.0
31	South Dakota	242.3
5	Tennessee	287.2
26	Texas	252.1
50	Utah	187.3
27	Vermont	250.3
13	Virginia	265.8
36	Washington	236.5
6	West Virginia	282.9
29	Wisconsin	244.8
42	Wyoming	232.6

RANK ORDER

RANK	STATE	RATE
1	Mississippi	306.7
2	Louisiana	303.8
3	Kentucky	298.9
4	Alabama	290.4
5	Tennessee	287.2
6	West Virginia	282.9
7	South Carolina	281.0
8	Arkansas	277.3
9	Indiana	274.2
10	North Carolina	272.7
11	Georgia	272.5
12	Ohio	269.3
13	Virginia	265.8
14	Delaware	265.5
15	Maryland	265.3
16	Oklahoma	265.2
17	Maine	264.7
18	Rhode Island	264.4
19	Illinois	263.5
20	Missouri	262.4
21	Pennsylvania	260.9
22	Massachusetts	258.3
23	New Hampshire	256.7
24	Michigan	255.7
25	New Jersey	255.2
26	Texas	252.1
27	Vermont	250.3
28	Nevada	249.5
29	Wisconsin	244.8
30	Montana	244.4
31	South Dakota	242.3
32	Iowa	241.2
33	Oregon	240.9
34	Kansas	239.2
35	New York	238.3
36	Washington	236.5
37	Florida	236.2
38	Alaska	235.5
39	Connecticut	234.7
40	Minnesota	234.2
41	North Dakota	234.0
42	Wyoming	232.6
43	Nebraska	231.6
44	California	221.3
45	Idaho	220.0
46	Arizona	212.3
47	Colorado	210.9
48	New Mexico	209.0
49	Hawaii	195.7
50	Utah	187.3
	District of Columbia	310.7

Source: American Cancer Society
   "Cancer Facts & Figures 2005" (Copyright 2005, American Cancer Society)
*For 1997 to 2001. Age-adjusted to the 2000 U.S. standard population.

Age-Adjusted Death Rate by Cancer for Females in 2001

National Rate = 166.7 Deaths per 100,000 Female Population*

ALPHA ORDER

RANK	STATE	RATE
28	Alabama	167.1
16	Alaska	172.4
46	Arizona	150.5
25	Arkansas	167.9
37	California	158.9
47	Colorado	148.0
29	Connecticut	165.5
1	Delaware	186.6
39	Florida	157.7
31	Georgia	164.1
49	Hawaii	127.7
44	Idaho	151.6
12	Illinois	175.3
10	Indiana	176.8
41	Iowa	157.4
40	Kansas	157.5
4	Kentucky	180.9
3	Louisiana	183.5
7	Maine	179.1
8	Maryland	177.1
14	Massachusetts	173.9
19	Michigan	171.4
38	Minnesota	157.9
23	Mississippi	169.2
15	Missouri	173.2
35	Montana	161.4
43	Nebraska	154.1
6	Nevada	179.3
17	New Hampshire	172.3
5	New Jersey	179.7
48	New Mexico	145.7
27	New York	167.2
32	North Carolina	163.4
45	North Dakota	151.5
9	Ohio	176.9
24	Oklahoma	168.1
19	Oregon	171.4
13	Pennsylvania	174.1
11	Rhode Island	175.9
30	South Carolina	164.8
42	South Dakota	155.6
18	Tennessee	171.5
36	Texas	160.6
50	Utah	126.3
22	Vermont	169.4
21	Virginia	171.3
26	Washington	167.7
2	West Virginia	186.0
34	Wisconsin	162.1
33	Wyoming	163.0

RANK ORDER

RANK	STATE	RATE
1	Delaware	186.6
2	West Virginia	186.0
3	Louisiana	183.5
4	Kentucky	180.9
5	New Jersey	179.7
6	Nevada	179.3
7	Maine	179.1
8	Maryland	177.1
9	Ohio	176.9
10	Indiana	176.8
11	Rhode Island	175.9
12	Illinois	175.3
13	Pennsylvania	174.1
14	Massachusetts	173.9
15	Missouri	173.2
16	Alaska	172.4
17	New Hampshire	172.3
18	Tennessee	171.5
19	Michigan	171.4
19	Oregon	171.4
21	Virginia	171.3
22	Vermont	169.4
23	Mississippi	169.2
24	Oklahoma	168.1
25	Arkansas	167.9
26	Washington	167.7
27	New York	167.2
28	Alabama	167.1
29	Connecticut	165.5
30	South Carolina	164.8
31	Georgia	164.1
32	North Carolina	163.4
33	Wyoming	163.0
34	Wisconsin	162.1
35	Montana	161.4
36	Texas	160.6
37	California	158.9
38	Minnesota	157.9
39	Florida	157.7
40	Kansas	157.5
41	Iowa	157.4
42	South Dakota	155.6
43	Nebraska	154.1
44	Idaho	151.6
45	North Dakota	151.5
46	Arizona	150.5
47	Colorado	148.0
48	New Mexico	145.7
49	Hawaii	127.7
50	Utah	126.3
	District of Columbia	198.7

Source: American Cancer Society
"Cancer Facts & Figures 2005" (Copyright 2005, American Cancer Society)
*For 1997 to 2001. Age-adjusted to the 2000 U.S. standard population.

Estimated Deaths by Brain Cancer in 2005

National Estimated Total = 12,760 Deaths

ALPHA ORDER

RANK	STATE	DEATHS	% of USA
21	Alabama	210	1.6%
NA	Alaska*	NA	NA
20	Arizona	240	1.9%
29	Arkansas	160	1.3%
1	California	1,460	11.4%
25	Colorado	180	1.4%
32	Connecticut	140	1.1%
NA	Delaware*	NA	NA
2	Florida	930	7.3%
14	Georgia	300	2.4%
NA	Hawaii*	NA	NA
39	Idaho	70	0.5%
7	Illinois	480	3.8%
11	Indiana	320	2.5%
29	Iowa	160	1.3%
33	Kansas	130	1.0%
29	Kentucky	160	1.3%
23	Louisiana	190	1.5%
38	Maine	80	0.6%
22	Maryland	200	1.6%
15	Massachusetts	280	2.2%
8	Michigan	450	3.5%
19	Minnesota	250	2.0%
27	Mississippi	170	1.3%
17	Missouri	260	2.0%
42	Montana	50	0.4%
34	Nebraska	90	0.7%
34	Nevada	90	0.7%
39	New Hampshire	70	0.5%
11	New Jersey	320	2.5%
39	New Mexico	70	0.5%
4	New York	720	5.6%
10	North Carolina	340	2.7%
NA	North Dakota*	NA	NA
5	Ohio	530	4.2%
27	Oklahoma	170	1.3%
23	Oregon	190	1.5%
6	Pennsylvania	520	4.1%
42	Rhode Island	50	0.4%
25	South Carolina	180	1.4%
42	South Dakota	50	0.4%
11	Tennessee	320	2.5%
3	Texas	910	7.1%
34	Utah	90	0.7%
NA	Vermont*	NA	NA
16	Virginia	270	2.1%
9	Washington	350	2.7%
34	West Virginia	90	0.7%
17	Wisconsin	260	2.0%
NA	Wyoming*	NA	NA

RANK ORDER

RANK	STATE	DEATHS	% of USA
1	California	1,460	11.4%
2	Florida	930	7.3%
3	Texas	910	7.1%
4	New York	720	5.6%
5	Ohio	530	4.2%
6	Pennsylvania	520	4.1%
7	Illinois	480	3.8%
8	Michigan	450	3.5%
9	Washington	350	2.7%
10	North Carolina	340	2.7%
11	Indiana	320	2.5%
11	New Jersey	320	2.5%
11	Tennessee	320	2.5%
14	Georgia	300	2.4%
15	Massachusetts	280	2.2%
16	Virginia	270	2.1%
17	Missouri	260	2.0%
17	Wisconsin	260	2.0%
19	Minnesota	250	2.0%
20	Arizona	240	1.9%
21	Alabama	210	1.6%
22	Maryland	200	1.6%
23	Louisiana	190	1.5%
23	Oregon	190	1.5%
25	Colorado	180	1.4%
25	South Carolina	180	1.4%
27	Mississippi	170	1.3%
27	Oklahoma	170	1.3%
29	Arkansas	160	1.3%
29	Iowa	160	1.3%
29	Kentucky	160	1.3%
32	Connecticut	140	1.1%
33	Kansas	130	1.0%
34	Nebraska	90	0.7%
34	Nevada	90	0.7%
34	Utah	90	0.7%
34	West Virginia	90	0.7%
38	Maine	80	0.6%
39	Idaho	70	0.5%
39	New Hampshire	70	0.5%
39	New Mexico	70	0.5%
42	Montana	50	0.4%
42	Rhode Island	50	0.4%
42	South Dakota	50	0.4%
NA	Alaska*	NA	NA
NA	Delaware*	NA	NA
NA	Hawaii*	NA	NA
NA	North Dakota*	NA	NA
NA	Vermont*	NA	NA
NA	Wyoming*	NA	NA
	District of Columbia*	NA	NA

Source: American Cancer Society
   "Cancer Facts & Figures 2005" (Copyright 2005, American Cancer Society)
*Fewer than 50 deaths.

Estimated Death Rate by Brain Cancer in 2005

National Estimated Rate = 4.3 Deaths per 100,000 Population*

ALPHA ORDER

RANK	STATE	RATE
20	Alabama	4.6
NA	Alaska**	NA
27	Arizona	4.2
4	Arkansas	5.8
30	California	4.1
34	Colorado	3.9
31	Connecticut	4.0
NA	Delaware**	NA
10	Florida	5.3
44	Georgia	3.4
NA	Hawaii**	NA
14	Idaho	5.0
37	Illinois	3.8
13	Indiana	5.1
6	Iowa	5.4
17	Kansas	4.8
34	Kentucky	3.9
27	Louisiana	4.2
2	Maine	6.1
42	Maryland	3.6
24	Massachusetts	4.4
24	Michigan	4.4
16	Minnesota	4.9
3	Mississippi	5.9
23	Missouri	4.5
6	Montana	5.4
12	Nebraska	5.2
34	Nevada	3.9
6	New Hampshire	5.4
39	New Jersey	3.7
39	New Mexico	3.7
39	New York	3.7
31	North Carolina	4.0
NA	North Dakota**	NA
20	Ohio	4.6
17	Oklahoma	4.8
10	Oregon	5.3
27	Pennsylvania	4.2
20	Rhode Island	4.6
26	South Carolina	4.3
1	South Dakota	6.5
6	Tennessee	5.4
31	Texas	4.0
37	Utah	3.8
NA	Vermont**	NA
42	Virginia	3.6
5	Washington	5.6
14	West Virginia	5.0
19	Wisconsin	4.7
NA	Wyoming**	NA

RANK ORDER

RANK	STATE	RATE
1	South Dakota	6.5
2	Maine	6.1
3	Mississippi	5.9
4	Arkansas	5.8
5	Washington	5.6
6	Iowa	5.4
6	Montana	5.4
6	New Hampshire	5.4
6	Tennessee	5.4
10	Florida	5.3
10	Oregon	5.3
12	Nebraska	5.2
13	Indiana	5.1
14	Idaho	5.0
14	West Virginia	5.0
16	Minnesota	4.9
17	Kansas	4.8
17	Oklahoma	4.8
19	Wisconsin	4.7
20	Alabama	4.6
20	Ohio	4.6
20	Rhode Island	4.6
23	Missouri	4.5
24	Massachusetts	4.4
24	Michigan	4.4
26	South Carolina	4.3
27	Arizona	4.2
27	Louisiana	4.2
27	Pennsylvania	4.2
30	California	4.1
31	Connecticut	4.0
31	North Carolina	4.0
31	Texas	4.0
34	Colorado	3.9
34	Kentucky	3.9
34	Nevada	3.9
37	Illinois	3.8
37	Utah	3.8
39	New Jersey	3.7
39	New Mexico	3.7
39	New York	3.7
42	Maryland	3.6
42	Virginia	3.6
44	Georgia	3.4
NA	Alaska**	NA
NA	Delaware**	NA
NA	Hawaii**	NA
NA	North Dakota**	NA
NA	Vermont**	NA
NA	Wyoming**	NA
	District of Columbia**	NA

Source: Morgan Quitno Press using data from American Cancer Society
     "Cancer Facts & Figures 2005" (Copyright 2005, American Cancer Society)
*Rates calculated using 2004 Census resident population estimates. Not age-adjusted.
**Fewer than 50 deaths.

Estimated Deaths by Female Breast Cancer in 2005

National Estimated Total = 40,410 Deaths

ALPHA ORDER

RANK	STATE	DEATHS	% of USA
21	Alabama	730	1.8%
49	Alaska	50	0.1%
22	Arizona	720	1.8%
32	Arkansas	400	1.0%
1	California	4,050	10.0%
29	Colorado	490	1.2%
27	Connecticut	520	1.3%
45	Delaware	120	0.3%
3	Florida	2,570	6.4%
12	Georgia	1,120	2.8%
43	Hawaii	130	0.3%
39	Idaho	180	0.4%
7	Illinois	1,780	4.4%
14	Indiana	880	2.2%
31	Iowa	440	1.1%
33	Kansas	380	0.9%
23	Kentucky	630	1.6%
20	Louisiana	740	1.8%
40	Maine	170	0.4%
16	Maryland	840	2.1%
13	Massachusetts	940	2.3%
9	Michigan	1,380	3.4%
25	Minnesota	620	1.5%
30	Mississippi	450	1.1%
15	Missouri	870	2.2%
43	Montana	130	0.3%
36	Nebraska	230	0.6%
34	Nevada	310	0.8%
40	New Hampshire	170	0.4%
8	New Jersey	1,480	3.7%
38	New Mexico	190	0.5%
2	New York	2,760	6.8%
10	North Carolina	1,210	3.0%
46	North Dakota	100	0.2%
6	Ohio	1,850	4.6%
26	Oklahoma	540	1.3%
28	Oregon	500	1.2%
5	Pennsylvania	2,170	5.4%
42	Rhode Island	150	0.4%
23	South Carolina	630	1.6%
46	South Dakota	100	0.2%
17	Tennessee	810	2.0%
4	Texas	2,460	6.1%
37	Utah	220	0.5%
48	Vermont	90	0.2%
11	Virginia	1,150	2.8%
19	Washington	750	1.9%
35	West Virginia	270	0.7%
18	Wisconsin	790	2.0%
49	Wyoming	50	0.1%

RANK ORDER

RANK	STATE	DEATHS	% of USA
1	California	4,050	10.0%
2	New York	2,760	6.8%
3	Florida	2,570	6.4%
4	Texas	2,460	6.1%
5	Pennsylvania	2,170	5.4%
6	Ohio	1,850	4.6%
7	Illinois	1,780	4.4%
8	New Jersey	1,480	3.7%
9	Michigan	1,380	3.4%
10	North Carolina	1,210	3.0%
11	Virginia	1,150	2.8%
12	Georgia	1,120	2.8%
13	Massachusetts	940	2.3%
14	Indiana	880	2.2%
15	Missouri	870	2.2%
16	Maryland	840	2.1%
17	Tennessee	810	2.0%
18	Wisconsin	790	2.0%
19	Washington	750	1.9%
20	Louisiana	740	1.8%
21	Alabama	730	1.8%
22	Arizona	720	1.8%
23	Kentucky	630	1.6%
23	South Carolina	630	1.6%
25	Minnesota	620	1.5%
26	Oklahoma	540	1.3%
27	Connecticut	520	1.3%
28	Oregon	500	1.2%
29	Colorado	490	1.2%
30	Mississippi	450	1.1%
31	Iowa	440	1.1%
32	Arkansas	400	1.0%
33	Kansas	380	0.9%
34	Nevada	310	0.8%
35	West Virginia	270	0.7%
36	Nebraska	230	0.6%
37	Utah	220	0.5%
38	New Mexico	190	0.5%
39	Idaho	180	0.4%
40	Maine	170	0.4%
40	New Hampshire	170	0.4%
42	Rhode Island	150	0.4%
43	Hawaii	130	0.3%
43	Montana	130	0.3%
45	Delaware	120	0.3%
46	North Dakota	100	0.2%
46	South Dakota	100	0.2%
48	Vermont	90	0.2%
49	Alaska	50	0.1%
49	Wyoming	50	0.1%
	District of Columbia	100	0.2%

Source: American Cancer Society
"Cancer Facts & Figures 2005" (Copyright 2005, American Cancer Society)

Age-Adjusted Death Rate by Female Breast Cancer in 2001

National Rate = 27.0 Deaths per 100,000 Female Population*

ALPHA ORDER

RANK	STATE	RATE
23	Alabama	26.6
44	Alaska	23.9
37	Arizona	25.2
38	Arkansas	25.1
32	California	25.7
45	Colorado	23.6
17	Connecticut	27.2
2	Delaware	30.0
42	Florida	24.7
24	Georgia	26.5
50	Hawaii	19.7
34	Idaho	25.5
4	Illinois	29.2
13	Indiana	27.4
34	Iowa	25.5
36	Kansas	25.3
19	Kentucky	27.1
3	Louisiana	29.9
38	Maine	25.1
7	Maryland	28.8
11	Massachusetts	27.8
12	Michigan	27.5
30	Minnesota	25.9
10	Mississippi	28.2
21	Missouri	26.9
45	Montana	23.6
43	Nebraska	24.4
26	Nevada	26.4
19	New Hampshire	27.1
1	New Jersey	30.5
47	New Mexico	23.4
6	New York	28.9
24	North Carolina	26.5
30	North Dakota	25.9
5	Ohio	29.0
26	Oklahoma	26.4
28	Oregon	26.3
7	Pennsylvania	28.8
17	Rhode Island	27.2
13	South Carolina	27.4
48	South Dakota	23.3
22	Tennessee	26.8
33	Texas	25.6
48	Utah	23.3
13	Vermont	27.4
9	Virginia	28.4
41	Washington	25.0
16	West Virginia	27.3
29	Wisconsin	26.2
38	Wyoming	25.1

RANK ORDER

RANK	STATE	RATE
1	New Jersey	30.5
2	Delaware	30.0
3	Louisiana	29.9
4	Illinois	29.2
5	Ohio	29.0
6	New York	28.9
7	Maryland	28.8
7	Pennsylvania	28.8
9	Virginia	28.4
10	Mississippi	28.2
11	Massachusetts	27.8
12	Michigan	27.5
13	Indiana	27.4
13	South Carolina	27.4
13	Vermont	27.4
16	West Virginia	27.3
17	Connecticut	27.2
17	Rhode Island	27.2
19	Kentucky	27.1
19	New Hampshire	27.1
21	Missouri	26.9
22	Tennessee	26.8
23	Alabama	26.6
24	Georgia	26.5
24	North Carolina	26.5
26	Nevada	26.4
26	Oklahoma	26.4
28	Oregon	26.3
29	Wisconsin	26.2
30	Minnesota	25.9
30	North Dakota	25.9
32	California	25.7
33	Texas	25.6
34	Idaho	25.5
34	Iowa	25.5
36	Kansas	25.3
37	Arizona	25.2
38	Arkansas	25.1
38	Maine	25.1
38	Wyoming	25.1
41	Washington	25.0
42	Florida	24.7
43	Nebraska	24.4
44	Alaska	23.9
45	Colorado	23.6
45	Montana	23.6
47	New Mexico	23.4
48	South Dakota	23.3
48	Utah	23.3
50	Hawaii	19.7

| | District of Columbia | 37.3 |

Source: American Cancer Society
    "Cancer Facts & Figures 2005" (Copyright 2005, American Cancer Society)
*For 1997 to 2001. Age-adjusted to the 2000 U.S. standard population.

Estimated Deaths by Colon and Rectum Cancer in 2005

National Estimated Total = 56,290 Deaths

ALPHA ORDER

RANK	STATE	DEATHS	% of USA
23	Alabama	890	1.6%
50	Alaska	80	0.1%
21	Arizona	970	1.7%
31	Arkansas	630	1.1%
1	California	5,450	9.7%
30	Colorado	640	1.1%
29	Connecticut	650	1.2%
46	Delaware	160	0.3%
2	Florida	3,820	6.8%
13	Georgia	1,350	2.4%
42	Hawaii	210	0.4%
42	Idaho	210	0.4%
6	Illinois	2,560	4.5%
14	Indiana	1,320	2.3%
28	Iowa	660	1.2%
33	Kansas	610	1.1%
22	Kentucky	910	1.6%
20	Louisiana	1,000	1.8%
38	Maine	310	0.6%
17	Maryland	1,070	1.9%
11	Massachusetts	1,380	2.5%
8	Michigan	1,870	3.3%
25	Minnesota	860	1.5%
31	Mississippi	630	1.1%
15	Missouri	1,250	2.2%
44	Montana	180	0.3%
36	Nebraska	400	0.7%
35	Nevada	480	0.9%
41	New Hampshire	240	0.4%
9	New Jersey	1,810	3.2%
37	New Mexico	340	0.6%
3	New York	3,760	6.7%
10	North Carolina	1,590	2.8%
47	North Dakota	140	0.2%
7	Ohio	2,520	4.5%
26	Oklahoma	780	1.4%
27	Oregon	680	1.2%
5	Pennsylvania	3,150	5.6%
40	Rhode Island	250	0.4%
23	South Carolina	890	1.6%
44	South Dakota	180	0.3%
16	Tennessee	1,220	2.2%
4	Texas	3,590	6.4%
39	Utah	260	0.5%
48	Vermont	130	0.2%
11	Virginia	1,380	2.5%
19	Washington	1,030	1.8%
34	West Virginia	490	0.9%
17	Wisconsin	1,070	1.9%
49	Wyoming	110	0.2%

RANK ORDER

RANK	STATE	DEATHS	% of USA
1	California	5,450	9.7%
2	Florida	3,820	6.8%
3	New York	3,760	6.7%
4	Texas	3,590	6.4%
5	Pennsylvania	3,150	5.6%
6	Illinois	2,560	4.5%
7	Ohio	2,520	4.5%
8	Michigan	1,870	3.3%
9	New Jersey	1,810	3.2%
10	North Carolina	1,590	2.8%
11	Massachusetts	1,380	2.5%
11	Virginia	1,380	2.5%
13	Georgia	1,350	2.4%
14	Indiana	1,320	2.3%
15	Missouri	1,250	2.2%
16	Tennessee	1,220	2.2%
17	Maryland	1,070	1.9%
17	Wisconsin	1,070	1.9%
19	Washington	1,030	1.8%
20	Louisiana	1,000	1.8%
21	Arizona	970	1.7%
22	Kentucky	910	1.6%
23	Alabama	890	1.6%
23	South Carolina	890	1.6%
25	Minnesota	860	1.5%
26	Oklahoma	780	1.4%
27	Oregon	680	1.2%
28	Iowa	660	1.2%
29	Connecticut	650	1.2%
30	Colorado	640	1.1%
31	Arkansas	630	1.1%
31	Mississippi	630	1.1%
33	Kansas	610	1.1%
34	West Virginia	490	0.9%
35	Nevada	480	0.9%
36	Nebraska	400	0.7%
37	New Mexico	340	0.6%
38	Maine	310	0.6%
39	Utah	260	0.5%
40	Rhode Island	250	0.4%
41	New Hampshire	240	0.4%
42	Hawaii	210	0.4%
42	Idaho	210	0.4%
44	Montana	180	0.3%
44	South Dakota	180	0.3%
46	Delaware	160	0.3%
47	North Dakota	140	0.2%
48	Vermont	130	0.2%
49	Wyoming	110	0.2%
50	Alaska	80	0.1%
	District of Columbia	130	0.2%

Source: American Cancer Society
  "Cancer Facts & Figures 2005" (Copyright 2005, American Cancer Society)

Estimated Death Rate by Colon and Rectum Cancer in 2005

National Estimated Rate = 19.2 Deaths per 100,000 Population*

ALPHA ORDER

RANK ORDER

RANK	STATE	RATE		RANK	STATE	RATE
27	Alabama	19.6		1	West Virginia	27.0
49	Alaska	12.2		2	Pennsylvania	25.4
40	Arizona	16.9		3	Maine	23.5
6	Arkansas	22.9		4	South Dakota	23.3
46	California	15.2		5	Rhode Island	23.1
48	Colorado	13.9		6	Arkansas	22.9
34	Connecticut	18.6		6	Nebraska	22.9
31	Delaware	19.3		8	Iowa	22.3
13	Florida	22.0		8	Kansas	22.3
45	Georgia	15.3		10	Louisiana	22.1
42	Hawaii	16.6		10	North Dakota	22.1
47	Idaho	15.1		10	Oklahoma	22.1
26	Illinois	20.1		13	Florida	22.0
20	Indiana	21.2		13	Ohio	22.0
8	Iowa	22.3		15	Kentucky	21.9
8	Kansas	22.3		16	Mississippi	21.7
15	Kentucky	21.9		16	Missouri	21.7
10	Louisiana	22.1		16	Wyoming	21.7
3	Maine	23.5		19	Massachusetts	21.5
31	Maryland	19.3		20	Indiana	21.2
19	Massachusetts	21.5		20	South Carolina	21.2
36	Michigan	18.5		22	Vermont	20.9
40	Minnesota	16.9		23	New Jersey	20.8
16	Mississippi	21.7		24	Tennessee	20.7
16	Missouri	21.7		25	Nevada	20.6
29	Montana	19.4		26	Illinois	20.1
6	Nebraska	22.9		27	Alabama	19.6
25	Nevada	20.6		27	New York	19.6
36	New Hampshire	18.5		29	Montana	19.4
23	New Jersey	20.8		29	Wisconsin	19.4
39	New Mexico	17.9		31	Delaware	19.3
27	New York	19.6		31	Maryland	19.3
34	North Carolina	18.6		33	Oregon	18.9
10	North Dakota	22.1		34	Connecticut	18.6
13	Ohio	22.0		34	North Carolina	18.6
10	Oklahoma	22.1		36	Michigan	18.5
33	Oregon	18.9		36	New Hampshire	18.5
2	Pennsylvania	25.4		36	Virginia	18.5
5	Rhode Island	23.1		39	New Mexico	17.9
20	South Carolina	21.2		40	Arizona	16.9
4	South Dakota	23.3		40	Minnesota	16.9
24	Tennessee	20.7		42	Hawaii	16.6
44	Texas	16.0		42	Washington	16.6
50	Utah	10.9		44	Texas	16.0
22	Vermont	20.9		45	Georgia	15.3
36	Virginia	18.5		46	California	15.2
42	Washington	16.6		47	Idaho	15.1
1	West Virginia	27.0		48	Colorado	13.9
29	Wisconsin	19.4		49	Alaska	12.2
16	Wyoming	21.7		50	Utah	10.9

District of Columbia   23.5

Source: Morgan Quitno Press using data from American Cancer Society
"Cancer Facts & Figures 2005" (Copyright 2005, American Cancer Society)
Rates calculated using 2004 Census resident population estimates. Not age-adjusted.

Estimated Deaths by Leukemia in 2005

National Estimated Total = 22,570 Deaths

ALPHA ORDER

RANK	STATE	DEATHS	% of USA
22	Alabama	360	1.6%
NA	Alaska*	NA	NA
21	Arizona	400	1.8%
30	Arkansas	260	1.2%
1	California	2,190	9.7%
27	Colorado	300	1.3%
30	Connecticut	260	1.2%
43	Delaware	80	0.4%
2	Florida	1,700	7.5%
13	Georgia	530	2.3%
43	Hawaii	80	0.4%
40	Idaho	100	0.4%
6	Illinois	1,050	4.7%
13	Indiana	530	2.3%
26	Iowa	310	1.4%
33	Kansas	230	1.0%
25	Kentucky	320	1.4%
23	Louisiana	350	1.6%
40	Maine	100	0.4%
19	Maryland	440	1.9%
15	Massachusetts	500	2.2%
8	Michigan	810	3.6%
20	Minnesota	430	1.9%
32	Mississippi	240	1.1%
11	Missouri	540	2.4%
42	Montana	90	0.4%
35	Nebraska	160	0.7%
34	Nevada	170	0.8%
38	New Hampshire	110	0.5%
9	New Jersey	710	3.1%
38	New Mexico	110	0.5%
4	New York	1,410	6.2%
10	North Carolina	640	2.8%
46	North Dakota	70	0.3%
7	Ohio	980	4.3%
27	Oklahoma	300	1.3%
29	Oregon	270	1.2%
5	Pennsylvania	1,060	4.7%
43	Rhode Island	80	0.4%
24	South Carolina	330	1.5%
46	South Dakota	70	0.3%
17	Tennessee	490	2.2%
3	Texas	1,460	6.5%
36	Utah	140	0.6%
48	Vermont	60	0.3%
11	Virginia	540	2.4%
18	Washington	470	2.1%
36	West Virginia	140	0.6%
15	Wisconsin	500	2.2%
NA	Wyoming*	NA	NA

RANK ORDER

RANK	STATE	DEATHS	% of USA
1	California	2,190	9.7%
2	Florida	1,700	7.5%
3	Texas	1,460	6.5%
4	New York	1,410	6.2%
5	Pennsylvania	1,060	4.7%
6	Illinois	1,050	4.7%
7	Ohio	980	4.3%
8	Michigan	810	3.6%
9	New Jersey	710	3.1%
10	North Carolina	640	2.8%
11	Missouri	540	2.4%
11	Virginia	540	2.4%
13	Georgia	530	2.3%
13	Indiana	530	2.3%
15	Massachusetts	500	2.2%
15	Wisconsin	500	2.2%
17	Tennessee	490	2.2%
18	Washington	470	2.1%
19	Maryland	440	1.9%
20	Minnesota	430	1.9%
21	Arizona	400	1.8%
22	Alabama	360	1.6%
23	Louisiana	350	1.6%
24	South Carolina	330	1.5%
25	Kentucky	320	1.4%
26	Iowa	310	1.4%
27	Colorado	300	1.3%
27	Oklahoma	300	1.3%
29	Oregon	270	1.2%
30	Arkansas	260	1.2%
30	Connecticut	260	1.2%
32	Mississippi	240	1.1%
33	Kansas	230	1.0%
34	Nevada	170	0.8%
35	Nebraska	160	0.7%
36	Utah	140	0.6%
36	West Virginia	140	0.6%
38	New Hampshire	110	0.5%
38	New Mexico	110	0.5%
40	Idaho	100	0.4%
40	Maine	100	0.4%
42	Montana	90	0.4%
43	Delaware	80	0.4%
43	Hawaii	80	0.4%
43	Rhode Island	80	0.4%
46	North Dakota	70	0.3%
46	South Dakota	70	0.3%
48	Vermont	60	0.3%
NA	Alaska*	NA	NA
NA	Wyoming*	NA	NA
	District of Columbia*	NA	NA

Source: American Cancer Society
   "Cancer Facts & Figures 2005" (Copyright 2005, American Cancer Society)
*Fewer than 50 deaths.

Estimated Death Rate by Leukemia in 2005

National Estimated Rate = 7.7 Deaths per 100,000 Population*

ALPHA ORDER

RANK	STATE	RATE
24	Alabama	7.9
NA	Alaska**	NA
41	Arizona	7.0
7	Arkansas	9.4
45	California	6.1
42	Colorado	6.5
35	Connecticut	7.4
6	Delaware	9.6
3	Florida	9.8
46	Georgia	6.0
44	Hawaii	6.3
39	Idaho	7.2
19	Illinois	8.3
13	Indiana	8.5
2	Iowa	10.5
17	Kansas	8.4
29	Kentucky	7.7
27	Louisiana	7.8
31	Maine	7.6
24	Maryland	7.9
27	Massachusetts	7.8
23	Michigan	8.0
17	Minnesota	8.4
19	Mississippi	8.3
7	Missouri	9.4
4	Montana	9.7
9	Nebraska	9.2
37	Nevada	7.3
13	New Hampshire	8.5
22	New Jersey	8.2
48	New Mexico	5.8
37	New York	7.3
33	North Carolina	7.5
1	North Dakota	11.0
12	Ohio	8.6
13	Oklahoma	8.5
33	Oregon	7.5
13	Pennsylvania	8.5
35	Rhode Island	7.4
24	South Carolina	7.9
10	South Dakota	9.1
19	Tennessee	8.3
42	Texas	6.5
47	Utah	5.9
4	Vermont	9.7
39	Virginia	7.2
31	Washington	7.6
29	West Virginia	7.7
10	Wisconsin	9.1
NA	Wyoming**	NA

RANK ORDER

RANK	STATE	RATE
1	North Dakota	11.0
2	Iowa	10.5
3	Florida	9.8
4	Montana	9.7
4	Vermont	9.7
6	Delaware	9.6
7	Arkansas	9.4
7	Missouri	9.4
9	Nebraska	9.2
10	South Dakota	9.1
10	Wisconsin	9.1
12	Ohio	8.6
13	Indiana	8.5
13	New Hampshire	8.5
13	Oklahoma	8.5
13	Pennsylvania	8.5
17	Kansas	8.4
17	Minnesota	8.4
19	Illinois	8.3
19	Mississippi	8.3
19	Tennessee	8.3
22	New Jersey	8.2
23	Michigan	8.0
24	Alabama	7.9
24	Maryland	7.9
24	South Carolina	7.9
27	Louisiana	7.8
27	Massachusetts	7.8
29	Kentucky	7.7
29	West Virginia	7.7
31	Maine	7.6
31	Washington	7.6
33	North Carolina	7.5
33	Oregon	7.5
35	Connecticut	7.4
35	Rhode Island	7.4
37	Nevada	7.3
37	New York	7.3
39	Idaho	7.2
39	Virginia	7.2
41	Arizona	7.0
42	Colorado	6.5
42	Texas	6.5
44	Hawaii	6.3
45	California	6.1
46	Georgia	6.0
47	Utah	5.9
48	New Mexico	5.8
NA	Alaska**	NA
NA	Wyoming**	NA
	District of Columbia**	NA

Source: Morgan Quitno Press using data from American Cancer Society
"Cancer Facts & Figures 2005" (Copyright 2005, American Cancer Society)
*Rates calculated using 2004 Census resident population estimates. Not age-adjusted.
**Fewer than 50 deaths.

Estimated Deaths by Liver Cancer in 2005

National Estimated Total = 15,420 Deaths

ALPHA ORDER

RANK	STATE	DEATHS	% of USA
17	Alabama	290	1.9%
NA	Alaska*	NA	NA
17	Arizona	290	1.9%
25	Arkansas	200	1.3%
1	California	2,070	13.4%
27	Colorado	170	1.1%
27	Connecticut	170	1.1%
NA	Delaware*	NA	NA
3	Florida	1,110	7.2%
12	Georgia	340	2.2%
37	Hawaii	100	0.6%
43	Idaho	50	0.3%
6	Illinois	680	4.4%
22	Indiana	250	1.6%
33	Iowa	120	0.8%
33	Kansas	120	0.8%
25	Kentucky	200	1.3%
15	Louisiana	310	2.0%
38	Maine	70	0.5%
21	Maryland	260	1.7%
11	Massachusetts	370	2.4%
8	Michigan	530	3.4%
24	Minnesota	210	1.4%
31	Mississippi	150	1.0%
17	Missouri	290	1.9%
43	Montana	50	0.3%
40	Nebraska	60	0.4%
33	Nevada	120	0.8%
38	New Hampshire	70	0.5%
9	New Jersey	410	2.7%
32	New Mexico	130	0.8%
4	New York	1,010	6.5%
10	North Carolina	380	2.5%
NA	North Dakota*	NA	NA
7	Ohio	570	3.7%
27	Oklahoma	170	1.1%
30	Oregon	160	1.0%
5	Pennsylvania	730	4.7%
40	Rhode Island	60	0.4%
23	South Carolina	220	1.4%
NA	South Dakota*	NA	NA
16	Tennessee	300	1.9%
2	Texas	1,280	8.3%
40	Utah	60	0.4%
NA	Vermont*	NA	NA
12	Virginia	340	2.2%
12	Washington	340	2.2%
36	West Virginia	110	0.7%
17	Wisconsin	290	1.9%
NA	Wyoming*	NA	NA

RANK ORDER

RANK	STATE	DEATHS	% of USA
1	California	2,070	13.4%
2	Texas	1,280	8.3%
3	Florida	1,110	7.2%
4	New York	1,010	6.5%
5	Pennsylvania	730	4.7%
6	Illinois	680	4.4%
7	Ohio	570	3.7%
8	Michigan	530	3.4%
9	New Jersey	410	2.7%
10	North Carolina	380	2.5%
11	Massachusetts	370	2.4%
12	Georgia	340	2.2%
12	Virginia	340	2.2%
12	Washington	340	2.2%
15	Louisiana	310	2.0%
16	Tennessee	300	1.9%
17	Alabama	290	1.9%
17	Arizona	290	1.9%
17	Missouri	290	1.9%
17	Wisconsin	290	1.9%
21	Maryland	260	1.7%
22	Indiana	250	1.6%
23	South Carolina	220	1.4%
24	Minnesota	210	1.4%
25	Arkansas	200	1.3%
25	Kentucky	200	1.3%
27	Colorado	170	1.1%
27	Connecticut	170	1.1%
27	Oklahoma	170	1.1%
30	Oregon	160	1.0%
31	Mississippi	150	1.0%
32	New Mexico	130	0.8%
33	Iowa	120	0.8%
33	Kansas	120	0.8%
33	Nevada	120	0.8%
36	West Virginia	110	0.7%
37	Hawaii	100	0.6%
38	Maine	70	0.5%
38	New Hampshire	70	0.5%
40	Nebraska	60	0.4%
40	Rhode Island	60	0.4%
40	Utah	60	0.4%
43	Idaho	50	0.3%
43	Montana	50	0.3%
NA	Alaska*	NA	NA
NA	Delaware*	NA	NA
NA	North Dakota*	NA	NA
NA	South Dakota*	NA	NA
NA	Vermont*	NA	NA
NA	Wyoming*	NA	NA
	District of Columbia*	NA	NA

Source: American Cancer Society
"Cancer Facts & Figures 2005" (Copyright 2005, American Cancer Society)
*Fewer than 50 deaths.

Estimated Death Rate by Liver Cancer in 2005

National Estimated Rate = 5.3 Deaths per 100,000 Population*

ALPHA ORDER

RANK	STATE	RATE
5	Alabama	6.4
NA	Alaska**	NA
25	Arizona	5.0
2	Arkansas	7.3
9	California	5.8
41	Colorado	3.7
28	Connecticut	4.9
NA	Delaware**	NA
5	Florida	6.4
40	Georgia	3.9
1	Hawaii	7.9
42	Idaho	3.6
16	Illinois	5.3
39	Indiana	4.0
37	Iowa	4.1
35	Kansas	4.4
29	Kentucky	4.8
3	Louisiana	6.9
16	Maine	5.3
31	Maryland	4.7
9	Massachusetts	5.8
20	Michigan	5.2
37	Minnesota	4.1
20	Mississippi	5.2
25	Missouri	5.0
14	Montana	5.4
43	Nebraska	3.4
23	Nevada	5.1
14	New Hampshire	5.4
31	New Jersey	4.7
4	New Mexico	6.8
16	New York	5.3
35	North Carolina	4.4
NA	North Dakota**	NA
25	Ohio	5.0
29	Oklahoma	4.8
34	Oregon	4.5
8	Pennsylvania	5.9
12	Rhode Island	5.6
20	South Carolina	5.2
NA	South Dakota**	NA
23	Tennessee	5.1
11	Texas	5.7
44	Utah	2.5
NA	Vermont**	NA
33	Virginia	4.6
13	Washington	5.5
7	West Virginia	6.1
16	Wisconsin	5.3
NA	Wyoming**	NA

RANK ORDER

RANK	STATE	RATE
1	Hawaii	7.9
2	Arkansas	7.3
3	Louisiana	6.9
4	New Mexico	6.8
5	Alabama	6.4
5	Florida	6.4
7	West Virginia	6.1
8	Pennsylvania	5.9
9	California	5.8
9	Massachusetts	5.8
11	Texas	5.7
12	Rhode Island	5.6
13	Washington	5.5
14	Montana	5.4
14	New Hampshire	5.4
16	Illinois	5.3
16	Maine	5.3
16	New York	5.3
16	Wisconsin	5.3
20	Michigan	5.2
20	Mississippi	5.2
20	South Carolina	5.2
23	Nevada	5.1
23	Tennessee	5.1
25	Arizona	5.0
25	Missouri	5.0
25	Ohio	5.0
28	Connecticut	4.9
29	Kentucky	4.8
29	Oklahoma	4.8
31	Maryland	4.7
31	New Jersey	4.7
33	Virginia	4.6
34	Oregon	4.5
35	Kansas	4.4
35	North Carolina	4.4
37	Iowa	4.1
37	Minnesota	4.1
39	Indiana	4.0
40	Georgia	3.9
41	Colorado	3.7
42	Idaho	3.6
43	Nebraska	3.4
44	Utah	2.5
NA	Alaska**	NA
NA	Delaware**	NA
NA	North Dakota**	NA
NA	South Dakota**	NA
NA	Vermont**	NA
NA	Wyoming**	NA
	District of Columbia**	NA

Source: Morgan Quitno Press using data from American Cancer Society
    "Cancer Facts & Figures 2005" (Copyright 2005, American Cancer Society)
*Rates calculated using 2004 Census resident population estimates. Not age-adjusted.
**Fewer than 50 deaths.

Estimated Deaths by Lung Cancer in 2005

National Estimated Total = 163,510 Deaths

ALPHA ORDER

RANK	STATE	DEATHS	% of USA
19	Alabama	3,160	1.9%
50	Alaska	210	0.1%
24	Arizona	2,720	1.7%
27	Arkansas	2,400	1.5%
1	California	14,350	8.8%
32	Colorado	1,660	1.0%
30	Connecticut	1,850	1.1%
44	Delaware	460	0.3%
2	Florida	12,440	7.6%
11	Georgia	4,550	2.8%
43	Hawaii	480	0.3%
41	Idaho	600	0.4%
7	Illinois	6,840	4.2%
13	Indiana	4,180	2.6%
31	Iowa	1,700	1.0%
34	Kansas	1,540	0.9%
17	Kentucky	3,490	2.1%
21	Louisiana	2,930	1.8%
37	Maine	940	0.6%
20	Maryland	3,040	1.9%
16	Massachusetts	3,800	2.3%
8	Michigan	5,790	3.5%
25	Minnesota	2,480	1.5%
28	Mississippi	2,070	1.3%
15	Missouri	3,860	2.4%
42	Montana	590	0.4%
36	Nebraska	950	0.6%
35	Nevada	1,450	0.9%
38	New Hampshire	750	0.5%
10	New Jersey	4,580	2.8%
39	New Mexico	720	0.4%
4	New York	9,350	5.7%
9	North Carolina	5,230	3.2%
48	North Dakota	310	0.2%
6	Ohio	7,380	4.5%
26	Oklahoma	2,440	1.5%
29	Oregon	2,050	1.3%
5	Pennsylvania	8,030	4.9%
40	Rhode Island	680	0.4%
23	South Carolina	2,730	1.7%
46	South Dakota	410	0.3%
12	Tennessee	4,390	2.7%
3	Texas	10,620	6.5%
45	Utah	440	0.3%
47	Vermont	370	0.2%
14	Virginia	4,170	2.6%
18	Washington	3,260	2.0%
33	West Virginia	1,610	1.0%
22	Wisconsin	2,900	1.8%
49	Wyoming	270	0.2%

RANK ORDER

RANK	STATE	DEATHS	% of USA
1	California	14,350	8.8%
2	Florida	12,440	7.6%
3	Texas	10,620	6.5%
4	New York	9,350	5.7%
5	Pennsylvania	8,030	4.9%
6	Ohio	7,380	4.5%
7	Illinois	6,840	4.2%
8	Michigan	5,790	3.5%
9	North Carolina	5,230	3.2%
10	New Jersey	4,580	2.8%
11	Georgia	4,550	2.8%
12	Tennessee	4,390	2.7%
13	Indiana	4,180	2.6%
14	Virginia	4,170	2.6%
15	Missouri	3,860	2.4%
16	Massachusetts	3,800	2.3%
17	Kentucky	3,490	2.1%
18	Washington	3,260	2.0%
19	Alabama	3,160	1.9%
20	Maryland	3,040	1.9%
21	Louisiana	2,930	1.8%
22	Wisconsin	2,900	1.8%
23	South Carolina	2,730	1.7%
24	Arizona	2,720	1.7%
25	Minnesota	2,480	1.5%
26	Oklahoma	2,440	1.5%
27	Arkansas	2,400	1.5%
28	Mississippi	2,070	1.3%
29	Oregon	2,050	1.3%
30	Connecticut	1,850	1.1%
31	Iowa	1,700	1.0%
32	Colorado	1,660	1.0%
33	West Virginia	1,610	1.0%
34	Kansas	1,540	0.9%
35	Nevada	1,450	0.9%
36	Nebraska	950	0.6%
37	Maine	940	0.6%
38	New Hampshire	750	0.5%
39	New Mexico	720	0.4%
40	Rhode Island	680	0.4%
41	Idaho	600	0.4%
42	Montana	590	0.4%
43	Hawaii	480	0.3%
44	Delaware	460	0.3%
45	Utah	440	0.3%
46	South Dakota	410	0.3%
47	Vermont	370	0.2%
48	North Dakota	310	0.2%
49	Wyoming	270	0.2%
50	Alaska	210	0.1%
	District of Columbia	290	0.2%

Source: American Cancer Society
"Cancer Facts & Figures 2005" (Copyright 2005, American Cancer Society)

Estimated Death Rate by Lung Cancer in 2005

National Estimated Rate = 55.7 Deaths per 100,000 Population*

ALPHA ORDER

RANK	STATE	RATE
8	Alabama	69.8
49	Alaska	32.0
42	Arizona	47.4
2	Arkansas	87.2
45	California	40.0
48	Colorado	36.1
34	Connecticut	52.8
28	Delaware	55.4
5	Florida	71.5
38	Georgia	51.5
46	Hawaii	38.0
44	Idaho	43.1
31	Illinois	53.8
11	Indiana	67.0
23	Iowa	57.5
26	Kansas	56.3
3	Kentucky	84.2
13	Louisiana	64.9
6	Maine	71.4
29	Maryland	54.7
21	Massachusetts	59.2
24	Michigan	57.3
40	Minnesota	48.6
7	Mississippi	71.3
10	Missouri	67.1
16	Montana	63.7
30	Nebraska	54.4
18	Nevada	62.1
22	New Hampshire	57.7
35	New Jersey	52.7
47	New Mexico	37.8
40	New York	48.6
19	North Carolina	61.2
39	North Dakota	48.9
15	Ohio	64.4
9	Oklahoma	69.2
25	Oregon	57.0
14	Pennsylvania	64.7
17	Rhode Island	62.9
12	South Carolina	65.0
33	South Dakota	53.2
4	Tennessee	74.4
43	Texas	47.2
50	Utah	18.4
20	Vermont	59.5
27	Virginia	55.9
37	Washington	52.5
1	West Virginia	88.7
36	Wisconsin	52.6
32	Wyoming	53.3

RANK ORDER

RANK	STATE	RATE
1	West Virginia	88.7
2	Arkansas	87.2
3	Kentucky	84.2
4	Tennessee	74.4
5	Florida	71.5
6	Maine	71.4
7	Mississippi	71.3
8	Alabama	69.8
9	Oklahoma	69.2
10	Missouri	67.1
11	Indiana	67.0
12	South Carolina	65.0
13	Louisiana	64.9
14	Pennsylvania	64.7
15	Ohio	64.4
16	Montana	63.7
17	Rhode Island	62.9
18	Nevada	62.1
19	North Carolina	61.2
20	Vermont	59.5
21	Massachusetts	59.2
22	New Hampshire	57.7
23	Iowa	57.5
24	Michigan	57.3
25	Oregon	57.0
26	Kansas	56.3
27	Virginia	55.9
28	Delaware	55.4
29	Maryland	54.7
30	Nebraska	54.4
31	Illinois	53.8
32	Wyoming	53.3
33	South Dakota	53.2
34	Connecticut	52.8
35	New Jersey	52.7
36	Wisconsin	52.6
37	Washington	52.5
38	Georgia	51.5
39	North Dakota	48.9
40	Minnesota	48.6
40	New York	48.6
42	Arizona	47.4
43	Texas	47.2
44	Idaho	43.1
45	California	40.0
46	Hawaii	38.0
47	New Mexico	37.8
48	Colorado	36.1
49	Alaska	32.0
50	Utah	18.4

	District of Columbia	52.4

Source: Morgan Quitno Press using data from American Cancer Society
"Cancer Facts & Figures 2005" (Copyright 2005, American Cancer Society)
*Rates calculated using 2004 Census resident population estimates. Not age-adjusted.

Estimated Deaths by Non-Hodgkin's Lymphoma in 2005

National Estimated Total = 19,200 Deaths

ALPHA ORDER

RANK	STATE	DEATHS	% of USA
25	Alabama	320	1.7%
NA	Alaska*	NA	NA
20	Arizona	360	1.9%
31	Arkansas	220	1.1%
1	California	1,940	10.1%
27	Colorado	300	1.6%
29	Connecticut	250	1.3%
44	Delaware	70	0.4%
2	Florida	1,180	6.1%
14	Georgia	470	2.4%
41	Hawaii	90	0.5%
44	Idaho	70	0.4%
6	Illinois	750	3.9%
12	Indiana	480	2.5%
28	Iowa	260	1.4%
31	Kansas	220	1.1%
24	Kentucky	330	1.7%
20	Louisiana	360	1.9%
41	Maine	90	0.5%
22	Maryland	350	1.8%
17	Massachusetts	430	2.2%
7	Michigan	730	3.8%
14	Minnesota	470	2.4%
33	Mississippi	180	0.9%
11	Missouri	520	2.7%
44	Montana	70	0.4%
36	Nebraska	130	0.7%
35	Nevada	150	0.8%
38	New Hampshire	110	0.6%
9	New Jersey	600	3.1%
38	New Mexico	110	0.6%
4	New York	1,000	5.2%
9	North Carolina	600	3.1%
47	North Dakota	60	0.3%
8	Ohio	670	3.5%
30	Oklahoma	230	1.2%
23	Oregon	340	1.8%
5	Pennsylvania	980	5.1%
40	Rhode Island	100	0.5%
25	South Carolina	320	1.7%
43	South Dakota	80	0.4%
16	Tennessee	460	2.4%
3	Texas	1,040	5.4%
36	Utah	130	0.7%
47	Vermont	60	0.3%
18	Virginia	400	2.1%
12	Washington	480	2.5%
34	West Virginia	170	0.9%
19	Wisconsin	380	2.0%
NA	Wyoming*	NA	NA

RANK ORDER

RANK	STATE	DEATHS	% of USA
1	California	1,940	10.1%
2	Florida	1,180	6.1%
3	Texas	1,040	5.4%
4	New York	1,000	5.2%
5	Pennsylvania	980	5.1%
6	Illinois	750	3.9%
7	Michigan	730	3.8%
8	Ohio	670	3.5%
9	New Jersey	600	3.1%
9	North Carolina	600	3.1%
11	Missouri	520	2.7%
12	Indiana	480	2.5%
12	Washington	480	2.5%
14	Georgia	470	2.4%
14	Minnesota	470	2.4%
16	Tennessee	460	2.4%
17	Massachusetts	430	2.2%
18	Virginia	400	2.1%
19	Wisconsin	380	2.0%
20	Arizona	360	1.9%
20	Louisiana	360	1.9%
22	Maryland	350	1.8%
23	Oregon	340	1.8%
24	Kentucky	330	1.7%
25	Alabama	320	1.7%
25	South Carolina	320	1.7%
27	Colorado	300	1.6%
28	Iowa	260	1.4%
29	Connecticut	250	1.3%
30	Oklahoma	230	1.2%
31	Arkansas	220	1.1%
31	Kansas	220	1.1%
33	Mississippi	180	0.9%
34	West Virginia	170	0.9%
35	Nevada	150	0.8%
36	Nebraska	130	0.7%
36	Utah	130	0.7%
38	New Hampshire	110	0.6%
38	New Mexico	110	0.6%
40	Rhode Island	100	0.5%
41	Hawaii	90	0.5%
41	Maine	90	0.5%
43	South Dakota	80	0.4%
44	Delaware	70	0.4%
44	Idaho	70	0.4%
44	Montana	70	0.4%
47	North Dakota	60	0.3%
47	Vermont	60	0.3%
NA	Alaska*	NA	NA
NA	Wyoming*	NA	NA
	District of Columbia*	NA	NA

Source: American Cancer Society
     "Cancer Facts & Figures 2005" (Copyright 2005, American Cancer Society)
*Fewer than 50 deaths.

121

Estimated Death Rate by Non-Hodgkin's Lymphoma in 2005

National Estimated Rate = 6.5 Deaths per 100,000 Population*

ALPHA ORDER

RANK	STATE	RATE
24	Alabama	7.1
NA	Alaska**	NA
36	Arizona	6.3
12	Arkansas	8.0
42	California	5.4
33	Colorado	6.5
24	Connecticut	7.1
11	Delaware	8.4
30	Florida	6.8
45	Georgia	5.3
24	Hawaii	7.1
47	Idaho	5.0
39	Illinois	5.9
18	Indiana	7.7
9	Iowa	8.8
12	Kansas	8.0
12	Kentucky	8.0
12	Louisiana	8.0
30	Maine	6.8
36	Maryland	6.3
32	Massachusetts	6.7
23	Michigan	7.2
7	Minnesota	9.2
38	Mississippi	6.2
8	Missouri	9.0
20	Montana	7.6
22	Nebraska	7.4
35	Nevada	6.4
10	New Hampshire	8.5
28	New Jersey	6.9
40	New Mexico	5.8
46	New York	5.2
27	North Carolina	7.0
3	North Dakota	9.5
40	Ohio	5.8
33	Oklahoma	6.5
3	Oregon	9.5
16	Pennsylvania	7.9
6	Rhode Island	9.3
20	South Carolina	7.6
1	South Dakota	10.4
17	Tennessee	7.8
48	Texas	4.6
42	Utah	5.4
2	Vermont	9.7
42	Virginia	5.4
18	Washington	7.7
5	West Virginia	9.4
28	Wisconsin	6.9
NA	Wyoming**	NA

RANK ORDER

RANK	STATE	RATE
1	South Dakota	10.4
2	Vermont	9.7
3	North Dakota	9.5
3	Oregon	9.5
5	West Virginia	9.4
6	Rhode Island	9.3
7	Minnesota	9.2
8	Missouri	9.0
9	Iowa	8.8
10	New Hampshire	8.5
11	Delaware	8.4
12	Arkansas	8.0
12	Kansas	8.0
12	Kentucky	8.0
12	Louisiana	8.0
16	Pennsylvania	7.9
17	Tennessee	7.8
18	Indiana	7.7
18	Washington	7.7
20	Montana	7.6
20	South Carolina	7.6
22	Nebraska	7.4
23	Michigan	7.2
24	Alabama	7.1
24	Connecticut	7.1
24	Hawaii	7.1
27	North Carolina	7.0
28	New Jersey	6.9
28	Wisconsin	6.9
30	Florida	6.8
30	Maine	6.8
32	Massachusetts	6.7
33	Colorado	6.5
33	Oklahoma	6.5
35	Nevada	6.4
36	Arizona	6.3
36	Maryland	6.3
38	Mississippi	6.2
39	Illinois	5.9
40	New Mexico	5.8
40	Ohio	5.8
42	California	5.4
42	Utah	5.4
42	Virginia	5.4
45	Georgia	5.3
46	New York	5.2
47	Idaho	5.0
48	Texas	4.6
NA	Alaska**	NA
NA	Wyoming**	NA
	District of Columbia**	NA

Source: Morgan Quitno Press using data from American Cancer Society
"Cancer Facts & Figures 2005" (Copyright 2005, American Cancer Society)
*Rates calculated using 2004 Census resident population estimates. Not age-adjusted.
**Fewer than 50 deaths.

Estimated Deaths by Pancreatic Cancer in 2005

National Estimated Total = 31,800 Deaths

ALPHA ORDER

RANK	STATE	DEATHS	% of USA
22	Alabama	530	1.7%
49	Alaska	50	0.2%
20	Arizona	550	1.7%
32	Arkansas	310	1.0%
1	California	3,150	9.9%
28	Colorado	400	1.3%
25	Connecticut	430	1.4%
44	Delaware	100	0.3%
3	Florida	2,250	7.1%
12	Georgia	770	2.4%
40	Hawaii	150	0.5%
43	Idaho	130	0.4%
6	Illinois	1,470	4.6%
14	Indiana	690	2.2%
29	Iowa	390	1.2%
33	Kansas	290	0.9%
26	Kentucky	420	1.3%
23	Louisiana	520	1.6%
36	Maine	180	0.6%
19	Maryland	590	1.9%
11	Massachusetts	850	2.7%
8	Michigan	1,140	3.6%
20	Minnesota	550	1.7%
31	Mississippi	330	1.0%
17	Missouri	670	2.1%
44	Montana	100	0.3%
36	Nebraska	180	0.6%
34	Nevada	230	0.7%
41	New Hampshire	140	0.4%
9	New Jersey	1,050	3.3%
36	New Mexico	180	0.6%
2	New York	2,270	7.1%
10	North Carolina	910	2.9%
47	North Dakota	80	0.3%
7	Ohio	1,300	4.1%
30	Oklahoma	360	1.1%
27	Oregon	410	1.3%
5	Pennsylvania	1,670	5.3%
41	Rhode Island	140	0.4%
24	South Carolina	510	1.6%
46	South Dakota	90	0.3%
16	Tennessee	680	2.1%
4	Texas	1,950	6.1%
39	Utah	170	0.5%
48	Vermont	70	0.2%
13	Virginia	750	2.4%
14	Washington	690	2.2%
35	West Virginia	200	0.6%
18	Wisconsin	650	2.0%
49	Wyoming	50	0.2%

RANK ORDER

RANK	STATE	DEATHS	% of USA
1	California	3,150	9.9%
2	New York	2,270	7.1%
3	Florida	2,250	7.1%
4	Texas	1,950	6.1%
5	Pennsylvania	1,670	5.3%
6	Illinois	1,470	4.6%
7	Ohio	1,300	4.1%
8	Michigan	1,140	3.6%
9	New Jersey	1,050	3.3%
10	North Carolina	910	2.9%
11	Massachusetts	850	2.7%
12	Georgia	770	2.4%
13	Virginia	750	2.4%
14	Indiana	690	2.2%
14	Washington	690	2.2%
16	Tennessee	680	2.1%
17	Missouri	670	2.1%
18	Wisconsin	650	2.0%
19	Maryland	590	1.9%
20	Arizona	550	1.7%
20	Minnesota	550	1.7%
22	Alabama	530	1.7%
23	Louisiana	520	1.6%
24	South Carolina	510	1.6%
25	Connecticut	430	1.4%
26	Kentucky	420	1.3%
27	Oregon	410	1.3%
28	Colorado	400	1.3%
29	Iowa	390	1.2%
30	Oklahoma	360	1.1%
31	Mississippi	330	1.0%
32	Arkansas	310	1.0%
33	Kansas	290	0.9%
34	Nevada	230	0.7%
35	West Virginia	200	0.6%
36	Maine	180	0.6%
36	Nebraska	180	0.6%
36	New Mexico	180	0.6%
39	Utah	170	0.5%
40	Hawaii	150	0.5%
41	New Hampshire	140	0.4%
41	Rhode Island	140	0.4%
43	Idaho	130	0.4%
44	Delaware	100	0.3%
44	Montana	100	0.3%
46	South Dakota	90	0.3%
47	North Dakota	80	0.3%
48	Vermont	70	0.2%
49	Alaska	50	0.2%
49	Wyoming	50	0.2%
	District of Columbia	60	0.2%

Source: American Cancer Society
"Cancer Facts & Figures 2005" (Copyright 2005, American Cancer Society)

Estimated Death Rate by Pancreatic Cancer in 2005

National Estimated Rate = 10.8 Deaths per 100,000 Population*

ALPHA ORDER

RANK	STATE	RATE
15	Alabama	11.7
49	Alaska	7.6
42	Arizona	9.6
23	Arkansas	11.3
45	California	8.8
46	Colorado	8.7
8	Connecticut	12.3
11	Delaware	12.0
6	Florida	12.9
46	Georgia	8.7
12	Hawaii	11.9
44	Idaho	9.3
17	Illinois	11.6
27	Indiana	11.1
3	Iowa	13.2
34	Kansas	10.6
38	Kentucky	10.1
19	Louisiana	11.5
1	Maine	13.7
34	Maryland	10.6
3	Massachusetts	13.2
23	Michigan	11.3
30	Minnesota	10.8
21	Mississippi	11.4
17	Missouri	11.6
30	Montana	10.8
36	Nebraska	10.3
40	Nevada	9.9
30	New Hampshire	10.8
9	New Jersey	12.1
43	New Mexico	9.5
13	New York	11.8
33	North Carolina	10.7
7	North Dakota	12.6
23	Ohio	11.3
37	Oklahoma	10.2
21	Oregon	11.4
2	Pennsylvania	13.5
5	Rhode Island	13.0
9	South Carolina	12.1
15	South Dakota	11.7
19	Tennessee	11.5
46	Texas	8.7
50	Utah	7.1
23	Vermont	11.3
38	Virginia	10.1
27	Washington	11.1
29	West Virginia	11.0
13	Wisconsin	11.8
40	Wyoming	9.9

RANK ORDER

RANK	STATE	RATE
1	Maine	13.7
2	Pennsylvania	13.5
3	Iowa	13.2
3	Massachusetts	13.2
5	Rhode Island	13.0
6	Florida	12.9
7	North Dakota	12.6
8	Connecticut	12.3
9	New Jersey	12.1
9	South Carolina	12.1
11	Delaware	12.0
12	Hawaii	11.9
13	New York	11.8
13	Wisconsin	11.8
15	Alabama	11.7
15	South Dakota	11.7
17	Illinois	11.6
17	Missouri	11.6
19	Louisiana	11.5
19	Tennessee	11.5
21	Mississippi	11.4
21	Oregon	11.4
23	Arkansas	11.3
23	Michigan	11.3
23	Ohio	11.3
23	Vermont	11.3
27	Indiana	11.1
27	Washington	11.1
29	West Virginia	11.0
30	Minnesota	10.8
30	Montana	10.8
30	New Hampshire	10.8
33	North Carolina	10.7
34	Kansas	10.6
34	Maryland	10.6
36	Nebraska	10.3
37	Oklahoma	10.2
38	Kentucky	10.1
38	Virginia	10.1
40	Nevada	9.9
40	Wyoming	9.9
42	Arizona	9.6
43	New Mexico	9.5
44	Idaho	9.3
45	California	8.8
46	Colorado	8.7
46	Georgia	8.7
46	Texas	8.7
49	Alaska	7.6
50	Utah	7.1

	District of Columbia	10.8

Source: Morgan Quitno Press using data from American Cancer Society
   "Cancer Facts & Figures 2005" (Copyright 2005, American Cancer Society)
*Rates calculated using 2004 Census resident population estimates. Not age-adjusted.

Estimated Deaths by Prostate Cancer in 2005

National Estimated Total = 30,350 Deaths

ALPHA ORDER

RANK	STATE	DEATHS	% of USA
16	Alabama	570	1.9%
NA	Alaska*	NA	NA
22	Arizona	510	1.7%
32	Arkansas	270	0.9%
1	California	3,270	10.8%
29	Colorado	350	1.2%
24	Connecticut	440	1.4%
46	Delaware	80	0.3%
2	Florida	2,570	8.5%
12	Georgia	740	2.4%
43	Hawaii	120	0.4%
39	Idaho	150	0.5%
7	Illinois	1,230	4.1%
15	Indiana	640	2.1%
26	Iowa	400	1.3%
32	Kansas	270	0.9%
30	Kentucky	330	1.1%
23	Louisiana	450	1.5%
38	Maine	170	0.6%
19	Maryland	550	1.8%
14	Massachusetts	700	2.3%
8	Michigan	1,000	3.3%
16	Minnesota	570	1.9%
25	Mississippi	420	1.4%
26	Missouri	400	1.3%
42	Montana	130	0.4%
37	Nebraska	180	0.6%
34	Nevada	260	0.9%
39	New Hampshire	150	0.5%
10	New Jersey	840	2.8%
35	New Mexico	220	0.7%
3	New York	1,860	6.1%
9	North Carolina	890	2.9%
46	North Dakota	80	0.3%
6	Ohio	1,420	4.7%
31	Oklahoma	320	1.1%
28	Oregon	390	1.3%
5	Pennsylvania	1,720	5.7%
45	Rhode Island	110	0.4%
19	South Carolina	550	1.8%
43	South Dakota	120	0.4%
18	Tennessee	560	1.8%
4	Texas	1,750	5.8%
39	Utah	150	0.5%
49	Vermont	60	0.2%
11	Virginia	750	2.5%
13	Washington	720	2.4%
36	West Virginia	190	0.6%
21	Wisconsin	530	1.7%
46	Wyoming	80	0.3%

RANK ORDER

RANK	STATE	DEATHS	% of USA
1	California	3,270	10.8%
2	Florida	2,570	8.5%
3	New York	1,860	6.1%
4	Texas	1,750	5.8%
5	Pennsylvania	1,720	5.7%
6	Ohio	1,420	4.7%
7	Illinois	1,230	4.1%
8	Michigan	1,000	3.3%
9	North Carolina	890	2.9%
10	New Jersey	840	2.8%
11	Virginia	750	2.5%
12	Georgia	740	2.4%
13	Washington	720	2.4%
14	Massachusetts	700	2.3%
15	Indiana	640	2.1%
16	Alabama	570	1.9%
16	Minnesota	570	1.9%
18	Tennessee	560	1.8%
19	Maryland	550	1.8%
19	South Carolina	550	1.8%
21	Wisconsin	530	1.7%
22	Arizona	510	1.7%
23	Louisiana	450	1.5%
24	Connecticut	440	1.4%
25	Mississippi	420	1.4%
26	Iowa	400	1.3%
26	Missouri	400	1.3%
28	Oregon	390	1.3%
29	Colorado	350	1.2%
30	Kentucky	330	1.1%
31	Oklahoma	320	1.1%
32	Arkansas	270	0.9%
32	Kansas	270	0.9%
34	Nevada	260	0.9%
35	New Mexico	220	0.7%
36	West Virginia	190	0.6%
37	Nebraska	180	0.6%
38	Maine	170	0.6%
39	Idaho	150	0.5%
39	New Hampshire	150	0.5%
39	Utah	150	0.5%
42	Montana	130	0.4%
43	Hawaii	120	0.4%
43	South Dakota	120	0.4%
45	Rhode Island	110	0.4%
46	Delaware	80	0.3%
46	North Dakota	80	0.3%
46	Wyoming	80	0.3%
49	Vermont	60	0.2%
NA	Alaska*	NA	NA
	District of Columbia	80	0.3%

Source: American Cancer Society
    "Cancer Facts & Figures 2005" (Copyright 2005, American Cancer Society)
*Fewer than 50 deaths.

Age-Adjusted Death Rate by Prostate Cancer in 2001

National Rate = 31.5 Deaths per 100,000 Male Population*

ALPHA ORDER

RANK	STATE	RATE
2	Alabama	40.1
49	Alaska	25.1
48	Arizona	26.7
12	Arkansas	33.6
46	California	28.0
39	Colorado	29.6
45	Connecticut	28.6
19	Delaware	32.4
47	Florida	26.9
5	Georgia	38.0
50	Hawaii	21.2
22	Idaho	32.3
12	Illinois	33.6
14	Indiana	33.5
30	Iowa	31.2
42	Kansas	28.8
22	Kentucky	32.3
4	Louisiana	38.1
33	Maine	30.3
9	Maryland	34.6
27	Massachusetts	31.7
16	Michigan	33.0
17	Minnesota	32.9
1	Mississippi	43.2
41	Missouri	29.4
11	Montana	34.2
43	Nebraska	28.7
37	Nevada	29.8
35	New Hampshire	30.0
29	New Jersey	31.5
38	New Mexico	29.7
32	New York	30.4
6	North Carolina	36.9
19	North Dakota	32.4
24	Ohio	32.2
39	Oklahoma	29.6
19	Oregon	32.4
26	Pennsylvania	31.8
25	Rhode Island	32.0
2	South Carolina	40.1
28	South Dakota	31.6
10	Tennessee	34.3
31	Texas	31.1
15	Utah	33.1
36	Vermont	29.9
8	Virginia	36.1
43	Washington	28.7
34	West Virginia	30.1
18	Wisconsin	32.6
7	Wyoming	36.3

RANK ORDER

RANK	STATE	RATE
1	Mississippi	43.2
2	Alabama	40.1
2	South Carolina	40.1
4	Louisiana	38.1
5	Georgia	38.0
6	North Carolina	36.9
7	Wyoming	36.3
8	Virginia	36.1
9	Maryland	34.6
10	Tennessee	34.3
11	Montana	34.2
12	Arkansas	33.6
12	Illinois	33.6
14	Indiana	33.5
15	Utah	33.1
16	Michigan	33.0
17	Minnesota	32.9
18	Wisconsin	32.6
19	Delaware	32.4
19	North Dakota	32.4
19	Oregon	32.4
22	Idaho	32.3
22	Kentucky	32.3
24	Ohio	32.2
25	Rhode Island	32.0
26	Pennsylvania	31.8
27	Massachusetts	31.7
28	South Dakota	31.6
29	New Jersey	31.5
30	Iowa	31.2
31	Texas	31.1
32	New York	30.4
33	Maine	30.3
34	West Virginia	30.1
35	New Hampshire	30.0
36	Vermont	29.9
37	Nevada	29.8
38	New Mexico	29.7
39	Colorado	29.6
39	Oklahoma	29.6
41	Missouri	29.4
42	Kansas	28.8
43	Nebraska	28.7
43	Washington	28.7
45	Connecticut	28.6
46	California	28.0
47	Florida	26.9
48	Arizona	26.7
49	Alaska	25.1
50	Hawaii	21.2
	District of Columbia	49.9

Source: American Cancer Society
    "Cancer Facts & Figures 2005" (Copyright 2005, American Cancer Society)
*For 1997 to 2001. Age-adjusted to the 2000 U.S. standard population.

Estimated Deaths by Ovarian Cancer in 2005

National Estimated Total = 16,210 Deaths

ALPHA ORDER

RANK	STATE	DEATHS	% of USA
20	Alabama	300	1.9%
NA	Alaska*	NA	NA
21	Arizona	290	1.8%
31	Arkansas	160	1.0%
1	California	1,720	10.6%
25	Colorado	220	1.4%
28	Connecticut	200	1.2%
45	Delaware	50	0.3%
2	Florida	1,120	6.9%
11	Georgia	420	2.6%
45	Hawaii	50	0.3%
40	Idaho	80	0.5%
7	Illinois	650	4.0%
14	Indiana	380	2.3%
27	Iowa	210	1.3%
31	Kansas	160	1.0%
24	Kentucky	230	1.4%
25	Louisiana	220	1.4%
36	Maine	100	0.6%
19	Maryland	310	1.9%
14	Massachusetts	380	2.3%
8	Michigan	590	3.6%
22	Minnesota	270	1.7%
31	Mississippi	160	1.0%
17	Missouri	340	2.1%
41	Montana	70	0.4%
36	Nebraska	100	0.6%
35	Nevada	120	0.7%
42	New Hampshire	60	0.4%
9	New Jersey	540	3.3%
38	New Mexico	90	0.6%
3	New York	1,080	6.7%
10	North Carolina	470	2.9%
NA	North Dakota*	NA	NA
6	Ohio	660	4.1%
30	Oklahoma	180	1.1%
23	Oregon	240	1.5%
5	Pennsylvania	880	5.4%
42	Rhode Island	60	0.4%
29	South Carolina	190	1.2%
42	South Dakota	60	0.4%
16	Tennessee	350	2.2%
4	Texas	960	5.9%
38	Utah	90	0.6%
NA	Vermont*	NA	NA
12	Virginia	400	2.5%
13	Washington	390	2.4%
34	West Virginia	140	0.9%
18	Wisconsin	320	2.0%
NA	Wyoming*	NA	NA

RANK ORDER

RANK	STATE	DEATHS	% of USA
1	California	1,720	10.6%
2	Florida	1,120	6.9%
3	New York	1,080	6.7%
4	Texas	960	5.9%
5	Pennsylvania	880	5.4%
6	Ohio	660	4.1%
7	Illinois	650	4.0%
8	Michigan	590	3.6%
9	New Jersey	540	3.3%
10	North Carolina	470	2.9%
11	Georgia	420	2.6%
12	Virginia	400	2.5%
13	Washington	390	2.4%
14	Indiana	380	2.3%
14	Massachusetts	380	2.3%
16	Tennessee	350	2.2%
17	Missouri	340	2.1%
18	Wisconsin	320	2.0%
19	Maryland	310	1.9%
20	Alabama	300	1.9%
21	Arizona	290	1.8%
22	Minnesota	270	1.7%
23	Oregon	240	1.5%
24	Kentucky	230	1.4%
25	Colorado	220	1.4%
25	Louisiana	220	1.4%
27	Iowa	210	1.3%
28	Connecticut	200	1.2%
29	South Carolina	190	1.2%
30	Oklahoma	180	1.1%
31	Arkansas	160	1.0%
31	Kansas	160	1.0%
31	Mississippi	160	1.0%
34	West Virginia	140	0.9%
35	Nevada	120	0.7%
36	Maine	100	0.6%
36	Nebraska	100	0.6%
38	New Mexico	90	0.6%
38	Utah	90	0.6%
40	Idaho	80	0.5%
41	Montana	70	0.4%
42	New Hampshire	60	0.4%
42	Rhode Island	60	0.4%
42	South Dakota	60	0.4%
45	Delaware	50	0.3%
45	Hawaii	50	0.3%
NA	Alaska*	NA	NA
NA	North Dakota*	NA	NA
NA	Vermont*	NA	NA
NA	Wyoming*	NA	NA
	District of Columbia*	NA	NA

Source: American Cancer Society
   "Cancer Facts & Figures 2005" (Copyright 2005, American Cancer Society)
*Fewer than 50 deaths.

Estimated Death Rate by Ovarian Cancer in 2005

National Estimated Rate = 11.3 Deaths per 100,000 Female Population*

ALPHA ORDER

RANK	STATE	RATE
7	Alabama	13.8
NA	Alaska**	NA
35	Arizona	10.4
17	Arkansas	12.0
40	California	9.7
41	Colorado	9.6
20	Connecticut	11.8
12	Delaware	12.6
9	Florida	13.4
38	Georgia	9.8
45	Hawaii	7.9
23	Idaho	11.7
33	Illinois	10.5
13	Indiana	12.5
6	Iowa	14.5
20	Kansas	11.8
29	Kentucky	11.4
37	Louisiana	10.1
3	Maine	15.7
24	Maryland	11.6
15	Massachusetts	12.2
18	Michigan	11.9
32	Minnesota	10.8
28	Mississippi	11.5
15	Missouri	12.2
4	Montana	15.3
24	Nebraska	11.6
33	Nevada	10.5
42	New Hampshire	9.5
10	New Jersey	12.8
38	New Mexico	9.8
24	New York	11.6
29	North Carolina	11.4
NA	North Dakota**	NA
18	Ohio	11.9
35	Oklahoma	10.4
8	Oregon	13.6
5	Pennsylvania	14.7
24	Rhode Island	11.6
43	South Carolina	9.4
2	South Dakota	15.8
14	Tennessee	12.3
44	Texas	8.7
46	Utah	7.6
NA	Vermont**	NA
31	Virginia	11.0
10	Washington	12.8
1	West Virginia	15.9
20	Wisconsin	11.8
NA	Wyoming**	NA

RANK ORDER

RANK	STATE	RATE
1	West Virginia	15.9
2	South Dakota	15.8
3	Maine	15.7
4	Montana	15.3
5	Pennsylvania	14.7
6	Iowa	14.5
7	Alabama	13.8
8	Oregon	13.6
9	Florida	13.4
10	New Jersey	12.8
10	Washington	12.8
12	Delaware	12.6
13	Indiana	12.5
14	Tennessee	12.3
15	Massachusetts	12.2
15	Missouri	12.2
17	Arkansas	12.0
18	Michigan	11.9
18	Ohio	11.9
20	Connecticut	11.8
20	Kansas	11.8
20	Wisconsin	11.8
23	Idaho	11.7
24	Maryland	11.6
24	Nebraska	11.6
24	New York	11.6
24	Rhode Island	11.6
28	Mississippi	11.5
29	Kentucky	11.4
29	North Carolina	11.4
31	Virginia	11.0
32	Minnesota	10.8
33	Illinois	10.5
33	Nevada	10.5
35	Arizona	10.4
35	Oklahoma	10.4
37	Louisiana	10.1
38	Georgia	9.8
38	New Mexico	9.8
40	California	9.7
41	Colorado	9.6
42	New Hampshire	9.5
43	South Carolina	9.4
44	Texas	8.7
45	Hawaii	7.9
46	Utah	7.6
NA	Alaska**	NA
NA	North Dakota**	NA
NA	Vermont**	NA
NA	Wyoming**	NA
	District of Columbia**	NA

Source: Morgan Quitno Press using data from American Cancer Society
"Cancer Facts & Figures 2005" (Copyright 2005, American Cancer Society)
Rates calculated using 2003 Census female population estimates. Not age-adjusted.
**Fewer than 50 deaths.*

Deaths by Alzheimer's Disease in 2002

National Total = 58,866 Deaths*

ALPHA ORDER

RANK	STATE	DEATHS	% of USA
20	Alabama	1,189	2.0%
50	Alaska	61	0.1%
15	Arizona	1,433	2.4%
33	Arkansas	551	0.9%
1	California	5,421	9.2%
26	Colorado	954	1.6%
32	Connecticut	570	1.0%
48	Delaware	128	0.2%
2	Florida	4,052	6.9%
12	Georgia	1,525	2.6%
47	Hawaii	141	0.2%
38	Idaho	318	0.5%
6	Illinois	2,398	4.1%
14	Indiana	1,475	2.5%
27	Iowa	899	1.5%
29	Kansas	755	1.3%
24	Kentucky	1,013	1.7%
23	Louisiana	1,111	1.9%
34	Maine	513	0.9%
28	Maryland	866	1.5%
11	Massachusetts	1,570	2.7%
9	Michigan	1,958	3.3%
19	Minnesota	1,192	2.0%
31	Mississippi	574	1.0%
21	Missouri	1,187	2.0%
42	Montana	285	0.5%
35	Nebraska	460	0.8%
44	Nevada	253	0.4%
39	New Hampshire	311	0.5%
13	New Jersey	1,522	2.6%
37	New Mexico	325	0.6%
10	New York	1,803	3.1%
8	North Carolina	1,962	3.3%
41	North Dakota	294	0.5%
5	Ohio	2,599	4.4%
30	Oklahoma	754	1.3%
22	Oregon	1,124	1.9%
4	Pennsylvania	2,823	4.8%
43	Rhode Island	264	0.4%
25	South Carolina	967	1.6%
45	South Dakota	167	0.3%
18	Tennessee	1,299	2.2%
3	Texas	3,793	6.4%
40	Utah	303	0.5%
46	Vermont	163	0.3%
16	Virginia	1,368	2.3%
7	Washington	2,195	3.7%
36	West Virginia	405	0.7%
17	Wisconsin	1,344	2.3%
49	Wyoming	122	0.2%

RANK ORDER

RANK	STATE	DEATHS	% of USA
1	California	5,421	9.2%
2	Florida	4,052	6.9%
3	Texas	3,793	6.4%
4	Pennsylvania	2,823	4.8%
5	Ohio	2,599	4.4%
6	Illinois	2,398	4.1%
7	Washington	2,195	3.7%
8	North Carolina	1,962	3.3%
9	Michigan	1,958	3.3%
10	New York	1,803	3.1%
11	Massachusetts	1,570	2.7%
12	Georgia	1,525	2.6%
13	New Jersey	1,522	2.6%
14	Indiana	1,475	2.5%
15	Arizona	1,433	2.4%
16	Virginia	1,368	2.3%
17	Wisconsin	1,344	2.3%
18	Tennessee	1,299	2.2%
19	Minnesota	1,192	2.0%
20	Alabama	1,189	2.0%
21	Missouri	1,187	2.0%
22	Oregon	1,124	1.9%
23	Louisiana	1,111	1.9%
24	Kentucky	1,013	1.7%
25	South Carolina	967	1.6%
26	Colorado	954	1.6%
27	Iowa	899	1.5%
28	Maryland	866	1.5%
29	Kansas	755	1.3%
30	Oklahoma	754	1.3%
31	Mississippi	574	1.0%
32	Connecticut	570	1.0%
33	Arkansas	551	0.9%
34	Maine	513	0.9%
35	Nebraska	460	0.8%
36	West Virginia	405	0.7%
37	New Mexico	325	0.6%
38	Idaho	318	0.5%
39	New Hampshire	311	0.5%
40	Utah	303	0.5%
41	North Dakota	294	0.5%
42	Montana	285	0.5%
43	Rhode Island	264	0.4%
44	Nevada	253	0.4%
45	South Dakota	167	0.3%
46	Vermont	163	0.3%
47	Hawaii	141	0.2%
48	Delaware	128	0.2%
49	Wyoming	122	0.2%
50	Alaska	61	0.1%
	District of Columbia	107	0.2%

Source: U.S. Department of Health and Human Services, National Center for Health Statistics
"National Vital Statistics Reports" (Vol. 53, No. 5, October 12, 2004)
*Final data by state of residence. A degenerative disease of the brain cells producing loss of memory and general intellectual impairment. It usually affects people over age 65. As the disease progresses, a variety of symptoms may become apparent, including confusion, irritability, and restlessness, as well as disorientation and impaired judgment and concentration.

Death Rate by Alzheimer's Disease in 2002

National Rate = 20.4 Deaths per 100,000 Population*

<table>
<tr><td colspan="3">ALPHA ORDER</td><td colspan="3">RANK ORDER</td></tr>
<tr><td>RANK</td><td>STATE</td><td>RATE</td><td>RANK</td><td>STATE</td><td>RATE</td></tr>
<tr><td>9</td><td>Alabama</td><td>26.5</td><td>1</td><td>North Dakota</td><td>46.4</td></tr>
<tr><td>49</td><td>Alaska</td><td>9.5</td><td>2</td><td>Maine</td><td>39.6</td></tr>
<tr><td>11</td><td>Arizona</td><td>26.3</td><td>3</td><td>Washington</td><td>36.2</td></tr>
<tr><td>33</td><td>Arkansas</td><td>20.3</td><td>4</td><td>Oregon</td><td>31.9</td></tr>
<tr><td>45</td><td>California</td><td>15.4</td><td>5</td><td>Montana</td><td>31.3</td></tr>
<tr><td>31</td><td>Colorado</td><td>21.2</td><td>6</td><td>Iowa</td><td>30.6</td></tr>
<tr><td>42</td><td>Connecticut</td><td>16.5</td><td>7</td><td>Kansas</td><td>27.8</td></tr>
<tr><td>43</td><td>Delaware</td><td>15.9</td><td>8</td><td>Nebraska</td><td>26.6</td></tr>
<tr><td>19</td><td>Florida</td><td>24.2</td><td>9</td><td>Alabama</td><td>26.5</td></tr>
<tr><td>38</td><td>Georgia</td><td>17.8</td><td>10</td><td>Vermont</td><td>26.4</td></tr>
<tr><td>48</td><td>Hawaii</td><td>11.3</td><td>11</td><td>Arizona</td><td>26.3</td></tr>
<tr><td>21</td><td>Idaho</td><td>23.7</td><td>12</td><td>Kentucky</td><td>24.8</td></tr>
<tr><td>36</td><td>Illinois</td><td>19.0</td><td>12</td><td>Louisiana</td><td>24.8</td></tr>
<tr><td>20</td><td>Indiana</td><td>23.9</td><td>14</td><td>Rhode Island</td><td>24.7</td></tr>
<tr><td>6</td><td>Iowa</td><td>30.6</td><td>14</td><td>Wisconsin</td><td>24.7</td></tr>
<tr><td>7</td><td>Kansas</td><td>27.8</td><td>16</td><td>Wyoming</td><td>24.5</td></tr>
<tr><td>12</td><td>Kentucky</td><td>24.8</td><td>17</td><td>Massachusetts</td><td>24.4</td></tr>
<tr><td>12</td><td>Louisiana</td><td>24.8</td><td>17</td><td>New Hampshire</td><td>24.4</td></tr>
<tr><td>2</td><td>Maine</td><td>39.6</td><td>19</td><td>Florida</td><td>24.2</td></tr>
<tr><td>43</td><td>Maryland</td><td>15.9</td><td>20</td><td>Indiana</td><td>23.9</td></tr>
<tr><td>17</td><td>Massachusetts</td><td>24.4</td><td>21</td><td>Idaho</td><td>23.7</td></tr>
<tr><td>35</td><td>Michigan</td><td>19.5</td><td>21</td><td>Minnesota</td><td>23.7</td></tr>
<tr><td>21</td><td>Minnesota</td><td>23.7</td><td>23</td><td>North Carolina</td><td>23.6</td></tr>
<tr><td>34</td><td>Mississippi</td><td>20.0</td><td>24</td><td>South Carolina</td><td>23.5</td></tr>
<tr><td>32</td><td>Missouri</td><td>20.9</td><td>25</td><td>Pennsylvania</td><td>22.9</td></tr>
<tr><td>5</td><td>Montana</td><td>31.3</td><td>26</td><td>Ohio</td><td>22.8</td></tr>
<tr><td>8</td><td>Nebraska</td><td>26.6</td><td>27</td><td>West Virginia</td><td>22.5</td></tr>
<tr><td>47</td><td>Nevada</td><td>11.6</td><td>28</td><td>Tennessee</td><td>22.4</td></tr>
<tr><td>17</td><td>New Hampshire</td><td>24.4</td><td>29</td><td>South Dakota</td><td>21.9</td></tr>
<tr><td>39</td><td>New Jersey</td><td>17.7</td><td>30</td><td>Oklahoma</td><td>21.6</td></tr>
<tr><td>40</td><td>New Mexico</td><td>17.5</td><td>31</td><td>Colorado</td><td>21.2</td></tr>
<tr><td>50</td><td>New York</td><td>9.4</td><td>32</td><td>Missouri</td><td>20.9</td></tr>
<tr><td>23</td><td>North Carolina</td><td>23.6</td><td>33</td><td>Arkansas</td><td>20.3</td></tr>
<tr><td>1</td><td>North Dakota</td><td>46.4</td><td>34</td><td>Mississippi</td><td>20.0</td></tr>
<tr><td>26</td><td>Ohio</td><td>22.8</td><td>35</td><td>Michigan</td><td>19.5</td></tr>
<tr><td>30</td><td>Oklahoma</td><td>21.6</td><td>36</td><td>Illinois</td><td>19.0</td></tr>
<tr><td>4</td><td>Oregon</td><td>31.9</td><td>37</td><td>Virginia</td><td>18.8</td></tr>
<tr><td>25</td><td>Pennsylvania</td><td>22.9</td><td>38</td><td>Georgia</td><td>17.8</td></tr>
<tr><td>14</td><td>Rhode Island</td><td>24.7</td><td>39</td><td>New Jersey</td><td>17.7</td></tr>
<tr><td>24</td><td>South Carolina</td><td>23.5</td><td>40</td><td>New Mexico</td><td>17.5</td></tr>
<tr><td>29</td><td>South Dakota</td><td>21.9</td><td>41</td><td>Texas</td><td>17.4</td></tr>
<tr><td>28</td><td>Tennessee</td><td>22.4</td><td>42</td><td>Connecticut</td><td>16.5</td></tr>
<tr><td>41</td><td>Texas</td><td>17.4</td><td>43</td><td>Delaware</td><td>15.9</td></tr>
<tr><td>46</td><td>Utah</td><td>13.1</td><td>43</td><td>Maryland</td><td>15.9</td></tr>
<tr><td>10</td><td>Vermont</td><td>26.4</td><td>45</td><td>California</td><td>15.4</td></tr>
<tr><td>37</td><td>Virginia</td><td>18.8</td><td>46</td><td>Utah</td><td>13.1</td></tr>
<tr><td>3</td><td>Washington</td><td>36.2</td><td>47</td><td>Nevada</td><td>11.6</td></tr>
<tr><td>27</td><td>West Virginia</td><td>22.5</td><td>48</td><td>Hawaii</td><td>11.3</td></tr>
<tr><td>14</td><td>Wisconsin</td><td>24.7</td><td>49</td><td>Alaska</td><td>9.5</td></tr>
<tr><td>16</td><td>Wyoming</td><td>24.5</td><td>50</td><td>New York</td><td>9.4</td></tr>
<tr><td></td><td></td><td></td><td></td><td>District of Columbia</td><td>18.7</td></tr>
</table>

Source: U.S. Department of Health and Human Services, National Center for Health Statistics
    "National Vital Statistics Reports" (Vol. 53, No. 5, October 12, 2004)
Final data by state of residence. A degenerative disease of the brain cells producing loss of memory and general intellectual impairment. It usually affects people over age 65. As the disease progresses, a variety of symptoms may become apparent, including confusion, irritability, and restlessness, as well as disorientation and impaired judgment and concentration. Not age-adjusted.

Age-Adjusted Death Rate by Alzheimer's Disease in 2002

National Rate = 20.2 Deaths per 100,000 Population*

ALPHA ORDER

RANK ORDER

RANK	STATE	RATE		RANK	STATE	RATE
10	Alabama	26.1		1	Washington	37.9
15	Alaska	25.4		2	North Dakota	33.2
8	Arizona	27.5		3	Maine	33.0
39	Arkansas	18.2		4	Oregon	29.0
40	California	18.0		5	Colorado	28.0
5	Colorado	28.0		6	Louisiana	27.8
48	Connecticut	13.4		7	Montana	27.6
46	Delaware	16.2		8	Arizona	27.5
42	Florida	17.5		9	Wyoming	26.3
16	Georgia	24.7		10	Alabama	26.1
49	Hawaii	10.6		10	South Carolina	26.1
13	Idaho	25.6		12	North Carolina	25.9
36	Illinois	18.8		13	Idaho	25.6
19	Indiana	23.7		13	Kentucky	25.6
23	Iowa	22.2		15	Alaska	25.4
20	Kansas	23.6		16	Georgia	24.7
13	Kentucky	25.6		16	New Hampshire	24.7
6	Louisiana	27.8		18	Vermont	24.6
3	Maine	33.0		19	Indiana	23.7
40	Maryland	18.0		20	Kansas	23.6
30	Massachusetts	20.6		21	Tennessee	23.3
32	Michigan	19.6		22	Texas	23.0
24	Minnesota	22.0		23	Iowa	22.2
29	Mississippi	21.0		24	Minnesota	22.0
37	Missouri	18.7		25	Nebraska	21.9
7	Montana	27.6		26	Virginia	21.7
25	Nebraska	21.9		27	Wisconsin	21.6
44	Nevada	16.7		28	Ohio	21.2
16	New Hampshire	24.7		29	Mississippi	21.0
46	New Jersey	16.2		30	Massachusetts	20.6
33	New Mexico	19.4		31	Oklahoma	20.5
50	New York	8.6		32	Michigan	19.6
12	North Carolina	25.9		33	New Mexico	19.4
2	North Dakota	33.2		33	Utah	19.4
28	Ohio	21.2		35	Rhode Island	19.0
31	Oklahoma	20.5		36	Illinois	18.8
4	Oregon	29.0		37	Missouri	18.7
43	Pennsylvania	17.3		37	West Virginia	18.7
35	Rhode Island	19.0		39	Arkansas	18.2
10	South Carolina	26.1		40	California	18.0
45	South Dakota	16.6		40	Maryland	18.0
21	Tennessee	23.3		42	Florida	17.5
22	Texas	23.0		43	Pennsylvania	17.3
33	Utah	19.4		44	Nevada	16.7
18	Vermont	24.6		45	South Dakota	16.6
26	Virginia	21.7		46	Delaware	16.2
1	Washington	37.9		46	New Jersey	16.2
37	West Virginia	18.7		48	Connecticut	13.4
27	Wisconsin	21.6		49	Hawaii	10.6
9	Wyoming	26.3		50	New York	8.6
					District of Columbia	18.3

Source: U.S. Department of Health and Human Services, National Center for Health Statistics
    "National Vital Statistics Reports" (Vol. 53, No. 5, October 12, 2004)
*Final data by state of residence. A degenerative disease of the brain cells producing loss of memory and general intellectual impairment. It usually affects people over age 65. As the disease progresses, a variety of symptoms may become apparent, including confusion, irritability, and restlessness, as well as disorientation and impaired judgment and concentration. Age-adjusted rates based on the year 2000 standard population.

Deaths by Cerebrovascular Diseases in 2002

National Total = 162,672 Deaths*

ALPHA ORDER

RANK	STATE	DEATHS	% of USA
19	Alabama	3,201	2.0%
50	Alaska	158	0.1%
26	Arizona	2,535	1.6%
28	Arkansas	2,232	1.4%
1	California	17,626	10.8%
31	Colorado	1,915	1.2%
32	Connecticut	1,861	1.1%
47	Delaware	405	0.2%
3	Florida	10,269	6.3%
10	Georgia	4,261	2.6%
39	Hawaii	812	0.5%
40	Idaho	736	0.5%
7	Illinois	7,183	4.4%
16	Indiana	3,717	2.3%
29	Iowa	2,226	1.4%
33	Kansas	1,845	1.1%
25	Kentucky	2,554	1.6%
24	Louisiana	2,595	1.6%
38	Maine	823	0.5%
21	Maryland	2,811	1.7%
17	Massachusetts	3,559	2.2%
8	Michigan	5,814	3.6%
22	Minnesota	2,706	1.7%
30	Mississippi	1,926	1.2%
14	Missouri	3,885	2.4%
42	Montana	639	0.4%
35	Nebraska	1,103	0.7%
36	Nevada	976	0.6%
43	New Hampshire	627	0.4%
11	New Jersey	4,016	2.5%
41	New Mexico	715	0.4%
5	New York	7,625	4.7%
9	North Carolina	5,259	3.2%
46	North Dakota	469	0.3%
6	Ohio	7,252	4.5%
27	Oklahoma	2,427	1.5%
23	Oregon	2,645	1.6%
4	Pennsylvania	8,579	5.3%
44	Rhode Island	605	0.4%
20	South Carolina	2,822	1.7%
45	South Dakota	518	0.3%
12	Tennessee	3,980	2.4%
2	Texas	10,548	6.5%
37	Utah	903	0.6%
48	Vermont	335	0.2%
13	Virginia	3,960	2.4%
15	Washington	3,753	2.3%
34	West Virginia	1,260	0.8%
18	Wisconsin	3,479	2.1%
49	Wyoming	243	0.1%

RANK ORDER

RANK	STATE	DEATHS	% of USA
1	California	17,626	10.8%
2	Texas	10,548	6.5%
3	Florida	10,269	6.3%
4	Pennsylvania	8,579	5.3%
5	New York	7,625	4.7%
6	Ohio	7,252	4.5%
7	Illinois	7,183	4.4%
8	Michigan	5,814	3.6%
9	North Carolina	5,259	3.2%
10	Georgia	4,261	2.6%
11	New Jersey	4,016	2.5%
12	Tennessee	3,980	2.4%
13	Virginia	3,960	2.4%
14	Missouri	3,885	2.4%
15	Washington	3,753	2.3%
16	Indiana	3,717	2.3%
17	Massachusetts	3,559	2.2%
18	Wisconsin	3,479	2.1%
19	Alabama	3,201	2.0%
20	South Carolina	2,822	1.7%
21	Maryland	2,811	1.7%
22	Minnesota	2,706	1.7%
23	Oregon	2,645	1.6%
24	Louisiana	2,595	1.6%
25	Kentucky	2,554	1.6%
26	Arizona	2,535	1.6%
27	Oklahoma	2,427	1.5%
28	Arkansas	2,232	1.4%
29	Iowa	2,226	1.4%
30	Mississippi	1,926	1.2%
31	Colorado	1,915	1.2%
32	Connecticut	1,861	1.1%
33	Kansas	1,845	1.1%
34	West Virginia	1,260	0.8%
35	Nebraska	1,103	0.7%
36	Nevada	976	0.6%
37	Utah	903	0.6%
38	Maine	823	0.5%
39	Hawaii	812	0.5%
40	Idaho	736	0.5%
41	New Mexico	715	0.4%
42	Montana	639	0.4%
43	New Hampshire	627	0.4%
44	Rhode Island	605	0.4%
45	South Dakota	518	0.3%
46	North Dakota	469	0.3%
47	Delaware	405	0.2%
48	Vermont	335	0.2%
49	Wyoming	243	0.1%
50	Alaska	158	0.1%
	District of Columbia	279	0.2%

Source: U.S. Department of Health and Human Services, National Center for Health Statistics
"National Vital Statistics Reports" (Vol. 53, No. 5, October 12, 2004)
Final data by state of residence. Cerebrovascular diseases include stroke and other disorders of the blood vessels of the brain.

Death Rate by Cerebrovascular Diseases in 2002

National Rate = 56.4 Deaths per 100,000 Population*

ALPHA ORDER

RANK	STATE	RATE
5	Alabama	71.3
50	Alaska	24.5
44	Arizona	46.5
1	Arkansas	82.4
37	California	50.2
46	Colorado	42.5
35	Connecticut	53.8
37	Delaware	50.2
24	Florida	61.4
39	Georgia	49.8
16	Hawaii	65.2
31	Idaho	54.9
28	Illinois	57.0
25	Indiana	60.4
2	Iowa	75.8
14	Kansas	67.9
22	Kentucky	62.4
26	Louisiana	57.9
19	Maine	63.6
36	Maryland	51.5
30	Massachusetts	55.4
27	Michigan	57.8
34	Minnesota	53.9
15	Mississippi	67.1
12	Missouri	68.5
6	Montana	70.3
18	Nebraska	63.8
45	Nevada	44.9
40	New Hampshire	49.2
43	New Jersey	46.8
49	New Mexico	38.5
47	New York	39.8
21	North Carolina	63.2
4	North Dakota	74.0
20	Ohio	63.5
8	Oklahoma	69.5
3	Oregon	75.1
8	Pennsylvania	69.5
29	Rhode Island	56.6
10	South Carolina	68.7
13	South Dakota	68.1
10	Tennessee	68.7
42	Texas	48.4
48	Utah	39.0
32	Vermont	54.3
32	Virginia	54.3
23	Washington	61.8
7	West Virginia	69.9
17	Wisconsin	63.9
41	Wyoming	48.7

RANK ORDER

RANK	STATE	RATE
1	Arkansas	82.4
2	Iowa	75.8
3	Oregon	75.1
4	North Dakota	74.0
5	Alabama	71.3
6	Montana	70.3
7	West Virginia	69.9
8	Oklahoma	69.5
8	Pennsylvania	69.5
10	South Carolina	68.7
10	Tennessee	68.7
12	Missouri	68.5
13	South Dakota	68.1
14	Kansas	67.9
15	Mississippi	67.1
16	Hawaii	65.2
17	Wisconsin	63.9
18	Nebraska	63.8
19	Maine	63.6
20	Ohio	63.5
21	North Carolina	63.2
22	Kentucky	62.4
23	Washington	61.8
24	Florida	61.4
25	Indiana	60.4
26	Louisiana	57.9
27	Michigan	57.8
28	Illinois	57.0
29	Rhode Island	56.6
30	Massachusetts	55.4
31	Idaho	54.9
32	Vermont	54.3
32	Virginia	54.3
34	Minnesota	53.9
35	Connecticut	53.8
36	Maryland	51.5
37	California	50.2
37	Delaware	50.2
39	Georgia	49.8
40	New Hampshire	49.2
41	Wyoming	48.7
42	Texas	48.4
43	New Jersey	46.8
44	Arizona	46.5
45	Nevada	44.9
46	Colorado	42.5
47	New York	39.8
48	Utah	39.0
49	New Mexico	38.5
50	Alaska	24.5
	District of Columbia	48.9

Source: U.S. Department of Health and Human Services, National Center for Health Statistics
  "National Vital Statistics Reports" (Vol. 53, No. 5, October 12, 2004)
*Final data by state of residence. Cerebrovascular diseases include stroke and other disorders of the blood vessels of the brain. Not age-adjusted.

Age-Adjusted Death Rate by Cerebrovascular Diseases in 2002

National Rate = 56.2 Deaths per 100,000 Population*

ALPHA ORDER

RANK	STATE	RATE
4	Alabama	69.6
31	Alaska	55.1
44	Arizona	47.7
1	Arkansas	74.3
24	California	58.0
34	Colorado	54.4
47	Connecticut	45.6
41	Delaware	50.4
45	Florida	46.0
9	Georgia	65.3
17	Hawaii	60.6
20	Idaho	59.4
27	Illinois	57.2
18	Indiana	60.1
25	Iowa	57.9
19	Kansas	59.5
11	Kentucky	63.5
12	Louisiana	63.0
37	Maine	53.7
30	Maryland	56.7
43	Massachusetts	48.1
23	Michigan	58.1
39	Minnesota	51.3
5	Mississippi	69.5
13	Missouri	62.5
14	Montana	62.4
32	Nebraska	54.7
28	Nevada	56.8
42	New Hampshire	50.1
48	New Jersey	43.4
49	New Mexico	41.5
50	New York	37.4
7	North Carolina	67.8
33	North Dakota	54.6
20	Ohio	59.4
8	Oklahoma	66.2
5	Oregon	69.5
34	Pennsylvania	54.4
46	Rhode Island	45.8
2	South Carolina	72.7
36	South Dakota	54.2
3	Tennessee	70.1
15	Texas	61.8
28	Utah	56.8
40	Vermont	50.9
16	Virginia	61.2
10	Washington	65.2
22	West Virginia	58.3
26	Wisconsin	57.7
38	Wyoming	51.5

RANK ORDER

RANK	STATE	RATE
1	Arkansas	74.3
2	South Carolina	72.7
3	Tennessee	70.1
4	Alabama	69.6
5	Mississippi	69.5
5	Oregon	69.5
7	North Carolina	67.8
8	Oklahoma	66.2
9	Georgia	65.3
10	Washington	65.2
11	Kentucky	63.5
12	Louisiana	63.0
13	Missouri	62.5
14	Montana	62.4
15	Texas	61.8
16	Virginia	61.2
17	Hawaii	60.6
18	Indiana	60.1
19	Kansas	59.5
20	Idaho	59.4
20	Ohio	59.4
22	West Virginia	58.3
23	Michigan	58.1
24	California	58.0
25	Iowa	57.9
26	Wisconsin	57.7
27	Illinois	57.2
28	Nevada	56.8
28	Utah	56.8
30	Maryland	56.7
31	Alaska	55.1
32	Nebraska	54.7
33	North Dakota	54.6
34	Colorado	54.4
34	Pennsylvania	54.4
36	South Dakota	54.2
37	Maine	53.7
38	Wyoming	51.5
39	Minnesota	51.3
40	Vermont	50.9
41	Delaware	50.4
42	New Hampshire	50.1
43	Massachusetts	48.1
44	Arizona	47.7
45	Florida	46.0
46	Rhode Island	45.8
47	Connecticut	45.6
48	New Jersey	43.4
49	New Mexico	41.5
50	New York	37.4
	District of Columbia	48.7

Source: U.S. Department of Health and Human Services, National Center for Health Statistics
   "National Vital Statistics Reports" (Vol. 53, No. 5, October 12, 2004)
*Final data by state of residence. Cerebrovascular diseases include stroke and other disorders of the blood vessels of the brain. Age-adjusted rates based on the year 2000 standard population.

Deaths by Chronic Liver Disease and Cirrhosis in 2002

National Total = 27,257 Deaths*

ALPHA ORDER

RANK	STATE	DEATHS	% of USA
22	Alabama	425	1.6%
50	Alaska	55	0.2%
12	Arizona	671	2.5%
33	Arkansas	222	0.8%
1	California	3,747	13.7%
23	Colorado	415	1.5%
29	Connecticut	318	1.2%
44	Delaware	88	0.3%
3	Florida	2,151	7.9%
11	Georgia	696	2.6%
45	Hawaii	79	0.3%
42	Idaho	105	0.4%
6	Illinois	1,068	3.9%
17	Indiana	514	1.9%
34	Iowa	220	0.8%
36	Kansas	187	0.7%
25	Kentucky	377	1.4%
27	Louisiana	365	1.3%
41	Maine	116	0.4%
18	Maryland	443	1.6%
14	Massachusetts	602	2.2%
8	Michigan	993	3.6%
28	Minnesota	320	1.2%
32	Mississippi	229	0.8%
20	Missouri	433	1.6%
39	Montana	127	0.5%
39	Nebraska	127	0.5%
31	Nevada	268	1.0%
42	New Hampshire	105	0.4%
10	New Jersey	730	2.7%
30	New Mexico	317	1.2%
4	New York	1,338	4.9%
9	North Carolina	735	2.7%
49	North Dakota	63	0.2%
7	Ohio	1,047	3.8%
21	Oklahoma	428	1.6%
26	Oregon	367	1.3%
5	Pennsylvania	1,156	4.2%
38	Rhode Island	128	0.5%
24	South Carolina	386	1.4%
46	South Dakota	75	0.3%
13	Tennessee	611	2.2%
2	Texas	2,284	8.4%
37	Utah	133	0.5%
48	Vermont	66	0.2%
15	Virginia	598	2.2%
16	Washington	525	1.9%
35	West Virginia	209	0.8%
19	Wisconsin	437	1.6%
47	Wyoming	70	0.3%

RANK ORDER

RANK	STATE	DEATHS	% of USA
1	California	3,747	13.7%
2	Texas	2,284	8.4%
3	Florida	2,151	7.9%
4	New York	1,338	4.9%
5	Pennsylvania	1,156	4.2%
6	Illinois	1,068	3.9%
7	Ohio	1,047	3.8%
8	Michigan	993	3.6%
9	North Carolina	735	2.7%
10	New Jersey	730	2.7%
11	Georgia	696	2.6%
12	Arizona	671	2.5%
13	Tennessee	611	2.2%
14	Massachusetts	602	2.2%
15	Virginia	598	2.2%
16	Washington	525	1.9%
17	Indiana	514	1.9%
18	Maryland	443	1.6%
19	Wisconsin	437	1.6%
20	Missouri	433	1.6%
21	Oklahoma	428	1.6%
22	Alabama	425	1.6%
23	Colorado	415	1.5%
24	South Carolina	386	1.4%
25	Kentucky	377	1.4%
26	Oregon	367	1.3%
27	Louisiana	365	1.3%
28	Minnesota	320	1.2%
29	Connecticut	318	1.2%
30	New Mexico	317	1.2%
31	Nevada	268	1.0%
32	Mississippi	229	0.8%
33	Arkansas	222	0.8%
34	Iowa	220	0.8%
35	West Virginia	209	0.8%
36	Kansas	187	0.7%
37	Utah	133	0.5%
38	Rhode Island	128	0.5%
39	Montana	127	0.5%
39	Nebraska	127	0.5%
41	Maine	116	0.4%
42	Idaho	105	0.4%
42	New Hampshire	105	0.4%
44	Delaware	88	0.3%
45	Hawaii	79	0.3%
46	South Dakota	75	0.3%
47	Wyoming	70	0.3%
48	Vermont	66	0.2%
49	North Dakota	63	0.2%
50	Alaska	55	0.2%
	District of Columbia	88	0.3%

Source: U.S. Department of Health and Human Services, National Center for Health Statistics
    "National Vital Statistics Reports" (Vol. 53, No. 5, October 12, 2004)
*Final data by state of residence. Cirrhosis of the liver is characterized by the replacement of normal tissue with fibrous tissue and the loss of functional liver cells. It can result from alcohol abuse, nutritional deprivation, or infection especially by the hepatitis virus.

Death Rate by Chronic Liver Disease and Cirrhosis in 2002

National Rate = 9.5 Deaths per 100,000 Population*

ALPHA ORDER

RANK	STATE	RATE
19	Alabama	9.5
30	Alaska	8.5
5	Arizona	12.3
34	Arkansas	8.2
11	California	10.7
23	Colorado	9.2
23	Connecticut	9.2
10	Delaware	10.9
4	Florida	12.9
37	Georgia	8.1
49	Hawaii	6.3
42	Idaho	7.8
30	Illinois	8.5
33	Indiana	8.3
44	Iowa	7.5
47	Kansas	6.9
23	Kentucky	9.2
37	Louisiana	8.1
27	Maine	9.0
37	Maryland	8.1
20	Massachusetts	9.4
16	Michigan	9.9
48	Minnesota	6.4
40	Mississippi	8.0
43	Missouri	7.6
2	Montana	14.0
45	Nebraska	7.3
5	Nevada	12.3
34	New Hampshire	8.2
30	New Jersey	8.5
1	New Mexico	17.1
46	New York	7.0
28	North Carolina	8.8
16	North Dakota	9.9
23	Ohio	9.2
5	Oklahoma	12.3
15	Oregon	10.4
20	Pennsylvania	9.4
8	Rhode Island	12.0
20	South Carolina	9.4
16	South Dakota	9.9
13	Tennessee	10.5
13	Texas	10.5
50	Utah	5.7
11	Vermont	10.7
34	Virginia	8.2
29	Washington	8.7
9	West Virginia	11.6
40	Wisconsin	8.0
2	Wyoming	14.0

RANK ORDER

RANK	STATE	RATE
1	New Mexico	17.1
2	Montana	14.0
2	Wyoming	14.0
4	Florida	12.9
5	Arizona	12.3
5	Nevada	12.3
5	Oklahoma	12.3
8	Rhode Island	12.0
9	West Virginia	11.6
10	Delaware	10.9
11	California	10.7
11	Vermont	10.7
13	Tennessee	10.5
13	Texas	10.5
15	Oregon	10.4
16	Michigan	9.9
16	North Dakota	9.9
16	South Dakota	9.9
19	Alabama	9.5
20	Massachusetts	9.4
20	Pennsylvania	9.4
20	South Carolina	9.4
23	Colorado	9.2
23	Connecticut	9.2
23	Kentucky	9.2
23	Ohio	9.2
27	Maine	9.0
28	North Carolina	8.8
29	Washington	8.7
30	Alaska	8.5
30	Illinois	8.5
30	New Jersey	8.5
33	Indiana	8.3
34	Arkansas	8.2
34	New Hampshire	8.2
34	Virginia	8.2
37	Georgia	8.1
37	Louisiana	8.1
37	Maryland	8.1
40	Mississippi	8.0
40	Wisconsin	8.0
42	Idaho	7.8
43	Missouri	7.6
44	Iowa	7.5
45	Nebraska	7.3
46	New York	7.0
47	Kansas	6.9
48	Minnesota	6.4
49	Hawaii	6.3
50	Utah	5.7

| | District of Columbia | 15.4 |

Source: U.S. Department of Health and Human Services, National Center for Health Statistics
    "National Vital Statistics Reports" (Vol. 53, No. 5, October 12, 2004)
*Final data by state of residence. Cirrhosis of the liver is characterized by the replacement of normal tissue with fibrous tissue and the loss of functional liver cells. It can result from alcohol abuse, nutritional deprivation, or infection especially by the hepatitis virus. Not age-adjusted.

Age-Adjusted Death Rate by Chronic Liver Disease and Cirrhosis in 2002

National Rate = 9.4 Deaths per 100,000 Population*

ALPHA ORDER

RANK	STATE	RATE
21	Alabama	9.1
19	Alaska	9.3
4	Arizona	12.6
42	Arkansas	7.7
8	California	11.6
15	Colorado	9.9
30	Connecticut	8.5
11	Delaware	10.4
9	Florida	11.2
23	Georgia	9.0
50	Hawaii	6.0
34	Idaho	8.2
29	Illinois	8.7
31	Indiana	8.4
46	Iowa	6.8
46	Kansas	6.8
24	Kentucky	8.8
31	Louisiana	8.4
40	Maine	7.9
37	Maryland	8.1
24	Massachusetts	8.8
17	Michigan	9.7
49	Minnesota	6.5
34	Mississippi	8.2
44	Missouri	7.3
3	Montana	12.8
44	Nebraska	7.3
5	Nevada	12.4
37	New Hampshire	8.1
39	New Jersey	8.0
1	New Mexico	17.1
48	New York	6.7
24	North Carolina	8.8
19	North Dakota	9.3
24	Ohio	8.8
6	Oklahoma	11.9
14	Oregon	10.0
34	Pennsylvania	8.2
10	Rhode Island	11.1
21	South Carolina	9.1
17	South Dakota	9.7
12	Tennessee	10.2
7	Texas	11.7
42	Utah	7.7
15	Vermont	9.9
31	Virginia	8.4
24	Washington	8.8
13	West Virginia	10.1
41	Wisconsin	7.8
2	Wyoming	13.4

RANK ORDER

RANK	STATE	RATE
1	New Mexico	17.1
2	Wyoming	13.4
3	Montana	12.8
4	Arizona	12.6
5	Nevada	12.4
6	Oklahoma	11.9
7	Texas	11.7
8	California	11.6
9	Florida	11.2
10	Rhode Island	11.1
11	Delaware	10.4
12	Tennessee	10.2
13	West Virginia	10.1
14	Oregon	10.0
15	Colorado	9.9
15	Vermont	9.9
17	Michigan	9.7
17	South Dakota	9.7
19	Alaska	9.3
19	North Dakota	9.3
21	Alabama	9.1
21	South Carolina	9.1
23	Georgia	9.0
24	Kentucky	8.8
24	Massachusetts	8.8
24	North Carolina	8.8
24	Ohio	8.8
24	Washington	8.8
29	Illinois	8.7
30	Connecticut	8.5
31	Indiana	8.4
31	Louisiana	8.4
31	Virginia	8.4
34	Idaho	8.2
34	Mississippi	8.2
34	Pennsylvania	8.2
37	Maryland	8.1
37	New Hampshire	8.1
39	New Jersey	8.0
40	Maine	7.9
41	Wisconsin	7.8
42	Arkansas	7.7
42	Utah	7.7
44	Missouri	7.3
44	Nebraska	7.3
46	Iowa	6.8
46	Kansas	6.8
48	New York	6.7
49	Minnesota	6.5
50	Hawaii	6.0

District of Columbia   15.5

Source: U.S. Department of Health and Human Services, National Center for Health Statistics
    "National Vital Statistics Reports" (Vol. 53, No. 5, October 12, 2004)
*Final data by state of residence. Cirrhosis of the liver is characterized by the replacement of normal tissue with fibrous tissue and the loss of functional liver cells. It can result from alcohol abuse, nutritional deprivation, or infection especially by the hepatitis virus. Age-adjusted rates based on the year 2000 standard population.

Deaths by Chronic Lower Respiratory Diseases in 2002

National Total = 124,816 Deaths*

ALPHA ORDER

RANK ORDER

RANK	STATE	DEATHS	% of USA
21	Alabama	2,328	1.9%
50	Alaska	142	0.1%
18	Arizona	2,575	2.1%
31	Arkansas	1,441	1.2%
1	California	12,684	10.2%
26	Colorado	1,848	1.5%
30	Connecticut	1,453	1.2%
45	Delaware	350	0.3%
2	Florida	9,062	7.3%
10	Georgia	3,163	2.5%
49	Hawaii	265	0.2%
40	Idaho	595	0.5%
7	Illinois	4,827	3.9%
11	Indiana	3,138	2.5%
29	Iowa	1,580	1.3%
33	Kansas	1,367	1.1%
19	Kentucky	2,401	1.9%
28	Louisiana	1,696	1.4%
38	Maine	791	0.6%
24	Maryland	1,944	1.6%
16	Massachusetts	2,745	2.2%
8	Michigan	4,431	3.6%
23	Minnesota	1,971	1.6%
32	Mississippi	1,378	1.1%
14	Missouri	2,867	2.3%
42	Montana	576	0.5%
36	Nebraska	934	0.7%
35	Nevada	1,174	0.9%
41	New Hampshire	577	0.5%
13	New Jersey	2,885	2.3%
37	New Mexico	857	0.7%
4	New York	6,966	5.6%
9	North Carolina	3,674	2.9%
47	North Dakota	322	0.3%
5	Ohio	6,063	4.9%
22	Oklahoma	1,988	1.6%
27	Oregon	1,845	1.5%
6	Pennsylvania	6,017	4.8%
43	Rhode Island	521	0.4%
25	South Carolina	1,889	1.5%
44	South Dakota	383	0.3%
12	Tennessee	3,011	2.4%
3	Texas	7,720	6.2%
39	Utah	603	0.5%
48	Vermont	276	0.2%
15	Virginia	2,752	2.2%
17	Washington	2,721	2.2%
34	West Virginia	1,228	1.0%
20	Wisconsin	2,335	1.9%
46	Wyoming	324	0.3%

RANK	STATE	DEATHS	% of USA
1	California	12,684	10.2%
2	Florida	9,062	7.3%
3	Texas	7,720	6.2%
4	New York	6,966	5.6%
5	Ohio	6,063	4.9%
6	Pennsylvania	6,017	4.8%
7	Illinois	4,827	3.9%
8	Michigan	4,431	3.6%
9	North Carolina	3,674	2.9%
10	Georgia	3,163	2.5%
11	Indiana	3,138	2.5%
12	Tennessee	3,011	2.4%
13	New Jersey	2,885	2.3%
14	Missouri	2,867	2.3%
15	Virginia	2,752	2.2%
16	Massachusetts	2,745	2.2%
17	Washington	2,721	2.2%
18	Arizona	2,575	2.1%
19	Kentucky	2,401	1.9%
20	Wisconsin	2,335	1.9%
21	Alabama	2,328	1.9%
22	Oklahoma	1,988	1.6%
23	Minnesota	1,971	1.6%
24	Maryland	1,944	1.6%
25	South Carolina	1,889	1.5%
26	Colorado	1,848	1.5%
27	Oregon	1,845	1.5%
28	Louisiana	1,696	1.4%
29	Iowa	1,580	1.3%
30	Connecticut	1,453	1.2%
31	Arkansas	1,441	1.2%
32	Mississippi	1,378	1.1%
33	Kansas	1,367	1.1%
34	West Virginia	1,228	1.0%
35	Nevada	1,174	0.9%
36	Nebraska	934	0.7%
37	New Mexico	857	0.7%
38	Maine	791	0.6%
39	Utah	603	0.5%
40	Idaho	595	0.5%
41	New Hampshire	577	0.5%
42	Montana	576	0.5%
43	Rhode Island	521	0.4%
44	South Dakota	383	0.3%
45	Delaware	350	0.3%
46	Wyoming	324	0.3%
47	North Dakota	322	0.3%
48	Vermont	276	0.2%
49	Hawaii	265	0.2%
50	Alaska	142	0.1%
	District of Columbia	133	0.1%

Source: U.S. Department of Health and Human Services, National Center for Health Statistics
"National Vital Statistics Reports" (Vol. 53, No. 5, October 12, 2004)
Final data by state of residence. Chronic lower respiratory diseases are diseases of the lungs including bronchitis, emphysema and asthma. Includes allied conditions.

Death Rate by Chronic Lower Respiratory Diseases in 2002

National Rate = 43.3 Deaths per 100,000 Population*

ALPHA ORDER

RANK	STATE	RATE
14	Alabama	51.9
49	Alaska	22.1
24	Arizona	47.2
11	Arkansas	53.2
44	California	36.1
37	Colorado	41.0
36	Connecticut	42.0
33	Delaware	43.3
7	Florida	54.2
42	Georgia	36.9
50	Hawaii	21.3
30	Idaho	44.4
39	Illinois	38.3
16	Indiana	50.9
10	Iowa	53.8
19	Kansas	50.3
5	Kentucky	58.7
40	Louisiana	37.8
4	Maine	61.1
45	Maryland	35.6
35	Massachusetts	42.7
32	Michigan	44.1
38	Minnesota	39.3
23	Mississippi	48.0
18	Missouri	50.5
3	Montana	63.3
8	Nebraska	54.0
8	Nevada	54.0
27	New Hampshire	45.3
47	New Jersey	33.6
25	New Mexico	46.2
43	New York	36.4
31	North Carolina	44.2
17	North Dakota	50.8
12	Ohio	53.1
6	Oklahoma	56.9
13	Oregon	52.4
21	Pennsylvania	48.8
22	Rhode Island	48.7
26	South Carolina	46.0
19	South Dakota	50.3
14	Tennessee	51.9
46	Texas	35.4
48	Utah	26.0
28	Vermont	44.8
41	Virginia	37.7
28	Washington	44.8
1	West Virginia	68.2
34	Wisconsin	42.9
2	Wyoming	65.0

RANK ORDER

RANK	STATE	RATE
1	West Virginia	68.2
2	Wyoming	65.0
3	Montana	63.3
4	Maine	61.1
5	Kentucky	58.7
6	Oklahoma	56.9
7	Florida	54.2
8	Nebraska	54.0
8	Nevada	54.0
10	Iowa	53.8
11	Arkansas	53.2
12	Ohio	53.1
13	Oregon	52.4
14	Alabama	51.9
14	Tennessee	51.9
16	Indiana	50.9
17	North Dakota	50.8
18	Missouri	50.5
19	Kansas	50.3
19	South Dakota	50.3
21	Pennsylvania	48.8
22	Rhode Island	48.7
23	Mississippi	48.0
24	Arizona	47.2
25	New Mexico	46.2
26	South Carolina	46.0
27	New Hampshire	45.3
28	Vermont	44.8
28	Washington	44.8
30	Idaho	44.4
31	North Carolina	44.2
32	Michigan	44.1
33	Delaware	43.3
34	Wisconsin	42.9
35	Massachusetts	42.7
36	Connecticut	42.0
37	Colorado	41.0
38	Minnesota	39.3
39	Illinois	38.3
40	Louisiana	37.8
41	Virginia	37.7
42	Georgia	36.9
43	New York	36.4
44	California	36.1
45	Maryland	35.6
46	Texas	35.4
47	New Jersey	33.6
48	Utah	26.0
49	Alaska	22.1
50	Hawaii	21.3

	District of Columbia	23.3

Source: U.S. Department of Health and Human Services, National Center for Health Statistics
   "National Vital Statistics Reports" (Vol. 53, No. 5, October 12, 2004)
*Final data by state of residence. Chronic lower respiratory diseases are diseases of the lungs including
bronchitis, emphysema and asthma. Includes allied conditions. Not age-adjusted.

Age-Adjusted Death Rate by Chronic Lower Respiratory Diseases in 2002

National Rate = 43.5 Deaths per 100,000 Population*

ALPHA ORDER

RANK ORDER

RANK	STATE	RATE	RANK	STATE	RATE
11	Alabama	50.3	1	Wyoming	67.7
24	Alaska	46.9	2	Nevada	65.5
21	Arizona	47.4	3	Kentucky	58.7
19	Arkansas	48.2	4	Montana	57.7
34	California	42.0	5	West Virginia	56.4
8	Colorado	52.2	6	Oklahoma	54.3
47	Connecticut	36.7	7	Maine	52.7
32	Delaware	42.7	8	Colorado	52.2
39	Florida	40.5	8	Tennessee	52.2
20	Georgia	47.8	10	Indiana	51.3
50	Hawaii	19.7	11	Alabama	50.3
17	Idaho	48.6	12	Oregon	50.2
41	Illinois	39.3	13	Mississippi	50.0
10	Indiana	51.3	14	Ohio	49.9
30	Iowa	44.3	15	New Mexico	49.3
24	Kansas	46.9	16	Nebraska	48.8
3	Kentucky	58.7	17	Idaho	48.6
37	Louisiana	41.0	18	Washington	48.3
7	Maine	52.7	19	Arkansas	48.2
42	Maryland	39.1	20	Georgia	47.8
45	Massachusetts	38.3	21	Arizona	47.4
29	Michigan	44.5	21	South Carolina	47.4
42	Minnesota	39.1	23	Missouri	47.1
13	Mississippi	50.0	24	Alaska	46.9
23	Missouri	47.1	24	Kansas	46.9
4	Montana	57.7	26	New Hampshire	46.6
16	Nebraska	48.8	27	North Carolina	46.5
2	Nevada	65.5	28	Texas	44.9
26	New Hampshire	46.6	29	Michigan	44.5
49	New Jersey	31.5	30	Iowa	44.3
15	New Mexico	49.3	31	South Dakota	43.0
48	New York	34.6	32	Delaware	42.7
27	North Carolina	46.5	33	Vermont	42.5
36	North Dakota	41.6	34	California	42.0
14	Ohio	49.9	35	Virginia	41.9
6	Oklahoma	54.3	36	North Dakota	41.6
12	Oregon	50.2	37	Louisiana	41.0
44	Pennsylvania	38.9	38	Rhode Island	40.9
38	Rhode Island	40.9	39	Florida	40.5
21	South Carolina	47.4	40	Wisconsin	40.1
31	South Dakota	43.0	41	Illinois	39.3
8	Tennessee	52.2	42	Maryland	39.1
28	Texas	44.9	42	Minnesota	39.1
46	Utah	37.7	44	Pennsylvania	38.9
33	Vermont	42.5	45	Massachusetts	38.3
35	Virginia	41.9	46	Utah	37.7
18	Washington	48.3	47	Connecticut	36.7
5	West Virginia	56.4	48	New York	34.6
40	Wisconsin	40.1	49	New Jersey	31.5
1	Wyoming	67.7	50	Hawaii	19.7

District of Columbia 23.5

Source: U.S. Department of Health and Human Services, National Center for Health Statistics
       "National Vital Statistics Reports" (Vol. 53, No. 5, October 12, 2004)
*Final data by state of residence. Chronic lower respiratory diseases are diseases of the lungs including bronchitis, emphysema and asthma. Includes allied conditions. Age-adjusted rates based on the year 2000 standard population.

Deaths by Diabetes Mellitus in 2002

National Total = 73,249 Deaths*

ALPHA ORDER

RANK	STATE	DEATHS	% of USA
19	Alabama	1,486	2.0%
50	Alaska	86	0.1%
24	Arizona	1,231	1.7%
29	Arkansas	793	1.1%
1	California	6,807	9.3%
34	Colorado	659	0.9%
32	Connecticut	675	0.9%
43	Delaware	215	0.3%
3	Florida	4,583	6.3%
15	Georgia	1,576	2.2%
46	Hawaii	204	0.3%
40	Idaho	322	0.4%
7	Illinois	3,011	4.1%
13	Indiana	1,688	2.3%
31	Iowa	734	1.0%
30	Kansas	765	1.0%
23	Kentucky	1,265	1.7%
11	Louisiana	1,774	2.4%
37	Maine	404	0.6%
17	Maryland	1,519	2.1%
20	Massachusetts	1,423	1.9%
8	Michigan	2,785	3.8%
22	Minnesota	1,317	1.8%
33	Mississippi	671	0.9%
14	Missouri	1,625	2.2%
45	Montana	210	0.3%
38	Nebraska	393	0.5%
39	Nevada	343	0.5%
41	New Hampshire	311	0.4%
9	New Jersey	2,532	3.5%
35	New Mexico	582	0.8%
4	New York	3,934	5.4%
10	North Carolina	2,205	3.0%
44	North Dakota	214	0.3%
5	Ohio	3,846	5.3%
26	Oklahoma	1,064	1.5%
27	Oregon	1,041	1.4%
6	Pennsylvania	3,708	5.1%
42	Rhode Island	263	0.4%
25	South Carolina	1,112	1.5%
47	South Dakota	195	0.3%
12	Tennessee	1,749	2.4%
2	Texas	5,654	7.7%
36	Utah	514	0.7%
48	Vermont	174	0.2%
16	Virginia	1,558	2.1%
18	Washington	1,494	2.0%
28	West Virginia	846	1.2%
21	Wisconsin	1,353	1.8%
49	Wyoming	145	0.2%

RANK ORDER

RANK	STATE	DEATHS	% of USA
1	California	6,807	9.3%
2	Texas	5,654	7.7%
3	Florida	4,583	6.3%
4	New York	3,934	5.4%
5	Ohio	3,846	5.3%
6	Pennsylvania	3,708	5.1%
7	Illinois	3,011	4.1%
8	Michigan	2,785	3.8%
9	New Jersey	2,532	3.5%
10	North Carolina	2,205	3.0%
11	Louisiana	1,774	2.4%
12	Tennessee	1,749	2.4%
13	Indiana	1,688	2.3%
14	Missouri	1,625	2.2%
15	Georgia	1,576	2.2%
16	Virginia	1,558	2.1%
17	Maryland	1,519	2.1%
18	Washington	1,494	2.0%
19	Alabama	1,486	2.0%
20	Massachusetts	1,423	1.9%
21	Wisconsin	1,353	1.8%
22	Minnesota	1,317	1.8%
23	Kentucky	1,265	1.7%
24	Arizona	1,231	1.7%
25	South Carolina	1,112	1.5%
26	Oklahoma	1,064	1.5%
27	Oregon	1,041	1.4%
28	West Virginia	846	1.2%
29	Arkansas	793	1.1%
30	Kansas	765	1.0%
31	Iowa	734	1.0%
32	Connecticut	675	0.9%
33	Mississippi	671	0.9%
34	Colorado	659	0.9%
35	New Mexico	582	0.8%
36	Utah	514	0.7%
37	Maine	404	0.6%
38	Nebraska	393	0.5%
39	Nevada	343	0.5%
40	Idaho	322	0.4%
41	New Hampshire	311	0.4%
42	Rhode Island	263	0.4%
43	Delaware	215	0.3%
44	North Dakota	214	0.3%
45	Montana	210	0.3%
46	Hawaii	204	0.3%
47	South Dakota	195	0.3%
48	Vermont	174	0.2%
49	Wyoming	145	0.2%
50	Alaska	86	0.1%
	District of Columbia	191	0.3%

Source: U.S. Department of Health and Human Services, National Center for Health Statistics
"National Vital Statistics Reports" (Vol. 53, No. 5, October 12, 2004)
*Final data by state of residence. A severe, chronic form of diabetes caused by insufficient production of insulin and resulting in abnormal metabolism of carbohydrates, fats, and proteins. The disease, which typically appears in childhood or adolescence, is characterized by increased sugar levels in the blood and urine, excessive thirst and frequent urination.

Death Rate by Diabetes Mellitus in 2002

National Rate = 25.4 Deaths per 100,000 Population*

ALPHA ORDER

RANK	STATE	RATE
5	Alabama	33.1
50	Alaska	13.4
39	Arizona	22.6
14	Arkansas	29.3
45	California	19.4
49	Colorado	14.6
44	Connecticut	19.5
24	Delaware	26.6
21	Florida	27.4
46	Georgia	18.4
47	Hawaii	16.4
34	Idaho	24.0
35	Illinois	23.9
21	Indiana	27.4
29	Iowa	25.0
17	Kansas	28.2
8	Kentucky	30.9
2	Louisiana	39.6
7	Maine	31.2
19	Maryland	27.8
41	Massachusetts	22.1
20	Michigan	27.7
26	Minnesota	26.2
36	Mississippi	23.4
16	Missouri	28.6
37	Montana	23.1
38	Nebraska	22.7
48	Nevada	15.8
33	New Hampshire	24.4
13	New Jersey	29.5
6	New Mexico	31.4
43	New York	20.5
25	North Carolina	26.5
3	North Dakota	33.7
3	Ohio	33.7
9	Oklahoma	30.5
12	Oregon	29.6
11	Pennsylvania	30.1
31	Rhode Island	24.6
23	South Carolina	27.1
28	South Dakota	25.6
10	Tennessee	30.2
27	Texas	26.0
40	Utah	22.2
17	Vermont	28.2
42	Virginia	21.4
31	Washington	24.6
1	West Virginia	47.0
30	Wisconsin	24.9
15	Wyoming	29.1

RANK ORDER

RANK	STATE	RATE
1	West Virginia	47.0
2	Louisiana	39.6
3	North Dakota	33.7
3	Ohio	33.7
5	Alabama	33.1
6	New Mexico	31.4
7	Maine	31.2
8	Kentucky	30.9
9	Oklahoma	30.5
10	Tennessee	30.2
11	Pennsylvania	30.1
12	Oregon	29.6
13	New Jersey	29.5
14	Arkansas	29.3
15	Wyoming	29.1
16	Missouri	28.6
17	Kansas	28.2
17	Vermont	28.2
19	Maryland	27.8
20	Michigan	27.7
21	Florida	27.4
21	Indiana	27.4
23	South Carolina	27.1
24	Delaware	26.6
25	North Carolina	26.5
26	Minnesota	26.2
27	Texas	26.0
28	South Dakota	25.6
29	Iowa	25.0
30	Wisconsin	24.9
31	Rhode Island	24.6
31	Washington	24.6
33	New Hampshire	24.4
34	Idaho	24.0
35	Illinois	23.9
36	Mississippi	23.4
37	Montana	23.1
38	Nebraska	22.7
39	Arizona	22.6
40	Utah	22.2
41	Massachusetts	22.1
42	Virginia	21.4
43	New York	20.5
44	Connecticut	19.5
45	California	19.4
46	Georgia	18.4
47	Hawaii	16.4
48	Nevada	15.8
49	Colorado	14.6
50	Alaska	13.4

| | District of Columbia | 33.5 |

Source: U.S. Department of Health and Human Services, National Center for Health Statistics
     "National Vital Statistics Reports" (Vol. 53, No. 5, October 12, 2004)

*Final data by state of residence. A severe, chronic form of diabetes caused by insufficient production of insulin and resulting in abnormal metabolism of carbohydrates, fats, and proteins. The disease, which typically appears in childhood or adolescence, is characterized by increased sugar levels in the blood and urine, excessive thirst and frequent urination. Not age-adjusted.

Age-Adjusted Death Rate by Diabetes Mellitus in 2002

National Rate = 25.4 Deaths per 100,000 Population*

ALPHA ORDER

RANK	STATE	RATE
4	Alabama	31.9
39	Alaska	21.7
36	Arizona	22.7
21	Arkansas	26.8
38	California	22.2
47	Colorado	17.7
49	Connecticut	17.2
27	Delaware	25.9
40	Florida	21.4
35	Georgia	22.9
50	Hawaii	15.2
26	Idaho	26.0
31	Illinois	24.4
16	Indiana	27.5
43	Iowa	20.7
24	Kansas	26.3
8	Kentucky	30.7
1	Louisiana	42.1
19	Maine	27.0
11	Maryland	29.9
45	Massachusetts	20.1
14	Michigan	27.8
27	Minnesota	25.9
32	Mississippi	24.2
22	Missouri	26.7
42	Montana	21.0
44	Nebraska	20.6
48	Nevada	17.5
29	New Hampshire	24.6
14	New Jersey	27.8
3	New Mexico	32.9
46	New York	19.6
16	North Carolina	27.5
20	North Dakota	26.9
5	Ohio	31.8
12	Oklahoma	29.2
13	Oregon	28.2
29	Pennsylvania	24.6
41	Rhode Island	21.2
18	South Carolina	27.4
37	South Dakota	22.6
9	Tennessee	30.1
6	Texas	31.7
7	Utah	31.4
23	Vermont	26.6
34	Virginia	23.1
25	Washington	26.2
2	West Virginia	39.3
33	Wisconsin	23.3
10	Wyoming	30.0

RANK ORDER

RANK	STATE	RATE
1	Louisiana	42.1
2	West Virginia	39.3
3	New Mexico	32.9
4	Alabama	31.9
5	Ohio	31.8
6	Texas	31.7
7	Utah	31.4
8	Kentucky	30.7
9	Tennessee	30.1
10	Wyoming	30.0
11	Maryland	29.9
12	Oklahoma	29.2
13	Oregon	28.2
14	Michigan	27.8
14	New Jersey	27.8
16	Indiana	27.5
16	North Carolina	27.5
18	South Carolina	27.4
19	Maine	27.0
20	North Dakota	26.9
21	Arkansas	26.8
22	Missouri	26.7
23	Vermont	26.6
24	Kansas	26.3
25	Washington	26.2
26	Idaho	26.0
27	Delaware	25.9
27	Minnesota	25.9
29	New Hampshire	24.6
29	Pennsylvania	24.6
31	Illinois	24.4
32	Mississippi	24.2
33	Wisconsin	23.3
34	Virginia	23.1
35	Georgia	22.9
36	Arizona	22.7
37	South Dakota	22.6
38	California	22.2
39	Alaska	21.7
40	Florida	21.4
41	Rhode Island	21.2
42	Montana	21.0
43	Iowa	20.7
44	Nebraska	20.6
45	Massachusetts	20.1
46	New York	19.6
47	Colorado	17.7
48	Nevada	17.5
49	Connecticut	17.2
50	Hawaii	15.2
	District of Columbia	33.7

Source: U.S. Department of Health and Human Services, National Center for Health Statistics
   "National Vital Statistics Reports" (Vol. 53, No. 5, October 12, 2004)
*Final data by state of residence. A severe, chronic form of diabetes caused by insufficient production of insulin and resulting in abnormal metabolism of carbohydrates, fats, and proteins. The disease, which typically appears in childhood or adolescence, is characterized by increased sugar levels in the blood and urine, excessive thirst and frequent urination. Age-adjusted rates based on the year 2000 standard population.

Deaths by Diseases of the Heart in 2002

National Total = 696,947 Deaths*

ALPHA ORDER

RANK	STATE	DEATHS	% of USA
17	Alabama	13,197	1.9%
50	Alaska	567	0.1%
24	Arizona	10,852	1.6%
29	Arkansas	8,330	1.2%
1	California	68,797	9.9%
33	Colorado	6,425	0.9%
27	Connecticut	8,815	1.3%
46	Delaware	1,918	0.3%
3	Florida	49,235	7.1%
11	Georgia	17,529	2.5%
43	Hawaii	2,512	0.4%
42	Idaho	2,532	0.4%
7	Illinois	30,821	4.4%
14	Indiana	15,321	2.2%
30	Iowa	8,181	1.2%
32	Kansas	6,680	1.0%
20	Kentucky	11,696	1.7%
22	Louisiana	11,185	1.6%
38	Maine	3,170	0.5%
19	Maryland	12,008	1.7%
16	Massachusetts	14,736	2.1%
8	Michigan	26,659	3.8%
28	Minnesota	8,602	1.2%
26	Mississippi	9,061	1.3%
12	Missouri	16,708	2.4%
44	Montana	1,944	0.3%
36	Nebraska	4,242	0.6%
35	Nevada	4,421	0.6%
41	New Hampshire	2,776	0.4%
9	New Jersey	22,510	3.2%
37	New Mexico	3,360	0.5%
2	New York	56,672	8.1%
10	North Carolina	18,524	2.7%
47	North Dakota	1,623	0.2%
6	Ohio	31,388	4.5%
21	Oklahoma	11,230	1.6%
31	Oregon	7,262	1.0%
5	Pennsylvania	38,852	5.6%
39	Rhode Island	3,109	0.4%
25	South Carolina	9,659	1.4%
45	South Dakota	1,937	0.3%
13	Tennessee	16,226	2.3%
4	Texas	43,452	6.2%
40	Utah	2,977	0.4%
48	Vermont	1,370	0.2%
15	Virginia	14,952	2.1%
23	Washington	11,141	1.6%
34	West Virginia	6,189	0.9%
18	Wisconsin	12,923	1.9%
49	Wyoming	1,005	0.1%

RANK ORDER

RANK	STATE	DEATHS	% of USA
1	California	68,797	9.9%
2	New York	56,672	8.1%
3	Florida	49,235	7.1%
4	Texas	43,452	6.2%
5	Pennsylvania	38,852	5.6%
6	Ohio	31,388	4.5%
7	Illinois	30,821	4.4%
8	Michigan	26,659	3.8%
9	New Jersey	22,510	3.2%
10	North Carolina	18,524	2.7%
11	Georgia	17,529	2.5%
12	Missouri	16,708	2.4%
13	Tennessee	16,226	2.3%
14	Indiana	15,321	2.2%
15	Virginia	14,952	2.1%
16	Massachusetts	14,736	2.1%
17	Alabama	13,197	1.9%
18	Wisconsin	12,923	1.9%
19	Maryland	12,008	1.7%
20	Kentucky	11,696	1.7%
21	Oklahoma	11,230	1.6%
22	Louisiana	11,185	1.6%
23	Washington	11,141	1.6%
24	Arizona	10,852	1.6%
25	South Carolina	9,659	1.4%
26	Mississippi	9,061	1.3%
27	Connecticut	8,815	1.3%
28	Minnesota	8,602	1.2%
29	Arkansas	8,330	1.2%
30	Iowa	8,181	1.2%
31	Oregon	7,262	1.0%
32	Kansas	6,680	1.0%
33	Colorado	6,425	0.9%
34	West Virginia	6,189	0.9%
35	Nevada	4,421	0.6%
36	Nebraska	4,242	0.6%
37	New Mexico	3,360	0.5%
38	Maine	3,170	0.5%
39	Rhode Island	3,109	0.4%
40	Utah	2,977	0.4%
41	New Hampshire	2,776	0.4%
42	Idaho	2,532	0.4%
43	Hawaii	2,512	0.4%
44	Montana	1,944	0.3%
45	South Dakota	1,937	0.3%
46	Delaware	1,918	0.3%
47	North Dakota	1,623	0.2%
48	Vermont	1,370	0.2%
49	Wyoming	1,005	0.1%
50	Alaska	567	0.1%
	District of Columbia	1,666	0.2%

Source: U.S. Department of Health and Human Services, National Center for Health Statistics "National Vital Statistics Reports" (Vol. 53, No. 5, October 12, 2004)
*Final data by state of residence.

Death Rate by Diseases of the Heart in 2002

National Rate = 241.7 Deaths per 100,000 Population*

ALPHA ORDER

RANK	STATE	RATE
9	Alabama	294.1
50	Alaska	88.1
42	Arizona	198.9
5	Arkansas	307.4
43	California	195.9
48	Colorado	142.6
18	Connecticut	254.7
26	Delaware	237.6
7	Florida	294.6
37	Georgia	204.8
39	Hawaii	201.8
44	Idaho	188.8
25	Illinois	244.6
21	Indiana	248.8
13	Iowa	278.6
22	Kansas	246.0
11	Kentucky	285.8
20	Louisiana	249.5
24	Maine	244.9
32	Maryland	220.0
29	Massachusetts	229.3
15	Michigan	265.3
47	Minnesota	171.4
3	Mississippi	315.5
8	Missouri	294.5
34	Montana	213.8
23	Nebraska	245.3
38	Nevada	203.4
33	New Hampshire	217.7
16	New Jersey	262.0
46	New Mexico	181.1
6	New York	295.8
30	North Carolina	222.6
17	North Dakota	255.9
14	Ohio	274.8
2	Oklahoma	321.4
35	Oregon	206.2
4	Pennsylvania	315.0
10	Rhode Island	290.6
28	South Carolina	235.2
19	South Dakota	254.5
12	Tennessee	279.9
41	Texas	199.5
49	Utah	128.5
31	Vermont	222.2
36	Virginia	205.0
45	Washington	183.6
1	West Virginia	343.5
27	Wisconsin	237.5
40	Wyoming	201.5

RANK ORDER

RANK	STATE	RATE
1	West Virginia	343.5
2	Oklahoma	321.4
3	Mississippi	315.5
4	Pennsylvania	315.0
5	Arkansas	307.4
6	New York	295.8
7	Florida	294.6
8	Missouri	294.5
9	Alabama	294.1
10	Rhode Island	290.6
11	Kentucky	285.8
12	Tennessee	279.9
13	Iowa	278.6
14	Ohio	274.8
15	Michigan	265.3
16	New Jersey	262.0
17	North Dakota	255.9
18	Connecticut	254.7
19	South Dakota	254.5
20	Louisiana	249.5
21	Indiana	248.8
22	Kansas	246.0
23	Nebraska	245.3
24	Maine	244.9
25	Illinois	244.6
26	Delaware	237.6
27	Wisconsin	237.5
28	South Carolina	235.2
29	Massachusetts	229.3
30	North Carolina	222.6
31	Vermont	222.2
32	Maryland	220.0
33	New Hampshire	217.7
34	Montana	213.8
35	Oregon	206.2
36	Virginia	205.0
37	Georgia	204.8
38	Nevada	203.4
39	Hawaii	201.8
40	Wyoming	201.5
41	Texas	199.5
42	Arizona	198.9
43	California	195.9
44	Idaho	188.8
45	Washington	183.6
46	New Mexico	181.1
47	Minnesota	171.4
48	Colorado	142.6
49	Utah	128.5
50	Alaska	88.1
	District of Columbia	291.8

Source: U.S. Department of Health and Human Services, National Center for Health Statistics
    "National Vital Statistics Reports" (Vol. 53, No. 5, October 12, 2004)
*Final data by state of residence. Not age-adjusted.

Age-Adjusted Death Rate by Diseases of the Heart in 2002

National Rate = 240.8 Deaths per 100,000 Population*

ALPHA ORDER

RANK	STATE	RATE
5	Alabama	285.8
49	Alaska	166.0
39	Arizona	202.9
7	Arkansas	278.7
26	California	225.7
48	Colorado	178.9
31	Connecticut	217.6
23	Delaware	236.0
27	Florida	222.0
12	Georgia	261.8
46	Hawaii	188.3
38	Idaho	203.0
17	Illinois	246.4
16	Indiana	248.4
30	Iowa	219.5
28	Kansas	220.6
4	Kentucky	287.0
10	Louisiana	269.6
36	Maine	208.5
21	Maryland	239.6
40	Massachusetts	201.3
11	Michigan	266.0
50	Minnesota	164.7
1	Mississippi	326.6
9	Missouri	270.3
45	Montana	191.6
33	Nebraska	213.5
18	Nevada	245.1
29	New Hampshire	220.2
20	New Jersey	243.5
42	New Mexico	193.3
8	New York	277.4
24	North Carolina	235.2
40	North Dakota	201.3
13	Ohio	258.2
2	Oklahoma	306.0
44	Oregon	192.3
14	Pennsylvania	250.1
22	Rhode Island	239.1
19	South Carolina	244.4
35	South Dakota	209.7
6	Tennessee	282.4
15	Texas	249.8
47	Utah	185.1
37	Vermont	208.3
25	Virginia	226.8
42	Washington	193.3
3	West Virginia	287.3
32	Wisconsin	216.5
34	Wyoming	210.0

RANK ORDER

RANK	STATE	RATE
1	Mississippi	326.6
2	Oklahoma	306.0
3	West Virginia	287.3
4	Kentucky	287.0
5	Alabama	285.8
6	Tennessee	282.4
7	Arkansas	278.7
8	New York	277.4
9	Missouri	270.3
10	Louisiana	269.6
11	Michigan	266.0
12	Georgia	261.8
13	Ohio	258.2
14	Pennsylvania	250.1
15	Texas	249.8
16	Indiana	248.4
17	Illinois	246.4
18	Nevada	245.1
19	South Carolina	244.4
20	New Jersey	243.5
21	Maryland	239.6
22	Rhode Island	239.1
23	Delaware	236.0
24	North Carolina	235.2
25	Virginia	226.8
26	California	225.7
27	Florida	222.0
28	Kansas	220.6
29	New Hampshire	220.2
30	Iowa	219.5
31	Connecticut	217.6
32	Wisconsin	216.5
33	Nebraska	213.5
34	Wyoming	210.0
35	South Dakota	209.7
36	Maine	208.5
37	Vermont	208.3
38	Idaho	203.0
39	Arizona	202.9
40	Massachusetts	201.3
40	North Dakota	201.3
42	New Mexico	193.3
42	Washington	193.3
44	Oregon	192.3
45	Montana	191.6
46	Hawaii	188.3
47	Utah	185.1
48	Colorado	178.9
49	Alaska	166.0
50	Minnesota	164.7

| | District of Columbia | 291.7 |

Source: U.S. Department of Health and Human Services, National Center for Health Statistics
"National Vital Statistics Reports" (Vol. 53, No. 5, October 12, 2004)
*Final data by state of residence. Age-adjusted rates based on the year 2000 standard population.

Deaths by Malignant Neoplasms in 2002

National Total = 557,271 Deaths*

ALPHA ORDER					RANK ORDER			
RANK	STATE	DEATHS	% of USA		RANK	STATE	DEATHS	% of USA
20	Alabama	9,698	1.7%		1	California	54,143	9.7%
50	Alaska	715	0.1%		2	Florida	39,140	7.0%
23	Arizona	9,359	1.7%		3	New York	36,661	6.6%
31	Arkansas	6,282	1.1%		4	Texas	34,164	6.1%
1	California	54,143	9.7%		5	Pennsylvania	29,849	5.4%
30	Colorado	6,384	1.1%		6	Ohio	25,173	4.5%
28	Connecticut	7,163	1.3%		7	Illinois	24,737	4.4%
45	Delaware	1,621	0.3%		8	Michigan	19,985	3.6%
2	Florida	39,140	7.0%		9	New Jersey	17,827	3.2%
11	Georgia	13,975	2.5%		10	North Carolina	16,210	2.9%
43	Hawaii	1,945	0.3%		11	Georgia	13,975	2.5%
42	Idaho	2,138	0.4%		12	Massachusetts	13,914	2.5%
7	Illinois	24,737	4.4%		13	Virginia	13,602	2.4%
14	Indiana	12,865	2.3%		14	Indiana	12,865	2.3%
29	Iowa	6,473	1.2%		15	Tennessee	12,518	2.2%
33	Kansas	5,362	1.0%		16	Missouri	12,322	2.2%
22	Kentucky	9,438	1.7%		17	Washington	10,858	1.9%
21	Louisiana	9,441	1.7%		18	Wisconsin	10,828	1.9%
37	Maine	3,206	0.6%		19	Maryland	10,395	1.9%
19	Maryland	10,395	1.9%		20	Alabama	9,698	1.7%
12	Massachusetts	13,914	2.5%		21	Louisiana	9,441	1.7%
8	Michigan	19,985	3.6%		22	Kentucky	9,438	1.7%
24	Minnesota	9,210	1.7%		23	Arizona	9,359	1.7%
32	Mississippi	6,069	1.1%		24	Minnesota	9,210	1.7%
16	Missouri	12,322	2.2%		25	South Carolina	8,333	1.5%
44	Montana	1,911	0.3%		26	Oklahoma	7,474	1.3%
36	Nebraska	3,433	0.6%		27	Oregon	7,249	1.3%
35	Nevada	3,937	0.7%		28	Connecticut	7,163	1.3%
39	New Hampshire	2,529	0.5%		29	Iowa	6,473	1.2%
9	New Jersey	17,827	3.2%		30	Colorado	6,384	1.1%
38	New Mexico	3,067	0.6%		31	Arkansas	6,282	1.1%
3	New York	36,661	6.6%		32	Mississippi	6,069	1.1%
10	North Carolina	16,210	2.9%		33	Kansas	5,362	1.0%
47	North Dakota	1,293	0.2%		34	West Virginia	4,652	0.8%
6	Ohio	25,173	4.5%		35	Nevada	3,937	0.7%
26	Oklahoma	7,474	1.3%		36	Nebraska	3,433	0.6%
27	Oregon	7,249	1.3%		37	Maine	3,206	0.6%
5	Pennsylvania	29,849	5.4%		38	New Mexico	3,067	0.6%
40	Rhode Island	2,404	0.4%		39	New Hampshire	2,529	0.5%
25	South Carolina	8,333	1.5%		40	Rhode Island	2,404	0.4%
46	South Dakota	1,562	0.3%		41	Utah	2,376	0.4%
15	Tennessee	12,518	2.2%		42	Idaho	2,138	0.4%
4	Texas	34,164	6.1%		43	Hawaii	1,945	0.3%
41	Utah	2,376	0.4%		44	Montana	1,911	0.3%
48	Vermont	1,224	0.2%		45	Delaware	1,621	0.3%
13	Virginia	13,602	2.4%		46	South Dakota	1,562	0.3%
17	Washington	10,858	1.9%		47	North Dakota	1,293	0.2%
34	West Virginia	4,652	0.8%		48	Vermont	1,224	0.2%
18	Wisconsin	10,828	1.9%		49	Wyoming	859	0.2%
49	Wyoming	859	0.2%		50	Alaska	715	0.1%
						District of Columbia	1,298	0.2%

Source: U.S. Department of Health and Human Services, National Center for Health Statistics
   "National Vital Statistics Reports" (Vol. 53, No. 5, October 12, 2004)
*Final data by state of residence. Neoplasms are abnormal tissue, tumors. Includes many cancers.

Death Rate by Malignant Neoplasms in 2002

National Rate = 193.2 Deaths per 100,000 Population*

ALPHA ORDER			RANK ORDER		
RANK	STATE	RATE	RANK	STATE	RATE
12	Alabama	216.2	1	West Virginia	258.2
49	Alaska	111.1	2	Maine	247.7
41	Arizona	171.5	3	Pennsylvania	242.0
5	Arkansas	231.8	4	Florida	234.2
47	California	154.2	5	Arkansas	231.8
48	Colorado	141.7	6	Kentucky	230.6
20	Connecticut	207.0	7	Rhode Island	224.7
25	Delaware	200.8	8	Iowa	220.4
4	Florida	234.2	8	Ohio	220.4
43	Georgia	163.3	10	Missouri	217.2
46	Hawaii	156.2	11	Massachusetts	216.5
44	Idaho	159.4	12	Alabama	216.2
32	Illinois	196.3	13	Tennessee	215.9
18	Indiana	208.9	14	Oklahoma	213.9
8	Iowa	220.4	15	Mississippi	211.3
31	Kansas	197.4	16	Louisiana	210.6
6	Kentucky	230.6	17	Montana	210.1
16	Louisiana	210.6	18	Indiana	208.9
2	Maine	247.7	19	New Jersey	207.5
35	Maryland	190.4	20	Connecticut	207.0
11	Massachusetts	216.5	21	Oregon	205.8
27	Michigan	198.8	22	South Dakota	205.2
37	Minnesota	183.5	23	North Dakota	203.9
15	Mississippi	211.3	24	South Carolina	202.9
10	Missouri	217.2	25	Delaware	200.8
17	Montana	210.1	26	Wisconsin	199.0
28	Nebraska	198.5	27	Michigan	198.8
38	Nevada	181.1	28	Nebraska	198.5
30	New Hampshire	198.3	28	Vermont	198.5
19	New Jersey	207.5	30	New Hampshire	198.3
42	New Mexico	165.3	31	Kansas	197.4
34	New York	191.4	32	Illinois	196.3
33	North Carolina	194.8	33	North Carolina	194.8
23	North Dakota	203.9	34	New York	191.4
8	Ohio	220.4	35	Maryland	190.4
14	Oklahoma	213.9	36	Virginia	186.5
21	Oregon	205.8	37	Minnesota	183.5
3	Pennsylvania	242.0	38	Nevada	181.1
7	Rhode Island	224.7	39	Washington	178.9
24	South Carolina	202.9	40	Wyoming	172.2
22	South Dakota	205.2	41	Arizona	171.5
13	Tennessee	215.9	42	New Mexico	165.3
45	Texas	156.9	43	Georgia	163.3
50	Utah	102.6	44	Idaho	159.4
28	Vermont	198.5	45	Texas	156.9
36	Virginia	186.5	46	Hawaii	156.2
39	Washington	178.9	47	California	154.2
1	West Virginia	258.2	48	Colorado	141.7
26	Wisconsin	199.0	49	Alaska	111.1
40	Wyoming	172.2	50	Utah	102.6
				District of Columbia	227.4

Source: U.S. Department of Health and Human Services, National Center for Health Statistics
   "National Vital Statistics Reports" (Vol. 53, No. 5, October 12, 2004)
*Final data by state of residence. Neoplasms are abnormal tissue, tumors. Includes many cancers. Not age-adjusted.

Age-Adjusted Death Rate by Malignant Neoplasms in 2002

National Rate = 193.5 Deaths per 100,000 Population*

ALPHA ORDER

RANK ORDER

RANK	STATE	RATE	RANK	STATE	RATE
10	Alabama	207.5	1	Kentucky	226.3
36	Alaska	185.9	2	Louisiana	222.9
48	Arizona	171.6	3	Mississippi	218.3
7	Arkansas	212.1	4	West Virginia	215.3
42	California	176.0	5	Maine	214.2
47	Colorado	171.8	6	Tennessee	213.6
35	Connecticut	186.4	7	Arkansas	212.1
27	Delaware	193.8	8	Indiana	209.8
40	Florida	183.4	9	Ohio	208.8
20	Georgia	199.6	10	Alabama	207.5
49	Hawaii	145.4	11	Missouri	204.3
46	Idaho	172.2	12	Oklahoma	204.2
15	Illinois	201.9	13	South Carolina	203.7
8	Indiana	209.8	14	Nevada	202.0
32	Iowa	189.0	15	Illinois	201.9
33	Kansas	188.1	16	Maryland	201.6
1	Kentucky	226.3	17	Pennsylvania	200.8
2	Louisiana	222.9	18	North Carolina	200.4
5	Maine	214.2	19	Virginia	199.8
16	Maryland	201.6	20	Georgia	199.6
22	Massachusetts	199.2	21	New Hampshire	199.5
22	Michigan	199.2	22	Massachusetts	199.2
38	Minnesota	185.0	22	Michigan	199.2
3	Mississippi	218.3	24	Oregon	197.8
11	Missouri	204.3	25	Rhode Island	196.9
28	Montana	190.7	26	New Jersey	196.3
36	Nebraska	185.9	27	Delaware	193.8
14	Nevada	202.0	28	Montana	190.7
21	New Hampshire	199.5	29	Washington	189.9
26	New Jersey	196.3	30	Texas	189.6
45	New Mexico	172.5	31	Wisconsin	189.5
39	New York	184.0	32	Iowa	189.0
18	North Carolina	200.4	33	Kansas	188.1
44	North Dakota	175.0	34	Vermont	186.7
9	Ohio	208.8	35	Connecticut	186.4
12	Oklahoma	204.2	36	Alaska	185.9
24	Oregon	197.8	36	Nebraska	185.9
17	Pennsylvania	200.8	38	Minnesota	185.0
25	Rhode Island	196.9	39	New York	184.0
13	South Carolina	203.7	40	Florida	183.4
41	South Dakota	182.4	41	South Dakota	182.4
6	Tennessee	213.6	42	California	176.0
30	Texas	189.6	43	Wyoming	175.1
50	Utah	143.3	44	North Dakota	175.0
34	Vermont	186.7	45	New Mexico	172.5
19	Virginia	199.8	46	Idaho	172.2
29	Washington	189.9	47	Colorado	171.8
4	West Virginia	215.3	48	Arizona	171.6
31	Wisconsin	189.5	49	Hawaii	145.4
43	Wyoming	175.1	50	Utah	143.3

District of Columbia   230.0

Source: U.S. Department of Health and Human Services, National Center for Health Statistics
    "National Vital Statistics Reports" (Vol. 53, No. 5, October 12, 2004)
*Final data by state of residence. Neoplasms are abnormal tissue, tumors. Includes many cancers. Age-adjusted
rates based on the year 2000 standard population.

Deaths by Nephritis and Other Kidney Diseases in 2002

National Total = 40,974 Deaths*

ALPHA ORDER

RANK	STATE	DEATHS	% of USA
16	Alabama	1,032	2.5%
50	Alaska	21	0.1%
23	Arizona	622	1.5%
24	Arkansas	601	1.5%
6	California	2,164	5.3%
31	Colorado	417	1.0%
27	Connecticut	554	1.4%
44	Delaware	117	0.3%
4	Florida	2,201	5.4%
11	Georgia	1,335	3.3%
42	Hawaii	136	0.3%
46	Idaho	86	0.2%
3	Illinois	2,328	5.7%
14	Indiana	1,222	3.0%
36	Iowa	261	0.6%
28	Kansas	517	1.3%
19	Kentucky	813	2.0%
17	Louisiana	983	2.4%
37	Maine	232	0.6%
22	Maryland	630	1.5%
12	Massachusetts	1,297	3.2%
9	Michigan	1,618	3.9%
21	Minnesota	649	1.6%
26	Mississippi	580	1.4%
15	Missouri	1,076	2.6%
45	Montana	105	0.3%
34	Nebraska	277	0.7%
32	Nevada	372	0.9%
41	New Hampshire	141	0.3%
8	New Jersey	1,662	4.1%
38	New Mexico	220	0.5%
2	New York	2,465	6.0%
10	North Carolina	1,437	3.5%
47	North Dakota	57	0.1%
7	Ohio	2,027	4.9%
29	Oklahoma	500	1.2%
35	Oregon	266	0.6%
1	Pennsylvania	2,944	7.2%
40	Rhode Island	142	0.3%
20	South Carolina	781	1.9%
43	South Dakota	128	0.3%
25	Tennessee	586	1.4%
5	Texas	2,166	5.3%
39	Utah	184	0.4%
48	Vermont	53	0.1%
13	Virginia	1,236	3.0%
33	Washington	306	0.7%
30	West Virginia	462	1.1%
18	Wisconsin	852	2.1%
49	Wyoming	43	0.1%

RANK ORDER

RANK	STATE	DEATHS	% of USA
1	Pennsylvania	2,944	7.2%
2	New York	2,465	6.0%
3	Illinois	2,328	5.7%
4	Florida	2,201	5.4%
5	Texas	2,166	5.3%
6	California	2,164	5.3%
7	Ohio	2,027	4.9%
8	New Jersey	1,662	4.1%
9	Michigan	1,618	3.9%
10	North Carolina	1,437	3.5%
11	Georgia	1,335	3.3%
12	Massachusetts	1,297	3.2%
13	Virginia	1,236	3.0%
14	Indiana	1,222	3.0%
15	Missouri	1,076	2.6%
16	Alabama	1,032	2.5%
17	Louisiana	983	2.4%
18	Wisconsin	852	2.1%
19	Kentucky	813	2.0%
20	South Carolina	781	1.9%
21	Minnesota	649	1.6%
22	Maryland	630	1.5%
23	Arizona	622	1.5%
24	Arkansas	601	1.5%
25	Tennessee	586	1.4%
26	Mississippi	580	1.4%
27	Connecticut	554	1.4%
28	Kansas	517	1.3%
29	Oklahoma	500	1.2%
30	West Virginia	462	1.1%
31	Colorado	417	1.0%
32	Nevada	372	0.9%
33	Washington	306	0.7%
34	Nebraska	277	0.7%
35	Oregon	266	0.6%
36	Iowa	261	0.6%
37	Maine	232	0.6%
38	New Mexico	220	0.5%
39	Utah	184	0.4%
40	Rhode Island	142	0.3%
41	New Hampshire	141	0.3%
42	Hawaii	136	0.3%
43	South Dakota	128	0.3%
44	Delaware	117	0.3%
45	Montana	105	0.3%
46	Idaho	86	0.2%
47	North Dakota	57	0.1%
48	Vermont	53	0.1%
49	Wyoming	43	0.1%
50	Alaska	21	0.1%
	District of Columbia	70	0.2%

Source: U.S. Department of Health and Human Services, National Center for Health Statistics
"National Vital Statistics Reports" (Vol. 53, No. 5, October 12, 2004)
*Final data by state of residence. Includes nephrotic syndrome and nephrosis.

Death Rate by Nephritis and Other Kidney Diseases in 2002

National Rate = 14.2 Deaths per 100,000 Population*

ALPHA ORDER

RANK	STATE	RATE
3	Alabama	23.0
50	Alaska	3.3
35	Arizona	11.4
4	Arkansas	22.2
48	California	6.2
40	Colorado	9.3
22	Connecticut	16.0
26	Delaware	14.5
29	Florida	13.2
25	Georgia	15.6
37	Hawaii	10.9
47	Idaho	6.4
14	Illinois	18.5
9	Indiana	19.8
42	Iowa	8.9
11	Kansas	19.0
8	Kentucky	19.9
5	Louisiana	21.9
15	Maine	17.9
33	Maryland	11.5
6	Massachusetts	20.2
21	Michigan	16.1
30	Minnesota	12.9
6	Mississippi	20.2
11	Missouri	19.0
33	Montana	11.5
22	Nebraska	16.0
18	Nevada	17.1
36	New Hampshire	11.1
10	New Jersey	19.3
32	New Mexico	11.9
30	New York	12.9
17	North Carolina	17.3
41	North Dakota	9.0
16	Ohio	17.7
27	Oklahoma	14.3
46	Oregon	7.6
2	Pennsylvania	23.9
28	Rhode Island	13.3
11	South Carolina	19.0
20	South Dakota	16.8
38	Tennessee	10.1
39	Texas	9.9
45	Utah	7.9
43	Vermont	8.6
19	Virginia	16.9
49	Washington	5.0
1	West Virginia	25.6
24	Wisconsin	15.7
43	Wyoming	8.6

RANK ORDER

RANK	STATE	RATE
1	West Virginia	25.6
2	Pennsylvania	23.9
3	Alabama	23.0
4	Arkansas	22.2
5	Louisiana	21.9
6	Massachusetts	20.2
6	Mississippi	20.2
8	Kentucky	19.9
9	Indiana	19.8
10	New Jersey	19.3
11	Kansas	19.0
11	Missouri	19.0
11	South Carolina	19.0
14	Illinois	18.5
15	Maine	17.9
16	Ohio	17.7
17	North Carolina	17.3
18	Nevada	17.1
19	Virginia	16.9
20	South Dakota	16.8
21	Michigan	16.1
22	Connecticut	16.0
22	Nebraska	16.0
24	Wisconsin	15.7
25	Georgia	15.6
26	Delaware	14.5
27	Oklahoma	14.3
28	Rhode Island	13.3
29	Florida	13.2
30	Minnesota	12.9
30	New York	12.9
32	New Mexico	11.9
33	Maryland	11.5
33	Montana	11.5
35	Arizona	11.4
36	New Hampshire	11.1
37	Hawaii	10.9
38	Tennessee	10.1
39	Texas	9.9
40	Colorado	9.3
41	North Dakota	9.0
42	Iowa	8.9
43	Vermont	8.6
43	Wyoming	8.6
45	Utah	7.9
46	Oregon	7.6
47	Idaho	6.4
48	California	6.2
49	Washington	5.0
50	Alaska	3.3
	District of Columbia	12.3

Source: U.S. Department of Health and Human Services, National Center for Health Statistics
        "National Vital Statistics Reports" (Vol. 53, No. 5, October 12, 2004)
*Final data by state of residence. Includes nephrotic syndrome and nephrosis.
Not age-adjusted.

Age-Adjusted Death Rate by Nephritis and Other Kidney Diseases in 2002

National Rate = 14.2 Deaths per 100,000 Population*

ALPHA ORDER

RANK ORDER

RANK	STATE	RATE
2	Alabama	22.4
49	Alaska	6.7
34	Arizona	11.6
6	Arkansas	20.2
44	California	7.1
33	Colorado	11.7
25	Connecticut	13.9
22	Delaware	14.3
41	Florida	10.0
7	Georgia	20.1
40	Hawaii	10.1
47	Idaho	6.9
13	Illinois	18.7
9	Indiana	19.8
46	Iowa	7.0
18	Kansas	17.1
7	Kentucky	20.1
1	Louisiana	23.7
21	Maine	15.3
29	Maryland	12.5
16	Massachusetts	17.8
20	Michigan	16.2
29	Minnesota	12.5
4	Mississippi	20.9
17	Missouri	17.4
38	Montana	10.4
24	Nebraska	14.1
5	Nevada	20.6
36	New Hampshire	11.3
15	New Jersey	18.1
28	New Mexico	12.7
32	New York	12.2
14	North Carolina	18.3
48	North Dakota	6.8
19	Ohio	16.7
26	Oklahoma	13.7
44	Oregon	7.1
11	Pennsylvania	19.0
37	Rhode Island	11.1
9	South Carolina	19.8
26	South Dakota	13.7
39	Tennessee	10.2
31	Texas	12.4
35	Utah	11.5
43	Vermont	8.2
12	Virginia	18.8
50	Washington	5.3
3	West Virginia	21.4
22	Wisconsin	14.3
42	Wyoming	9.0

RANK	STATE	RATE
1	Louisiana	23.7
2	Alabama	22.4
3	West Virginia	21.4
4	Mississippi	20.9
5	Nevada	20.6
6	Arkansas	20.2
7	Georgia	20.1
7	Kentucky	20.1
9	Indiana	19.8
9	South Carolina	19.8
11	Pennsylvania	19.0
12	Virginia	18.8
13	Illinois	18.7
14	North Carolina	18.3
15	New Jersey	18.1
16	Massachusetts	17.8
17	Missouri	17.4
18	Kansas	17.1
19	Ohio	16.7
20	Michigan	16.2
21	Maine	15.3
22	Delaware	14.3
22	Wisconsin	14.3
24	Nebraska	14.1
25	Connecticut	13.9
26	Oklahoma	13.7
26	South Dakota	13.7
28	New Mexico	12.7
29	Maryland	12.5
29	Minnesota	12.5
31	Texas	12.4
32	New York	12.2
33	Colorado	11.7
34	Arizona	11.6
35	Utah	11.5
36	New Hampshire	11.3
37	Rhode Island	11.1
38	Montana	10.4
39	Tennessee	10.2
40	Hawaii	10.1
41	Florida	10.0
42	Wyoming	9.0
43	Vermont	8.2
44	California	7.1
44	Oregon	7.1
46	Iowa	7.0
47	Idaho	6.9
48	North Dakota	6.8
49	Alaska	6.7
50	Washington	5.3
	District of Columbia	12.4

Source: U.S. Department of Health and Human Services, National Center for Health Statistics
"National Vital Statistics Reports" (Vol. 53, No. 5, October 12, 2004)
*Final data by state of residence. Includes nephrotic syndrome and nephrosis.
Age-adjusted rates based on the year 2000 standard population.

Deaths by Pneumonia and Influenza in 2002

National Total = 65,681 Deaths*

ALPHA ORDER

RANK	STATE	DEATHS	% of USA
20	Alabama	1,218	1.9%
50	Alaska	51	0.1%
17	Arizona	1,319	2.0%
30	Arkansas	776	1.2%
1	California	8,128	12.4%
31	Colorado	752	1.1%
28	Connecticut	888	1.4%
46	Delaware	168	0.3%
4	Florida	3,290	5.0%
12	Georgia	1,791	2.7%
43	Hawaii	246	0.4%
41	Idaho	265	0.4%
6	Illinois	2,940	4.5%
16	Indiana	1,360	2.1%
23	Iowa	942	1.4%
32	Kansas	698	1.1%
19	Kentucky	1,236	1.9%
22	Louisiana	956	1.5%
40	Maine	317	0.5%
21	Maryland	1,121	1.7%
8	Massachusetts	2,087	3.2%
9	Michigan	2,029	3.1%
27	Minnesota	900	1.4%
29	Mississippi	801	1.2%
14	Missouri	1,619	2.5%
42	Montana	255	0.4%
36	Nebraska	418	0.6%
38	Nevada	368	0.6%
45	New Hampshire	237	0.4%
10	New Jersey	1,973	3.0%
37	New Mexico	372	0.6%
2	New York	5,368	8.2%
11	North Carolina	1,898	2.9%
47	North Dakota	162	0.2%
7	Ohio	2,487	3.8%
24	Oklahoma	914	1.4%
33	Oregon	666	1.0%
5	Pennsylvania	2,957	4.5%
39	Rhode Island	319	0.5%
25	South Carolina	910	1.4%
44	South Dakota	240	0.4%
13	Tennessee	1,710	2.6%
3	Texas	3,673	5.6%
35	Utah	424	0.6%
49	Vermont	111	0.2%
15	Virginia	1,480	2.3%
26	Washington	907	1.4%
34	West Virginia	427	0.7%
18	Wisconsin	1,291	2.0%
48	Wyoming	135	0.2%

RANK ORDER

RANK	STATE	DEATHS	% of USA
1	California	8,128	12.4%
2	New York	5,368	8.2%
3	Texas	3,673	5.6%
4	Florida	3,290	5.0%
5	Pennsylvania	2,957	4.5%
6	Illinois	2,940	4.5%
7	Ohio	2,487	3.8%
8	Massachusetts	2,087	3.2%
9	Michigan	2,029	3.1%
10	New Jersey	1,973	3.0%
11	North Carolina	1,898	2.9%
12	Georgia	1,791	2.7%
13	Tennessee	1,710	2.6%
14	Missouri	1,619	2.5%
15	Virginia	1,480	2.3%
16	Indiana	1,360	2.1%
17	Arizona	1,319	2.0%
18	Wisconsin	1,291	2.0%
19	Kentucky	1,236	1.9%
20	Alabama	1,218	1.9%
21	Maryland	1,121	1.7%
22	Louisiana	956	1.5%
23	Iowa	942	1.4%
24	Oklahoma	914	1.4%
25	South Carolina	910	1.4%
26	Washington	907	1.4%
27	Minnesota	900	1.4%
28	Connecticut	888	1.4%
29	Mississippi	801	1.2%
30	Arkansas	776	1.2%
31	Colorado	752	1.1%
32	Kansas	698	1.1%
33	Oregon	666	1.0%
34	West Virginia	427	0.7%
35	Utah	424	0.6%
36	Nebraska	418	0.6%
37	New Mexico	372	0.6%
38	Nevada	368	0.6%
39	Rhode Island	319	0.5%
40	Maine	317	0.5%
41	Idaho	265	0.4%
42	Montana	255	0.4%
43	Hawaii	246	0.4%
44	South Dakota	240	0.4%
45	New Hampshire	237	0.4%
46	Delaware	168	0.3%
47	North Dakota	162	0.2%
48	Wyoming	135	0.2%
49	Vermont	111	0.2%
50	Alaska	51	0.1%
	District of Columbia	81	0.1%

Source: U.S. Department of Health and Human Services, National Center for Health Statistics
"National Vital Statistics Reports" (Vol. 53, No. 5, October 12, 2004)
*Final data by state of residence.

Death Rate by Pneumonia and Influenza in 2002

National Rate = 22.8 Deaths per 100,000 Population*

ALPHA ORDER

RANK	STATE	RATE
12	Alabama	27.1
50	Alaska	7.9
19	Arizona	24.2
7	Arkansas	28.6
25	California	23.1
48	Colorado	16.7
15	Connecticut	25.7
33	Delaware	20.8
40	Florida	19.7
32	Georgia	20.9
38	Hawaii	19.8
38	Idaho	19.8
24	Illinois	23.3
29	Indiana	22.1
2	Iowa	32.1
15	Kansas	25.7
4	Kentucky	30.2
31	Louisiana	21.3
18	Maine	24.5
34	Maryland	20.5
1	Massachusetts	32.5
36	Michigan	20.2
45	Minnesota	17.9
11	Mississippi	27.9
8	Missouri	28.5
9	Montana	28.0
19	Nebraska	24.2
46	Nevada	16.9
42	New Hampshire	18.6
26	New Jersey	23.0
37	New Mexico	20.1
9	New York	28.0
27	North Carolina	22.8
17	North Dakota	25.5
30	Ohio	21.8
14	Oklahoma	26.2
41	Oregon	18.9
21	Pennsylvania	24.0
5	Rhode Island	29.8
28	South Carolina	22.2
3	South Dakota	31.5
6	Tennessee	29.5
46	Texas	16.9
43	Utah	18.3
44	Vermont	18.0
35	Virginia	20.3
49	Washington	14.9
22	West Virginia	23.7
22	Wisconsin	23.7
12	Wyoming	27.1

RANK ORDER

RANK	STATE	RATE
1	Massachusetts	32.5
2	Iowa	32.1
3	South Dakota	31.5
4	Kentucky	30.2
5	Rhode Island	29.8
6	Tennessee	29.5
7	Arkansas	28.6
8	Missouri	28.5
9	Montana	28.0
9	New York	28.0
11	Mississippi	27.9
12	Alabama	27.1
12	Wyoming	27.1
14	Oklahoma	26.2
15	Connecticut	25.7
15	Kansas	25.7
17	North Dakota	25.5
18	Maine	24.5
19	Arizona	24.2
19	Nebraska	24.2
21	Pennsylvania	24.0
22	West Virginia	23.7
22	Wisconsin	23.7
24	Illinois	23.3
25	California	23.1
26	New Jersey	23.0
27	North Carolina	22.8
28	South Carolina	22.2
29	Indiana	22.1
30	Ohio	21.8
31	Louisiana	21.3
32	Georgia	20.9
33	Delaware	20.8
34	Maryland	20.5
35	Virginia	20.3
36	Michigan	20.2
37	New Mexico	20.1
38	Hawaii	19.8
38	Idaho	19.8
40	Florida	19.7
41	Oregon	18.9
42	New Hampshire	18.6
43	Utah	18.3
44	Vermont	18.0
45	Minnesota	17.9
46	Nevada	16.9
46	Texas	16.9
48	Colorado	16.7
49	Washington	14.9
50	Alaska	7.9
	District of Columbia	14.2

Source: U.S. Department of Health and Human Services, National Center for Health Statistics
"National Vital Statistics Reports" (Vol. 53, No. 5, October 12, 2004)
*Final data by state of residence. Not age-adjusted.

Age-Adjusted Death Rate by Pneumonia and Influenza in 2002

National Rate = 22.6 Deaths per 100,000 Population*

ALPHA ORDER

RANK ORDER

RANK	STATE	RATE		RANK	STATE	RATE
8	Alabama	26.6		1	Kentucky	30.8
41	Alaska	19.2		2	Tennessee	30.2
15	Arizona	24.9		3	Mississippi	28.9
12	Arkansas	25.7		4	Wyoming	28.5
7	California	26.8		5	Georgia	27.8
30	Colorado	21.3		5	Massachusetts	27.8
33	Connecticut	21.2		7	California	26.8
35	Delaware	20.9		8	Alabama	26.6
50	Florida	14.8		8	Utah	26.6
5	Georgia	27.8		10	New York	26.1
44	Hawaii	18.4		11	Missouri	25.9
30	Idaho	21.3		12	Arkansas	25.7
22	Illinois	23.2		13	Montana	25.0
27	Indiana	21.9		13	South Dakota	25.0
18	Iowa	24.0		15	Arizona	24.9
25	Kansas	22.3		15	Oklahoma	24.9
1	Kentucky	30.8		17	North Carolina	24.6
21	Louisiana	23.5		18	Iowa	24.0
36	Maine	20.5		19	Rhode Island	23.9
24	Maryland	22.7		20	South Carolina	23.8
5	Massachusetts	27.8		21	Louisiana	23.5
39	Michigan	20.3		22	Illinois	23.2
47	Minnesota	16.7		23	Virginia	23.1
3	Mississippi	28.9		24	Maryland	22.7
11	Missouri	25.9		25	Kansas	22.3
13	Montana	25.0		26	Nevada	22.1
37	Nebraska	20.4		27	Indiana	21.9
26	Nevada	22.1		28	New Mexico	21.7
42	New Hampshire	18.9		29	Texas	21.6
30	New Jersey	21.3		30	Colorado	21.3
28	New Mexico	21.7		30	Idaho	21.3
10	New York	26.1		30	New Jersey	21.3
17	North Carolina	24.6		33	Connecticut	21.2
44	North Dakota	18.4		34	Wisconsin	21.0
37	Ohio	20.4		35	Delaware	20.9
15	Oklahoma	24.9		36	Maine	20.5
46	Oregon	17.3		37	Nebraska	20.4
43	Pennsylvania	18.6		37	Ohio	20.4
19	Rhode Island	23.9		39	Michigan	20.3
20	South Carolina	23.8		40	West Virginia	19.8
13	South Dakota	25.0		41	Alaska	19.2
2	Tennessee	30.2		42	New Hampshire	18.9
29	Texas	21.6		43	Pennsylvania	18.6
8	Utah	26.6		44	Hawaii	18.4
47	Vermont	16.7		44	North Dakota	18.4
23	Virginia	23.1		46	Oregon	17.3
49	Washington	15.6		47	Minnesota	16.7
40	West Virginia	19.8		47	Vermont	16.7
34	Wisconsin	21.0		49	Washington	15.6
4	Wyoming	28.5		50	Florida	14.8
					District of Columbia	14.1

Source: U.S. Department of Health and Human Services, National Center for Health Statistics
      "National Vital Statistics Reports" (Vol. 53, No. 5, October 12, 2004)
Final data by state of residence. Age-adjusted rates based on the year 2000 standard population.

Deaths by Injury in 2001

National Total = 157,078 Deaths*

ALPHA ORDER				RANK ORDER			
RANK	STATE	DEATHS	% of USA	RANK	STATE	DEATHS	% of USA
17	Alabama	3,178	2.0%	1	California	13,353	8.5%
46	Alaska	496	0.3%	2	Texas	11,759	7.5%
13	Arizona	3,839	2.4%	3	Florida	10,399	6.6%
30	Arkansas	1,919	1.2%	4	New York	9,224	5.9%
1	California	13,353	8.5%	5	Pennsylvania	6,609	4.2%
25	Colorado	2,727	1.7%	6	Illinois	6,438	4.1%
32	Connecticut	1,555	1.0%	7	Ohio	5,695	3.6%
47	Delaware	447	0.3%	8	Michigan	5,265	3.4%
3	Florida	10,399	6.6%	9	Georgia	5,121	3.3%
9	Georgia	5,121	3.3%	10	North Carolina	5,071	3.2%
43	Hawaii	580	0.4%	11	New Jersey	4,123	2.6%
39	Idaho	844	0.5%	12	Tennessee	3,951	2.5%
6	Illinois	6,438	4.1%	13	Arizona	3,839	2.4%
16	Indiana	3,454	2.2%	14	Virginia	3,789	2.4%
34	Iowa	1,446	0.9%	15	Missouri	3,716	2.4%
31	Kansas	1,613	1.0%	16	Indiana	3,454	2.2%
24	Kentucky	2,748	1.7%	17	Alabama	3,178	2.0%
18	Louisiana	3,109	2.0%	18	Louisiana	3,109	2.0%
41	Maine	677	0.4%	19	Washington	3,098	2.0%
21	Maryland	2,947	1.9%	20	Wisconsin	3,006	1.9%
23	Massachusetts	2,784	1.8%	21	Maryland	2,947	1.9%
8	Michigan	5,265	3.4%	22	South Carolina	2,806	1.8%
27	Minnesota	2,461	1.6%	23	Massachusetts	2,784	1.8%
28	Mississippi	2,277	1.4%	24	Kentucky	2,748	1.7%
15	Missouri	3,716	2.4%	25	Colorado	2,727	1.7%
40	Montana	700	0.4%	26	Oklahoma	2,482	1.6%
38	Nebraska	903	0.6%	27	Minnesota	2,461	1.6%
35	Nevada	1,376	0.9%	28	Mississippi	2,277	1.4%
42	New Hampshire	583	0.4%	29	Oregon	2,000	1.3%
11	New Jersey	4,123	2.6%	30	Arkansas	1,919	1.2%
33	New Mexico	1,530	1.0%	31	Kansas	1,613	1.0%
4	New York	9,224	5.9%	32	Connecticut	1,555	1.0%
10	North Carolina	5,071	3.2%	33	New Mexico	1,530	1.0%
49	North Dakota	330	0.2%	34	Iowa	1,446	0.9%
7	Ohio	5,695	3.6%	35	Nevada	1,376	0.9%
26	Oklahoma	2,482	1.6%	36	West Virginia	1,266	0.8%
29	Oregon	2,000	1.3%	37	Utah	1,183	0.8%
5	Pennsylvania	6,609	4.2%	38	Nebraska	903	0.6%
45	Rhode Island	510	0.3%	39	Idaho	844	0.5%
22	South Carolina	2,806	1.8%	40	Montana	700	0.4%
44	South Dakota	515	0.3%	41	Maine	677	0.4%
12	Tennessee	3,951	2.5%	42	New Hampshire	583	0.4%
2	Texas	11,759	7.5%	43	Hawaii	580	0.4%
37	Utah	1,183	0.8%	44	South Dakota	515	0.3%
50	Vermont	326	0.2%	45	Rhode Island	510	0.3%
14	Virginia	3,789	2.4%	46	Alaska	496	0.3%
19	Washington	3,098	2.0%	47	Delaware	447	0.3%
36	West Virginia	1,266	0.8%	48	Wyoming	377	0.2%
20	Wisconsin	3,006	1.9%	49	North Dakota	330	0.2%
48	Wyoming	377	0.2%	50	Vermont	326	0.2%
					District of Columbia	473	0.3%

*Source: U.S. Department of Health and Human Services, National Center for Health Statistics
(http://wonder.cdc.gov)*
By state of residence. Injury as used here includes Accidents (including motor vehicle), Suicides, Homicides and "Other" undetermined.

Death Rate by Injury in 2001

National Rate = 55.1 Deaths per 100,000 Population*

<table>
<thead>
<tr><th colspan="3">ALPHA ORDER</th><th colspan="3">RANK ORDER</th></tr>
<tr><th>RANK</th><th>STATE</th><th>RATE</th><th>RANK</th><th>STATE</th><th>RATE</th></tr>
</thead>
<tbody>
<tr><td>9</td><td>Alabama</td><td>71.1</td><td>1</td><td>New Mexico</td><td>83.6</td></tr>
<tr><td>3</td><td>Alaska</td><td>78.3</td><td>2</td><td>Mississippi</td><td>79.7</td></tr>
<tr><td>6</td><td>Arizona</td><td>72.3</td><td>3</td><td>Alaska</td><td>78.3</td></tr>
<tr><td>8</td><td>Arkansas</td><td>71.2</td><td>4</td><td>Montana</td><td>77.3</td></tr>
<tr><td>50</td><td>California</td><td>38.6</td><td>5</td><td>Wyoming</td><td>76.3</td></tr>
<tr><td>21</td><td>Colorado</td><td>61.5</td><td>6</td><td>Arizona</td><td>72.3</td></tr>
<tr><td>48</td><td>Connecticut</td><td>45.3</td><td>7</td><td>Oklahoma</td><td>71.5</td></tr>
<tr><td>26</td><td>Delaware</td><td>56.1</td><td>8</td><td>Arkansas</td><td>71.2</td></tr>
<tr><td>19</td><td>Florida</td><td>63.5</td><td>9</td><td>Alabama</td><td>71.1</td></tr>
<tr><td>22</td><td>Georgia</td><td>61.0</td><td>10</td><td>West Virginia</td><td>70.2</td></tr>
<tr><td>46</td><td>Hawaii</td><td>47.3</td><td>11</td><td>Louisiana</td><td>69.6</td></tr>
<tr><td>18</td><td>Idaho</td><td>63.9</td><td>12</td><td>South Carolina</td><td>69.1</td></tr>
<tr><td>39</td><td>Illinois</td><td>51.4</td><td>13</td><td>Tennessee</td><td>68.7</td></tr>
<tr><td>25</td><td>Indiana</td><td>56.4</td><td>14</td><td>South Dakota</td><td>67.9</td></tr>
<tr><td>41</td><td>Iowa</td><td>49.3</td><td>15</td><td>Kentucky</td><td>67.5</td></tr>
<tr><td>23</td><td>Kansas</td><td>59.7</td><td>16</td><td>Missouri</td><td>65.9</td></tr>
<tr><td>15</td><td>Kentucky</td><td>67.5</td><td>17</td><td>Nevada</td><td>65.6</td></tr>
<tr><td>11</td><td>Louisiana</td><td>69.6</td><td>18</td><td>Idaho</td><td>63.9</td></tr>
<tr><td>32</td><td>Maine</td><td>52.7</td><td>19</td><td>Florida</td><td>63.5</td></tr>
<tr><td>29</td><td>Maryland</td><td>54.7</td><td>20</td><td>North Carolina</td><td>61.8</td></tr>
<tr><td>49</td><td>Massachusetts</td><td>43.5</td><td>21</td><td>Colorado</td><td>61.5</td></tr>
<tr><td>34</td><td>Michigan</td><td>52.6</td><td>22</td><td>Georgia</td><td>61.0</td></tr>
<tr><td>41</td><td>Minnesota</td><td>49.3</td><td>23</td><td>Kansas</td><td>59.7</td></tr>
<tr><td>2</td><td>Mississippi</td><td>79.7</td><td>24</td><td>Oregon</td><td>57.6</td></tr>
<tr><td>16</td><td>Missouri</td><td>65.9</td><td>25</td><td>Indiana</td><td>56.4</td></tr>
<tr><td>4</td><td>Montana</td><td>77.3</td><td>26</td><td>Delaware</td><td>56.1</td></tr>
<tr><td>35</td><td>Nebraska</td><td>52.5</td><td>27</td><td>Wisconsin</td><td>55.6</td></tr>
<tr><td>17</td><td>Nevada</td><td>65.6</td><td>28</td><td>Texas</td><td>55.0</td></tr>
<tr><td>47</td><td>New Hampshire</td><td>46.3</td><td>29</td><td>Maryland</td><td>54.7</td></tr>
<tr><td>43</td><td>New Jersey</td><td>48.4</td><td>30</td><td>Pennsylvania</td><td>53.7</td></tr>
<tr><td>1</td><td>New Mexico</td><td>83.6</td><td>31</td><td>Vermont</td><td>53.2</td></tr>
<tr><td>44</td><td>New York</td><td>48.3</td><td>32</td><td>Maine</td><td>52.7</td></tr>
<tr><td>20</td><td>North Carolina</td><td>61.8</td><td>32</td><td>Virginia</td><td>52.7</td></tr>
<tr><td>37</td><td>North Dakota</td><td>51.8</td><td>34</td><td>Michigan</td><td>52.6</td></tr>
<tr><td>40</td><td>Ohio</td><td>50.0</td><td>35</td><td>Nebraska</td><td>52.5</td></tr>
<tr><td>7</td><td>Oklahoma</td><td>71.5</td><td>36</td><td>Utah</td><td>51.9</td></tr>
<tr><td>24</td><td>Oregon</td><td>57.6</td><td>37</td><td>North Dakota</td><td>51.8</td></tr>
<tr><td>30</td><td>Pennsylvania</td><td>53.7</td><td>38</td><td>Washington</td><td>51.7</td></tr>
<tr><td>45</td><td>Rhode Island</td><td>48.1</td><td>39</td><td>Illinois</td><td>51.4</td></tr>
<tr><td>12</td><td>South Carolina</td><td>69.1</td><td>40</td><td>Ohio</td><td>50.0</td></tr>
<tr><td>14</td><td>South Dakota</td><td>67.9</td><td>41</td><td>Iowa</td><td>49.3</td></tr>
<tr><td>13</td><td>Tennessee</td><td>68.7</td><td>41</td><td>Minnesota</td><td>49.3</td></tr>
<tr><td>28</td><td>Texas</td><td>55.0</td><td>43</td><td>New Jersey</td><td>48.4</td></tr>
<tr><td>36</td><td>Utah</td><td>51.9</td><td>44</td><td>New York</td><td>48.3</td></tr>
<tr><td>31</td><td>Vermont</td><td>53.2</td><td>45</td><td>Rhode Island</td><td>48.1</td></tr>
<tr><td>32</td><td>Virginia</td><td>52.7</td><td>46</td><td>Hawaii</td><td>47.3</td></tr>
<tr><td>38</td><td>Washington</td><td>51.7</td><td>47</td><td>New Hampshire</td><td>46.3</td></tr>
<tr><td>10</td><td>West Virginia</td><td>70.2</td><td>48</td><td>Connecticut</td><td>45.3</td></tr>
<tr><td>27</td><td>Wisconsin</td><td>55.6</td><td>49</td><td>Massachusetts</td><td>43.5</td></tr>
<tr><td>5</td><td>Wyoming</td><td>76.3</td><td>50</td><td>California</td><td>38.6</td></tr>
<tr><td></td><td></td><td></td><td></td><td>District of Columbia</td><td>82.5</td></tr>
</tbody>
</table>

Source: U.S. Department of Health and Human Services, National Center for Health Statistics
(http://wonder.cdc.gov)

By state of residence. Injury as used here includes Accidents (including motor vehicle), Suicides, Homicides and "Other" undetermined. Not age-adjusted.

Age-Adjusted Death Rate by Injury in 2001

National Rate = 54.9 Deaths per 100,000 Population*

ALPHA ORDER

RANK	STATE	RATE
7	Alabama	70.8
2	Alaska	83.7
6	Arizona	73.3
10	Arkansas	70.5
50	California	39.6
19	Colorado	64.2
48	Connecticut	44.0
28	Delaware	55.7
22	Florida	61.0
20	Georgia	64.1
44	Hawaii	46.4
16	Idaho	65.3
35	Illinois	51.5
26	Indiana	56.5
46	Iowa	45.5
23	Kansas	58.2
15	Kentucky	66.9
9	Louisiana	70.7
38	Maine	49.9
29	Maryland	55.2
49	Massachusetts	41.4
32	Michigan	52.8
41	Minnesota	48.4
3	Mississippi	80.6
17	Missouri	64.6
5	Montana	75.4
37	Nebraska	50.4
13	Nevada	68.0
45	New Hampshire	46.3
42	New Jersey	47.6
1	New Mexico	85.9
43	New York	47.4
21	North Carolina	62.3
40	North Dakota	48.6
39	Ohio	49.4
7	Oklahoma	70.8
27	Oregon	56.3
36	Pennsylvania	51.1
47	Rhode Island	45.1
11	South Carolina	69.3
18	South Dakota	64.5
12	Tennessee	68.5
25	Texas	57.7
24	Utah	58.1
34	Vermont	51.7
31	Virginia	53.7
33	Washington	52.1
14	West Virginia	67.7
30	Wisconsin	53.8
4	Wyoming	76.3

RANK ORDER

RANK	STATE	RATE
1	New Mexico	85.9
2	Alaska	83.7
3	Mississippi	80.6
4	Wyoming	76.3
5	Montana	75.4
6	Arizona	73.3
7	Alabama	70.8
7	Oklahoma	70.8
9	Louisiana	70.7
10	Arkansas	70.5
11	South Carolina	69.3
12	Tennessee	68.5
13	Nevada	68.0
14	West Virginia	67.7
15	Kentucky	66.9
16	Idaho	65.3
17	Missouri	64.6
18	South Dakota	64.5
19	Colorado	64.2
20	Georgia	64.1
21	North Carolina	62.3
22	Florida	61.0
23	Kansas	58.2
24	Utah	58.1
25	Texas	57.7
26	Indiana	56.5
27	Oregon	56.3
28	Delaware	55.7
29	Maryland	55.2
30	Wisconsin	53.8
31	Virginia	53.7
32	Michigan	52.8
33	Washington	52.1
34	Vermont	51.7
35	Illinois	51.5
36	Pennsylvania	51.1
37	Nebraska	50.4
38	Maine	49.9
39	Ohio	49.4
40	North Dakota	48.6
41	Minnesota	48.4
42	New Jersey	47.6
43	New York	47.4
44	Hawaii	46.4
45	New Hampshire	46.3
46	Iowa	45.5
47	Rhode Island	45.1
48	Connecticut	44.0
49	Massachusetts	41.4
50	California	39.6

| | District of Columbia | 78.3 |

Source: U.S. Department of Health and Human Services, National Center for Health Statistics
    (http://wonder.cdc.gov)
*By state of residence. Injury as used here includes Accidents (including motor vehicle), Suicides, Homicides and
"Other" undetermined. Age-adjusted rates based on the year 2000 standard population.

Deaths by Accidents in 2002

National Total = 106,742 Deaths*

ALPHA ORDER

RANK	STATE	DEATHS	% of USA
17	Alabama	2,228	2.1%
45	Alaska	346	0.3%
14	Arizona	2,577	2.4%
30	Arkansas	1,311	1.2%
1	California	10,107	9.5%
24	Colorado	1,812	1.7%
31	Connecticut	1,182	1.1%
46	Delaware	292	0.3%
3	Florida	7,396	6.9%
9	Georgia	3,333	3.1%
42	Hawaii	393	0.4%
39	Idaho	611	0.6%
6	Illinois	4,222	4.0%
19	Indiana	2,148	2.0%
34	Iowa	1,093	1.0%
32	Kansas	1,139	1.1%
21	Kentucky	2,090	2.0%
20	Louisiana	2,115	2.0%
41	Maine	511	0.5%
29	Maryland	1,332	1.2%
27	Massachusetts	1,413	1.3%
10	Michigan	3,285	3.1%
23	Minnesota	1,928	1.8%
25	Mississippi	1,642	1.5%
12	Missouri	2,641	2.5%
40	Montana	524	0.5%
37	Nebraska	762	0.7%
36	Nevada	860	0.8%
43	New Hampshire	357	0.3%
13	New Jersey	2,599	2.4%
33	New Mexico	1,105	1.0%
5	New York	4,663	4.4%
8	North Carolina	3,700	3.5%
49	North Dakota	246	0.2%
7	Ohio	4,146	3.9%
26	Oklahoma	1,580	1.5%
28	Oregon	1,397	1.3%
4	Pennsylvania	4,728	4.4%
48	Rhode Island	277	0.3%
22	South Carolina	1,972	1.8%
44	South Dakota	348	0.3%
11	Tennessee	2,744	2.6%
2	Texas	8,232	7.7%
38	Utah	714	0.7%
50	Vermont	240	0.2%
15	Virginia	2,479	2.3%
18	Washington	2,203	2.1%
35	West Virginia	956	0.9%
16	Wisconsin	2,274	2.1%
47	Wyoming	289	0.3%

RANK ORDER

RANK	STATE	DEATHS	% of USA
1	California	10,107	9.5%
2	Texas	8,232	7.7%
3	Florida	7,396	6.9%
4	Pennsylvania	4,728	4.4%
5	New York	4,663	4.4%
6	Illinois	4,222	4.0%
7	Ohio	4,146	3.9%
8	North Carolina	3,700	3.5%
9	Georgia	3,333	3.1%
10	Michigan	3,285	3.1%
11	Tennessee	2,744	2.6%
12	Missouri	2,641	2.5%
13	New Jersey	2,599	2.4%
14	Arizona	2,577	2.4%
15	Virginia	2,479	2.3%
16	Wisconsin	2,274	2.1%
17	Alabama	2,228	2.1%
18	Washington	2,203	2.1%
19	Indiana	2,148	2.0%
20	Louisiana	2,115	2.0%
21	Kentucky	2,090	2.0%
22	South Carolina	1,972	1.8%
23	Minnesota	1,928	1.8%
24	Colorado	1,812	1.7%
25	Mississippi	1,642	1.5%
26	Oklahoma	1,580	1.5%
27	Massachusetts	1,413	1.3%
28	Oregon	1,397	1.3%
29	Maryland	1,332	1.2%
30	Arkansas	1,311	1.2%
31	Connecticut	1,182	1.1%
32	Kansas	1,139	1.1%
33	New Mexico	1,105	1.0%
34	Iowa	1,093	1.0%
35	West Virginia	956	0.9%
36	Nevada	860	0.8%
37	Nebraska	762	0.7%
38	Utah	714	0.7%
39	Idaho	611	0.6%
40	Montana	524	0.5%
41	Maine	511	0.5%
42	Hawaii	393	0.4%
43	New Hampshire	357	0.3%
44	South Dakota	348	0.3%
45	Alaska	346	0.3%
46	Delaware	292	0.3%
47	Wyoming	289	0.3%
48	Rhode Island	277	0.3%
49	North Dakota	246	0.2%
50	Vermont	240	0.2%
	District of Columbia	200	0.2%

Source: U.S. Department of Health and Human Services, National Center for Health Statistics
    "National Vital Statistics Reports" (Vol. 53, No. 5, October 12, 2004)
*Final data by state of residence. Includes motor vehicle deaths, poisoning, falls, drowning and other accidents.

Death Rate by Accidents in 2002

National Rate = 37.0 Deaths per 100,000 Population*

ALPHA ORDER

RANK	STATE	RATE
8	Alabama	49.7
5	Alaska	53.7
12	Arizona	47.2
9	Arkansas	48.4
45	California	28.8
23	Colorado	40.2
38	Connecticut	34.2
36	Delaware	36.2
19	Florida	44.3
27	Georgia	38.9
42	Hawaii	31.6
16	Idaho	45.6
40	Illinois	33.5
37	Indiana	34.9
33	Iowa	37.2
21	Kansas	41.9
7	Kentucky	51.1
12	Louisiana	47.2
26	Maine	39.5
48	Maryland	24.4
50	Massachusetts	22.0
41	Michigan	32.7
30	Minnesota	38.4
4	Mississippi	57.2
14	Missouri	46.6
3	Montana	57.6
20	Nebraska	44.1
25	Nevada	39.6
46	New Hampshire	28.0
44	New Jersey	30.3
1	New Mexico	59.6
49	New York	24.3
18	North Carolina	44.5
29	North Dakota	38.8
34	Ohio	36.3
17	Oklahoma	45.2
24	Oregon	39.7
31	Pennsylvania	38.3
47	Rhode Island	25.9
10	South Carolina	48.0
15	South Dakota	45.7
11	Tennessee	47.3
32	Texas	37.8
43	Utah	30.8
27	Vermont	38.9
39	Virginia	34.0
34	Washington	36.3
6	West Virginia	53.1
22	Wisconsin	41.8
2	Wyoming	58.0

RANK ORDER

RANK	STATE	RATE
1	New Mexico	59.6
2	Wyoming	58.0
3	Montana	57.6
4	Mississippi	57.2
5	Alaska	53.7
6	West Virginia	53.1
7	Kentucky	51.1
8	Alabama	49.7
9	Arkansas	48.4
10	South Carolina	48.0
11	Tennessee	47.3
12	Arizona	47.2
12	Louisiana	47.2
14	Missouri	46.6
15	South Dakota	45.7
16	Idaho	45.6
17	Oklahoma	45.2
18	North Carolina	44.5
19	Florida	44.3
20	Nebraska	44.1
21	Kansas	41.9
22	Wisconsin	41.8
23	Colorado	40.2
24	Oregon	39.7
25	Nevada	39.6
26	Maine	39.5
27	Georgia	38.9
27	Vermont	38.9
29	North Dakota	38.8
30	Minnesota	38.4
31	Pennsylvania	38.3
32	Texas	37.8
33	Iowa	37.2
34	Ohio	36.3
34	Washington	36.3
36	Delaware	36.2
37	Indiana	34.9
38	Connecticut	34.2
39	Virginia	34.0
40	Illinois	33.5
41	Michigan	32.7
42	Hawaii	31.6
43	Utah	30.8
44	New Jersey	30.3
45	California	28.8
46	New Hampshire	28.0
47	Rhode Island	25.9
48	Maryland	24.4
49	New York	24.3
50	Massachusetts	22.0
	District of Columbia	35.0

Source: U.S. Department of Health and Human Services, National Center for Health Statistics
    "National Vital Statistics Reports" (Vol. 53, No. 5, October 12, 2004)
*Final data by state of residence. Includes motor vehicle deaths, poisoning, falls, drowning and other accidents.
Not age-adjusted.

Age-Adjusted Death Rate by Accidents in 2002

National Rate = 36.9 Deaths per 100,000 Population*

ALPHA ORDER

RANK	STATE	RATE
8	Alabama	49.2
2	Alaska	59.0
10	Arizona	48.1
13	Arkansas	47.3
44	California	29.9
19	Colorado	42.8
42	Connecticut	32.5
32	Delaware	35.9
20	Florida	41.9
22	Georgia	41.8
43	Hawaii	30.4
14	Idaho	46.8
39	Illinois	33.5
38	Indiana	34.8
40	Iowa	33.3
24	Kansas	40.6
7	Kentucky	50.5
11	Louisiana	48.0
28	Maine	37.6
47	Maryland	25.1
50	Massachusetts	20.5
41	Michigan	32.7
29	Minnesota	37.3
3	Mississippi	57.9
15	Missouri	45.3
5	Montana	55.2
23	Nebraska	41.4
20	Nevada	41.9
46	New Hampshire	28.1
45	New Jersey	29.5
1	New Mexico	61.1
48	New York	23.7
16	North Carolina	45.2
36	North Dakota	35.0
33	Ohio	35.6
17	Oklahoma	44.6
27	Oregon	38.1
33	Pennsylvania	35.6
49	Rhode Island	23.1
9	South Carolina	48.2
18	South Dakota	43.3
12	Tennessee	47.4
25	Texas	40.1
33	Utah	35.6
30	Vermont	37.2
36	Virginia	35.0
31	Washington	36.5
6	West Virginia	50.7
26	Wisconsin	39.7
3	Wyoming	57.9

RANK ORDER

RANK	STATE	RATE
1	New Mexico	61.1
2	Alaska	59.0
3	Mississippi	57.9
3	Wyoming	57.9
5	Montana	55.2
6	West Virginia	50.7
7	Kentucky	50.5
8	Alabama	49.2
9	South Carolina	48.2
10	Arizona	48.1
11	Louisiana	48.0
12	Tennessee	47.4
13	Arkansas	47.3
14	Idaho	46.8
15	Missouri	45.3
16	North Carolina	45.2
17	Oklahoma	44.6
18	South Dakota	43.3
19	Colorado	42.8
20	Florida	41.9
20	Nevada	41.9
22	Georgia	41.8
23	Nebraska	41.4
24	Kansas	40.6
25	Texas	40.1
26	Wisconsin	39.7
27	Oregon	38.1
28	Maine	37.6
29	Minnesota	37.3
30	Vermont	37.2
31	Washington	36.5
32	Delaware	35.9
33	Ohio	35.6
33	Pennsylvania	35.6
33	Utah	35.6
36	North Dakota	35.0
36	Virginia	35.0
38	Indiana	34.8
39	Illinois	33.5
40	Iowa	33.3
41	Michigan	32.7
42	Connecticut	32.5
43	Hawaii	30.4
44	California	29.9
45	New Jersey	29.5
46	New Hampshire	28.1
47	Maryland	25.1
48	New York	23.7
49	Rhode Island	23.1
50	Massachusetts	20.5

District of Columbia	34.5

Source: U.S. Department of Health and Human Services, National Center for Health Statistics
    "National Vital Statistics Reports" (Vol. 53, No. 5, October 12, 2004)
*Final data by state of residence. Includes motor vehicle deaths, poisoning, falls, drowning and other accidents.
Age-adjusted rates based on the year 2000 standard population.

Deaths by Motor Vehicle Accidents in 2002

National Total = 45,380 Deaths*

ALPHA ORDER

RANK	STATE	DEATHS	% of USA
13	Alabama	1,115	2.5%
47	Alaska	112	0.2%
14	Arizona	1,105	2.4%
28	Arkansas	693	1.5%
1	California	4,248	9.4%
23	Colorado	781	1.7%
36	Connecticut	348	0.8%
45	Delaware	121	0.3%
3	Florida	3,196	7.0%
9	Georgia	1,526	3.4%
45	Hawaii	121	0.3%
39	Idaho	296	0.7%
8	Illinois	1,579	3.5%
16	Indiana	963	2.1%
32	Iowa	426	0.9%
30	Kansas	563	1.2%
19	Kentucky	923	2.0%
18	Louisiana	959	2.1%
41	Maine	215	0.5%
27	Maryland	718	1.6%
29	Massachusetts	565	1.2%
10	Michigan	1,386	3.1%
26	Minnesota	744	1.6%
20	Mississippi	879	1.9%
12	Missouri	1,213	2.7%
40	Montana	255	0.6%
37	Nebraska	337	0.7%
35	Nevada	386	0.9%
44	New Hampshire	125	0.3%
22	New Jersey	786	1.7%
33	New Mexico	423	0.9%
5	New York	1,695	3.7%
6	North Carolina	1,690	3.7%
48	North Dakota	111	0.2%
7	Ohio	1,602	3.5%
24	Oklahoma	766	1.7%
31	Oregon	462	1.0%
4	Pennsylvania	1,739	3.8%
49	Rhode Island	95	0.2%
15	South Carolina	1,024	2.3%
42	South Dakota	186	0.4%
11	Tennessee	1,250	2.8%
2	Texas	4,024	8.9%
38	Utah	329	0.7%
50	Vermont	78	0.2%
16	Virginia	963	2.1%
25	Washington	760	1.7%
34	West Virginia	414	0.9%
21	Wisconsin	870	1.9%
43	Wyoming	157	0.3%

RANK ORDER

RANK	STATE	DEATHS	% of USA
1	California	4,248	9.4%
2	Texas	4,024	8.9%
3	Florida	3,196	7.0%
4	Pennsylvania	1,739	3.8%
5	New York	1,695	3.7%
6	North Carolina	1,690	3.7%
7	Ohio	1,602	3.5%
8	Illinois	1,579	3.5%
9	Georgia	1,526	3.4%
10	Michigan	1,386	3.1%
11	Tennessee	1,250	2.8%
12	Missouri	1,213	2.7%
13	Alabama	1,115	2.5%
14	Arizona	1,105	2.4%
15	South Carolina	1,024	2.3%
16	Indiana	963	2.1%
16	Virginia	963	2.1%
18	Louisiana	959	2.1%
19	Kentucky	923	2.0%
20	Mississippi	879	1.9%
21	Wisconsin	870	1.9%
22	New Jersey	786	1.7%
23	Colorado	781	1.7%
24	Oklahoma	766	1.7%
25	Washington	760	1.7%
26	Minnesota	744	1.6%
27	Maryland	718	1.6%
28	Arkansas	693	1.5%
29	Massachusetts	565	1.2%
30	Kansas	563	1.2%
31	Oregon	462	1.0%
32	Iowa	426	0.9%
33	New Mexico	423	0.9%
34	West Virginia	414	0.9%
35	Nevada	386	0.9%
36	Connecticut	348	0.8%
37	Nebraska	337	0.7%
38	Utah	329	0.7%
39	Idaho	296	0.7%
40	Montana	255	0.6%
41	Maine	215	0.5%
42	South Dakota	186	0.4%
43	Wyoming	157	0.3%
44	New Hampshire	125	0.3%
45	Delaware	121	0.3%
45	Hawaii	121	0.3%
47	Alaska	112	0.2%
48	North Dakota	111	0.2%
49	Rhode Island	95	0.2%
50	Vermont	78	0.2%
	District of Columbia	58	0.1%

Source: U.S. Department of Health and Human Services, National Center for Health Statistics
    "National Vital Statistics Reports" (Vol. 53, No. 5, October 12, 2004)
*Final data by state of residence. These numbers are compiled from death certificates by the Centers for Disease Control and Prevention. They may differ from motor vehicle deaths collected by the U.S. Department of Transportation from other sources.

Death Rate by Motor Vehicle Accidents in 2002

National Rate = 15.7 Deaths per 100,000 Population*

ALPHA ORDER

RANK	STATE	RATE
5	Alabama	24.9
25	Alaska	17.4
17	Arizona	20.3
4	Arkansas	25.6
43	California	12.1
26	Colorado	17.3
44	Connecticut	10.1
30	Delaware	15.0
20	Florida	19.1
22	Georgia	17.8
46	Hawaii	9.7
11	Idaho	22.1
41	Illinois	12.5
29	Indiana	15.6
32	Iowa	14.5
16	Kansas	20.7
10	Kentucky	22.6
14	Louisiana	21.4
27	Maine	16.6
37	Maryland	13.2
49	Massachusetts	8.8
36	Michigan	13.8
31	Minnesota	14.8
2	Mississippi	30.6
14	Missouri	21.4
3	Montana	28.0
19	Nebraska	19.5
22	Nevada	17.8
45	New Hampshire	9.8
47	New Jersey	9.1
9	New Mexico	22.8
49	New York	8.8
17	North Carolina	20.3
24	North Dakota	17.5
35	Ohio	14.0
12	Oklahoma	21.9
39	Oregon	13.1
34	Pennsylvania	14.1
48	Rhode Island	8.9
5	South Carolina	24.9
7	South Dakota	24.4
13	Tennessee	21.6
21	Texas	18.5
33	Utah	14.2
40	Vermont	12.7
37	Virginia	13.2
41	Washington	12.5
8	West Virginia	23.0
28	Wisconsin	16.0
1	Wyoming	31.5

RANK ORDER

RANK	STATE	RATE
1	Wyoming	31.5
2	Mississippi	30.6
3	Montana	28.0
4	Arkansas	25.6
5	Alabama	24.9
5	South Carolina	24.9
7	South Dakota	24.4
8	West Virginia	23.0
9	New Mexico	22.8
10	Kentucky	22.6
11	Idaho	22.1
12	Oklahoma	21.9
13	Tennessee	21.6
14	Louisiana	21.4
14	Missouri	21.4
16	Kansas	20.7
17	Arizona	20.3
17	North Carolina	20.3
19	Nebraska	19.5
20	Florida	19.1
21	Texas	18.5
22	Georgia	17.8
22	Nevada	17.8
24	North Dakota	17.5
25	Alaska	17.4
26	Colorado	17.3
27	Maine	16.6
28	Wisconsin	16.0
29	Indiana	15.6
30	Delaware	15.0
31	Minnesota	14.8
32	Iowa	14.5
33	Utah	14.2
34	Pennsylvania	14.1
35	Ohio	14.0
36	Michigan	13.8
37	Maryland	13.2
37	Virginia	13.2
39	Oregon	13.1
40	Vermont	12.7
41	Illinois	12.5
41	Washington	12.5
43	California	12.1
44	Connecticut	10.1
45	New Hampshire	9.8
46	Hawaii	9.7
47	New Jersey	9.1
48	Rhode Island	8.9
49	Massachusetts	8.8
49	New York	8.8

District of Columbia   10.2

Source: U.S. Department of Health and Human Services, National Center for Health Statistics
     "National Vital Statistics Reports" (Vol. 53, No. 5, October 12, 2004)
*Final data by state of residence. These numbers are compiled from death certificates by the Centers for Disease Control and Prevention. They may differ from motor vehicle deaths collected by the U.S. Department of Transportation from other sources. Not age-adjusted.

Age-Adjusted Death Rate by Motor Vehicle Accidents in 2002

National Rate = 15.7 Deaths per 100,000 Population*

ALPHA ORDER			RANK ORDER		
RANK	STATE	RATE	RANK	STATE	RATE
5	Alabama	24.7	1	Wyoming	31.2
19	Alaska	19.1	2	Mississippi	30.6
16	Arizona	20.5	3	Montana	27.4
4	Arkansas	25.4	4	Arkansas	25.4
43	California	12.2	5	Alabama	24.7
25	Colorado	17.4	6	South Carolina	24.6
44	Connecticut	10.2	7	South Dakota	23.9
30	Delaware	14.8	8	New Mexico	22.7
20	Florida	18.9	9	West Virginia	22.4
24	Georgia	18.1	10	Idaho	22.2
46	Hawaii	9.5	11	Kentucky	22.1
10	Idaho	22.2	12	Oklahoma	21.6
40	Illinois	12.5	13	Tennessee	21.5
29	Indiana	15.5	14	Louisiana	21.3
33	Iowa	13.9	15	Missouri	21.1
17	Kansas	20.3	16	Arizona	20.5
11	Kentucky	22.1	17	Kansas	20.3
14	Louisiana	21.3	17	North Carolina	20.3
27	Maine	16.1	19	Alaska	19.1
37	Maryland	13.3	20	Florida	18.9
49	Massachusetts	8.6	20	Nebraska	18.9
35	Michigan	13.8	22	Texas	18.7
32	Minnesota	14.6	23	Nevada	18.3
2	Mississippi	30.6	24	Georgia	18.1
15	Missouri	21.1	25	Colorado	17.4
3	Montana	27.4	26	North Dakota	16.6
20	Nebraska	18.9	27	Maine	16.1
23	Nevada	18.3	28	Wisconsin	15.6
45	New Hampshire	9.8	29	Indiana	15.5
47	New Jersey	9.2	30	Delaware	14.8
8	New Mexico	22.7	31	Utah	14.7
48	New York	8.7	32	Minnesota	14.6
17	North Carolina	20.3	33	Iowa	13.9
26	North Dakota	16.6	33	Ohio	13.9
33	Ohio	13.9	35	Michigan	13.8
12	Oklahoma	21.6	35	Pennsylvania	13.8
39	Oregon	12.8	37	Maryland	13.3
35	Pennsylvania	13.8	38	Virginia	13.2
50	Rhode Island	8.5	39	Oregon	12.8
6	South Carolina	24.6	40	Illinois	12.5
7	South Dakota	23.9	40	Vermont	12.5
13	Tennessee	21.5	40	Washington	12.5
22	Texas	18.7	43	California	12.2
31	Utah	14.7	44	Connecticut	10.2
40	Vermont	12.5	45	New Hampshire	9.8
38	Virginia	13.2	46	Hawaii	9.5
40	Washington	12.5	47	New Jersey	9.2
9	West Virginia	22.4	48	New York	8.7
28	Wisconsin	15.6	49	Massachusetts	8.6
1	Wyoming	31.2	50	Rhode Island	8.5
				District of Columbia	9.4

Source: U.S. Department of Health and Human Services, National Center for Health Statistics
    "National Vital Statistics Reports" (Vol. 52, No. 3, September 18, 2003)
*Final data by state of residence. These numbers are compiled from death certificates by the Centers for Disease Control and Prevention. They may differ from motor vehicle deaths collected by the U.S. Department of Transportation from other sources. Age-adjusted rates based on the year 2000 standard population.

Deaths by Firearm Injury in 2002

National Total = 30,242 Deaths*

ALPHA ORDER

RANK	STATE	DEATHS	% of USA
15	Alabama	724	2.4%
41	Alaska	127	0.4%
11	Arizona	968	3.2%
26	Arkansas	441	1.5%
1	California	3,410	11.3%
22	Colorado	517	1.7%
38	Connecticut	147	0.5%
45	Delaware	74	0.2%
3	Florida	1,886	6.2%
7	Georgia	1,133	3.7%
50	Hawaii	36	0.1%
37	Idaho	163	0.5%
4	Illinois	1,231	4.1%
16	Indiana	723	2.4%
36	Iowa	201	0.7%
33	Kansas	268	0.9%
21	Kentucky	544	1.8%
13	Louisiana	876	2.9%
43	Maine	88	0.3%
18	Maryland	615	2.0%
35	Massachusetts	204	0.7%
8	Michigan	1,092	3.6%
30	Minnesota	306	1.0%
23	Mississippi	492	1.6%
17	Missouri	696	2.3%
40	Montana	134	0.4%
39	Nebraska	140	0.5%
29	Nevada	370	1.2%
44	New Hampshire	76	0.3%
27	New Jersey	415	1.4%
31	New Mexico	304	1.0%
10	New York	994	3.3%
6	North Carolina	1,136	3.8%
48	North Dakota	58	0.2%
9	Ohio	1,069	3.5%
24	Oklahoma	452	1.5%
28	Oregon	374	1.2%
5	Pennsylvania	1,220	4.0%
49	Rhode Island	55	0.2%
20	South Carolina	566	1.9%
47	South Dakota	61	0.2%
12	Tennessee	905	3.0%
2	Texas	2,301	7.6%
34	Utah	207	0.7%
46	Vermont	62	0.2%
14	Virginia	806	2.7%
19	Washington	568	1.9%
32	West Virginia	271	0.9%
25	Wisconsin	446	1.5%
42	Wyoming	95	0.3%

RANK ORDER

RANK	STATE	DEATHS	% of USA
1	California	3,410	11.3%
2	Texas	2,301	7.6%
3	Florida	1,886	6.2%
4	Illinois	1,231	4.1%
5	Pennsylvania	1,220	4.0%
6	North Carolina	1,136	3.8%
7	Georgia	1,133	3.7%
8	Michigan	1,092	3.6%
9	Ohio	1,069	3.5%
10	New York	994	3.3%
11	Arizona	968	3.2%
12	Tennessee	905	3.0%
13	Louisiana	876	2.9%
14	Virginia	806	2.7%
15	Alabama	724	2.4%
16	Indiana	723	2.4%
17	Missouri	696	2.3%
18	Maryland	615	2.0%
19	Washington	568	1.9%
20	South Carolina	566	1.9%
21	Kentucky	544	1.8%
22	Colorado	517	1.7%
23	Mississippi	492	1.6%
24	Oklahoma	452	1.5%
25	Wisconsin	446	1.5%
26	Arkansas	441	1.5%
27	New Jersey	415	1.4%
28	Oregon	374	1.2%
29	Nevada	370	1.2%
30	Minnesota	306	1.0%
31	New Mexico	304	1.0%
32	West Virginia	271	0.9%
33	Kansas	268	0.9%
34	Utah	207	0.7%
35	Massachusetts	204	0.7%
36	Iowa	201	0.7%
37	Idaho	163	0.5%
38	Connecticut	147	0.5%
39	Nebraska	140	0.5%
40	Montana	134	0.4%
41	Alaska	127	0.4%
42	Wyoming	95	0.3%
43	Maine	88	0.3%
44	New Hampshire	76	0.3%
45	Delaware	74	0.2%
46	Vermont	62	0.2%
47	South Dakota	61	0.2%
48	North Dakota	58	0.2%
49	Rhode Island	55	0.2%
50	Hawaii	36	0.1%
	District of Columbia	195	0.6%

Source: U.S. Department of Health and Human Services, National Center for Health Statistics
"National Vital Statistics Reports" (Vol. 53, No. 5, October 12, 2004)
*Final data by state of residence.

Death Rate by Firearm Injury in 2002

National Rate = 10.5 Deaths per 100,000 Population*

ALPHA ORDER				RANK ORDER		
RANK	STATE	RATE		RANK	STATE	RATE
9	Alabama	16.1		1	Alaska	19.7
1	Alaska	19.7		2	Louisiana	19.5
4	Arizona	17.7		3	Wyoming	19.0
8	Arkansas	16.3		4	Arizona	17.7
32	California	9.7		5	Mississippi	17.1
21	Colorado	11.5		6	Nevada	17.0
48	Connecticut	4.2		7	New Mexico	16.4
35	Delaware	9.2		8	Arkansas	16.3
22	Florida	11.3		9	Alabama	16.1
16	Georgia	13.2		10	Tennessee	15.6
50	Hawaii	2.9		11	West Virginia	15.0
19	Idaho	12.2		12	Montana	14.7
31	Illinois	9.8		13	South Carolina	13.8
20	Indiana	11.7		14	North Carolina	13.7
41	Iowa	6.8		15	Kentucky	13.3
29	Kansas	9.9		16	Georgia	13.2
15	Kentucky	13.3		17	Oklahoma	12.9
2	Louisiana	19.5		18	Missouri	12.3
41	Maine	6.8		19	Idaho	12.2
22	Maryland	11.3		20	Indiana	11.7
49	Massachusetts	3.2		21	Colorado	11.5
25	Michigan	10.9		22	Florida	11.3
43	Minnesota	6.1		22	Maryland	11.3
5	Mississippi	17.1		24	Virginia	11.1
18	Missouri	12.3		25	Michigan	10.9
12	Montana	14.7		26	Oregon	10.6
39	Nebraska	8.1		26	Texas	10.6
6	Nevada	17.0		28	Vermont	10.1
44	New Hampshire	6.0		29	Kansas	9.9
47	New Jersey	4.8		29	Pennsylvania	9.9
7	New Mexico	16.4		31	Illinois	9.8
45	New York	5.2		32	California	9.7
14	North Carolina	13.7		33	Ohio	9.4
36	North Dakota	9.1		33	Washington	9.4
33	Ohio	9.4		35	Delaware	9.2
17	Oklahoma	12.9		36	North Dakota	9.1
26	Oregon	10.6		37	Utah	8.9
29	Pennsylvania	9.9		38	Wisconsin	8.2
46	Rhode Island	5.1		39	Nebraska	8.1
13	South Carolina	13.8		40	South Dakota	8.0
40	South Dakota	8.0		41	Iowa	6.8
10	Tennessee	15.6		41	Maine	6.8
26	Texas	10.6		43	Minnesota	6.1
37	Utah	8.9		44	New Hampshire	6.0
28	Vermont	10.1		45	New York	5.2
24	Virginia	11.1		46	Rhode Island	5.1
33	Washington	9.4		47	New Jersey	4.8
11	West Virginia	15.0		48	Connecticut	4.2
38	Wisconsin	8.2		49	Massachusetts	3.2
3	Wyoming	19.0		50	Hawaii	2.9
					District of Columbia	34.2

Source: U.S. Department of Health and Human Services, National Center for Health Statistics
"National Vital Statistics Reports" (Vol. 53, No. 5, October 12, 2004)
Final data by state of residence. Not age-adjusted.

Age-Adjusted Death Rate by Firearm Injury in 2002

National Rate = 10.4 Deaths per 100,000 Population*

ALPHA ORDER

RANK	STATE	RATE
9	Alabama	16.0
1	Alaska	20.0
4	Arizona	17.9
8	Arkansas	16.3
29	California	9.7
21	Colorado	11.5
48	Connecticut	4.3
36	Delaware	9.0
23	Florida	11.1
15	Georgia	13.4
50	Hawaii	2.8
18	Idaho	12.4
29	Illinois	9.7
20	Indiana	11.7
41	Iowa	6.7
29	Kansas	9.7
16	Kentucky	12.9
2	Louisiana	19.4
42	Maine	6.5
22	Maryland	11.4
49	Massachusetts	3.1
25	Michigan	10.9
43	Minnesota	6.0
6	Mississippi	17.2
19	Missouri	12.2
12	Montana	14.5
38	Nebraska	8.1
5	Nevada	17.3
44	New Hampshire	5.8
47	New Jersey	4.9
7	New Mexico	16.6
45	New York	5.1
13	North Carolina	13.6
36	North Dakota	9.0
35	Ohio	9.3
17	Oklahoma	12.8
27	Oregon	10.5
28	Pennsylvania	9.9
46	Rhode Island	5.0
13	South Carolina	13.6
40	South Dakota	7.9
10	Tennessee	15.4
26	Texas	10.8
32	Utah	9.6
32	Vermont	9.6
24	Virginia	11.0
34	Washington	9.4
11	West Virginia	14.7
39	Wisconsin	8.0
3	Wyoming	18.8

RANK ORDER

RANK	STATE	RATE
1	Alaska	20.0
2	Louisiana	19.4
3	Wyoming	18.8
4	Arizona	17.9
5	Nevada	17.3
6	Mississippi	17.2
7	New Mexico	16.6
8	Arkansas	16.3
9	Alabama	16.0
10	Tennessee	15.4
11	West Virginia	14.7
12	Montana	14.5
13	North Carolina	13.6
13	South Carolina	13.6
15	Georgia	13.4
16	Kentucky	12.9
17	Oklahoma	12.8
18	Idaho	12.4
19	Missouri	12.2
20	Indiana	11.7
21	Colorado	11.5
22	Maryland	11.4
23	Florida	11.1
24	Virginia	11.0
25	Michigan	10.9
26	Texas	10.8
27	Oregon	10.5
28	Pennsylvania	9.9
29	California	9.7
29	Illinois	9.7
29	Kansas	9.7
32	Utah	9.6
32	Vermont	9.6
34	Washington	9.4
35	Ohio	9.3
36	Delaware	9.0
36	North Dakota	9.0
38	Nebraska	8.1
39	Wisconsin	8.0
40	South Dakota	7.9
41	Iowa	6.7
42	Maine	6.5
43	Minnesota	6.0
44	New Hampshire	5.8
45	New York	5.1
46	Rhode Island	5.0
47	New Jersey	4.9
48	Connecticut	4.3
49	Massachusetts	3.1
50	Hawaii	2.8
	District of Columbia	31.3

Source: U.S. Department of Health and Human Services, National Center for Health Statistics
"National Vital Statistics Reports" (Vol. 53, No. 5, October 12, 2004)
*Final data by state of residence. Age-adjusted rates based on the year 2000 standard population.

Deaths by Homicide in 2002

National Total = 17,638 Homicides*

RANK	STATE	HOMICIDES	% of USA
15	Alabama	416	2.4%
40	Alaska	40	0.2%
13	Arizona	504	2.9%
25	Arkansas	194	1.1%
1	California	2,485	14.1%
28	Colorado	184	1.0%
34	Connecticut	98	0.6%
41	Delaware	38	0.2%
4	Florida	1,008	5.7%
7	Georgia	672	3.8%
41	Hawaii	38	0.2%
43	Idaho	32	0.2%
3	Illinois	1,016	5.8%
17	Indiana	385	2.2%
36	Iowa	56	0.3%
31	Kansas	129	0.7%
24	Kentucky	195	1.1%
10	Louisiana	607	3.4%
47	Maine	11	0.1%
12	Maryland	540	3.1%
27	Massachusetts	185	1.0%
6	Michigan	696	3.9%
32	Minnesota	127	0.7%
21	Mississippi	305	1.7%
18	Missouri	366	2.1%
44	Montana	23	0.1%
38	Nebraska	50	0.3%
29	Nevada	175	1.0%
48	New Hampshire	9	0.1%
19	New Jersey	333	1.9%
30	New Mexico	161	0.9%
5	New York	929	5.3%
8	North Carolina	644	3.7%
50	North Dakota	7	0.0%
11	Ohio	549	3.1%
23	Oklahoma	196	1.1%
33	Oregon	106	0.6%
9	Pennsylvania	640	3.6%
39	Rhode Island	43	0.2%
20	South Carolina	326	1.8%
46	South Dakota	22	0.1%
14	Tennessee	467	2.6%
2	Texas	1,421	8.1%
37	Utah	54	0.3%
49	Vermont	8	0.0%
16	Virginia	397	2.3%
22	Washington	213	1.2%
35	West Virginia	95	0.5%
26	Wisconsin	191	1.1%
44	Wyoming	23	0.1%

RANK	STATE	HOMICIDES	% of USA
1	California	2,485	14.1%
2	Texas	1,421	8.1%
3	Illinois	1,016	5.8%
4	Florida	1,008	5.7%
5	New York	929	5.3%
6	Michigan	696	3.9%
7	Georgia	672	3.8%
8	North Carolina	644	3.7%
9	Pennsylvania	640	3.6%
10	Louisiana	607	3.4%
11	Ohio	549	3.1%
12	Maryland	540	3.1%
13	Arizona	504	2.9%
14	Tennessee	467	2.6%
15	Alabama	416	2.4%
16	Virginia	397	2.3%
17	Indiana	385	2.2%
18	Missouri	366	2.1%
19	New Jersey	333	1.9%
20	South Carolina	326	1.8%
21	Mississippi	305	1.7%
22	Washington	213	1.2%
23	Oklahoma	196	1.1%
24	Kentucky	195	1.1%
25	Arkansas	194	1.1%
26	Wisconsin	191	1.1%
27	Massachusetts	185	1.0%
28	Colorado	184	1.0%
29	Nevada	175	1.0%
30	New Mexico	161	0.9%
31	Kansas	129	0.7%
32	Minnesota	127	0.7%
33	Oregon	106	0.6%
34	Connecticut	98	0.6%
35	West Virginia	95	0.5%
36	Iowa	56	0.3%
37	Utah	54	0.3%
38	Nebraska	50	0.3%
39	Rhode Island	43	0.2%
40	Alaska	40	0.2%
41	Delaware	38	0.2%
41	Hawaii	38	0.2%
43	Idaho	32	0.2%
44	Montana	23	0.1%
44	Wyoming	23	0.1%
46	South Dakota	22	0.1%
47	Maine	11	0.1%
48	New Hampshire	9	0.1%
49	Vermont	8	0.0%
50	North Dakota	7	0.0%
	District of Columbia	229	1.3%

Source: U.S. Department of Health and Human Services, National Center for Health Statistics
"National Vital Statistics Reports" (Vol. 53, No. 5, October 12, 2004)
By state of residence. Includes legal intervention. Homicide data shown here are collected by the Centers for Disease Control and Prevention based on death certificates and differ from murder data collected by the F.B.I. from other sources.

Death Rate by Homicide in 2002

National Rate = 6.1 Deaths per 100,000 Population*

ALPHA ORDER

RANK	STATE	RATE
4	Alabama	9.3
19	Alaska	6.2
5	Arizona	9.2
13	Arkansas	7.2
14	California	7.1
31	Colorado	4.1
41	Connecticut	2.8
28	Delaware	4.7
20	Florida	6.0
10	Georgia	7.9
36	Hawaii	3.1
44	Idaho	2.4
7	Illinois	8.1
18	Indiana	6.3
46	Iowa	1.9
28	Kansas	4.7
25	Kentucky	4.8
1	Louisiana	13.5
NA	Maine**	NA
3	Maryland	9.9
38	Massachusetts	2.9
15	Michigan	6.9
42	Minnesota	2.5
2	Mississippi	10.6
16	Missouri	6.5
42	Montana	2.5
38	Nebraska	2.9
7	Nevada	8.1
NA	New Hampshire**	NA
33	New Jersey	3.9
6	New Mexico	8.7
25	New York	4.8
12	North Carolina	7.7
NA	North Dakota**	NA
25	Ohio	4.8
21	Oklahoma	5.6
37	Oregon	3.0
24	Pennsylvania	5.2
32	Rhode Island	4.0
10	South Carolina	7.9
38	South Dakota	2.9
7	Tennessee	8.1
16	Texas	6.5
45	Utah	2.3
NA	Vermont**	NA
22	Virginia	5.4
34	Washington	3.5
23	West Virginia	5.3
34	Wisconsin	3.5
30	Wyoming	4.6

RANK ORDER

RANK	STATE	RATE
1	Louisiana	13.5
2	Mississippi	10.6
3	Maryland	9.9
4	Alabama	9.3
5	Arizona	9.2
6	New Mexico	8.7
7	Illinois	8.1
7	Nevada	8.1
7	Tennessee	8.1
10	Georgia	7.9
10	South Carolina	7.9
12	North Carolina	7.7
13	Arkansas	7.2
14	California	7.1
15	Michigan	6.9
16	Missouri	6.5
16	Texas	6.5
18	Indiana	6.3
19	Alaska	6.2
20	Florida	6.0
21	Oklahoma	5.6
22	Virginia	5.4
23	West Virginia	5.3
24	Pennsylvania	5.2
25	Kentucky	4.8
25	New York	4.8
25	Ohio	4.8
28	Delaware	4.7
28	Kansas	4.7
30	Wyoming	4.6
31	Colorado	4.1
32	Rhode Island	4.0
33	New Jersey	3.9
34	Washington	3.5
34	Wisconsin	3.5
36	Hawaii	3.1
37	Oregon	3.0
38	Massachusetts	2.9
38	Nebraska	2.9
38	South Dakota	2.9
41	Connecticut	2.8
42	Minnesota	2.5
42	Montana	2.5
44	Idaho	2.4
45	Utah	2.3
46	Iowa	1.9
NA	Maine**	NA
NA	New Hampshire**	NA
NA	North Dakota**	NA
NA	Vermont**	NA

District of Columbia	40.1

Source: U.S. Department of Health and Human Services, National Center for Health Statistics
    "National Vital Statistics Reports" (Vol. 53, No. 5, October 12, 2004)
*By state of residence. Includes legal intervention. Homicide data shown here are collected by the Centers for Disease Control and Prevention based on death certificates and differ from murder data collected by the F.B.I. from other sources. Not age-adjusted.
**Insufficient data to determine a reliable rate.

Age-Adjusted Death Rate by Homicide in 2002

National Rate = 6.1 Deaths per 100,000 Population*

ALPHA ORDER

RANK	STATE	RATE
4	Alabama	9.2
20	Alaska	6.0
4	Arizona	9.2
13	Arkansas	7.2
15	California	6.8
31	Colorado	4.0
38	Connecticut	3.0
27	Delaware	4.7
18	Florida	6.3
12	Georgia	7.5
36	Hawaii	3.1
44	Idaho	2.4
9	Illinois	7.9
19	Indiana	6.2
46	Iowa	1.9
27	Kansas	4.7
27	Kentucky	4.7
1	Louisiana	13.3
NA	Maine**	NA
3	Maryland	10.0
40	Massachusetts	2.9
14	Michigan	7.0
42	Minnesota	2.5
2	Mississippi	10.7
16	Missouri	6.5
42	Montana	2.5
40	Nebraska	2.9
7	Nevada	8.1
NA	New Hampshire**	NA
31	New Jersey	4.0
6	New Mexico	8.7
26	New York	4.8
11	North Carolina	7.6
NA	North Dakota**	NA
25	Ohio	4.9
21	Oklahoma	5.6
36	Oregon	3.1
23	Pennsylvania	5.4
31	Rhode Island	4.0
10	South Carolina	7.8
38	South Dakota	3.0
8	Tennessee	8.0
17	Texas	6.4
45	Utah	2.3
NA	Vermont**	NA
23	Virginia	5.4
34	Washington	3.5
22	West Virginia	5.5
34	Wisconsin	3.5
27	Wyoming	4.7

RANK ORDER

RANK	STATE	RATE
1	Louisiana	13.3
2	Mississippi	10.7
3	Maryland	10.0
4	Alabama	9.2
4	Arizona	9.2
6	New Mexico	8.7
7	Nevada	8.1
8	Tennessee	8.0
9	Illinois	7.9
10	South Carolina	7.8
11	North Carolina	7.6
12	Georgia	7.5
13	Arkansas	7.2
14	Michigan	7.0
15	California	6.8
16	Missouri	6.5
17	Texas	6.4
18	Florida	6.3
19	Indiana	6.2
20	Alaska	6.0
21	Oklahoma	5.6
22	West Virginia	5.5
23	Pennsylvania	5.4
23	Virginia	5.4
25	Ohio	4.9
26	New York	4.8
27	Delaware	4.7
27	Kansas	4.7
27	Kentucky	4.7
27	Wyoming	4.7
31	Colorado	4.0
31	New Jersey	4.0
31	Rhode Island	4.0
34	Washington	3.5
34	Wisconsin	3.5
36	Hawaii	3.1
36	Oregon	3.1
38	Connecticut	3.0
38	South Dakota	3.0
40	Massachusetts	2.9
40	Nebraska	2.9
42	Minnesota	2.5
42	Montana	2.5
44	Idaho	2.4
45	Utah	2.3
46	Iowa	1.9
NA	Maine**	NA
NA	New Hampshire**	NA
NA	North Dakota**	NA
NA	Vermont**	NA

District of Columbia 37.2

Source: U.S. Department of Health and Human Services, National Center for Health Statistics
"National Vital Statistics Reports" (Vol. 52, No. 3, September 18, 2003)
By state of residence. Includes legal intervention. Homicide data shown here are collected by the Centers for Disease Control and Prevention based on death certificates and differ from murder data collected by the F.B.I. from other sources. Age-adjusted rates based on the year 2000 standard population.
**Insufficient data to determine a reliable rate.*

Deaths by Suicide in 2002

National Total = 31,655 Suicides*

ALPHA ORDER

RANK ORDER

RANK	STATE	SUICIDES	% of USA
22	Alabama	514	1.6%
42	Alaska	132	0.4%
11	Arizona	886	2.8%
30	Arkansas	377	1.2%
1	California	3,228	10.2%
16	Colorado	727	2.3%
37	Connecticut	260	0.8%
50	Delaware	74	0.2%
2	Florida	2,338	7.4%
10	Georgia	909	2.9%
44	Hawaii	120	0.4%
38	Idaho	202	0.6%
7	Illinois	1,145	3.6%
15	Indiana	743	2.3%
35	Iowa	314	1.0%
32	Kansas	345	1.1%
20	Kentucky	540	1.7%
24	Louisiana	499	1.6%
41	Maine	166	0.5%
26	Maryland	477	1.5%
28	Massachusetts	436	1.4%
8	Michigan	1,106	3.5%
25	Minnesota	497	1.6%
33	Mississippi	343	1.1%
17	Missouri	693	2.2%
40	Montana	184	0.6%
39	Nebraska	201	0.6%
29	Nevada	423	1.3%
42	New Hampshire	132	0.4%
19	New Jersey	553	1.7%
31	New Mexico	349	1.1%
6	New York	1,228	3.9%
9	North Carolina	986	3.1%
48	North Dakota	91	0.3%
5	Ohio	1,287	4.1%
23	Oklahoma	501	1.6%
21	Oregon	518	1.6%
4	Pennsylvania	1,341	4.2%
49	Rhode Island	86	0.3%
27	South Carolina	440	1.4%
46	South Dakota	94	0.3%
14	Tennessee	778	2.5%
3	Texas	2,311	7.3%
34	Utah	340	1.1%
47	Vermont	92	0.3%
13	Virginia	799	2.5%
12	Washington	811	2.6%
36	West Virginia	276	0.9%
18	Wisconsin	627	2.0%
45	Wyoming	105	0.3%

RANK	STATE	SUICIDES	% of USA
1	California	3,228	10.2%
2	Florida	2,338	7.4%
3	Texas	2,311	7.3%
4	Pennsylvania	1,341	4.2%
5	Ohio	1,287	4.1%
6	New York	1,228	3.9%
7	Illinois	1,145	3.6%
8	Michigan	1,106	3.5%
9	North Carolina	986	3.1%
10	Georgia	909	2.9%
11	Arizona	886	2.8%
12	Washington	811	2.6%
13	Virginia	799	2.5%
14	Tennessee	778	2.5%
15	Indiana	743	2.3%
16	Colorado	727	2.3%
17	Missouri	693	2.2%
18	Wisconsin	627	2.0%
19	New Jersey	553	1.7%
20	Kentucky	540	1.7%
21	Oregon	518	1.6%
22	Alabama	514	1.6%
23	Oklahoma	501	1.6%
24	Louisiana	499	1.6%
25	Minnesota	497	1.6%
26	Maryland	477	1.5%
27	South Carolina	440	1.4%
28	Massachusetts	436	1.4%
29	Nevada	423	1.3%
30	Arkansas	377	1.2%
31	New Mexico	349	1.1%
32	Kansas	345	1.1%
33	Mississippi	343	1.1%
34	Utah	340	1.1%
35	Iowa	314	1.0%
36	West Virginia	276	0.9%
37	Connecticut	260	0.8%
38	Idaho	202	0.6%
39	Nebraska	201	0.6%
40	Montana	184	0.6%
41	Maine	166	0.5%
42	Alaska	132	0.4%
42	New Hampshire	132	0.4%
44	Hawaii	120	0.4%
45	Wyoming	105	0.3%
46	South Dakota	94	0.3%
47	Vermont	92	0.3%
48	North Dakota	91	0.3%
49	Rhode Island	86	0.3%
50	Delaware	74	0.2%
	District of Columbia	31	0.1%

Source: U.S. Department of Health and Human Services, National Center for Health Statistics
"National Vital Statistics Reports" (Vol. 53, No. 5, October 12, 2004)
*Final data by state of residence.

Death Rate by Suicide in 2002

National Rate = 11.0 Deaths per 100,000 Population*

ALPHA ORDER

RANK	STATE	RATE
28	Alabama	11.5
2	Alaska	20.5
6	Arizona	16.2
16	Arkansas	13.9
42	California	9.2
7	Colorado	16.1
47	Connecticut	7.5
42	Delaware	9.2
15	Florida	14.0
37	Georgia	10.6
41	Hawaii	9.6
9	Idaho	15.1
44	Illinois	9.1
24	Indiana	12.1
35	Iowa	10.7
21	Kansas	12.7
19	Kentucky	13.2
31	Louisiana	11.1
20	Maine	12.8
45	Maryland	8.7
48	Massachusetts	6.8
32	Michigan	11.0
40	Minnesota	9.9
25	Mississippi	11.9
23	Missouri	12.2
3	Montana	20.2
27	Nebraska	11.6
4	Nevada	19.5
39	New Hampshire	10.4
49	New Jersey	6.4
5	New Mexico	18.8
49	New York	6.4
25	North Carolina	11.9
13	North Dakota	14.4
30	Ohio	11.3
14	Oklahoma	14.3
11	Oregon	14.7
34	Pennsylvania	10.9
46	Rhode Island	8.0
35	South Carolina	10.7
22	South Dakota	12.4
17	Tennessee	13.4
37	Texas	10.6
11	Utah	14.7
10	Vermont	14.9
32	Virginia	11.0
17	Washington	13.4
8	West Virginia	15.3
28	Wisconsin	11.5
1	Wyoming	21.1

RANK ORDER

RANK	STATE	RATE
1	Wyoming	21.1
2	Alaska	20.5
3	Montana	20.2
4	Nevada	19.5
5	New Mexico	18.8
6	Arizona	16.2
7	Colorado	16.1
8	West Virginia	15.3
9	Idaho	15.1
10	Vermont	14.9
11	Oregon	14.7
11	Utah	14.7
13	North Dakota	14.4
14	Oklahoma	14.3
15	Florida	14.0
16	Arkansas	13.9
17	Tennessee	13.4
17	Washington	13.4
19	Kentucky	13.2
20	Maine	12.8
21	Kansas	12.7
22	South Dakota	12.4
23	Missouri	12.2
24	Indiana	12.1
25	Mississippi	11.9
25	North Carolina	11.9
27	Nebraska	11.6
28	Alabama	11.5
28	Wisconsin	11.5
30	Ohio	11.3
31	Louisiana	11.1
32	Michigan	11.0
32	Virginia	11.0
34	Pennsylvania	10.9
35	Iowa	10.7
35	South Carolina	10.7
37	Georgia	10.6
37	Texas	10.6
39	New Hampshire	10.4
40	Minnesota	9.9
41	Hawaii	9.6
42	California	9.2
42	Delaware	9.2
44	Illinois	9.1
45	Maryland	8.7
46	Rhode Island	8.0
47	Connecticut	7.5
48	Massachusetts	6.8
49	New Jersey	6.4
49	New York	6.4
	District of Columbia	5.4

Source: U.S. Department of Health and Human Services, National Center for Health Statistics
    "National Vital Statistics Reports" (Vol. 53, No. 5, October 12, 2004)
*Final data by state of residence. Not age-adjusted.

Age-Adjusted Death Rate by Suicide in 2002

National Rate = 10.9 Deaths per 100,000 Population*

ALPHA ORDER

RANK ORDER

RANK	STATE	RATE	RANK	STATE	RATE
28	Alabama	11.4	1	Alaska	21.0
1	Alaska	21.0	2	Wyoming	20.7
6	Arizona	16.5	3	Montana	19.9
15	Arkansas	14.0	4	Nevada	19.8
41	California	9.6	5	New Mexico	19.1
7	Colorado	16.2	6	Arizona	16.5
47	Connecticut	7.4	7	Colorado	16.2
44	Delaware	9.0	8	Utah	16.1
16	Florida	13.4	9	Idaho	15.5
32	Georgia	11.0	10	West Virginia	14.8
42	Hawaii	9.5	11	Oregon	14.4
9	Idaho	15.5	12	Oklahoma	14.3
43	Illinois	9.1	13	North Dakota	14.2
23	Indiana	12.1	14	Vermont	14.1
38	Iowa	10.5	15	Arkansas	14.0
20	Kansas	12.6	16	Florida	13.4
19	Kentucky	12.8	17	Washington	13.3
30	Louisiana	11.2	18	Tennessee	13.2
21	Maine	12.3	19	Kentucky	12.8
45	Maryland	8.7	20	Kansas	12.6
48	Massachusetts	6.5	21	Maine	12.3
32	Michigan	11.0	22	South Dakota	12.2
40	Minnesota	9.7	23	Indiana	12.1
23	Mississippi	12.1	23	Mississippi	12.1
23	Missouri	12.1	23	Missouri	12.1
3	Montana	19.9	26	North Carolina	11.8
27	Nebraska	11.7	27	Nebraska	11.7
4	Nevada	19.8	28	Alabama	11.4
39	New Hampshire	10.2	29	Wisconsin	11.3
49	New Jersey	6.3	30	Louisiana	11.2
5	New Mexico	19.1	30	Ohio	11.2
49	New York	6.3	32	Georgia	11.0
26	North Carolina	11.8	32	Michigan	11.0
13	North Dakota	14.2	32	Texas	11.0
30	Ohio	11.2	35	Virginia	10.9
12	Oklahoma	14.3	36	Pennsylvania	10.7
11	Oregon	14.4	37	South Carolina	10.6
36	Pennsylvania	10.7	38	Iowa	10.5
46	Rhode Island	7.9	39	New Hampshire	10.2
37	South Carolina	10.6	40	Minnesota	9.7
22	South Dakota	12.2	41	California	9.6
18	Tennessee	13.2	42	Hawaii	9.5
32	Texas	11.0	43	Illinois	9.1
8	Utah	16.1	44	Delaware	9.0
14	Vermont	14.1	45	Maryland	8.7
35	Virginia	10.9	46	Rhode Island	7.9
17	Washington	13.3	47	Connecticut	7.4
10	West Virginia	14.8	48	Massachusetts	6.5
29	Wisconsin	11.3	49	New Jersey	6.3
2	Wyoming	20.7	49	New York	6.3
				District of Columbia	5.1

Source: U.S. Department of Health and Human Services, National Center for Health Statistics
     "National Vital Statistics Reports" (Vol. 53, No. 5, October 12, 2004)
*Final data by state of residence. Age-adjusted rates based on the year 2000 standard population.

Alcohol-Induced Deaths in 2001

National Total = 19,817 Deaths*

RANK	STATE	DEATHS	% of USA
29	Alabama	227	1.1%
39	Alaska	119	0.6%
14	Arizona	447	2.3%
35	Arkansas	154	0.8%
1	California	3,364	17.0%
10	Colorado	508	2.6%
32	Connecticut	157	0.8%
45	Delaware	68	0.3%
2	Florida	1,391	7.0%
13	Georgia	486	2.5%
50	Hawaii	35	0.2%
38	Idaho	121	0.6%
7	Illinois	622	3.1%
24	Indiana	306	1.5%
32	Iowa	157	0.8%
32	Kansas	157	0.8%
26	Kentucky	253	1.3%
28	Louisiana	228	1.2%
42	Maine	94	0.5%
25	Maryland	276	1.4%
20	Massachusetts	340	1.7%
5	Michigan	703	3.5%
23	Minnesota	319	1.6%
31	Mississippi	158	0.8%
17	Missouri	366	1.8%
41	Montana	107	0.5%
43	Nebraska	86	0.4%
27	Nevada	248	1.3%
37	New Hampshire	122	0.6%
11	New Jersey	493	2.5%
21	New Mexico	328	1.7%
4	New York	1,152	5.8%
6	North Carolina	624	3.1%
46	North Dakota	67	0.3%
8	Ohio	608	3.1%
30	Oklahoma	222	1.1%
18	Oregon	365	1.8%
12	Pennsylvania	488	2.5%
47	Rhode Island	62	0.3%
21	South Carolina	328	1.7%
44	South Dakota	74	0.4%
15	Tennessee	402	2.0%
3	Texas	1,209	6.1%
40	Utah	113	0.6%
49	Vermont	38	0.2%
19	Virginia	346	1.7%
9	Washington	603	3.0%
36	West Virginia	130	0.7%
16	Wisconsin	384	1.9%
48	Wyoming	55	0.3%

RANK	STATE	DEATHS	% of USA
1	California	3,364	17.0%
2	Florida	1,391	7.0%
3	Texas	1,209	6.1%
4	New York	1,152	5.8%
5	Michigan	703	3.5%
6	North Carolina	624	3.1%
7	Illinois	622	3.1%
8	Ohio	608	3.1%
9	Washington	603	3.0%
10	Colorado	508	2.6%
11	New Jersey	493	2.5%
12	Pennsylvania	488	2.5%
13	Georgia	486	2.5%
14	Arizona	447	2.3%
15	Tennessee	402	2.0%
16	Wisconsin	384	1.9%
17	Missouri	366	1.8%
18	Oregon	365	1.8%
19	Virginia	346	1.7%
20	Massachusetts	340	1.7%
21	New Mexico	328	1.7%
21	South Carolina	328	1.7%
23	Minnesota	319	1.6%
24	Indiana	306	1.5%
25	Maryland	276	1.4%
26	Kentucky	253	1.3%
27	Nevada	248	1.3%
28	Louisiana	228	1.2%
29	Alabama	227	1.1%
30	Oklahoma	222	1.1%
31	Mississippi	158	0.8%
32	Connecticut	157	0.8%
32	Iowa	157	0.8%
32	Kansas	157	0.8%
35	Arkansas	154	0.8%
36	West Virginia	130	0.7%
37	New Hampshire	122	0.6%
38	Idaho	121	0.6%
39	Alaska	119	0.6%
40	Utah	113	0.6%
41	Montana	107	0.5%
42	Maine	94	0.5%
43	Nebraska	86	0.4%
44	South Dakota	74	0.4%
45	Delaware	68	0.3%
46	North Dakota	67	0.3%
47	Rhode Island	62	0.3%
48	Wyoming	55	0.3%
49	Vermont	38	0.2%
50	Hawaii	35	0.2%
	District of Columbia	107	0.5%

Source: U.S. Department of Health and Human Services, National Center for Health Statistics (http://wonder.cdc.gov)

By state of residence. Includes excessive blood level of alcohol, accidental poisoning by alcohol and the following alcohol-related causes: psychoses, dependence syndrome, polyneuropathy, cardiomyopathy, gastritis, chronic liver disease and cirrhosis. Excludes accidents, homicides and other causes indirectly related to alcohol use.

Death Rate by Alcohol-Induced Deaths in 2001

National Rate = 6.9 Deaths per 100,000 Population*

ALPHA ORDER

RANK	STATE	RATE
40	Alabama	5.1
1	Alaska	18.8
16	Arizona	8.4
34	Arkansas	5.7
11	California	9.7
5	Colorado	11.5
48	Connecticut	4.6
14	Delaware	8.5
14	Florida	8.5
30	Georgia	5.8
50	Hawaii	2.9
13	Idaho	9.2
43	Illinois	5.0
43	Indiana	5.0
37	Iowa	5.4
30	Kansas	5.8
27	Kentucky	6.2
40	Louisiana	5.1
19	Maine	7.3
40	Maryland	5.1
38	Massachusetts	5.3
22	Michigan	7.0
25	Minnesota	6.4
36	Mississippi	5.5
24	Missouri	6.5
3	Montana	11.8
43	Nebraska	5.0
3	Nevada	11.8
11	New Hampshire	9.7
30	New Jersey	5.8
2	New Mexico	17.9
29	New York	6.0
18	North Carolina	7.6
7	North Dakota	10.5
38	Ohio	5.3
25	Oklahoma	6.4
7	Oregon	10.5
49	Pennsylvania	4.0
30	Rhode Island	5.8
17	South Carolina	8.1
10	South Dakota	9.8
22	Tennessee	7.0
34	Texas	5.7
43	Utah	5.0
27	Vermont	6.2
47	Virginia	4.8
9	Washington	10.1
20	West Virginia	7.2
21	Wisconsin	7.1
6	Wyoming	11.1

RANK ORDER

RANK	STATE	RATE
1	Alaska	18.8
2	New Mexico	17.9
3	Montana	11.8
3	Nevada	11.8
5	Colorado	11.5
6	Wyoming	11.1
7	North Dakota	10.5
7	Oregon	10.5
9	Washington	10.1
10	South Dakota	9.8
11	California	9.7
11	New Hampshire	9.7
13	Idaho	9.2
14	Delaware	8.5
14	Florida	8.5
16	Arizona	8.4
17	South Carolina	8.1
18	North Carolina	7.6
19	Maine	7.3
20	West Virginia	7.2
21	Wisconsin	7.1
22	Michigan	7.0
22	Tennessee	7.0
24	Missouri	6.5
25	Minnesota	6.4
25	Oklahoma	6.4
27	Kentucky	6.2
27	Vermont	6.2
29	New York	6.0
30	Georgia	5.8
30	Kansas	5.8
30	New Jersey	5.8
30	Rhode Island	5.8
34	Arkansas	5.7
34	Texas	5.7
36	Mississippi	5.5
37	Iowa	5.4
38	Massachusetts	5.3
38	Ohio	5.3
40	Alabama	5.1
40	Louisiana	5.1
40	Maryland	5.1
43	Illinois	5.0
43	Indiana	5.0
43	Nebraska	5.0
43	Utah	5.0
47	Virginia	4.8
48	Connecticut	4.6
49	Pennsylvania	4.0
50	Hawaii	2.9

	District of Columbia	18.7

Source: U.S. Department of Health and Human Services, National Center for Health Statistics
       (http://wonder.cdc.gov)
*By state of residence. Includes excessive blood level of alcohol, accidental poisoning by alcohol and the following alcohol-related causes: psychoses, dependence syndrome, polyneuropathy, cardiomyopathy, gastritis, chronic liver disease and cirrhosis. Excludes accidents, homicides and other causes indirectly related to alcohol use. Not age-adjusted.

175

Occupational Fatalities in 2003

National Total = 5,559 Deaths*

ALPHA ORDER

RANK	STATE	DEATHS	% of USA
16	Alabama	121	2.2%
42	Alaska	28	0.5%
27	Arizona	80	1.4%
25	Arkansas	87	1.6%
2	California	456	8.2%
20	Colorado	102	1.8%
41	Connecticut	36	0.6%
50	Delaware	6	0.1%
3	Florida	347	6.2%
8	Georgia	199	3.6%
46	Hawaii	21	0.4%
38	Idaho	43	0.8%
7	Illinois	200	3.6%
15	Indiana	132	2.4%
30	Iowa	76	1.4%
28	Kansas	78	1.4%
13	Kentucky	145	2.6%
23	Louisiana	95	1.7%
45	Maine	23	0.4%
24	Maryland	92	1.7%
29	Massachusetts	77	1.4%
12	Michigan	151	2.7%
32	Minnesota	72	1.3%
21	Mississippi	100	1.8%
11	Missouri	154	2.8%
39	Montana	39	0.7%
35	Nebraska	51	0.9%
34	Nevada	52	0.9%
47	New Hampshire	19	0.3%
18	New Jersey	104	1.9%
37	New Mexico	46	0.8%
4	New York	227	4.1%
9	North Carolina	182	3.3%
44	North Dakota	26	0.5%
6	Ohio	206	3.7%
21	Oklahoma	100	1.8%
31	Oregon	75	1.3%
5	Pennsylvania	208	3.7%
48	Rhode Island	18	0.3%
17	South Carolina	114	2.1%
42	South Dakota	28	0.5%
14	Tennessee	136	2.4%
1	Texas	491	8.8%
33	Utah	54	1.0%
49	Vermont	14	0.3%
10	Virginia	155	2.8%
26	Washington	82	1.5%
35	West Virginia	51	0.9%
19	Wisconsin	103	1.9%
40	Wyoming	37	0.7%

RANK ORDER

RANK	STATE	DEATHS	% of USA
1	Texas	491	8.8%
2	California	456	8.2%
3	Florida	347	6.2%
4	New York	227	4.1%
5	Pennsylvania	208	3.7%
6	Ohio	206	3.7%
7	Illinois	200	3.6%
8	Georgia	199	3.6%
9	North Carolina	182	3.3%
10	Virginia	155	2.8%
11	Missouri	154	2.8%
12	Michigan	151	2.7%
13	Kentucky	145	2.6%
14	Tennessee	136	2.4%
15	Indiana	132	2.4%
16	Alabama	121	2.2%
17	South Carolina	114	2.1%
18	New Jersey	104	1.9%
19	Wisconsin	103	1.9%
20	Colorado	102	1.8%
21	Mississippi	100	1.8%
21	Oklahoma	100	1.8%
23	Louisiana	95	1.7%
24	Maryland	92	1.7%
25	Arkansas	87	1.6%
26	Washington	82	1.5%
27	Arizona	80	1.4%
28	Kansas	78	1.4%
29	Massachusetts	77	1.4%
30	Iowa	76	1.4%
31	Oregon	75	1.3%
32	Minnesota	72	1.3%
33	Utah	54	1.0%
34	Nevada	52	0.9%
35	Nebraska	51	0.9%
35	West Virginia	51	0.9%
37	New Mexico	46	0.8%
38	Idaho	43	0.8%
39	Montana	39	0.7%
40	Wyoming	37	0.7%
41	Connecticut	36	0.6%
42	Alaska	28	0.5%
42	South Dakota	28	0.5%
44	North Dakota	26	0.5%
45	Maine	23	0.4%
46	Hawaii	21	0.4%
47	New Hampshire	19	0.3%
48	Rhode Island	18	0.3%
49	Vermont	14	0.3%
50	Delaware	6	0.1%
	District of Columbia	19	0.3%

Source: U.S. Department of Labor, Bureau of Labor Statistics
   "National Census of Fatal Occupational Injuries, 2003" (press release, September 22, 2004)
*Includes one fatality that occurred within the territorial boundaries of the United States but for which a state of incident could not be determined.

Occupational Fatality Rate in 2003

National Rate = 4.0 Deaths per 100,000 Workers*

ALPHA ORDER

RANK	STATE	RATE
12	Alabama	6.0
2	Alaska	8.7
40	Arizona	3.2
7	Arkansas	7.0
42	California	2.8
27	Colorado	4.4
49	Connecticut	2.1
50	Delaware	1.5
26	Florida	4.5
22	Georgia	4.8
33	Hawaii	3.6
10	Idaho	6.6
38	Illinois	3.3
29	Indiana	4.3
19	Iowa	4.9
14	Kansas	5.5
5	Kentucky	7.7
19	Louisiana	4.9
34	Maine	3.5
38	Maryland	3.3
48	Massachusetts	2.4
40	Michigan	3.2
45	Minnesota	2.6
4	Mississippi	8.0
15	Missouri	5.4
3	Montana	8.6
15	Nebraska	5.4
19	Nevada	4.9
42	New Hampshire	2.8
47	New Jersey	2.5
15	New Mexico	5.4
45	New York	2.6
24	North Carolina	4.6
6	North Dakota	7.6
32	Ohio	3.7
11	Oklahoma	6.2
27	Oregon	4.4
34	Pennsylvania	3.5
37	Rhode Island	3.4
12	South Carolina	6.0
8	South Dakota	6.8
18	Tennessee	5.0
22	Texas	4.8
24	Utah	4.6
31	Vermont	4.1
30	Virginia	4.2
42	Washington	2.8
8	West Virginia	6.8
34	Wisconsin	3.5
1	Wyoming	13.9

RANK ORDER

RANK	STATE	RATE
1	Wyoming	13.9
2	Alaska	8.7
3	Montana	8.6
4	Mississippi	8.0
5	Kentucky	7.7
6	North Dakota	7.6
7	Arkansas	7.0
8	South Dakota	6.8
8	West Virginia	6.8
10	Idaho	6.6
11	Oklahoma	6.2
12	Alabama	6.0
12	South Carolina	6.0
14	Kansas	5.5
15	Missouri	5.4
15	Nebraska	5.4
15	New Mexico	5.4
18	Tennessee	5.0
19	Iowa	4.9
19	Louisiana	4.9
19	Nevada	4.9
22	Georgia	4.8
22	Texas	4.8
24	North Carolina	4.6
24	Utah	4.6
26	Florida	4.5
27	Colorado	4.4
27	Oregon	4.4
29	Indiana	4.3
30	Virginia	4.2
31	Vermont	4.1
32	Ohio	3.7
33	Hawaii	3.6
34	Maine	3.5
34	Pennsylvania	3.5
34	Wisconsin	3.5
37	Rhode Island	3.4
38	Illinois	3.3
38	Maryland	3.3
40	Arizona	3.2
40	Michigan	3.2
42	California	2.8
42	New Hampshire	2.8
42	Washington	2.8
45	Minnesota	2.6
45	New York	2.6
47	New Jersey	2.5
48	Massachusetts	2.4
49	Connecticut	2.1
50	Delaware	1.5
	District of Columbia	6.6

Source: Morgan Quitno Press using data from U.S. Department of Labor, Bureau of Labor Statistics
   "National Census of Fatal Occupational Injuries, 2003" (press release, September 22, 2004)
*Based on employed civilian labor force.

Years Lost by Premature Death in 2001

National Average = 7,521 Years Lost per 100,000 Population*

ALPHA ORDER

RANK	STATE	YEARS
3	Alabama	9,814
15	Alaska	8,147
20	Arizona	7,826
5	Arkansas	9,325
40	California	6,470
39	Colorado	6,476
42	Connecticut	6,297
11	Delaware	8,361
18	Florida	8,023
9	Georgia	8,794
48	Hawaii	6,076
33	Idaho	6,691
24	Illinois	7,585
19	Indiana	7,882
47	Iowa	6,086
27	Kansas	7,244
10	Kentucky	8,665
2	Louisiana	10,279
41	Maine	6,421
17	Maryland	8,071
45	Massachusetts	6,142
22	Michigan	7,731
50	Minnesota	5,595
1	Mississippi	10,713
14	Missouri	8,149
29	Montana	7,163
37	Nebraska	6,491
13	Nevada	8,162
49	New Hampshire	5,706
30	New Jersey	7,126
16	New Mexico	8,127
32	New York	7,065
12	North Carolina	8,359
38	North Dakota	6,486
25	Ohio	7,575
8	Oklahoma	8,828
35	Oregon	6,596
26	Pennsylvania	7,565
34	Rhode Island	6,615
4	South Carolina	9,479
31	South Dakota	7,124
6	Tennessee	9,196
23	Texas	7,612
44	Utah	6,169
46	Vermont	6,130
28	Virginia	7,175
43	Washington	6,216
7	West Virginia	8,923
36	Wisconsin	6,535
21	Wyoming	7,755

RANK ORDER

RANK	STATE	YEARS
1	Mississippi	10,713
2	Louisiana	10,279
3	Alabama	9,814
4	South Carolina	9,479
5	Arkansas	9,325
6	Tennessee	9,196
7	West Virginia	8,923
8	Oklahoma	8,828
9	Georgia	8,794
10	Kentucky	8,665
11	Delaware	8,361
12	North Carolina	8,359
13	Nevada	8,162
14	Missouri	8,149
15	Alaska	8,147
16	New Mexico	8,127
17	Maryland	8,071
18	Florida	8,023
19	Indiana	7,882
20	Arizona	7,826
21	Wyoming	7,755
22	Michigan	7,731
23	Texas	7,612
24	Illinois	7,585
25	Ohio	7,575
26	Pennsylvania	7,565
27	Kansas	7,244
28	Virginia	7,175
29	Montana	7,163
30	New Jersey	7,126
31	South Dakota	7,124
32	New York	7,065
33	Idaho	6,691
34	Rhode Island	6,615
35	Oregon	6,596
36	Wisconsin	6,535
37	Nebraska	6,491
38	North Dakota	6,486
39	Colorado	6,476
40	California	6,470
41	Maine	6,421
42	Connecticut	6,297
43	Washington	6,216
44	Utah	6,169
45	Massachusetts	6,142
46	Vermont	6,130
47	Iowa	6,086
48	Hawaii	6,076
49	New Hampshire	5,706
50	Minnesota	5,595

	District of Columbia	13,080

Source: U.S. Department of Health and Human Services, National Center for Health Statistics
       unpublished data
Age-adjusted years of potential life lost due to death before age 75.

Years Lost by Premature Death from Cancer in 2001

National Average = 1,650 Years Lost per 100,000 Population*

ALPHA ORDER

RANK	STATE	YEARS
6	Alabama	1,879
48	Alaska	1,352
41	Arizona	1,479
7	Arkansas	1,864
39	California	1,485
49	Colorado	1,299
38	Connecticut	1,490
15	Delaware	1,734
16	Florida	1,711
12	Georgia	1,763
44	Hawaii	1,419
47	Idaho	1,377
18	Illinois	1,701
11	Indiana	1,811
33	Iowa	1,531
29	Kansas	1,576
3	Kentucky	2,024
1	Louisiana	2,044
23	Maine	1,657
20	Maryland	1,681
26	Massachusetts	1,594
21	Michigan	1,680
45	Minnesota	1,408
2	Mississippi	2,033
10	Missouri	1,815
43	Montana	1,430
40	Nebraska	1,482
28	Nevada	1,584
35	New Hampshire	1,503
24	New Jersey	1,634
46	New Mexico	1,385
27	New York	1,593
12	North Carolina	1,763
34	North Dakota	1,514
14	Ohio	1,747
8	Oklahoma	1,833
30	Oregon	1,574
17	Pennsylvania	1,705
19	Rhode Island	1,699
9	South Carolina	1,824
36	South Dakota	1,497
4	Tennessee	1,901
25	Texas	1,619
50	Utah	1,139
32	Vermont	1,542
22	Virginia	1,671
37	Washington	1,493
5	West Virginia	1,898
31	Wisconsin	1,549
42	Wyoming	1,456

RANK ORDER

RANK	STATE	YEARS
1	Louisiana	2,044
2	Mississippi	2,033
3	Kentucky	2,024
4	Tennessee	1,901
5	West Virginia	1,898
6	Alabama	1,879
7	Arkansas	1,864
8	Oklahoma	1,833
9	South Carolina	1,824
10	Missouri	1,815
11	Indiana	1,811
12	Georgia	1,763
12	North Carolina	1,763
14	Ohio	1,747
15	Delaware	1,734
16	Florida	1,711
17	Pennsylvania	1,705
18	Illinois	1,701
19	Rhode Island	1,699
20	Maryland	1,681
21	Michigan	1,680
22	Virginia	1,671
23	Maine	1,657
24	New Jersey	1,634
25	Texas	1,619
26	Massachusetts	1,594
27	New York	1,593
28	Nevada	1,584
29	Kansas	1,576
30	Oregon	1,574
31	Wisconsin	1,549
32	Vermont	1,542
33	Iowa	1,531
34	North Dakota	1,514
35	New Hampshire	1,503
36	South Dakota	1,497
37	Washington	1,493
38	Connecticut	1,490
39	California	1,485
40	Nebraska	1,482
41	Arizona	1,479
42	Wyoming	1,456
43	Montana	1,430
44	Hawaii	1,419
45	Minnesota	1,408
46	New Mexico	1,385
47	Idaho	1,377
48	Alaska	1,352
49	Colorado	1,299
50	Utah	1,139
	District of Columbia	2,062

Source: U.S. Department of Health and Human Services, National Center for Health Statistics
    unpublished data
*Age-adjusted years of potential life lost due to death before age 75.

Years Lost by Premature Death from Heart Disease in 2001

National Average = 1,220 Years Lost per 100,000 Population*

ALPHA ORDER

RANK	STATE	YEARS
2	Alabama	1,829
30	Alaska	1,059
31	Arizona	1,050
4	Arkansas	1,644
43	California	930
48	Colorado	810
34	Connecticut	1,031
20	Delaware	1,252
23	Florida	1,190
10	Georgia	1,513
26	Hawaii	1,087
38	Idaho	962
17	Illinois	1,333
16	Indiana	1,345
27	Iowa	1,074
29	Kansas	1,066
5	Kentucky	1,637
3	Louisiana	1,726
37	Maine	986
19	Maryland	1,293
41	Massachusetts	939
14	Michigan	1,363
49	Minnesota	809
1	Mississippi	1,999
12	Missouri	1,389
42	Montana	934
39	Nebraska	959
11	Nevada	1,470
46	New Hampshire	910
32	New Jersey	1,049
40	New Mexico	942
24	New York	1,160
15	North Carolina	1,362
33	North Dakota	1,037
13	Ohio	1,385
8	Oklahoma	1,566
47	Oregon	862
21	Pennsylvania	1,244
25	Rhode Island	1,104
9	South Carolina	1,551
28	South Dakota	1,070
6	Tennessee	1,607
18	Texas	1,320
50	Utah	800
44	Vermont	919
22	Virginia	1,200
45	Washington	918
7	West Virginia	1,570
36	Wisconsin	1,021
35	Wyoming	1,022

RANK ORDER

RANK	STATE	YEARS
1	Mississippi	1,999
2	Alabama	1,829
3	Louisiana	1,726
4	Arkansas	1,644
5	Kentucky	1,637
6	Tennessee	1,607
7	West Virginia	1,570
8	Oklahoma	1,566
9	South Carolina	1,551
10	Georgia	1,513
11	Nevada	1,470
12	Missouri	1,389
13	Ohio	1,385
14	Michigan	1,363
15	North Carolina	1,362
16	Indiana	1,345
17	Illinois	1,333
18	Texas	1,320
19	Maryland	1,293
20	Delaware	1,252
21	Pennsylvania	1,244
22	Virginia	1,200
23	Florida	1,190
24	New York	1,160
25	Rhode Island	1,104
26	Hawaii	1,087
27	Iowa	1,074
28	South Dakota	1,070
29	Kansas	1,066
30	Alaska	1,059
31	Arizona	1,050
32	New Jersey	1,049
33	North Dakota	1,037
34	Connecticut	1,031
35	Wyoming	1,022
36	Wisconsin	1,021
37	Maine	986
38	Idaho	962
39	Nebraska	959
40	New Mexico	942
41	Massachusetts	939
42	Montana	934
43	California	930
44	Vermont	919
45	Washington	918
46	New Hampshire	910
47	Oregon	862
48	Colorado	810
49	Minnesota	809
50	Utah	800
	District of Columbia	1,865

Source: U.S. Department of Health and Human Services, National Center for Health Statistics
unpublished data
Age-adjusted years of potential life lost due to death before age 75.

Years Lost by Premature Death from Homicide in 2001

National Average = 273 Years Lost per 100,000 Population*

ALPHA ORDER

RANK	STATE	YEARS
6	Alabama	399
24	Alaska	246
4	Arizona	427
15	Arkansas	310
18	California	281
31	Colorado	171
33	Connecticut	154
30	Delaware	176
19	Florida	260
10	Georgia	344
43	Hawaii	106
38	Idaho	126
5	Illinois	402
12	Indiana	322
44	Iowa	88
25	Kansas	230
26	Kentucky	219
1	Louisiana	548
NA	Maine**	NA
3	Maryland	457
40	Massachusetts	117
13	Michigan	318
42	Minnesota	107
2	Mississippi	488
7	Missouri	366
32	Montana	159
39	Nebraska	120
9	Nevada	352
NA	New Hampshire**	NA
28	New Jersey	197
16	New Mexico	309
23	New York	250
14	North Carolina	316
NA	North Dakota**	NA
27	Ohio	209
20	Oklahoma	259
40	Oregon	117
21	Pennsylvania	253
35	Rhode Island	138
8	South Carolina	363
NA	South Dakota**	NA
11	Tennessee	326
17	Texas	282
37	Utah	135
NA	Vermont**	NA
21	Virginia	253
35	Washington	138
34	West Virginia	140
29	Wisconsin	190
NA	Wyoming**	NA

RANK ORDER

RANK	STATE	YEARS
1	Louisiana	548
2	Mississippi	488
3	Maryland	457
4	Arizona	427
5	Illinois	402
6	Alabama	399
7	Missouri	366
8	South Carolina	363
9	Nevada	352
10	Georgia	344
11	Tennessee	326
12	Indiana	322
13	Michigan	318
14	North Carolina	316
15	Arkansas	310
16	New Mexico	309
17	Texas	282
18	California	281
19	Florida	260
20	Oklahoma	259
21	Pennsylvania	253
21	Virginia	253
23	New York	250
24	Alaska	246
25	Kansas	230
26	Kentucky	219
27	Ohio	209
28	New Jersey	197
29	Wisconsin	190
30	Delaware	176
31	Colorado	171
32	Montana	159
33	Connecticut	154
34	West Virginia	140
35	Rhode Island	138
35	Washington	138
37	Utah	135
38	Idaho	126
39	Nebraska	120
40	Massachusetts	117
40	Oregon	117
42	Minnesota	107
43	Hawaii	106
44	Iowa	88
NA	Maine**	NA
NA	New Hampshire**	NA
NA	North Dakota**	NA
NA	South Dakota**	NA
NA	Vermont**	NA
NA	Wyoming**	NA

	District of Columbia	1,383

*Source: U.S. Department of Health and Human Services, National Center for Health Statistics
    unpublished data*
Age-adjusted years of potential life lost due to death before age 75.
**Data for states with fewer than 20 deaths from homicide for persons under 75 years of age are considered
unreliable and are not shown.*

Years Lost by Premature Death from Suicide in 2001

National Average = 342 Years Lost per 100,000 Population*

<table>
<tr><td colspan="3">ALPHA ORDER</td><td colspan="3">RANK ORDER</td></tr>
<tr><td>RANK</td><td>STATE</td><td>YEARS</td><td>RANK</td><td>STATE</td><td>YEARS</td></tr>
<tr><td>29</td><td>Alabama</td><td>367</td><td>1</td><td>New Mexico</td><td>638</td></tr>
<tr><td>3</td><td>Alaska</td><td>602</td><td>2</td><td>Montana</td><td>617</td></tr>
<tr><td>13</td><td>Arizona</td><td>471</td><td>3</td><td>Alaska</td><td>602</td></tr>
<tr><td>10</td><td>Arkansas</td><td>483</td><td>4</td><td>Wyoming</td><td>598</td></tr>
<tr><td>47</td><td>California</td><td>242</td><td>5</td><td>Nevada</td><td>535</td></tr>
<tr><td>9</td><td>Colorado</td><td>516</td><td>6</td><td>Idaho</td><td>534</td></tr>
<tr><td>46</td><td>Connecticut</td><td>269</td><td>7</td><td>Utah</td><td>524</td></tr>
<tr><td>15</td><td>Delaware</td><td>446</td><td>8</td><td>South Dakota</td><td>521</td></tr>
<tr><td>19</td><td>Florida</td><td>411</td><td>9</td><td>Colorado</td><td>516</td></tr>
<tr><td>34</td><td>Georgia</td><td>361</td><td>10</td><td>Arkansas</td><td>483</td></tr>
<tr><td>29</td><td>Hawaii</td><td>367</td><td>10</td><td>Oklahoma</td><td>483</td></tr>
<tr><td>6</td><td>Idaho</td><td>534</td><td>12</td><td>New Hampshire</td><td>476</td></tr>
<tr><td>44</td><td>Illinois</td><td>293</td><td>13</td><td>Arizona</td><td>471</td></tr>
<tr><td>28</td><td>Indiana</td><td>372</td><td>14</td><td>Oregon</td><td>447</td></tr>
<tr><td>36</td><td>Iowa</td><td>353</td><td>15</td><td>Delaware</td><td>446</td></tr>
<tr><td>20</td><td>Kansas</td><td>396</td><td>16</td><td>West Virginia</td><td>443</td></tr>
<tr><td>25</td><td>Kentucky</td><td>384</td><td>17</td><td>North Dakota</td><td>442</td></tr>
<tr><td>35</td><td>Louisiana</td><td>354</td><td>18</td><td>Missouri</td><td>425</td></tr>
<tr><td>21</td><td>Maine</td><td>391</td><td>19</td><td>Florida</td><td>411</td></tr>
<tr><td>45</td><td>Maryland</td><td>273</td><td>20</td><td>Kansas</td><td>396</td></tr>
<tr><td>48</td><td>Massachusetts</td><td>218</td><td>21</td><td>Maine</td><td>391</td></tr>
<tr><td>37</td><td>Michigan</td><td>346</td><td>22</td><td>Mississippi</td><td>390</td></tr>
<tr><td>42</td><td>Minnesota</td><td>326</td><td>22</td><td>Tennessee</td><td>390</td></tr>
<tr><td>22</td><td>Mississippi</td><td>390</td><td>24</td><td>Wisconsin</td><td>388</td></tr>
<tr><td>18</td><td>Missouri</td><td>425</td><td>25</td><td>Kentucky</td><td>384</td></tr>
<tr><td>2</td><td>Montana</td><td>617</td><td>26</td><td>North Carolina</td><td>382</td></tr>
<tr><td>29</td><td>Nebraska</td><td>367</td><td>27</td><td>South Carolina</td><td>377</td></tr>
<tr><td>5</td><td>Nevada</td><td>535</td><td>28</td><td>Indiana</td><td>372</td></tr>
<tr><td>12</td><td>New Hampshire</td><td>476</td><td>29</td><td>Alabama</td><td>367</td></tr>
<tr><td>48</td><td>New Jersey</td><td>218</td><td>29</td><td>Hawaii</td><td>367</td></tr>
<tr><td>1</td><td>New Mexico</td><td>638</td><td>29</td><td>Nebraska</td><td>367</td></tr>
<tr><td>50</td><td>New York</td><td>209</td><td>32</td><td>Washington</td><td>363</td></tr>
<tr><td>26</td><td>North Carolina</td><td>382</td><td>33</td><td>Vermont</td><td>362</td></tr>
<tr><td>17</td><td>North Dakota</td><td>442</td><td>34</td><td>Georgia</td><td>361</td></tr>
<tr><td>40</td><td>Ohio</td><td>342</td><td>35</td><td>Louisiana</td><td>354</td></tr>
<tr><td>10</td><td>Oklahoma</td><td>483</td><td>36</td><td>Iowa</td><td>353</td></tr>
<tr><td>14</td><td>Oregon</td><td>447</td><td>37</td><td>Michigan</td><td>346</td></tr>
<tr><td>37</td><td>Pennsylvania</td><td>346</td><td>37</td><td>Pennsylvania</td><td>346</td></tr>
<tr><td>43</td><td>Rhode Island</td><td>295</td><td>39</td><td>Virginia</td><td>345</td></tr>
<tr><td>27</td><td>South Carolina</td><td>377</td><td>40</td><td>Ohio</td><td>342</td></tr>
<tr><td>8</td><td>South Dakota</td><td>521</td><td>41</td><td>Texas</td><td>340</td></tr>
<tr><td>22</td><td>Tennessee</td><td>390</td><td>42</td><td>Minnesota</td><td>326</td></tr>
<tr><td>41</td><td>Texas</td><td>340</td><td>43</td><td>Rhode Island</td><td>295</td></tr>
<tr><td>7</td><td>Utah</td><td>524</td><td>44</td><td>Illinois</td><td>293</td></tr>
<tr><td>33</td><td>Vermont</td><td>362</td><td>45</td><td>Maryland</td><td>273</td></tr>
<tr><td>39</td><td>Virginia</td><td>345</td><td>46</td><td>Connecticut</td><td>269</td></tr>
<tr><td>32</td><td>Washington</td><td>363</td><td>47</td><td>California</td><td>242</td></tr>
<tr><td>16</td><td>West Virginia</td><td>443</td><td>48</td><td>Massachusetts</td><td>218</td></tr>
<tr><td>24</td><td>Wisconsin</td><td>388</td><td>48</td><td>New Jersey</td><td>218</td></tr>
<tr><td>4</td><td>Wyoming</td><td>598</td><td>50</td><td>New York</td><td>209</td></tr>
<tr><td></td><td></td><td></td><td></td><td>District of Columbia</td><td>227</td></tr>
</table>

Source: U.S. Department of Health and Human Services, National Center for Health Statistics unpublished data

*Age-adjusted years of potential life lost due to death before age 75.

Years Lost by Premature Death from Unintentional Injuries in 2001

National Average = 1,035 Years Lost per 100,000 Population*

ALPHA ORDER

RANK	STATE	YEARS
6	Alabama	1,537
1	Alaska	1,977
10	Arizona	1,453
7	Arkansas	1,527
48	California	712
23	Colorado	1,125
39	Connecticut	854
25	Delaware	1,082
16	Florida	1,352
20	Georgia	1,227
43	Hawaii	816
17	Idaho	1,292
32	Illinois	949
27	Indiana	1,005
40	Iowa	851
18	Kansas	1,258
8	Kentucky	1,490
9	Louisiana	1,488
26	Maine	1,034
46	Maryland	740
50	Massachusetts	498
35	Michigan	925
41	Minnesota	844
2	Mississippi	1,781
19	Missouri	1,239
14	Montana	1,410
37	Nebraska	894
23	Nevada	1,125
45	New Hampshire	774
44	New Jersey	805
4	New Mexico	1,702
47	New York	716
20	North Carolina	1,227
29	North Dakota	962
34	Ohio	942
13	Oklahoma	1,419
31	Oregon	953
27	Pennsylvania	1,005
49	Rhode Island	601
5	South Carolina	1,552
15	South Dakota	1,392
12	Tennessee	1,431
22	Texas	1,158
42	Utah	836
36	Vermont	911
38	Virginia	890
30	Washington	959
11	West Virginia	1,447
33	Wisconsin	945
3	Wyoming	1,760

RANK ORDER

RANK	STATE	YEARS
1	Alaska	1,977
2	Mississippi	1,781
3	Wyoming	1,760
4	New Mexico	1,702
5	South Carolina	1,552
6	Alabama	1,537
7	Arkansas	1,527
8	Kentucky	1,490
9	Louisiana	1,488
10	Arizona	1,453
11	West Virginia	1,447
12	Tennessee	1,431
13	Oklahoma	1,419
14	Montana	1,410
15	South Dakota	1,392
16	Florida	1,352
17	Idaho	1,292
18	Kansas	1,258
19	Missouri	1,239
20	Georgia	1,227
20	North Carolina	1,227
22	Texas	1,158
23	Colorado	1,125
23	Nevada	1,125
25	Delaware	1,082
26	Maine	1,034
27	Indiana	1,005
27	Pennsylvania	1,005
29	North Dakota	962
30	Washington	959
31	Oregon	953
32	Illinois	949
33	Wisconsin	945
34	Ohio	942
35	Michigan	925
36	Vermont	911
37	Nebraska	894
38	Virginia	890
39	Connecticut	854
40	Iowa	851
41	Minnesota	844
42	Utah	836
43	Hawaii	816
44	New Jersey	805
45	New Hampshire	774
46	Maryland	740
47	New York	716
48	California	712
49	Rhode Island	601
50	Massachusetts	498
	District of Columbia	1,133

Source: U.S. Department of Health and Human Services, National Center for Health Statistics
    unpublished data
*Age-adjusted years of potential life lost due to death before age 75. Includes such subcategories as falls, drowning, fires/burns, poisonings and motor vehicle injuries.

III. FACILITIES

Community Hospitals in 2003

National Total = 4,895 Hospitals*

ALPHA ORDER

RANK	STATE	HOSPITALS	% of USA
20	Alabama	107	2.2%
47	Alaska	19	0.4%
30	Arizona	61	1.2%
23	Arkansas	88	1.8%
2	California	370	7.6%
29	Colorado	68	1.4%
42	Connecticut	34	0.7%
50	Delaware	6	0.1%
4	Florida	203	4.1%
8	Georgia	146	3.0%
45	Hawaii	24	0.5%
39	Idaho	39	0.8%
6	Illinois	192	3.9%
18	Indiana	112	2.3%
16	Iowa	116	2.4%
10	Kansas	134	2.7%
21	Kentucky	103	2.1%
12	Louisiana	127	2.6%
40	Maine	37	0.8%
35	Maryland	51	1.0%
27	Massachusetts	79	1.6%
9	Michigan	144	2.9%
11	Minnesota	131	2.7%
22	Mississippi	92	1.9%
15	Missouri	119	2.4%
34	Montana	53	1.1%
24	Nebraska	85	1.7%
44	Nevada	25	0.5%
43	New Hampshire	28	0.6%
28	New Jersey	78	1.6%
40	New Mexico	37	0.8%
3	New York	207	4.2%
17	North Carolina	113	2.3%
38	North Dakota	40	0.8%
7	Ohio	163	3.3%
19	Oklahoma	108	2.2%
32	Oregon	58	1.2%
5	Pennsylvania	201	4.1%
49	Rhode Island	11	0.2%
30	South Carolina	61	1.2%
36	South Dakota	50	1.0%
13	Tennessee	125	2.6%
1	Texas	414	8.5%
37	Utah	42	0.9%
48	Vermont	14	0.3%
26	Virginia	84	1.7%
24	Washington	85	1.7%
33	West Virginia	57	1.2%
14	Wisconsin	121	2.5%
46	Wyoming	23	0.5%

RANK ORDER

RANK	STATE	HOSPITALS	% of USA
1	Texas	414	8.5%
2	California	370	7.6%
3	New York	207	4.2%
4	Florida	203	4.1%
5	Pennsylvania	201	4.1%
6	Illinois	192	3.9%
7	Ohio	163	3.3%
8	Georgia	146	3.0%
9	Michigan	144	2.9%
10	Kansas	134	2.7%
11	Minnesota	131	2.7%
12	Louisiana	127	2.6%
13	Tennessee	125	2.6%
14	Wisconsin	121	2.5%
15	Missouri	119	2.4%
16	Iowa	116	2.4%
17	North Carolina	113	2.3%
18	Indiana	112	2.3%
19	Oklahoma	108	2.2%
20	Alabama	107	2.2%
21	Kentucky	103	2.1%
22	Mississippi	92	1.9%
23	Arkansas	88	1.8%
24	Nebraska	85	1.7%
24	Washington	85	1.7%
26	Virginia	84	1.7%
27	Massachusetts	79	1.6%
28	New Jersey	78	1.6%
29	Colorado	68	1.4%
30	Arizona	61	1.2%
30	South Carolina	61	1.2%
32	Oregon	58	1.2%
33	West Virginia	57	1.2%
34	Montana	53	1.1%
35	Maryland	51	1.0%
36	South Dakota	50	1.0%
37	Utah	42	0.9%
38	North Dakota	40	0.8%
39	Idaho	39	0.8%
40	Maine	37	0.8%
40	New Mexico	37	0.8%
42	Connecticut	34	0.7%
43	New Hampshire	28	0.6%
44	Nevada	25	0.5%
45	Hawaii	24	0.5%
46	Wyoming	23	0.5%
47	Alaska	19	0.4%
48	Vermont	14	0.3%
49	Rhode Island	11	0.2%
50	Delaware	6	0.1%
	District of Columbia	10	0.2%

Source: American Hospital Association (Chicago, IL)
"Hospital Statistics" (2005 edition)

**Community hospitals are all nonfederal, short-term, general and special hospitals whose facilities and services are available to the public.*

Rate of Community Hospitals in 2003

National Rate = 1.7 Community Hospitals per 100,000 Population*

ALPHA ORDER

RANK	STATE	RATE
18	Alabama	2.4
12	Alaska	2.9
41	Arizona	1.1
8	Arkansas	3.2
45	California	1.0
32	Colorado	1.5
45	Connecticut	1.0
50	Delaware	0.7
39	Florida	1.2
29	Georgia	1.7
25	Hawaii	1.9
12	Idaho	2.9
32	Illinois	1.5
27	Indiana	1.8
7	Iowa	3.9
4	Kansas	4.9
17	Kentucky	2.5
14	Louisiana	2.8
14	Maine	2.8
48	Maryland	0.9
39	Massachusetts	1.2
35	Michigan	1.4
16	Minnesota	2.6
8	Mississippi	3.2
22	Missouri	2.1
3	Montana	5.8
4	Nebraska	4.9
41	Nevada	1.1
20	New Hampshire	2.2
48	New Jersey	0.9
24	New Mexico	2.0
41	New York	1.1
38	North Carolina	1.3
2	North Dakota	6.3
35	Ohio	1.4
10	Oklahoma	3.1
30	Oregon	1.6
30	Pennsylvania	1.6
45	Rhode Island	1.0
32	South Carolina	1.5
1	South Dakota	6.5
22	Tennessee	2.1
25	Texas	1.9
27	Utah	1.8
19	Vermont	2.3
41	Virginia	1.1
35	Washington	1.4
10	West Virginia	3.1
20	Wisconsin	2.2
6	Wyoming	4.6

RANK ORDER

RANK	STATE	RATE
1	South Dakota	6.5
2	North Dakota	6.3
3	Montana	5.8
4	Kansas	4.9
4	Nebraska	4.9
6	Wyoming	4.6
7	Iowa	3.9
8	Arkansas	3.2
8	Mississippi	3.2
10	Oklahoma	3.1
10	West Virginia	3.1
12	Alaska	2.9
12	Idaho	2.9
14	Louisiana	2.8
14	Maine	2.8
16	Minnesota	2.6
17	Kentucky	2.5
18	Alabama	2.4
19	Vermont	2.3
20	New Hampshire	2.2
20	Wisconsin	2.2
22	Missouri	2.1
22	Tennessee	2.1
24	New Mexico	2.0
25	Hawaii	1.9
25	Texas	1.9
27	Indiana	1.8
27	Utah	1.8
29	Georgia	1.7
30	Oregon	1.6
30	Pennsylvania	1.6
32	Colorado	1.5
32	Illinois	1.5
32	South Carolina	1.5
35	Michigan	1.4
35	Ohio	1.4
35	Washington	1.4
38	North Carolina	1.3
39	Florida	1.2
39	Massachusetts	1.2
41	Arizona	1.1
41	Nevada	1.1
41	New York	1.1
41	Virginia	1.1
45	California	1.0
45	Connecticut	1.0
45	Rhode Island	1.0
48	Maryland	0.9
48	New Jersey	0.9
50	Delaware	0.7

District of Columbia	1.8

Source: Morgan Quitno Press using data from American Hospital Association (Chicago, IL)
     "Hospital Statistics" (2005 edition)
Community hospitals are all nonfederal, short-term, general and special hospitals whose facilities and services are available to the public.

Community Hospitals per 1,000 Square Miles in 2003

National Rate = 1.3 Community Hospitals*

ALPHA ORDER

RANK	STATE	RATE
23	Alabama	2.0
50	Alaska**	0.0
43	Arizona	0.5
28	Arkansas	1.7
20	California	2.3
39	Colorado	0.7
4	Connecticut	6.1
16	Delaware	2.5
10	Florida	3.4
16	Georgia	2.5
8	Hawaii	3.7
43	Idaho	0.5
11	Illinois	3.3
12	Indiana	3.1
21	Iowa	2.1
30	Kansas	1.6
16	Kentucky	2.5
15	Louisiana	2.6
37	Maine	1.1
6	Maryland	4.1
3	Massachusetts	8.5
31	Michigan	1.5
31	Minnesota	1.5
26	Mississippi	1.9
28	Missouri	1.7
46	Montana	0.4
37	Nebraska	1.1
48	Nevada	0.2
13	New Hampshire	3.0
1	New Jersey	9.5
47	New Mexico	0.3
7	New York	3.8
21	North Carolina	2.1
40	North Dakota	0.6
9	Ohio	3.6
31	Oklahoma	1.5
40	Oregon	0.6
5	Pennsylvania	4.4
2	Rhode Island	8.9
23	South Carolina	2.0
40	South Dakota	0.6
13	Tennessee	3.0
31	Texas	1.5
43	Utah	0.5
31	Vermont	1.5
23	Virginia	2.0
36	Washington	1.2
19	West Virginia	2.4
27	Wisconsin	1.8
48	Wyoming	0.2

RANK ORDER

RANK	STATE	RATE
1	New Jersey	9.5
2	Rhode Island	8.9
3	Massachusetts	8.5
4	Connecticut	6.1
5	Pennsylvania	4.4
6	Maryland	4.1
7	New York	3.8
8	Hawaii	3.7
9	Ohio	3.6
10	Florida	3.4
11	Illinois	3.3
12	Indiana	3.1
13	New Hampshire	3.0
13	Tennessee	3.0
15	Louisiana	2.6
16	Delaware	2.5
16	Georgia	2.5
16	Kentucky	2.5
19	West Virginia	2.4
20	California	2.3
21	Iowa	2.1
21	North Carolina	2.1
23	Alabama	2.0
23	South Carolina	2.0
23	Virginia	2.0
26	Mississippi	1.9
27	Wisconsin	1.8
28	Arkansas	1.7
28	Missouri	1.7
30	Kansas	1.6
31	Michigan	1.5
31	Minnesota	1.5
31	Oklahoma	1.5
31	Texas	1.5
31	Vermont	1.5
36	Washington	1.2
37	Maine	1.1
37	Nebraska	1.1
39	Colorado	0.7
40	North Dakota	0.6
40	Oregon	0.6
40	South Dakota	0.6
43	Arizona	0.5
43	Idaho	0.5
43	Utah	0.5
46	Montana	0.4
47	New Mexico	0.3
48	Nevada	0.2
48	Wyoming	0.2
50	Alaska**	0.0
	District of Columbia***	NA

Source: Morgan Quitno Press using data from American Hospital Association (Chicago, IL)
"Hospital Statistics" (2005 edition)
Based on 2000 Census land and water area figures. Community hospitals are nonfederal short-term general and other special hospitals, whose facilities and services are available to the public.
**Alaska has 19 community hospitals for its 616,240 square miles.*
***The District of Columbia has 10 community hospitals for its 68 square miles.*

Community Hospitals in Urban Areas in 2003

National Total = 2,729 Hospitals*

RANK	STATE	HOSPITALS	% of USA
16	Alabama	57	2.1%
48	Alaska	3	0.1%
20	Arizona	46	1.7%
26	Arkansas	32	1.2%
1	California	330	12.1%
26	Colorado	32	1.2%
29	Connecticut	28	1.0%
47	Delaware	4	0.1%
3	Florida	170	6.2%
13	Georgia	63	2.3%
38	Hawaii	13	0.5%
43	Idaho	6	0.2%
6	Illinois	120	4.4%
12	Indiana	67	2.5%
32	Iowa	21	0.8%
30	Kansas	27	1.0%
26	Kentucky	32	1.2%
9	Louisiana	78	2.9%
42	Maine	8	0.3%
23	Maryland	41	1.5%
11	Massachusetts	68	2.5%
8	Michigan	85	3.1%
21	Minnesota	45	1.6%
34	Mississippi	19	0.7%
14	Missouri	61	2.2%
46	Montana	5	0.2%
38	Nebraska	13	0.5%
36	Nevada	16	0.6%
40	New Hampshire	10	0.4%
9	New Jersey	78	2.9%
37	New Mexico	15	0.5%
3	New York	170	6.2%
18	North Carolina	51	1.9%
43	North Dakota	6	0.2%
7	Ohio	113	4.1%
23	Oklahoma	41	1.5%
30	Oregon	27	1.0%
5	Pennsylvania	158	5.8%
40	Rhode Island	10	0.4%
25	South Carolina	35	1.3%
43	South Dakota	6	0.2%
14	Tennessee	61	2.2%
2	Texas	253	9.3%
33	Utah	20	0.7%
49	Vermont	2	0.1%
19	Virginia	50	1.8%
21	Washington	45	1.6%
35	West Virginia	18	0.7%
16	Wisconsin	57	2.1%
49	Wyoming	2	0.1%

RANK	STATE	HOSPITALS	% of USA
1	California	330	12.1%
2	Texas	253	9.3%
3	Florida	170	6.2%
3	New York	170	6.2%
5	Pennsylvania	158	5.8%
6	Illinois	120	4.4%
7	Ohio	113	4.1%
8	Michigan	85	3.1%
9	Louisiana	78	2.9%
9	New Jersey	78	2.9%
11	Massachusetts	68	2.5%
12	Indiana	67	2.5%
13	Georgia	63	2.3%
14	Missouri	61	2.2%
14	Tennessee	61	2.2%
16	Alabama	57	2.1%
16	Wisconsin	57	2.1%
18	North Carolina	51	1.9%
19	Virginia	50	1.8%
20	Arizona	46	1.7%
21	Minnesota	45	1.6%
21	Washington	45	1.6%
23	Maryland	41	1.5%
23	Oklahoma	41	1.5%
25	South Carolina	35	1.3%
26	Arkansas	32	1.2%
26	Colorado	32	1.2%
26	Kentucky	32	1.2%
29	Connecticut	28	1.0%
30	Kansas	27	1.0%
30	Oregon	27	1.0%
32	Iowa	21	0.8%
33	Utah	20	0.7%
34	Mississippi	19	0.7%
35	West Virginia	18	0.7%
36	Nevada	16	0.6%
37	New Mexico	15	0.5%
38	Hawaii	13	0.5%
38	Nebraska	13	0.5%
40	New Hampshire	10	0.4%
40	Rhode Island	10	0.4%
42	Maine	8	0.3%
43	Idaho	6	0.2%
43	North Dakota	6	0.2%
43	South Dakota	6	0.2%
46	Montana	5	0.2%
47	Delaware	4	0.1%
48	Alaska	3	0.1%
49	Vermont	2	0.1%
49	Wyoming	2	0.1%
	District of Columbia	10	0.4%

Source: American Hospital Association (Chicago, IL)
"Hospital Statistics" (2005 edition)

*Community hospitals are all nonfederal, short-term, general and special hospitals whose facilities and services are available to the public. Urban is defined as any area inside a metropolitan statistical area as defined by the U.S. Office of Management and Budget.

Percent of Community Hospitals in Urban Areas in 2003

National Percent = 55.8% of Community Hospitals*

ALPHA ORDER

RANK ORDER

RANK	STATE	PERCENT	RANK	STATE	PERCENT
22	Alabama	53.3	1	New Jersey	100.0
43	Alaska	15.8	2	Rhode Island	90.9
10	Arizona	75.4	3	California	89.2
34	Arkansas	36.4	4	Massachusetts	86.1
3	California	89.2	5	Florida	83.7
27	Colorado	47.1	6	Connecticut	82.4
6	Connecticut	82.4	7	New York	82.1
12	Delaware	66.7	8	Maryland	80.4
5	Florida	83.7	9	Pennsylvania	78.6
31	Georgia	43.2	10	Arizona	75.4
21	Hawaii	54.2	11	Ohio	69.3
44	Idaho	15.4	12	Delaware	66.7
14	Illinois	62.5	13	Nevada	64.0
17	Indiana	59.8	14	Illinois	62.5
42	Iowa	18.1	15	Louisiana	61.4
41	Kansas	20.1	16	Texas	61.1
38	Kentucky	31.1	17	Indiana	59.8
15	Louisiana	61.4	18	Virginia	59.5
39	Maine	21.6	19	Michigan	59.0
8	Maryland	80.4	20	South Carolina	57.4
4	Massachusetts	86.1	21	Hawaii	54.2
19	Michigan	59.0	22	Alabama	53.3
36	Minnesota	34.4	23	Washington	52.9
40	Mississippi	20.7	24	Missouri	51.3
24	Missouri	51.3	25	Tennessee	48.8
49	Montana	9.4	26	Utah	47.6
45	Nebraska	15.3	27	Colorado	47.1
13	Nevada	64.0	27	Wisconsin	47.1
35	New Hampshire	35.7	29	Oregon	46.6
1	New Jersey	100.0	30	North Carolina	45.1
32	New Mexico	40.5	31	Georgia	43.2
7	New York	82.1	32	New Mexico	40.5
30	North Carolina	45.1	33	Oklahoma	38.0
46	North Dakota	15.0	34	Arkansas	36.4
11	Ohio	69.3	35	New Hampshire	35.7
33	Oklahoma	38.0	36	Minnesota	34.4
29	Oregon	46.6	37	West Virginia	31.6
9	Pennsylvania	78.6	38	Kentucky	31.1
2	Rhode Island	90.9	39	Maine	21.6
20	South Carolina	57.4	40	Mississippi	20.7
48	South Dakota	12.0	41	Kansas	20.1
25	Tennessee	48.8	42	Iowa	18.1
16	Texas	61.1	43	Alaska	15.8
26	Utah	47.6	44	Idaho	15.4
47	Vermont	14.3	45	Nebraska	15.3
18	Virginia	59.5	46	North Dakota	15.0
23	Washington	52.9	47	Vermont	14.3
37	West Virginia	31.6	48	South Dakota	12.0
27	Wisconsin	47.1	49	Montana	9.4
50	Wyoming	8.7	50	Wyoming	8.7

District of Columbia   100.0

*Source: Morgan Quitno Press using data from American Hospital Association (Chicago, IL)
"Hospital Statistics" (2005 edition)*
*Community hospitals are all nonfederal, short-term, general and special hospitals whose facilities and services are available to the public. Urban is defined as any area inside a metropolitan statistical area as defined by the U.S. Office of Management and Budget.

Community Hospitals in Rural Areas in 2003

National Total = 2,166 Hospitals*

ALPHA ORDER

RANK ORDER

RANK	STATE	HOSPITALS	% of USA
17	Alabama	50	2.3%
40	Alaska	16	0.7%
41	Arizona	15	0.7%
16	Arkansas	56	2.6%
24	California	40	1.8%
28	Colorado	36	1.7%
47	Connecticut	6	0.3%
48	Delaware	2	0.1%
31	Florida	33	1.5%
5	Georgia	83	3.8%
43	Hawaii	11	0.5%
31	Idaho	33	1.5%
7	Illinois	72	3.3%
21	Indiana	45	2.1%
3	Iowa	95	4.4%
2	Kansas	107	4.9%
9	Kentucky	71	3.3%
19	Louisiana	49	2.3%
34	Maine	29	1.3%
45	Maryland	10	0.5%
43	Massachusetts	11	0.5%
14	Michigan	59	2.7%
4	Minnesota	86	4.0%
6	Mississippi	73	3.4%
15	Missouri	58	2.7%
20	Montana	48	2.2%
7	Nebraska	72	3.3%
46	Nevada	9	0.4%
39	New Hampshire	18	0.8%
50	New Jersey	0	0.0%
36	New Mexico	22	1.0%
27	New York	37	1.7%
13	North Carolina	62	2.9%
29	North Dakota	34	1.6%
17	Ohio	50	2.3%
10	Oklahoma	67	3.1%
33	Oregon	31	1.4%
23	Pennsylvania	43	2.0%
49	Rhode Island	1	0.0%
35	South Carolina	26	1.2%
22	South Dakota	44	2.0%
11	Tennessee	64	3.0%
1	Texas	161	7.4%
36	Utah	22	1.0%
42	Vermont	12	0.6%
29	Virginia	34	1.6%
24	Washington	40	1.8%
26	West Virginia	39	1.8%
11	Wisconsin	64	3.0%
38	Wyoming	21	1.0%

RANK	STATE	HOSPITALS	% of USA
1	Texas	161	7.4%
2	Kansas	107	4.9%
3	Iowa	95	4.4%
4	Minnesota	86	4.0%
5	Georgia	83	3.8%
6	Mississippi	73	3.4%
7	Illinois	72	3.3%
7	Nebraska	72	3.3%
9	Kentucky	71	3.3%
10	Oklahoma	67	3.1%
11	Tennessee	64	3.0%
11	Wisconsin	64	3.0%
13	North Carolina	62	2.9%
14	Michigan	59	2.7%
15	Missouri	58	2.7%
16	Arkansas	56	2.6%
17	Alabama	50	2.3%
17	Ohio	50	2.3%
19	Louisiana	49	2.3%
20	Montana	48	2.2%
21	Indiana	45	2.1%
22	South Dakota	44	2.0%
23	Pennsylvania	43	2.0%
24	California	40	1.8%
24	Washington	40	1.8%
26	West Virginia	39	1.8%
27	New York	37	1.7%
28	Colorado	36	1.7%
29	North Dakota	34	1.6%
29	Virginia	34	1.6%
31	Florida	33	1.5%
31	Idaho	33	1.5%
33	Oregon	31	1.4%
34	Maine	29	1.3%
35	South Carolina	26	1.2%
36	New Mexico	22	1.0%
36	Utah	22	1.0%
38	Wyoming	21	1.0%
39	New Hampshire	18	0.8%
40	Alaska	16	0.7%
41	Arizona	15	0.7%
42	Vermont	12	0.6%
43	Hawaii	11	0.5%
43	Massachusetts	11	0.5%
45	Maryland	10	0.5%
46	Nevada	9	0.4%
47	Connecticut	6	0.3%
48	Delaware	2	0.1%
49	Rhode Island	1	0.0%
50	New Jersey	0	0.0%
	District of Columbia	0	0.0%

Source: American Hospital Association (Chicago, IL)
        "Hospital Statistics" (2005 edition)

Community hospitals are all nonfederal, short-term, general and special hospitals whose facilities and services are available to the public. Rural is defined as any area outside a metropolitan statistical area as defined by the U.S. Office of Management and Budget.

Percent of Community Hospitals in Rural Areas in 2003

National Percent = 44.2% of Community Hospitals*

ALPHA ORDER RANK	STATE	PERCENT	RANK ORDER RANK	STATE	PERCENT
29	Alabama	46.7	1	Wyoming	91.3
8	Alaska	84.2	2	Montana	90.6
41	Arizona	24.6	3	South Dakota	88.0
17	Arkansas	63.6	4	Vermont	85.7
48	California	10.8	5	North Dakota	85.0
23	Colorado	52.9	6	Nebraska	84.7
45	Connecticut	17.6	7	Idaho	84.6
39	Delaware	33.3	8	Alaska	84.2
46	Florida	16.3	9	Iowa	81.9
20	Georgia	56.8	10	Kansas	79.9
30	Hawaii	45.8	11	Mississippi	79.3
7	Idaho	84.6	12	Maine	78.4
37	Illinois	37.5	13	Kentucky	68.9
34	Indiana	40.2	14	West Virginia	68.4
9	Iowa	81.9	15	Minnesota	65.6
10	Kansas	79.9	16	New Hampshire	64.3
13	Kentucky	68.9	17	Arkansas	63.6
36	Louisiana	38.6	18	Oklahoma	62.0
12	Maine	78.4	19	New Mexico	59.5
43	Maryland	19.6	20	Georgia	56.8
47	Massachusetts	13.9	21	North Carolina	54.9
32	Michigan	41.0	22	Oregon	53.4
15	Minnesota	65.6	23	Colorado	52.9
11	Mississippi	79.3	23	Wisconsin	52.9
27	Missouri	48.7	25	Utah	52.4
2	Montana	90.6	26	Tennessee	51.2
6	Nebraska	84.7	27	Missouri	48.7
38	Nevada	36.0	28	Washington	47.1
16	New Hampshire	64.3	29	Alabama	46.7
50	New Jersey	0.0	30	Hawaii	45.8
19	New Mexico	59.5	31	South Carolina	42.6
44	New York	17.9	32	Michigan	41.0
21	North Carolina	54.9	33	Virginia	40.5
5	North Dakota	85.0	34	Indiana	40.2
40	Ohio	30.7	35	Texas	38.9
18	Oklahoma	62.0	36	Louisiana	38.6
22	Oregon	53.4	37	Illinois	37.5
42	Pennsylvania	21.4	38	Nevada	36.0
49	Rhode Island	9.1	39	Delaware	33.3
31	South Carolina	42.6	40	Ohio	30.7
3	South Dakota	88.0	41	Arizona	24.6
26	Tennessee	51.2	42	Pennsylvania	21.4
35	Texas	38.9	43	Maryland	19.6
25	Utah	52.4	44	New York	17.9
4	Vermont	85.7	45	Connecticut	17.6
33	Virginia	40.5	46	Florida	16.3
28	Washington	47.1	47	Massachusetts	13.9
14	West Virginia	68.4	48	California	10.8
23	Wisconsin	52.9	49	Rhode Island	9.1
1	Wyoming	91.3	50	New Jersey	0.0
				District of Columbia	0.0

Source: Morgan Quitno Press using data from American Hospital Association (Chicago, IL)
        "Hospital Statistics" (2005 edition)
*Community hospitals are all nonfederal, short-term, general and special hospitals whose facilities and services are available to the public. Rural is defined as any area outside a metropolitan statistical area as defined by the U.S. Office of Management and Budget.

Nongovernment Not-For-Profit Hospitals in 2003

National Total = 2,984 Hospitals*

ALPHA ORDER

RANK	STATE	HOSPITALS	% of USA
32	Alabama	35	1.2%
47	Alaska	10	0.3%
31	Arizona	38	1.3%
22	Arkansas	52	1.7%
1	California	207	6.9%
35	Colorado	32	1.1%
35	Connecticut	32	1.1%
49	Delaware	6	0.2%
10	Florida	88	2.9%
18	Georgia	62	2.1%
43	Hawaii	18	0.6%
45	Idaho	13	0.4%
4	Illinois	154	5.2%
20	Indiana	59	2.0%
21	Iowa	57	1.9%
19	Kansas	60	2.0%
13	Kentucky	73	2.4%
33	Louisiana	34	1.1%
33	Maine	34	1.1%
23	Maryland	47	1.6%
14	Massachusetts	68	2.3%
7	Michigan	122	4.1%
9	Minnesota	89	3.0%
38	Mississippi	26	0.9%
15	Missouri	67	2.2%
26	Montana	43	1.4%
25	Nebraska	44	1.5%
48	Nevada	9	0.3%
39	New Hampshire	24	0.8%
12	New Jersey	74	2.5%
42	New Mexico	19	0.6%
2	New York	178	6.0%
11	North Carolina	76	2.5%
30	North Dakota	40	1.3%
6	Ohio	136	4.6%
24	Oklahoma	46	1.5%
26	Oregon	43	1.4%
3	Pennsylvania	177	5.9%
46	Rhode Island	11	0.4%
40	South Carolina	23	0.8%
26	South Dakota	43	1.4%
16	Tennessee	63	2.1%
5	Texas	152	5.1%
41	Utah	22	0.7%
44	Vermont	14	0.5%
16	Virginia	63	2.1%
29	Washington	41	1.4%
37	West Virginia	31	1.0%
8	Wisconsin	117	3.9%
50	Wyoming	5	0.2%

RANK ORDER

RANK	STATE	HOSPITALS	% of USA
1	California	207	6.9%
2	New York	178	6.0%
3	Pennsylvania	177	5.9%
4	Illinois	154	5.2%
5	Texas	152	5.1%
6	Ohio	136	4.6%
7	Michigan	122	4.1%
8	Wisconsin	117	3.9%
9	Minnesota	89	3.0%
10	Florida	88	2.9%
11	North Carolina	76	2.5%
12	New Jersey	74	2.5%
13	Kentucky	73	2.4%
14	Massachusetts	68	2.3%
15	Missouri	67	2.2%
16	Tennessee	63	2.1%
16	Virginia	63	2.1%
18	Georgia	62	2.1%
19	Kansas	60	2.0%
20	Indiana	59	2.0%
21	Iowa	57	1.9%
22	Arkansas	52	1.7%
23	Maryland	47	1.6%
24	Oklahoma	46	1.5%
25	Nebraska	44	1.5%
26	Montana	43	1.4%
26	Oregon	43	1.4%
26	South Dakota	43	1.4%
29	Washington	41	1.4%
30	North Dakota	40	1.3%
31	Arizona	38	1.3%
32	Alabama	35	1.2%
33	Louisiana	34	1.1%
33	Maine	34	1.1%
35	Colorado	32	1.1%
35	Connecticut	32	1.1%
37	West Virginia	31	1.0%
38	Mississippi	26	0.9%
39	New Hampshire	24	0.8%
40	South Carolina	23	0.8%
41	Utah	22	0.7%
42	New Mexico	19	0.6%
43	Hawaii	18	0.6%
44	Vermont	14	0.5%
45	Idaho	13	0.4%
46	Rhode Island	11	0.4%
47	Alaska	10	0.3%
48	Nevada	9	0.3%
49	Delaware	6	0.2%
50	Wyoming	5	0.2%
	District of Columbia	7	0.2%

Source: American Hospital Association (Chicago, IL)
     "Hospital Statistics" (2005 edition)
*Nongovernment not-for-profit hospitals are a subset of community hospitals.

Investor-Owned (For-Profit) Hospitals in 2003

National Total = 790 Hospitals*

ALPHA ORDER

RANK	STATE	HOSPITALS	% of USA
6	Alabama	35	4.4%
36	Alaska	2	0.3%
11	Arizona	18	2.3%
10	Arkansas	21	2.7%
3	California	92	11.6%
22	Colorado	9	1.1%
40	Connecticut	1	0.1%
43	Delaware	0	0.0%
2	Florida	95	12.0%
7	Georgia	30	3.8%
43	Hawaii	0	0.0%
36	Idaho	2	0.3%
21	Illinois	10	1.3%
17	Indiana	15	1.9%
43	Iowa	0	0.0%
20	Kansas	13	1.6%
13	Kentucky	17	2.2%
4	Louisiana	43	5.4%
40	Maine	1	0.1%
31	Maryland	3	0.4%
25	Massachusetts	8	1.0%
28	Michigan	4	0.5%
43	Minnesota	0	0.0%
8	Mississippi	24	3.0%
15	Missouri	16	2.0%
43	Montana	0	0.0%
36	Nebraska	2	0.3%
22	Nevada	9	1.1%
28	New Hampshire	4	0.5%
31	New Jersey	3	0.4%
22	New Mexico	9	1.1%
31	New York	3	0.4%
25	North Carolina	8	1.0%
43	North Dakota	0	0.0%
28	Ohio	4	0.5%
17	Oklahoma	15	1.9%
31	Oregon	3	0.4%
9	Pennsylvania	22	2.8%
43	Rhode Island	0	0.0%
11	South Carolina	18	2.3%
40	South Dakota	1	0.1%
5	Tennessee	37	4.7%
1	Texas	133	16.8%
19	Utah	14	1.8%
43	Vermont	0	0.0%
13	Virginia	17	2.2%
27	Washington	5	0.6%
15	West Virginia	16	2.0%
36	Wisconsin	2	0.3%
31	Wyoming	3	0.4%

RANK ORDER

RANK	STATE	HOSPITALS	% of USA
1	Texas	133	16.8%
2	Florida	95	12.0%
3	California	92	11.6%
4	Louisiana	43	5.4%
5	Tennessee	37	4.7%
6	Alabama	35	4.4%
7	Georgia	30	3.8%
8	Mississippi	24	3.0%
9	Pennsylvania	22	2.8%
10	Arkansas	21	2.7%
11	Arizona	18	2.3%
11	South Carolina	18	2.3%
13	Kentucky	17	2.2%
13	Virginia	17	2.2%
15	Missouri	16	2.0%
15	West Virginia	16	2.0%
17	Indiana	15	1.9%
17	Oklahoma	15	1.9%
19	Utah	14	1.8%
20	Kansas	13	1.6%
21	Illinois	10	1.3%
22	Colorado	9	1.1%
22	Nevada	9	1.1%
22	New Mexico	9	1.1%
25	Massachusetts	8	1.0%
25	North Carolina	8	1.0%
27	Washington	5	0.6%
28	Michigan	4	0.5%
28	New Hampshire	4	0.5%
28	Ohio	4	0.5%
31	Maryland	3	0.4%
31	New Jersey	3	0.4%
31	New York	3	0.4%
31	Oregon	3	0.4%
31	Wyoming	3	0.4%
36	Alaska	2	0.3%
36	Idaho	2	0.3%
36	Nebraska	2	0.3%
36	Wisconsin	2	0.3%
40	Connecticut	1	0.1%
40	Maine	1	0.1%
40	South Dakota	1	0.1%
43	Delaware	0	0.0%
43	Hawaii	0	0.0%
43	Iowa	0	0.0%
43	Minnesota	0	0.0%
43	Montana	0	0.0%
43	North Dakota	0	0.0%
43	Rhode Island	0	0.0%
43	Vermont	0	0.0%
	District of Columbia	3	0.4%

Source: American Hospital Association (Chicago, IL)
   "Hospital Statistics" (2005 edition)
Investor-owned (for-profit) hospitals are a subset of community hospitals.

State and Local Government-Owned Hospitals in 2003

National Total = 1,121 Hospitals*

RANK	STATE	HOSPITALS	% of USA
13	Alabama	37	3.3%
32	Alaska	7	0.6%
37	Arizona	5	0.4%
25	Arkansas	15	1.3%
2	California	71	6.3%
17	Colorado	27	2.4%
43	Connecticut	1	0.1%
46	Delaware	0	0.0%
22	Florida	20	1.8%
5	Georgia	54	4.8%
34	Hawaii	6	0.5%
20	Idaho	24	2.1%
16	Illinois	28	2.5%
12	Indiana	38	3.4%
4	Iowa	59	5.3%
3	Kansas	61	5.4%
27	Kentucky	13	1.2%
6	Louisiana	50	4.5%
40	Maine	2	0.2%
43	Maryland	1	0.1%
39	Massachusetts	3	0.3%
24	Michigan	18	1.6%
8	Minnesota	42	3.7%
8	Mississippi	42	3.7%
14	Missouri	36	3.2%
29	Montana	10	0.9%
10	Nebraska	39	3.5%
32	Nevada	7	0.6%
46	New Hampshire	0	0.0%
43	New Jersey	1	0.1%
31	New Mexico	9	0.8%
18	New York	26	2.3%
15	North Carolina	29	2.6%
46	North Dakota	0	0.0%
21	Ohio	23	2.1%
7	Oklahoma	47	4.2%
28	Oregon	12	1.1%
40	Pennsylvania	2	0.2%
46	Rhode Island	0	0.0%
22	South Carolina	20	1.8%
34	South Dakota	6	0.5%
19	Tennessee	25	2.2%
1	Texas	129	11.5%
34	Utah	6	0.5%
46	Vermont	0	0.0%
38	Virginia	4	0.4%
10	Washington	39	3.5%
29	West Virginia	10	0.9%
40	Wisconsin	2	0.2%
25	Wyoming	15	1.3%

RANK ORDER

RANK	STATE	HOSPITALS	% of USA
1	Texas	129	11.5%
2	California	71	6.3%
3	Kansas	61	5.4%
4	Iowa	59	5.3%
5	Georgia	54	4.8%
6	Louisiana	50	4.5%
7	Oklahoma	47	4.2%
8	Minnesota	42	3.7%
8	Mississippi	42	3.7%
10	Nebraska	39	3.5%
10	Washington	39	3.5%
12	Indiana	38	3.4%
13	Alabama	37	3.3%
14	Missouri	36	3.2%
15	North Carolina	29	2.6%
16	Illinois	28	2.5%
17	Colorado	27	2.4%
18	New York	26	2.3%
19	Tennessee	25	2.2%
20	Idaho	24	2.1%
21	Ohio	23	2.1%
22	Florida	20	1.8%
22	South Carolina	20	1.8%
24	Michigan	18	1.6%
25	Arkansas	15	1.3%
25	Wyoming	15	1.3%
27	Kentucky	13	1.2%
28	Oregon	12	1.1%
29	Montana	10	0.9%
29	West Virginia	10	0.9%
31	New Mexico	9	0.8%
32	Alaska	7	0.6%
32	Nevada	7	0.6%
34	Hawaii	6	0.5%
34	South Dakota	6	0.5%
34	Utah	6	0.5%
37	Arizona	5	0.4%
38	Virginia	4	0.4%
39	Massachusetts	3	0.3%
40	Maine	2	0.2%
40	Pennsylvania	2	0.2%
40	Wisconsin	2	0.2%
43	Connecticut	1	0.1%
43	Maryland	1	0.1%
43	New Jersey	1	0.1%
46	Delaware	0	0.0%
46	New Hampshire	0	0.0%
46	North Dakota	0	0.0%
46	Rhode Island	0	0.0%
46	Vermont	0	0.0%
	District of Columbia	0	0.0%

Source: American Hospital Association (Chicago, IL)
"Hospital Statistics" (2005 edition)
*State and local government-owned hospitals are a subset of community hospitals.

Beds in Community Hospitals in 2003

National Total = 813,307 Beds*

ALPHA ORDER

RANK	STATE	BEDS	% of USA
19	Alabama	15,666	1.9%
50	Alaska	1,456	0.2%
28	Arizona	10,801	1.3%
30	Arkansas	9,909	1.2%
1	California	74,330	9.1%
31	Colorado	9,479	1.2%
34	Connecticut	7,185	0.9%
47	Delaware	2,051	0.3%
4	Florida	50,687	6.2%
9	Georgia	24,624	3.0%
44	Hawaii	3,121	0.4%
43	Idaho	3,412	0.4%
6	Illinois	35,048	4.3%
14	Indiana	18,932	2.3%
27	Iowa	11,002	1.4%
29	Kansas	10,554	1.3%
20	Kentucky	14,940	1.8%
15	Louisiana	17,829	2.2%
40	Maine	3,702	0.5%
23	Maryland	11,613	1.4%
18	Massachusetts	16,001	2.0%
8	Michigan	25,820	3.2%
17	Minnesota	16,439	2.0%
22	Mississippi	13,040	1.6%
13	Missouri	19,346	2.4%
38	Montana	4,326	0.5%
33	Nebraska	7,467	0.9%
39	Nevada	4,282	0.5%
45	New Hampshire	2,796	0.3%
11	New Jersey	22,807	2.8%
41	New Mexico	3,680	0.5%
2	New York	64,705	8.0%
10	North Carolina	23,285	2.9%
42	North Dakota	3,595	0.4%
7	Ohio	32,981	4.1%
26	Oklahoma	11,018	1.4%
35	Oregon	6,757	0.8%
5	Pennsylvania	40,908	5.0%
46	Rhode Island	2,410	0.3%
25	South Carolina	11,115	1.4%
36	South Dakota	4,418	0.5%
12	Tennessee	20,313	2.5%
3	Texas	57,374	7.1%
37	Utah	4,406	0.5%
49	Vermont	1,506	0.2%
16	Virginia	17,225	2.1%
24	Washington	11,190	1.4%
32	West Virginia	7,779	1.0%
21	Wisconsin	14,829	1.8%
48	Wyoming	1,773	0.2%

RANK ORDER

RANK	STATE	BEDS	% of USA
1	California	74,330	9.1%
2	New York	64,705	8.0%
3	Texas	57,374	7.1%
4	Florida	50,687	6.2%
5	Pennsylvania	40,908	5.0%
6	Illinois	35,048	4.3%
7	Ohio	32,981	4.1%
8	Michigan	25,820	3.2%
9	Georgia	24,624	3.0%
10	North Carolina	23,285	2.9%
11	New Jersey	22,807	2.8%
12	Tennessee	20,313	2.5%
13	Missouri	19,346	2.4%
14	Indiana	18,932	2.3%
15	Louisiana	17,829	2.2%
16	Virginia	17,225	2.1%
17	Minnesota	16,439	2.0%
18	Massachusetts	16,001	2.0%
19	Alabama	15,666	1.9%
20	Kentucky	14,940	1.8%
21	Wisconsin	14,829	1.8%
22	Mississippi	13,040	1.6%
23	Maryland	11,613	1.4%
24	Washington	11,190	1.4%
25	South Carolina	11,115	1.4%
26	Oklahoma	11,018	1.4%
27	Iowa	11,002	1.4%
28	Arizona	10,801	1.3%
29	Kansas	10,554	1.3%
30	Arkansas	9,909	1.2%
31	Colorado	9,479	1.2%
32	West Virginia	7,779	1.0%
33	Nebraska	7,467	0.9%
34	Connecticut	7,185	0.9%
35	Oregon	6,757	0.8%
36	South Dakota	4,418	0.5%
37	Utah	4,406	0.5%
38	Montana	4,326	0.5%
39	Nevada	4,282	0.5%
40	Maine	3,702	0.5%
41	New Mexico	3,680	0.5%
42	North Dakota	3,595	0.4%
43	Idaho	3,412	0.4%
44	Hawaii	3,121	0.4%
45	New Hampshire	2,796	0.3%
46	Rhode Island	2,410	0.3%
47	Delaware	2,051	0.3%
48	Wyoming	1,773	0.2%
49	Vermont	1,506	0.2%
50	Alaska	1,456	0.2%
	District of Columbia	3,375	0.4%

Source: American Hospital Association (Chicago, IL)
    "Hospital Statistics" (2005 edition)
*All nonfederal short-term general and other special hospitals, whose facilities and services are available to the public. Includes beds in hospital and nursing home units.

Rate of Beds in Community Hospitals in 2003

National Rate = 280 Beds per 100,000 Population*

ALPHA ORDER

RANK	STATE	RATE
13	Alabama	348
38	Alaska	225
46	Arizona	194
10	Arkansas	363
42	California	210
43	Colorado	208
44	Connecticut	206
32	Delaware	251
21	Florida	298
23	Georgia	284
33	Hawaii	250
33	Idaho	250
25	Illinois	277
20	Indiana	305
9	Iowa	374
8	Kansas	387
10	Kentucky	363
7	Louisiana	397
24	Maine	283
41	Maryland	211
35	Massachusetts	249
31	Michigan	256
18	Minnesota	325
4	Mississippi	452
15	Missouri	338
3	Montana	471
5	Nebraska	430
47	Nevada	191
40	New Hampshire	217
29	New Jersey	264
45	New Mexico	196
16	New York	337
25	North Carolina	277
2	North Dakota	568
22	Ohio	288
19	Oklahoma	314
48	Oregon	190
17	Pennsylvania	331
39	Rhode Island	224
28	South Carolina	268
1	South Dakota	578
13	Tennessee	348
30	Texas	260
49	Utah	187
36	Vermont	243
37	Virginia	234
50	Washington	183
6	West Virginia	429
27	Wisconsin	271
12	Wyoming	353

RANK ORDER

RANK	STATE	RATE
1	South Dakota	578
2	North Dakota	568
3	Montana	471
4	Mississippi	452
5	Nebraska	430
6	West Virginia	429
7	Louisiana	397
8	Kansas	387
9	Iowa	374
10	Arkansas	363
10	Kentucky	363
12	Wyoming	353
13	Alabama	348
13	Tennessee	348
15	Missouri	338
16	New York	337
17	Pennsylvania	331
18	Minnesota	325
19	Oklahoma	314
20	Indiana	305
21	Florida	298
22	Ohio	288
23	Georgia	284
24	Maine	283
25	Illinois	277
25	North Carolina	277
27	Wisconsin	271
28	South Carolina	268
29	New Jersey	264
30	Texas	260
31	Michigan	256
32	Delaware	251
33	Hawaii	250
33	Idaho	250
35	Massachusetts	249
36	Vermont	243
37	Virginia	234
38	Alaska	225
39	Rhode Island	224
40	New Hampshire	217
41	Maryland	211
42	California	210
43	Colorado	208
44	Connecticut	206
45	New Mexico	196
46	Arizona	194
47	Nevada	191
48	Oregon	190
49	Utah	187
50	Washington	183

District of Columbia   605

Source: Morgan Quitno Press using data from American Hospital Association (Chicago, IL)
    "Hospital Statistics" (2005 edition)

*All nonfederal short-term general and other special hospitals, whose facilities and services are available to the public. Includes beds in hospital and nursing home units.

Average Number of Beds per Community Hospital in 2003

National Average = 166 Beds per Community Hospital*

ALPHA ORDER

RANK	STATE	BEDS
23	Alabama	146
49	Alaska	77
17	Arizona	177
35	Arkansas	113
13	California	201
27	Colorado	139
7	Connecticut	211
1	Delaware	342
4	Florida	250
19	Georgia	169
31	Hawaii	130
46	Idaho	87
14	Illinois	183
19	Indiana	169
42	Iowa	95
48	Kansas	79
24	Kentucky	145
26	Louisiana	140
39	Maine	100
5	Maryland	228
11	Massachusetts	203
16	Michigan	179
32	Minnesota	125
25	Mississippi	142
21	Missouri	163
47	Montana	82
44	Nebraska	88
18	Nevada	171
39	New Hampshire	100
3	New Jersey	292
41	New Mexico	99
2	New York	313
8	North Carolina	206
43	North Dakota	90
12	Ohio	202
38	Oklahoma	102
34	Oregon	117
10	Pennsylvania	204
6	Rhode Island	219
15	South Carolina	182
44	South Dakota	88
21	Tennessee	163
27	Texas	139
37	Utah	105
36	Vermont	108
9	Virginia	205
30	Washington	132
29	West Virginia	136
33	Wisconsin	123
49	Wyoming	77

RANK ORDER

RANK	STATE	BEDS
1	Delaware	342
2	New York	313
3	New Jersey	292
4	Florida	250
5	Maryland	228
6	Rhode Island	219
7	Connecticut	211
8	North Carolina	206
9	Virginia	205
10	Pennsylvania	204
11	Massachusetts	203
12	Ohio	202
13	California	201
14	Illinois	183
15	South Carolina	182
16	Michigan	179
17	Arizona	177
18	Nevada	171
19	Georgia	169
19	Indiana	169
21	Missouri	163
21	Tennessee	163
23	Alabama	146
24	Kentucky	145
25	Mississippi	142
26	Louisiana	140
27	Colorado	139
27	Texas	139
29	West Virginia	136
30	Washington	132
31	Hawaii	130
32	Minnesota	125
33	Wisconsin	123
34	Oregon	117
35	Arkansas	113
36	Vermont	108
37	Utah	105
38	Oklahoma	102
39	Maine	100
39	New Hampshire	100
41	New Mexico	99
42	Iowa	95
43	North Dakota	90
44	Nebraska	88
44	South Dakota	88
46	Idaho	87
47	Montana	82
48	Kansas	79
49	Alaska	77
49	Wyoming	77

| | District of Columbia | 338 |

Source: Morgan Quitno Press using data from American Hospital Association (Chicago, IL) "Hospital Statistics" (2005 edition)

All nonfederal short-term general and other special hospitals, whose facilities and services are available to the public. Includes beds in hospital and nursing home units.

Admissions to Community Hospitals in 2003

National Total = 34,782,742 Admissions*

ALPHA ORDER

RANK	STATE	ADMISSIONS	% of USA
17	Alabama	708,995	2.0%
50	Alaska	45,982	0.1%
21	Arizona	603,310	1.7%
29	Arkansas	388,046	1.1%
1	California	3,473,879	10.0%
27	Colorado	443,773	1.3%
30	Connecticut	372,630	1.1%
46	Delaware	97,074	0.3%
4	Florida	2,296,184	6.6%
11	Georgia	925,681	2.7%
43	Hawaii	111,713	0.3%
40	Idaho	135,920	0.4%
6	Illinois	1,594,007	4.6%
16	Indiana	712,151	2.0%
31	Iowa	363,008	1.0%
33	Kansas	331,244	1.0%
22	Kentucky	600,454	1.7%
18	Louisiana	690,246	2.0%
39	Maine	148,517	0.4%
19	Maryland	645,158	1.9%
14	Massachusetts	784,618	2.3%
8	Michigan	1,168,359	3.4%
20	Minnesota	614,867	1.8%
28	Mississippi	415,909	1.2%
12	Missouri	831,210	2.4%
44	Montana	107,024	0.3%
37	Nebraska	211,567	0.6%
36	Nevada	212,821	0.6%
42	New Hampshire	117,814	0.3%
9	New Jersey	1,107,659	3.2%
38	New Mexico	165,709	0.5%
3	New York	2,499,137	7.2%
10	North Carolina	987,209	2.8%
47	North Dakota	88,132	0.3%
7	Ohio	1,457,933	4.2%
26	Oklahoma	449,936	1.3%
32	Oregon	342,282	1.0%
5	Pennsylvania	1,824,132	5.2%
41	Rhode Island	122,692	0.4%
25	South Carolina	506,488	1.5%
45	South Dakota	102,984	0.3%
13	Tennessee	812,915	2.3%
2	Texas	2,550,314	7.3%
35	Utah	215,158	0.6%
49	Vermont	51,852	0.1%
15	Virginia	758,258	2.2%
24	Washington	515,939	1.5%
34	West Virginia	296,089	0.9%
23	Wisconsin	588,466	1.7%
48	Wyoming	52,612	0.2%

RANK ORDER

RANK	STATE	ADMISSIONS	% of USA
1	California	3,473,879	10.0%
2	Texas	2,550,314	7.3%
3	New York	2,499,137	7.2%
4	Florida	2,296,184	6.6%
5	Pennsylvania	1,824,132	5.2%
6	Illinois	1,594,007	4.6%
7	Ohio	1,457,933	4.2%
8	Michigan	1,168,359	3.4%
9	New Jersey	1,107,659	3.2%
10	North Carolina	987,209	2.8%
11	Georgia	925,681	2.7%
12	Missouri	831,210	2.4%
13	Tennessee	812,915	2.3%
14	Massachusetts	784,618	2.3%
15	Virginia	758,258	2.2%
16	Indiana	712,151	2.0%
17	Alabama	708,995	2.0%
18	Louisiana	690,246	2.0%
19	Maryland	645,158	1.9%
20	Minnesota	614,867	1.8%
21	Arizona	603,310	1.7%
22	Kentucky	600,454	1.7%
23	Wisconsin	588,466	1.7%
24	Washington	515,939	1.5%
25	South Carolina	506,488	1.5%
26	Oklahoma	449,936	1.3%
27	Colorado	443,773	1.3%
28	Mississippi	415,909	1.2%
29	Arkansas	388,046	1.1%
30	Connecticut	372,630	1.1%
31	Iowa	363,008	1.0%
32	Oregon	342,282	1.0%
33	Kansas	331,244	1.0%
34	West Virginia	296,089	0.9%
35	Utah	215,158	0.6%
36	Nevada	212,821	0.6%
37	Nebraska	211,567	0.6%
38	New Mexico	165,709	0.5%
39	Maine	148,517	0.4%
40	Idaho	135,920	0.4%
41	Rhode Island	122,692	0.4%
42	New Hampshire	117,814	0.3%
43	Hawaii	111,713	0.3%
44	Montana	107,024	0.3%
45	South Dakota	102,984	0.3%
46	Delaware	97,074	0.3%
47	North Dakota	88,132	0.3%
48	Wyoming	52,612	0.2%
49	Vermont	51,852	0.1%
50	Alaska	45,982	0.1%
	District of Columbia	134,685	0.4%

Source: American Hospital Association (Chicago, IL)
"Hospital Statistics" (2005 edition)

*Admissions to all nonfederal short-term general and other special hospitals, whose facilities and services are available to the public. Includes admissions to hospital and nursing home units.

Inpatient Days in Community Hospitals in 2003

National Total = 196,649,769 Inpatient Days*

ALPHA ORDER

RANK	STATE	DAYS	% of USA
19	Alabama	3,547,203	1.8%
50	Alaska	287,351	0.1%
25	Arizona	2,669,152	1.4%
31	Arkansas	2,088,391	1.1%
1	California	18,814,783	9.6%
29	Colorado	2,252,174	1.1%
32	Connecticut	2,029,059	1.0%
47	Delaware	606,183	0.3%
4	Florida	11,966,726	6.1%
11	Georgia	6,024,083	3.1%
41	Hawaii	815,796	0.4%
44	Idaho	698,748	0.4%
6	Illinois	8,174,779	4.2%
17	Indiana	3,997,353	2.0%
28	Iowa	2,369,769	1.2%
30	Kansas	2,148,111	1.1%
20	Kentucky	3,394,239	1.7%
18	Louisiana	3,872,912	2.0%
40	Maine	816,332	0.4%
22	Maryland	3,167,111	1.6%
13	Massachusetts	4,372,515	2.2%
8	Michigan	6,223,908	3.2%
16	Minnesota	4,113,264	2.1%
24	Mississippi	2,696,522	1.4%
15	Missouri	4,342,987	2.2%
37	Montana	1,049,607	0.5%
34	Nebraska	1,593,254	0.8%
36	Nevada	1,111,624	0.6%
46	New Hampshire	637,803	0.3%
9	New Jersey	6,154,335	3.1%
42	New Mexico	780,895	0.4%
2	New York	18,455,619	9.4%
10	North Carolina	6,053,100	3.1%
43	North Dakota	774,175	0.4%
7	Ohio	7,501,323	3.8%
27	Oklahoma	2,380,232	1.2%
35	Oregon	1,455,069	0.7%
5	Pennsylvania	10,300,758	5.2%
45	Rhode Island	657,057	0.3%
23	South Carolina	2,949,736	1.5%
38	South Dakota	994,529	0.5%
12	Tennessee	4,533,373	2.3%
3	Texas	13,296,596	6.8%
39	Utah	921,001	0.5%
49	Vermont	341,581	0.2%
14	Virginia	4,367,997	2.2%
26	Washington	2,477,079	1.3%
33	West Virginia	1,770,290	0.9%
21	Wisconsin	3,355,918	1.7%
48	Wyoming	342,260	0.2%

RANK ORDER

RANK	STATE	DAYS	% of USA
1	California	18,814,783	9.6%
2	New York	18,455,619	9.4%
3	Texas	13,296,596	6.8%
4	Florida	11,966,726	6.1%
5	Pennsylvania	10,300,758	5.2%
6	Illinois	8,174,779	4.2%
7	Ohio	7,501,323	3.8%
8	Michigan	6,223,908	3.2%
9	New Jersey	6,154,335	3.1%
10	North Carolina	6,053,100	3.1%
11	Georgia	6,024,083	3.1%
12	Tennessee	4,533,373	2.3%
13	Massachusetts	4,372,515	2.2%
14	Virginia	4,367,997	2.2%
15	Missouri	4,342,987	2.2%
16	Minnesota	4,113,264	2.1%
17	Indiana	3,997,353	2.0%
18	Louisiana	3,872,912	2.0%
19	Alabama	3,547,203	1.8%
20	Kentucky	3,394,239	1.7%
21	Wisconsin	3,355,918	1.7%
22	Maryland	3,167,111	1.6%
23	South Carolina	2,949,736	1.5%
24	Mississippi	2,696,522	1.4%
25	Arizona	2,669,152	1.4%
26	Washington	2,477,079	1.3%
27	Oklahoma	2,380,232	1.2%
28	Iowa	2,369,769	1.2%
29	Colorado	2,252,174	1.1%
30	Kansas	2,148,111	1.1%
31	Arkansas	2,088,391	1.1%
32	Connecticut	2,029,059	1.0%
33	West Virginia	1,770,290	0.9%
34	Nebraska	1,593,254	0.8%
35	Oregon	1,455,069	0.7%
36	Nevada	1,111,624	0.6%
37	Montana	1,049,607	0.5%
38	South Dakota	994,529	0.5%
39	Utah	921,001	0.5%
40	Maine	816,332	0.4%
41	Hawaii	815,796	0.4%
42	New Mexico	780,895	0.4%
43	North Dakota	774,175	0.4%
44	Idaho	698,748	0.4%
45	Rhode Island	657,057	0.3%
46	New Hampshire	637,803	0.3%
47	Delaware	606,183	0.3%
48	Wyoming	342,260	0.2%
49	Vermont	341,581	0.2%
50	Alaska	287,351	0.1%
	District of Columbia	905,107	0.5%

Source: American Hospital Association (Chicago, IL)
"Hospital Statistics" (2005 edition)

*Inpatient days in all nonfederal short-term general and other special hospitals, whose facilities and services are available to the public. Includes days in hospital and nursing home units.

Average Daily Census in Community Hospitals in 2003

National Average = 538,766 Inpatients*

ALPHA ORDER

RANK ORDER

RANK	STATE	INPATIENTS	RANK	STATE	INPATIENTS
19	Alabama	9,718	1	California	51,547
50	Alaska	787	2	New York	50,563
25	Arizona	7,313	3	Texas	36,429
31	Arkansas	5,722	4	Florida	32,786
1	California	51,547	5	Pennsylvania	28,221
29	Colorado	6,170	6	Illinois	22,397
32	Connecticut	5,559	7	Ohio	20,552
47	Delaware	1,661	8	Michigan	17,052
4	Florida	32,786	9	New Jersey	16,861
11	Georgia	16,504	10	North Carolina	16,584
41	Hawaii	2,235	11	Georgia	16,504
44	Idaho	1,914	12	Tennessee	12,420
6	Illinois	22,397	13	Massachusetts	11,979
17	Indiana	10,952	14	Virginia	11,967
28	Iowa	6,493	15	Missouri	11,899
30	Kansas	5,885	16	Minnesota	11,269
20	Kentucky	9,299	17	Indiana	10,952
18	Louisiana	10,611	18	Louisiana	10,611
40	Maine	2,237	19	Alabama	9,718
22	Maryland	8,677	20	Kentucky	9,299
13	Massachusetts	11,979	21	Wisconsin	9,194
8	Michigan	17,052	22	Maryland	8,677
16	Minnesota	11,269	23	South Carolina	8,081
24	Mississippi	7,388	24	Mississippi	7,388
15	Missouri	11,899	25	Arizona	7,313
37	Montana	2,876	26	Washington	6,787
34	Nebraska	4,365	27	Oklahoma	6,521
36	Nevada	3,046	28	Iowa	6,493
46	New Hampshire	1,747	29	Colorado	6,170
9	New Jersey	16,861	30	Kansas	5,885
42	New Mexico	2,139	31	Arkansas	5,722
2	New York	50,563	32	Connecticut	5,559
10	North Carolina	16,584	33	West Virginia	4,850
43	North Dakota	2,121	34	Nebraska	4,365
7	Ohio	20,552	35	Oregon	3,986
27	Oklahoma	6,521	36	Nevada	3,046
35	Oregon	3,986	37	Montana	2,876
5	Pennsylvania	28,221	38	South Dakota	2,725
45	Rhode Island	1,800	39	Utah	2,523
23	South Carolina	8,081	40	Maine	2,237
38	South Dakota	2,725	41	Hawaii	2,235
12	Tennessee	12,420	42	New Mexico	2,139
3	Texas	36,429	43	North Dakota	2,121
39	Utah	2,523	44	Idaho	1,914
49	Vermont	936	45	Rhode Island	1,800
14	Virginia	11,967	46	New Hampshire	1,747
26	Washington	6,787	47	Delaware	1,661
33	West Virginia	4,850	48	Wyoming	938
21	Wisconsin	9,194	49	Vermont	936
48	Wyoming	938	50	Alaska	787
				District of Columbia	2,480

Source: Morgan Quitno Press using data from American Hospital Association (Chicago, IL)
    "Hospital Statistics" (2005 edition)
*Average total of inpatients receiving care in all nonfederal short-term general and other special hospitals, whose facilities and services are available to the public. Excludes newborns.

Average Stay in Community Hospitals in 2003

National Average = 5.7 Days*

RANK	STATE	DAYS
44	Alabama	5.0
14	Alaska	6.2
48	Arizona	4.4
29	Arkansas	5.4
29	California	5.4
40	Colorado	5.1
29	Connecticut	5.4
14	Delaware	6.2
36	Florida	5.2
9	Georgia	6.5
6	Hawaii	7.3
40	Idaho	5.1
40	Illinois	5.1
22	Indiana	5.6
9	Iowa	6.5
9	Kansas	6.5
20	Kentucky	5.7
22	Louisiana	5.6
28	Maine	5.5
45	Maryland	4.9
22	Massachusetts	5.6
34	Michigan	5.3
7	Minnesota	6.7
9	Mississippi	6.5
36	Missouri	5.2
1	Montana	9.8
4	Nebraska	7.5
36	Nevada	5.2
29	New Hampshire	5.4
22	New Jersey	5.6
47	New Mexico	4.7
5	New York	7.4
16	North Carolina	6.1
3	North Dakota	8.8
40	Ohio	5.1
34	Oklahoma	5.3
49	Oregon	4.3
22	Pennsylvania	5.6
29	Rhode Island	5.4
18	South Carolina	5.8
2	South Dakota	9.7
22	Tennessee	5.6
36	Texas	5.2
49	Utah	4.3
8	Vermont	6.6
18	Virginia	5.8
46	Washington	4.8
17	West Virginia	6.0
20	Wisconsin	5.7
9	Wyoming	6.5

RANK	STATE	DAYS
1	Montana	9.8
2	South Dakota	9.7
3	North Dakota	8.8
4	Nebraska	7.5
5	New York	7.4
6	Hawaii	7.3
7	Minnesota	6.7
8	Vermont	6.6
9	Georgia	6.5
9	Iowa	6.5
9	Kansas	6.5
9	Mississippi	6.5
9	Wyoming	6.5
14	Alaska	6.2
14	Delaware	6.2
16	North Carolina	6.1
17	West Virginia	6.0
18	South Carolina	5.8
18	Virginia	5.8
20	Kentucky	5.7
20	Wisconsin	5.7
22	Indiana	5.6
22	Louisiana	5.6
22	Massachusetts	5.6
22	New Jersey	5.6
22	Pennsylvania	5.6
22	Tennessee	5.6
28	Maine	5.5
29	Arkansas	5.4
29	California	5.4
29	Connecticut	5.4
29	New Hampshire	5.4
29	Rhode Island	5.4
34	Michigan	5.3
34	Oklahoma	5.3
36	Florida	5.2
36	Missouri	5.2
36	Nevada	5.2
36	Texas	5.2
40	Colorado	5.1
40	Idaho	5.1
40	Illinois	5.1
40	Ohio	5.1
44	Alabama	5.0
45	Maryland	4.9
46	Washington	4.8
47	New Mexico	4.7
48	Arizona	4.4
49	Oregon	4.3
49	Utah	4.3
	District of Columbia	6.7

Source: American Hospital Association (Chicago, IL)
   "Hospital Statistics" (2005 edition)
*All nonfederal short-term general and other special hospitals, whose facilities and services are available to the public.

Occupancy Rate in Community Hospitals in 2003

National Rate = 66.2% of Community Hospital Beds Occupied*

ALPHA ORDER

RANK	STATE	PERCENT
29	Alabama	62.0
49	Alaska	54.1
16	Arizona	67.7
44	Arkansas	57.7
13	California	69.3
20	Colorado	65.1
3	Connecticut	77.4
1	Delaware	81.0
21	Florida	64.7
17	Georgia	67.0
9	Hawaii	71.6
47	Idaho	56.1
22	Illinois	63.9
43	Indiana	57.8
38	Iowa	59.0
48	Kansas	55.8
27	Kentucky	62.2
36	Louisiana	59.5
35	Maine	60.4
5	Maryland	74.7
4	Massachusetts	74.9
19	Michigan	66.0
15	Minnesota	68.6
46	Mississippi	56.7
32	Missouri	61.5
18	Montana	66.5
41	Nebraska	58.5
11	Nevada	71.1
24	New Hampshire	62.5
7	New Jersey	73.9
42	New Mexico	58.1
2	New York	78.1
10	North Carolina	71.2
38	North Dakota	59.0
25	Ohio	62.3
37	Oklahoma	59.2
38	Oregon	59.0
14	Pennsylvania	69.0
5	Rhode Island	74.7
8	South Carolina	72.7
31	South Dakota	61.7
33	Tennessee	61.1
23	Texas	63.5
45	Utah	57.3
27	Vermont	62.2
12	Virginia	69.5
34	Washington	60.7
25	West Virginia	62.3
29	Wisconsin	62.0
50	Wyoming	52.9

RANK ORDER

RANK	STATE	PERCENT
1	Delaware	81.0
2	New York	78.1
3	Connecticut	77.4
4	Massachusetts	74.9
5	Maryland	74.7
5	Rhode Island	74.7
7	New Jersey	73.9
8	South Carolina	72.7
9	Hawaii	71.6
10	North Carolina	71.2
11	Nevada	71.1
12	Virginia	69.5
13	California	69.3
14	Pennsylvania	69.0
15	Minnesota	68.6
16	Arizona	67.7
17	Georgia	67.0
18	Montana	66.5
19	Michigan	66.0
20	Colorado	65.1
21	Florida	64.7
22	Illinois	63.9
23	Texas	63.5
24	New Hampshire	62.5
25	Ohio	62.3
25	West Virginia	62.3
27	Kentucky	62.2
27	Vermont	62.2
29	Alabama	62.0
29	Wisconsin	62.0
31	South Dakota	61.7
32	Missouri	61.5
33	Tennessee	61.1
34	Washington	60.7
35	Maine	60.4
36	Louisiana	59.5
37	Oklahoma	59.2
38	Iowa	59.0
38	North Dakota	59.0
38	Oregon	59.0
41	Nebraska	58.5
42	New Mexico	58.1
43	Indiana	57.8
44	Arkansas	57.7
45	Utah	57.3
46	Mississippi	56.7
47	Idaho	56.1
48	Kansas	55.8
49	Alaska	54.1
50	Wyoming	52.9

| | District of Columbia | 73.5 |

Source: Morgan Quitno Press using data from American Hospital Association (Chicago, IL)
    "Hospital Statistics" (2005 edition)
*Average daily census compared to number of community hospital beds.

Outpatient Visits to Community Hospitals in 2003

National Total = 563,186,046 Visits*

ALPHA ORDER

RANK	STATE	VISITS	% of USA
22	Alabama	8,899,175	1.6%
49	Alaska	1,443,409	0.3%
28	Arizona	6,706,717	1.2%
33	Arkansas	4,582,352	0.8%
2	California	48,036,139	8.5%
26	Colorado	6,987,293	1.2%
27	Connecticut	6,862,798	1.2%
45	Delaware	2,021,860	0.4%
8	Florida	22,023,554	3.9%
14	Georgia	12,849,345	2.3%
46	Hawaii	1,917,741	0.3%
40	Idaho	2,769,604	0.5%
6	Illinois	27,225,201	4.8%
11	Indiana	14,997,896	2.7%
20	Iowa	9,735,379	1.7%
30	Kansas	5,950,038	1.1%
23	Kentucky	8,543,109	1.5%
17	Louisiana	10,824,010	1.9%
37	Maine	3,925,464	0.7%
29	Maryland	6,522,366	1.2%
9	Massachusetts	19,633,146	3.5%
7	Michigan	27,175,040	4.8%
21	Minnesota	9,184,368	1.6%
36	Mississippi	3,998,966	0.7%
10	Missouri	15,668,704	2.8%
41	Montana	2,737,734	0.5%
38	Nebraska	3,676,098	0.7%
42	Nevada	2,283,973	0.4%
39	New Hampshire	3,071,130	0.5%
12	New Jersey	14,686,429	2.6%
35	New Mexico	4,502,569	0.8%
1	New York	48,235,916	8.6%
13	North Carolina	14,540,747	2.6%
47	North Dakota	1,812,996	0.3%
5	Ohio	30,022,353	5.3%
32	Oklahoma	5,489,728	1.0%
24	Oregon	8,187,084	1.5%
3	Pennsylvania	33,285,280	5.9%
44	Rhode Island	2,111,605	0.4%
25	South Carolina	7,401,406	1.3%
48	South Dakota	1,536,724	0.3%
19	Tennessee	10,156,452	1.8%
4	Texas	32,695,035	5.8%
34	Utah	4,545,669	0.8%
43	Vermont	2,211,564	0.4%
16	Virginia	11,191,378	2.0%
18	Washington	10,291,753	1.8%
31	West Virginia	5,757,228	1.0%
15	Wisconsin	11,815,201	2.1%
50	Wyoming	868,044	0.2%

RANK ORDER

RANK	STATE	VISITS	% of USA
1	New York	48,235,916	8.6%
2	California	48,036,139	8.5%
3	Pennsylvania	33,285,280	5.9%
4	Texas	32,695,035	5.8%
5	Ohio	30,022,353	5.3%
6	Illinois	27,225,201	4.8%
7	Michigan	27,175,040	4.8%
8	Florida	22,023,554	3.9%
9	Massachusetts	19,633,146	3.5%
10	Missouri	15,668,704	2.8%
11	Indiana	14,997,896	2.7%
12	New Jersey	14,686,429	2.6%
13	North Carolina	14,540,747	2.6%
14	Georgia	12,849,345	2.3%
15	Wisconsin	11,815,201	2.1%
16	Virginia	11,191,378	2.0%
17	Louisiana	10,824,010	1.9%
18	Washington	10,291,753	1.8%
19	Tennessee	10,156,452	1.8%
20	Iowa	9,735,379	1.7%
21	Minnesota	9,184,368	1.6%
22	Alabama	8,899,175	1.6%
23	Kentucky	8,543,109	1.5%
24	Oregon	8,187,084	1.5%
25	South Carolina	7,401,406	1.3%
26	Colorado	6,987,293	1.2%
27	Connecticut	6,862,798	1.2%
28	Arizona	6,706,717	1.2%
29	Maryland	6,522,366	1.2%
30	Kansas	5,950,038	1.1%
31	West Virginia	5,757,228	1.0%
32	Oklahoma	5,489,728	1.0%
33	Arkansas	4,582,352	0.8%
34	Utah	4,545,669	0.8%
35	New Mexico	4,502,569	0.8%
36	Mississippi	3,998,966	0.7%
37	Maine	3,925,464	0.7%
38	Nebraska	3,676,098	0.7%
39	New Hampshire	3,071,130	0.5%
40	Idaho	2,769,604	0.5%
41	Montana	2,737,734	0.5%
42	Nevada	2,283,973	0.4%
43	Vermont	2,211,564	0.4%
44	Rhode Island	2,111,605	0.4%
45	Delaware	2,021,860	0.4%
46	Hawaii	1,917,741	0.3%
47	North Dakota	1,812,996	0.3%
48	South Dakota	1,536,724	0.3%
49	Alaska	1,443,409	0.3%
50	Wyoming	868,044	0.2%
	District of Columbia	1,588,276	0.3%

Source: American Hospital Association (Chicago, IL)
   "Hospital Statistics" (2005 edition)
*All nonfederal short-term general and other special hospitals, whose facilities and services are available to the public. Includes emergency and other visits.

Emergency Outpatient Visits to Community Hospitals in 2003

National Total = 111,069,871 Visits*

ALPHA ORDER

RANK	STATE	VISITS	% of USA
18	Alabama	2,145,885	1.9%
49	Alaska	213,380	0.2%
24	Arizona	1,781,590	1.6%
30	Arkansas	1,251,391	1.1%
1	California	9,260,312	8.3%
28	Colorado	1,384,544	1.2%
29	Connecticut	1,372,015	1.2%
45	Delaware	300,450	0.3%
4	Florida	6,668,184	6.0%
9	Georgia	3,542,261	3.2%
43	Hawaii	330,034	0.3%
41	Idaho	468,818	0.4%
7	Illinois	4,867,066	4.4%
17	Indiana	2,492,597	2.2%
33	Iowa	1,066,268	1.0%
34	Kansas	945,208	0.9%
19	Kentucky	2,137,500	1.9%
16	Louisiana	2,498,935	2.2%
36	Maine	710,201	0.6%
20	Maryland	2,079,674	1.9%
12	Massachusetts	2,929,681	2.6%
8	Michigan	3,990,117	3.6%
26	Minnesota	1,581,734	1.4%
25	Mississippi	1,597,509	1.4%
15	Missouri	2,624,926	2.4%
44	Montana	301,772	0.3%
40	Nebraska	532,934	0.5%
38	Nevada	626,686	0.6%
39	New Hampshire	547,870	0.5%
13	New Jersey	2,922,644	2.6%
37	New Mexico	675,058	0.6%
3	New York	7,483,787	6.7%
10	North Carolina	3,433,432	3.1%
46	North Dakota	261,714	0.2%
5	Ohio	5,354,136	4.8%
27	Oklahoma	1,386,848	1.2%
31	Oregon	1,113,166	1.0%
6	Pennsylvania	5,160,713	4.6%
42	Rhode Island	463,961	0.4%
23	South Carolina	1,807,580	1.6%
48	South Dakota	214,831	0.2%
11	Tennessee	2,947,003	2.7%
2	Texas	8,315,483	7.5%
35	Utah	740,160	0.7%
47	Vermont	251,346	0.2%
14	Virginia	2,759,886	2.5%
21	Washington	2,030,209	1.8%
32	West Virginia	1,112,496	1.0%
22	Wisconsin	1,813,690	1.6%
50	Wyoming	212,562	0.2%

RANK ORDER

RANK	STATE	VISITS	% of USA
1	California	9,260,312	8.3%
2	Texas	8,315,483	7.5%
3	New York	7,483,787	6.7%
4	Florida	6,668,184	6.0%
5	Ohio	5,354,136	4.8%
6	Pennsylvania	5,160,713	4.6%
7	Illinois	4,867,066	4.4%
8	Michigan	3,990,117	3.6%
9	Georgia	3,542,261	3.2%
10	North Carolina	3,433,432	3.1%
11	Tennessee	2,947,003	2.7%
12	Massachusetts	2,929,681	2.6%
13	New Jersey	2,922,644	2.6%
14	Virginia	2,759,886	2.5%
15	Missouri	2,624,926	2.4%
16	Louisiana	2,498,935	2.2%
17	Indiana	2,492,597	2.2%
18	Alabama	2,145,885	1.9%
19	Kentucky	2,137,500	1.9%
20	Maryland	2,079,674	1.9%
21	Washington	2,030,209	1.8%
22	Wisconsin	1,813,690	1.6%
23	South Carolina	1,807,580	1.6%
24	Arizona	1,781,590	1.6%
25	Mississippi	1,597,509	1.4%
26	Minnesota	1,581,734	1.4%
27	Oklahoma	1,386,848	1.2%
28	Colorado	1,384,544	1.2%
29	Connecticut	1,372,015	1.2%
30	Arkansas	1,251,391	1.1%
31	Oregon	1,113,166	1.0%
32	West Virginia	1,112,496	1.0%
33	Iowa	1,066,268	1.0%
34	Kansas	945,208	0.9%
35	Utah	740,160	0.7%
36	Maine	710,201	0.6%
37	New Mexico	675,058	0.6%
38	Nevada	626,686	0.6%
39	New Hampshire	547,870	0.5%
40	Nebraska	532,934	0.5%
41	Idaho	468,818	0.4%
42	Rhode Island	463,961	0.4%
43	Hawaii	330,034	0.3%
44	Montana	301,772	0.3%
45	Delaware	300,450	0.3%
46	North Dakota	261,714	0.2%
47	Vermont	251,346	0.2%
48	South Dakota	214,831	0.2%
49	Alaska	213,380	0.2%
50	Wyoming	212,562	0.2%
	District of Columbia	359,624	0.3%

Source: American Hospital Association (Chicago, IL)
     "Hospital Statistics" (2005 edition)

*All nonfederal short-term general and other special hospitals, whose facilities and services are available to the public.

Surgical Operations in Community Hospitals in 2003

National Total = 27,106,538 Surgical Operations*

ALPHA ORDER

RANK	STATE	OPERATIONS	% of USA
19	Alabama	533,892	2.0%
49	Alaska	51,561	0.2%
25	Arizona	382,257	1.4%
32	Arkansas	268,834	1.0%
1	California	2,172,734	8.0%
28	Colorado	306,193	1.1%
29	Connecticut	305,871	1.1%
43	Delaware	94,600	0.3%
5	Florida	1,475,371	5.4%
10	Georgia	784,509	2.9%
44	Hawaii	86,735	0.3%
42	Idaho	103,656	0.4%
8	Illinois	1,130,538	4.2%
14	Indiana	653,550	2.4%
26	Iowa	373,046	1.4%
34	Kansas	252,472	0.9%
18	Kentucky	540,303	2.0%
24	Louisiana	425,841	1.6%
37	Maine	160,726	0.6%
20	Maryland	533,408	2.0%
13	Massachusetts	696,404	2.6%
7	Michigan	1,148,122	4.2%
22	Minnesota	463,903	1.7%
33	Mississippi	265,824	1.0%
17	Missouri	598,437	2.2%
47	Montana	73,990	0.3%
36	Nebraska	205,294	0.8%
38	Nevada	138,400	0.5%
41	New Hampshire	121,330	0.4%
12	New Jersey	716,802	2.6%
40	New Mexico	132,597	0.5%
2	New York	1,994,417	7.4%
9	North Carolina	852,249	3.1%
46	North Dakota	76,294	0.3%
6	Ohio	1,215,557	4.5%
30	Oklahoma	297,393	1.1%
27	Oregon	310,475	1.1%
4	Pennsylvania	1,497,939	5.5%
39	Rhode Island	137,271	0.5%
21	South Carolina	468,877	1.7%
45	South Dakota	84,748	0.3%
15	Tennessee	627,935	2.3%
3	Texas	1,865,016	6.9%
35	Utah	215,667	0.8%
48	Vermont	69,356	0.3%
11	Virginia	722,658	2.7%
23	Washington	441,054	1.6%
31	West Virginia	278,535	1.0%
16	Wisconsin	606,257	2.2%
50	Wyoming	42,090	0.2%

RANK ORDER

RANK	STATE	OPERATIONS	% of USA
1	California	2,172,734	8.0%
2	New York	1,994,417	7.4%
3	Texas	1,865,016	6.9%
4	Pennsylvania	1,497,939	5.5%
5	Florida	1,475,371	5.4%
6	Ohio	1,215,557	4.5%
7	Michigan	1,148,122	4.2%
8	Illinois	1,130,538	4.2%
9	North Carolina	852,249	3.1%
10	Georgia	784,509	2.9%
11	Virginia	722,658	2.7%
12	New Jersey	716,802	2.6%
13	Massachusetts	696,404	2.6%
14	Indiana	653,550	2.4%
15	Tennessee	627,935	2.3%
16	Wisconsin	606,257	2.2%
17	Missouri	598,437	2.2%
18	Kentucky	540,303	2.0%
19	Alabama	533,892	2.0%
20	Maryland	533,408	2.0%
21	South Carolina	468,877	1.7%
22	Minnesota	463,903	1.7%
23	Washington	441,054	1.6%
24	Louisiana	425,841	1.6%
25	Arizona	382,257	1.4%
26	Iowa	373,046	1.4%
27	Oregon	310,475	1.1%
28	Colorado	306,193	1.1%
29	Connecticut	305,871	1.1%
30	Oklahoma	297,393	1.1%
31	West Virginia	278,535	1.0%
32	Arkansas	268,834	1.0%
33	Mississippi	265,824	1.0%
34	Kansas	252,472	0.9%
35	Utah	215,667	0.8%
36	Nebraska	205,294	0.8%
37	Maine	160,726	0.6%
38	Nevada	138,400	0.5%
39	Rhode Island	137,271	0.5%
40	New Mexico	132,597	0.5%
41	New Hampshire	121,330	0.4%
42	Idaho	103,656	0.4%
43	Delaware	94,600	0.3%
44	Hawaii	86,735	0.3%
45	South Dakota	84,748	0.3%
46	North Dakota	76,294	0.3%
47	Montana	73,990	0.3%
48	Vermont	69,356	0.3%
49	Alaska	51,561	0.2%
50	Wyoming	42,090	0.2%
	District of Columbia	105,550	0.4%

Source: American Hospital Association (Chicago, IL)
   "Hospital Statistics" (2005 edition)
*Includes inpatient and outpatient surgeries.

Medicare and Medicaid Certified Facilities in 2005

National Total = 247,964 Facilities*

ALPHA ORDER

RANK	STATE	FACILITIES	% of USA
19	Alabama	4,341	1.8%
48	Alaska	576	0.2%
27	Arizona	3,660	1.5%
32	Arkansas	2,775	1.1%
1	California	23,962	9.7%
29	Colorado	3,278	1.3%
30	Connecticut	3,235	1.3%
47	Delaware	805	0.3%
3	Florida	16,162	6.5%
9	Georgia	7,588	3.1%
45	Hawaii	955	0.4%
40	Idaho	1,203	0.5%
6	Illinois	10,691	4.3%
11	Indiana	6,497	2.6%
26	Iowa	3,699	1.5%
28	Kansas	3,326	1.3%
22	Kentucky	4,009	1.6%
15	Louisiana	5,501	2.2%
39	Maine	1,328	0.5%
18	Maryland	4,383	1.8%
17	Massachusetts	4,568	1.8%
8	Michigan	8,004	3.2%
25	Minnesota	3,769	1.5%
31	Mississippi	2,897	1.2%
13	Missouri	6,007	2.4%
43	Montana	1,020	0.4%
35	Nebraska	2,072	0.8%
38	Nevada	1,412	0.6%
41	New Hampshire	1,153	0.5%
12	New Jersey	6,237	2.5%
36	New Mexico	1,663	0.7%
4	New York	12,572	5.1%
10	North Carolina	7,318	3.0%
46	North Dakota	872	0.4%
5	Ohio	11,610	4.7%
21	Oklahoma	4,014	1.6%
33	Oregon	2,655	1.1%
7	Pennsylvania	9,854	4.0%
44	Rhode Island	970	0.4%
23	South Carolina	3,987	1.6%
42	South Dakota	1,033	0.4%
14	Tennessee	5,566	2.2%
2	Texas	21,867	8.8%
37	Utah	1,539	0.6%
49	Vermont	551	0.2%
16	Virginia	5,366	2.2%
24	Washington	3,943	1.6%
34	West Virginia	2,170	0.9%
20	Wisconsin	4,119	1.7%
50	Wyoming	535	0.2%

RANK ORDER

RANK	STATE	FACILITIES	% of USA
1	California	23,962	9.7%
2	Texas	21,867	8.8%
3	Florida	16,162	6.5%
4	New York	12,572	5.1%
5	Ohio	11,610	4.7%
6	Illinois	10,691	4.3%
7	Pennsylvania	9,854	4.0%
8	Michigan	8,004	3.2%
9	Georgia	7,588	3.1%
10	North Carolina	7,318	3.0%
11	Indiana	6,497	2.6%
12	New Jersey	6,237	2.5%
13	Missouri	6,007	2.4%
14	Tennessee	5,566	2.2%
15	Louisiana	5,501	2.2%
16	Virginia	5,366	2.2%
17	Massachusetts	4,568	1.8%
18	Maryland	4,383	1.8%
19	Alabama	4,341	1.8%
20	Wisconsin	4,119	1.7%
21	Oklahoma	4,014	1.6%
22	Kentucky	4,009	1.6%
23	South Carolina	3,987	1.6%
24	Washington	3,943	1.6%
25	Minnesota	3,769	1.5%
26	Iowa	3,699	1.5%
27	Arizona	3,660	1.5%
28	Kansas	3,326	1.3%
29	Colorado	3,278	1.3%
30	Connecticut	3,235	1.3%
31	Mississippi	2,897	1.2%
32	Arkansas	2,775	1.1%
33	Oregon	2,655	1.1%
34	West Virginia	2,170	0.9%
35	Nebraska	2,072	0.8%
36	New Mexico	1,663	0.7%
37	Utah	1,539	0.6%
38	Nevada	1,412	0.6%
39	Maine	1,328	0.5%
40	Idaho	1,203	0.5%
41	New Hampshire	1,153	0.5%
42	South Dakota	1,033	0.4%
43	Montana	1,020	0.4%
44	Rhode Island	970	0.4%
45	Hawaii	955	0.4%
46	North Dakota	872	0.4%
47	Delaware	805	0.3%
48	Alaska	576	0.2%
49	Vermont	551	0.2%
50	Wyoming	535	0.2%
	District of Columbia	647	0.3%

Source: U.S. Department of Health and Human Services, Centers for Medicare and Medicaid Services
OSCAR Report 10 (January 10, 2005)

Certified by CMS to participate in the Medicare/Medicaid programs. All provider groups including hospitals, home health agencies, rural health centers, community mental health centers, nursing facilities, outpatient physical therapy facilities, hospices and laboratories. National total does not include 1,352 certified facilities in U.S. territories.

Medicare and Medicaid Certified Hospitals in 2005

National Total = 6,052 Hospitals*

ALPHA ORDER

RANK	STATE	HOSPITALS	% of USA
19	Alabama	126	2.1%
47	Alaska	24	0.4%
29	Arizona	91	1.5%
26	Arkansas	105	1.7%
2	California	433	7.2%
30	Colorado	86	1.4%
41	Connecticut	45	0.7%
50	Delaware	10	0.2%
5	Florida	237	3.9%
9	Georgia	178	2.9%
46	Hawaii	27	0.4%
39	Idaho	48	0.8%
7	Illinois	220	3.6%
11	Indiana	156	2.6%
20	Iowa	119	2.0%
13	Kansas	152	2.5%
20	Kentucky	119	2.0%
6	Louisiana	221	3.7%
42	Maine	43	0.7%
35	Maryland	65	1.1%
22	Massachusetts	112	1.9%
10	Michigan	175	2.9%
15	Minnesota	146	2.4%
23	Mississippi	111	1.8%
17	Missouri	138	2.3%
33	Montana	66	1.1%
28	Nebraska	96	1.6%
42	Nevada	43	0.7%
44	New Hampshire	33	0.5%
24	New Jersey	109	1.8%
37	New Mexico	51	0.8%
3	New York	248	4.1%
18	North Carolina	137	2.3%
38	North Dakota	50	0.8%
8	Ohio	215	3.6%
14	Oklahoma	151	2.5%
36	Oregon	59	1.0%
4	Pennsylvania	247	4.1%
49	Rhode Island	15	0.2%
31	South Carolina	76	1.3%
33	South Dakota	66	1.1%
12	Tennessee	153	2.5%
1	Texas	520	8.6%
39	Utah	48	0.8%
48	Vermont	16	0.3%
24	Virginia	109	1.8%
27	Washington	101	1.7%
32	West Virginia	69	1.1%
16	Wisconsin	143	2.4%
45	Wyoming	30	0.5%

RANK ORDER

RANK	STATE	HOSPITALS	% of USA
1	Texas	520	8.6%
2	California	433	7.2%
3	New York	248	4.1%
4	Pennsylvania	247	4.1%
5	Florida	237	3.9%
6	Louisiana	221	3.7%
7	Illinois	220	3.6%
8	Ohio	215	3.6%
9	Georgia	178	2.9%
10	Michigan	175	2.9%
11	Indiana	156	2.6%
12	Tennessee	153	2.5%
13	Kansas	152	2.5%
14	Oklahoma	151	2.5%
15	Minnesota	146	2.4%
16	Wisconsin	143	2.4%
17	Missouri	138	2.3%
18	North Carolina	137	2.3%
19	Alabama	126	2.1%
20	Iowa	119	2.0%
20	Kentucky	119	2.0%
22	Massachusetts	112	1.9%
23	Mississippi	111	1.8%
24	New Jersey	109	1.8%
24	Virginia	109	1.8%
26	Arkansas	105	1.7%
27	Washington	101	1.7%
28	Nebraska	96	1.6%
29	Arizona	91	1.5%
30	Colorado	86	1.4%
31	South Carolina	76	1.3%
32	West Virginia	69	1.1%
33	Montana	66	1.1%
33	South Dakota	66	1.1%
35	Maryland	65	1.1%
36	Oregon	59	1.0%
37	New Mexico	51	0.8%
38	North Dakota	50	0.8%
39	Idaho	48	0.8%
39	Utah	48	0.8%
41	Connecticut	45	0.7%
42	Maine	43	0.7%
42	Nevada	43	0.7%
44	New Hampshire	33	0.5%
45	Wyoming	30	0.5%
46	Hawaii	27	0.4%
47	Alaska	24	0.4%
48	Vermont	16	0.3%
49	Rhode Island	15	0.2%
50	Delaware	10	0.2%
	District of Columbia	14	0.2%

*Source: U.S. Department of Health and Human Services, Centers for Medicare and Medicaid Services
OSCAR Database (January 10, 2005)*
*Certified by CMS to participate in the Medicare/Medicaid programs. Excludes licensed facilities that do not accept federal funding and facilities managed by the Department of Veterans Affairs. National total does not include 64 certified hospitals in U.S. territories.

Beds in Medicare and Medicaid Certified Hospitals in 2005

National Total = 937,884 Beds*

<table>
<tr><td colspan="4">ALPHA ORDER</td><td colspan="4">RANK ORDER</td></tr>
<tr><td>RANK</td><td>STATE</td><td>BEDS</td><td>% of USA</td><td>RANK</td><td>STATE</td><td>BEDS</td><td>% of USA</td></tr>
<tr><td>17</td><td>Alabama</td><td>19,700</td><td>2.1%</td><td>1</td><td>California</td><td>82,040</td><td>8.7%</td></tr>
<tr><td>49</td><td>Alaska</td><td>1,528</td><td>0.2%</td><td>2</td><td>New York</td><td>72,334</td><td>7.7%</td></tr>
<tr><td>26</td><td>Arizona</td><td>13,013</td><td>1.4%</td><td>3</td><td>Texas</td><td>65,097</td><td>6.9%</td></tr>
<tr><td>30</td><td>Arkansas</td><td>11,134</td><td>1.2%</td><td>4</td><td>Florida</td><td>54,387</td><td>5.8%</td></tr>
<tr><td>1</td><td>California</td><td>82,040</td><td>8.7%</td><td>5</td><td>Illinois</td><td>46,559</td><td>5.0%</td></tr>
<tr><td>28</td><td>Colorado</td><td>11,745</td><td>1.3%</td><td>6</td><td>Ohio</td><td>45,063</td><td>4.8%</td></tr>
<tr><td>32</td><td>Connecticut</td><td>10,243</td><td>1.1%</td><td>7</td><td>Pennsylvania</td><td>40,466</td><td>4.3%</td></tr>
<tr><td>47</td><td>Delaware</td><td>2,261</td><td>0.2%</td><td>8</td><td>New Jersey</td><td>30,547</td><td>3.3%</td></tr>
<tr><td>4</td><td>Florida</td><td>54,387</td><td>5.8%</td><td>9</td><td>Michigan</td><td>29,096</td><td>3.1%</td></tr>
<tr><td>12</td><td>Georgia</td><td>24,681</td><td>2.6%</td><td>10</td><td>North Carolina</td><td>25,781</td><td>2.7%</td></tr>
<tr><td>46</td><td>Hawaii</td><td>2,710</td><td>0.3%</td><td>11</td><td>Tennessee</td><td>24,805</td><td>2.6%</td></tr>
<tr><td>43</td><td>Idaho</td><td>3,281</td><td>0.3%</td><td>12</td><td>Georgia</td><td>24,681</td><td>2.6%</td></tr>
<tr><td>5</td><td>Illinois</td><td>46,559</td><td>5.0%</td><td>13</td><td>Missouri</td><td>24,096</td><td>2.6%</td></tr>
<tr><td>15</td><td>Indiana</td><td>21,152</td><td>2.3%</td><td>14</td><td>Louisiana</td><td>22,501</td><td>2.4%</td></tr>
<tr><td>29</td><td>Iowa</td><td>11,655</td><td>1.2%</td><td>15</td><td>Indiana</td><td>21,152</td><td>2.3%</td></tr>
<tr><td>31</td><td>Kansas</td><td>11,117</td><td>1.2%</td><td>16</td><td>Virginia</td><td>20,785</td><td>2.2%</td></tr>
<tr><td>20</td><td>Kentucky</td><td>17,378</td><td>1.9%</td><td>17</td><td>Alabama</td><td>19,700</td><td>2.1%</td></tr>
<tr><td>14</td><td>Louisiana</td><td>22,501</td><td>2.4%</td><td>18</td><td>Massachusetts</td><td>19,489</td><td>2.1%</td></tr>
<tr><td>39</td><td>Maine</td><td>4,144</td><td>0.4%</td><td>19</td><td>Wisconsin</td><td>18,677</td><td>2.0%</td></tr>
<tr><td>22</td><td>Maryland</td><td>16,081</td><td>1.7%</td><td>20</td><td>Kentucky</td><td>17,378</td><td>1.9%</td></tr>
<tr><td>18</td><td>Massachusetts</td><td>19,489</td><td>2.1%</td><td>21</td><td>Minnesota</td><td>16,480</td><td>1.8%</td></tr>
<tr><td>9</td><td>Michigan</td><td>29,096</td><td>3.1%</td><td>22</td><td>Maryland</td><td>16,081</td><td>1.7%</td></tr>
<tr><td>21</td><td>Minnesota</td><td>16,480</td><td>1.8%</td><td>23</td><td>Oklahoma</td><td>14,663</td><td>1.6%</td></tr>
<tr><td>25</td><td>Mississippi</td><td>13,014</td><td>1.4%</td><td>24</td><td>Washington</td><td>13,678</td><td>1.5%</td></tr>
<tr><td>13</td><td>Missouri</td><td>24,096</td><td>2.6%</td><td>25</td><td>Mississippi</td><td>13,014</td><td>1.4%</td></tr>
<tr><td>45</td><td>Montana</td><td>2,951</td><td>0.3%</td><td>26</td><td>Arizona</td><td>13,013</td><td>1.4%</td></tr>
<tr><td>35</td><td>Nebraska</td><td>6,533</td><td>0.7%</td><td>27</td><td>South Carolina</td><td>12,607</td><td>1.3%</td></tr>
<tr><td>36</td><td>Nevada</td><td>5,598</td><td>0.6%</td><td>28</td><td>Colorado</td><td>11,745</td><td>1.3%</td></tr>
<tr><td>41</td><td>New Hampshire</td><td>3,424</td><td>0.4%</td><td>29</td><td>Iowa</td><td>11,655</td><td>1.2%</td></tr>
<tr><td>8</td><td>New Jersey</td><td>30,547</td><td>3.3%</td><td>30</td><td>Arkansas</td><td>11,134</td><td>1.2%</td></tr>
<tr><td>38</td><td>New Mexico</td><td>4,832</td><td>0.5%</td><td>31</td><td>Kansas</td><td>11,117</td><td>1.2%</td></tr>
<tr><td>2</td><td>New York</td><td>72,334</td><td>7.7%</td><td>32</td><td>Connecticut</td><td>10,243</td><td>1.1%</td></tr>
<tr><td>10</td><td>North Carolina</td><td>25,781</td><td>2.7%</td><td>33</td><td>West Virginia</td><td>9,801</td><td>1.0%</td></tr>
<tr><td>44</td><td>North Dakota</td><td>3,276</td><td>0.3%</td><td>34</td><td>Oregon</td><td>7,441</td><td>0.8%</td></tr>
<tr><td>6</td><td>Ohio</td><td>45,063</td><td>4.8%</td><td>35</td><td>Nebraska</td><td>6,533</td><td>0.7%</td></tr>
<tr><td>23</td><td>Oklahoma</td><td>14,663</td><td>1.6%</td><td>36</td><td>Nevada</td><td>5,598</td><td>0.6%</td></tr>
<tr><td>34</td><td>Oregon</td><td>7,441</td><td>0.8%</td><td>37</td><td>Utah</td><td>5,090</td><td>0.5%</td></tr>
<tr><td>7</td><td>Pennsylvania</td><td>40,466</td><td>4.3%</td><td>38</td><td>New Mexico</td><td>4,832</td><td>0.5%</td></tr>
<tr><td>40</td><td>Rhode Island</td><td>3,785</td><td>0.4%</td><td>39</td><td>Maine</td><td>4,144</td><td>0.4%</td></tr>
<tr><td>27</td><td>South Carolina</td><td>12,607</td><td>1.3%</td><td>40</td><td>Rhode Island</td><td>3,785</td><td>0.4%</td></tr>
<tr><td>42</td><td>South Dakota</td><td>3,384</td><td>0.4%</td><td>41</td><td>New Hampshire</td><td>3,424</td><td>0.4%</td></tr>
<tr><td>11</td><td>Tennessee</td><td>24,805</td><td>2.6%</td><td>42</td><td>South Dakota</td><td>3,384</td><td>0.4%</td></tr>
<tr><td>3</td><td>Texas</td><td>65,097</td><td>6.9%</td><td>43</td><td>Idaho</td><td>3,281</td><td>0.3%</td></tr>
<tr><td>37</td><td>Utah</td><td>5,090</td><td>0.5%</td><td>44</td><td>North Dakota</td><td>3,276</td><td>0.3%</td></tr>
<tr><td>48</td><td>Vermont</td><td>1,996</td><td>0.2%</td><td>45</td><td>Montana</td><td>2,951</td><td>0.3%</td></tr>
<tr><td>16</td><td>Virginia</td><td>20,785</td><td>2.2%</td><td>46</td><td>Hawaii</td><td>2,710</td><td>0.3%</td></tr>
<tr><td>24</td><td>Washington</td><td>13,678</td><td>1.5%</td><td>47</td><td>Delaware</td><td>2,261</td><td>0.2%</td></tr>
<tr><td>33</td><td>West Virginia</td><td>9,801</td><td>1.0%</td><td>48</td><td>Vermont</td><td>1,996</td><td>0.2%</td></tr>
<tr><td>19</td><td>Wisconsin</td><td>18,677</td><td>2.0%</td><td>49</td><td>Alaska</td><td>1,528</td><td>0.2%</td></tr>
<tr><td>50</td><td>Wyoming</td><td>1,479</td><td>0.2%</td><td>50</td><td>Wyoming</td><td>1,479</td><td>0.2%</td></tr>
<tr><td></td><td></td><td></td><td></td><td></td><td>District of Columbia</td><td>4,306</td><td>0.5%</td></tr>
</table>

Source: U.S. Department of Health and Human Services, Centers for Medicare and Medicaid Services
    OSCAR Database (January 10, 2005)
*Beds in hospitals certified by CMS to participate in the Medicare/Medicaid programs. Excludes licensed facilities
that do not accept federal funding and facilities managed by the Department of Veterans Affairs. National total
does not include 11,133 beds in U.S. territories.

Medicare and Medicaid Certified Children's Hospitals in 2005

National Total = 79 Hospitals*

ALPHA ORDER

RANK	STATE	HOSPITALS	% of USA
9	Alabama	2	2.5%
34	Alaska	0	0.0%
9	Arizona	2	2.5%
20	Arkansas	1	1.3%
1	California	9	11.4%
20	Colorado	1	1.3%
20	Connecticut	1	1.3%
20	Delaware	1	1.3%
9	Florida	2	2.5%
9	Georgia	2	2.5%
20	Hawaii	1	1.3%
34	Idaho	0	0.0%
9	Illinois	2	2.5%
20	Indiana	1	1.3%
34	Iowa	0	0.0%
20	Kansas	1	1.3%
34	Kentucky	0	0.0%
20	Louisiana	1	1.3%
34	Maine	0	0.0%
9	Maryland	2	2.5%
9	Massachusetts	2	2.5%
20	Michigan	1	1.3%
5	Minnesota	3	3.8%
34	Mississippi	0	0.0%
5	Missouri	3	3.8%
34	Montana	0	0.0%
9	Nebraska	2	2.5%
34	Nevada	0	0.0%
34	New Hampshire	0	0.0%
20	New Jersey	1	1.3%
20	New Mexico	1	1.3%
20	New York	1	1.3%
34	North Carolina	0	0.0%
34	North Dakota	0	0.0%
3	Ohio	7	8.9%
9	Oklahoma	2	2.5%
34	Oregon	0	0.0%
4	Pennsylvania	6	7.6%
34	Rhode Island	0	0.0%
34	South Carolina	0	0.0%
20	South Dakota	1	1.3%
9	Tennessee	2	2.5%
2	Texas	8	10.1%
20	Utah	1	1.3%
34	Vermont	0	0.0%
5	Virginia	3	3.8%
9	Washington	2	2.5%
34	West Virginia	0	0.0%
5	Wisconsin	3	3.8%
34	Wyoming	0	0.0%

RANK ORDER

RANK	STATE	HOSPITALS	% of USA
1	California	9	11.4%
2	Texas	8	10.1%
3	Ohio	7	8.9%
4	Pennsylvania	6	7.6%
5	Minnesota	3	3.8%
5	Missouri	3	3.8%
5	Virginia	3	3.8%
5	Wisconsin	3	3.8%
9	Alabama	2	2.5%
9	Arizona	2	2.5%
9	Florida	2	2.5%
9	Georgia	2	2.5%
9	Illinois	2	2.5%
9	Maryland	2	2.5%
9	Massachusetts	2	2.5%
9	Nebraska	2	2.5%
9	Oklahoma	2	2.5%
9	Tennessee	2	2.5%
9	Washington	2	2.5%
20	Arkansas	1	1.3%
20	Colorado	1	1.3%
20	Connecticut	1	1.3%
20	Delaware	1	1.3%
20	Hawaii	1	1.3%
20	Indiana	1	1.3%
20	Kansas	1	1.3%
20	Louisiana	1	1.3%
20	Michigan	1	1.3%
20	New Jersey	1	1.3%
20	New Mexico	1	1.3%
20	New York	1	1.3%
20	South Dakota	1	1.3%
20	Utah	1	1.3%
34	Alaska	0	0.0%
34	Idaho	0	0.0%
34	Iowa	0	0.0%
34	Kentucky	0	0.0%
34	Maine	0	0.0%
34	Mississippi	0	0.0%
34	Montana	0	0.0%
34	Nevada	0	0.0%
34	New Hampshire	0	0.0%
34	North Carolina	0	0.0%
34	North Dakota	0	0.0%
34	Oregon	0	0.0%
34	Rhode Island	0	0.0%
34	South Carolina	0	0.0%
34	Vermont	0	0.0%
34	West Virginia	0	0.0%
34	Wyoming	0	0.0%
	District of Columbia	1	1.3%

Source: U.S. Department of Health and Human Services, Centers for Medicare and Medicaid Services
OSCAR Database (January 10, 2005)
*Certified by CMS to participate in the Medicare/Medicaid programs. National total does not include one facility in U.S. territories. Excludes licensed facilities that do not accept federal funding and facilities managed by the Department of Veterans Affairs.

Beds in Medicare and Medicaid Certified Children's Hospitals in 2005

National Total = 11,886 Beds*

ALPHA ORDER

RANK	STATE	BEDS	% of USA
8	Alabama	424	3.6%
34	Alaska	0	0.0%
19	Arizona	223	1.9%
13	Arkansas	280	2.4%
1	California	1,605	13.5%
16	Colorado	253	2.1%
26	Connecticut	97	0.8%
26	Delaware	97	0.8%
8	Florida	424	3.6%
5	Georgia	435	3.7%
20	Hawaii	201	1.7%
34	Idaho	0	0.0%
10	Illinois	351	3.0%
33	Indiana	20	0.2%
34	Iowa	0	0.0%
31	Kansas	34	0.3%
34	Kentucky	0	0.0%
21	Louisiana	188	1.6%
34	Maine	0	0.0%
24	Maryland	150	1.3%
7	Massachusetts	425	3.6%
18	Michigan	228	1.9%
11	Minnesota	339	2.9%
34	Mississippi	0	0.0%
6	Missouri	432	3.6%
34	Montana	0	0.0%
24	Nebraska	150	1.3%
34	Nevada	0	0.0%
34	New Hampshire	0	0.0%
30	New Jersey	74	0.6%
32	New Mexico	28	0.2%
29	New York	92	0.8%
34	North Carolina	0	0.0%
34	North Dakota	0	0.0%
3	Ohio	1,419	11.9%
23	Oklahoma	160	1.3%
34	Oregon	0	0.0%
4	Pennsylvania	679	5.7%
34	Rhode Island	0	0.0%
34	South Carolina	0	0.0%
28	South Dakota	96	0.8%
22	Tennessee	175	1.5%
2	Texas	1,494	12.6%
17	Utah	232	2.0%
34	Vermont	0	0.0%
12	Virginia	286	2.4%
14	Washington	276	2.3%
34	West Virginia	0	0.0%
14	Wisconsin	276	2.3%
34	Wyoming	0	0.0%

RANK ORDER

RANK	STATE	BEDS	% of USA
1	California	1,605	13.5%
2	Texas	1,494	12.6%
3	Ohio	1,419	11.9%
4	Pennsylvania	679	5.7%
5	Georgia	435	3.7%
6	Missouri	432	3.6%
7	Massachusetts	425	3.6%
8	Alabama	424	3.6%
8	Florida	424	3.6%
10	Illinois	351	3.0%
11	Minnesota	339	2.9%
12	Virginia	286	2.4%
13	Arkansas	280	2.4%
14	Washington	276	2.3%
14	Wisconsin	276	2.3%
16	Colorado	253	2.1%
17	Utah	232	2.0%
18	Michigan	228	1.9%
19	Arizona	223	1.9%
20	Hawaii	201	1.7%
21	Louisiana	188	1.6%
22	Tennessee	175	1.5%
23	Oklahoma	160	1.3%
24	Maryland	150	1.3%
24	Nebraska	150	1.3%
26	Connecticut	97	0.8%
26	Delaware	97	0.8%
28	South Dakota	96	0.8%
29	New York	92	0.8%
30	New Jersey	74	0.6%
31	Kansas	34	0.3%
32	New Mexico	28	0.2%
33	Indiana	20	0.2%
34	Alaska	0	0.0%
34	Idaho	0	0.0%
34	Iowa	0	0.0%
34	Kentucky	0	0.0%
34	Maine	0	0.0%
34	Mississippi	0	0.0%
34	Montana	0	0.0%
34	Nevada	0	0.0%
34	New Hampshire	0	0.0%
34	North Carolina	0	0.0%
34	North Dakota	0	0.0%
34	Oregon	0	0.0%
34	Rhode Island	0	0.0%
34	South Carolina	0	0.0%
34	Vermont	0	0.0%
34	West Virginia	0	0.0%
34	Wyoming	0	0.0%
	District of Columbia	243	2.0%

Source: U.S. Department of Health and Human Services, Centers for Medicare and Medicaid Services
    OSCAR Database (January 10, 2005)
*Certified by CMS to participate in the Medicare/Medicaid programs. National total does not include 215 beds in one facility in U.S. territories. Excludes licensed facilities that do not accept federal funding and facilities managed by the Department of Veterans Affairs.

Medicare and Medicaid Certified Rehabilitation Hospitals in 2005

National Total = 217 Hospitals*

ALPHA ORDER

RANK	STATE	HOSPITALS	% of USA
6	Alabama	7	3.2%
41	Alaska	0	0.0%
14	Arizona	5	2.3%
10	Arkansas	6	2.8%
6	California	7	3.2%
25	Colorado	2	0.9%
31	Connecticut	1	0.5%
41	Delaware	0	0.0%
4	Florida	14	6.5%
25	Georgia	2	0.9%
31	Hawaii	1	0.5%
31	Idaho	1	0.5%
17	Illinois	4	1.8%
6	Indiana	7	3.2%
41	Iowa	0	0.0%
17	Kansas	4	1.8%
10	Kentucky	6	2.8%
2	Louisiana	26	12.0%
31	Maine	1	0.5%
25	Maryland	2	0.9%
6	Massachusetts	7	3.2%
14	Michigan	5	2.3%
31	Minnesota	1	0.5%
41	Mississippi	0	0.0%
22	Missouri	3	1.4%
41	Montana	0	0.0%
31	Nebraska	1	0.5%
22	Nevada	3	1.4%
25	New Hampshire	2	0.9%
5	New Jersey	10	4.6%
17	New Mexico	4	1.8%
17	New York	4	1.8%
25	North Carolina	2	0.9%
41	North Dakota	0	0.0%
25	Ohio	2	0.9%
22	Oklahoma	3	1.4%
41	Oregon	0	0.0%
3	Pennsylvania	18	8.3%
31	Rhode Island	1	0.5%
14	South Carolina	5	2.3%
41	South Dakota	0	0.0%
10	Tennessee	6	2.8%
1	Texas	30	13.8%
31	Utah	1	0.5%
41	Vermont	0	0.0%
17	Virginia	4	1.8%
31	Washington	1	0.5%
10	West Virginia	6	2.8%
31	Wisconsin	1	0.5%
41	Wyoming	0	0.0%

RANK ORDER

RANK	STATE	HOSPITALS	% of USA
1	Texas	30	13.8%
2	Louisiana	26	12.0%
3	Pennsylvania	18	8.3%
4	Florida	14	6.5%
5	New Jersey	10	4.6%
6	Alabama	7	3.2%
6	California	7	3.2%
6	Indiana	7	3.2%
6	Massachusetts	7	3.2%
10	Arkansas	6	2.8%
10	Kentucky	6	2.8%
10	Tennessee	6	2.8%
10	West Virginia	6	2.8%
14	Arizona	5	2.3%
14	Michigan	5	2.3%
14	South Carolina	5	2.3%
17	Illinois	4	1.8%
17	Kansas	4	1.8%
17	New Mexico	4	1.8%
17	New York	4	1.8%
17	Virginia	4	1.8%
22	Missouri	3	1.4%
22	Nevada	3	1.4%
22	Oklahoma	3	1.4%
25	Colorado	2	0.9%
25	Georgia	2	0.9%
25	Maryland	2	0.9%
25	New Hampshire	2	0.9%
25	North Carolina	2	0.9%
25	Ohio	2	0.9%
31	Connecticut	1	0.5%
31	Hawaii	1	0.5%
31	Idaho	1	0.5%
31	Maine	1	0.5%
31	Minnesota	1	0.5%
31	Nebraska	1	0.5%
31	Rhode Island	1	0.5%
31	Utah	1	0.5%
31	Washington	1	0.5%
31	Wisconsin	1	0.5%
41	Alaska	0	0.0%
41	Delaware	0	0.0%
41	Iowa	0	0.0%
41	Mississippi	0	0.0%
41	Montana	0	0.0%
41	North Dakota	0	0.0%
41	Oregon	0	0.0%
41	South Dakota	0	0.0%
41	Vermont	0	0.0%
41	Wyoming	0	0.0%
	District of Columbia	1	0.5%

Source: U.S. Department of Health and Human Services, Centers for Medicare and Medicaid Services
    OSCAR Database (January 10, 2005)

*Certified by CMS to participate in the Medicare/Medicaid programs. Excludes licensed facilities that do not accept federal funding and facilities managed by the Department of Veterans Affairs. National total does not include one certified hospital in U.S. territories.

Beds in Medicare and Medicaid Certified Rehabilitation Hospitals in 2005

National Total = 14,033 Beds*

ALPHA ORDER

RANK	STATE	BEDS	% of USA
13	Alabama	371	2.6%
41	Alaska	0	0.0%
18	Arizona	269	1.9%
7	Arkansas	459	3.3%
11	California	411	2.9%
23	Colorado	186	1.3%
38	Connecticut	60	0.4%
41	Delaware	0	0.0%
3	Florida	1,076	7.7%
29	Georgia	116	0.8%
31	Hawaii	100	0.7%
39	Idaho	59	0.4%
12	Illinois	408	2.9%
9	Indiana	430	3.1%
41	Iowa	0	0.0%
19	Kansas	257	1.8%
15	Kentucky	328	2.3%
6	Louisiana	628	4.5%
31	Maine	100	0.7%
33	Maryland	99	0.7%
5	Massachusetts	742	5.3%
17	Michigan	285	2.0%
40	Minnesota	15	0.1%
41	Mississippi	0	0.0%
21	Missouri	220	1.6%
41	Montana	0	0.0%
37	Nebraska	66	0.5%
24	Nevada	169	1.2%
28	New Hampshire	130	0.9%
4	New Jersey	786	5.6%
26	New Mexico	156	1.1%
10	New York	428	3.0%
20	North Carolina	233	1.7%
41	North Dakota	0	0.0%
27	Ohio	149	1.1%
25	Oklahoma	167	1.2%
41	Oregon	0	0.0%
2	Pennsylvania	1,565	11.2%
35	Rhode Island	82	0.6%
16	South Carolina	294	2.1%
41	South Dakota	0	0.0%
14	Tennessee	370	2.6%
1	Texas	1,737	12.4%
34	Utah	84	0.6%
41	Vermont	0	0.0%
22	Virginia	205	1.5%
30	Washington	102	0.7%
8	West Virginia	450	3.2%
36	Wisconsin	81	0.6%
41	Wyoming	0	0.0%

RANK ORDER

RANK	STATE	BEDS	% of USA
1	Texas	1,737	12.4%
2	Pennsylvania	1,565	11.2%
3	Florida	1,076	7.7%
4	New Jersey	786	5.6%
5	Massachusetts	742	5.3%
6	Louisiana	628	4.5%
7	Arkansas	459	3.3%
8	West Virginia	450	3.2%
9	Indiana	430	3.1%
10	New York	428	3.0%
11	California	411	2.9%
12	Illinois	408	2.9%
13	Alabama	371	2.6%
14	Tennessee	370	2.6%
15	Kentucky	328	2.3%
16	South Carolina	294	2.1%
17	Michigan	285	2.0%
18	Arizona	269	1.9%
19	Kansas	257	1.8%
20	North Carolina	233	1.7%
21	Missouri	220	1.6%
22	Virginia	205	1.5%
23	Colorado	186	1.3%
24	Nevada	169	1.2%
25	Oklahoma	167	1.2%
26	New Mexico	156	1.1%
27	Ohio	149	1.1%
28	New Hampshire	130	0.9%
29	Georgia	116	0.8%
30	Washington	102	0.7%
31	Hawaii	100	0.7%
31	Maine	100	0.7%
33	Maryland	99	0.7%
34	Utah	84	0.6%
35	Rhode Island	82	0.6%
36	Wisconsin	81	0.6%
37	Nebraska	66	0.5%
38	Connecticut	60	0.4%
39	Idaho	59	0.4%
40	Minnesota	15	0.1%
41	Alaska	0	0.0%
41	Delaware	0	0.0%
41	Iowa	0	0.0%
41	Mississippi	0	0.0%
41	Montana	0	0.0%
41	North Dakota	0	0.0%
41	Oregon	0	0.0%
41	South Dakota	0	0.0%
41	Vermont	0	0.0%
41	Wyoming	0	0.0%
	District of Columbia	160	1.1%

Source: U.S. Department of Health and Human Services, Centers for Medicare and Medicaid Services OSCAR Database (January 10, 2005)

*Beds in hospitals certified by CMS to participate in the Medicare/Medicaid programs. Excludes licensed facilities that do not accept federal funding and facilities managed by the Department of Veterans Affairs. National total does not include 30 beds in U.S. territories.

Medicare and Medicaid Certified Psychiatric Hospitals in 2005

National Total = 465 Psychiatric Hospitals*

ALPHA ORDER					RANK ORDER			

RANK	STATE	HOSPITALS	% of USA		RANK	STATE	HOSPITALS	% of USA
17	Alabama	10	2.2%		1	Texas	32	6.9%
41	Alaska	2	0.4%		2	California	31	6.7%
27	Arizona	6	1.3%		3	New York	29	6.2%
17	Arkansas	10	2.2%		4	Pennsylvania	24	5.2%
2	California	31	6.7%		5	Florida	20	4.3%
29	Colorado	5	1.1%		6	Indiana	19	4.1%
25	Connecticut	7	1.5%		7	Louisiana	18	3.9%
37	Delaware	3	0.6%		8	Massachusetts	17	3.7%
5	Florida	20	4.3%		9	Illinois	16	3.4%
11	Georgia	14	3.0%		9	New Jersey	16	3.4%
49	Hawaii	1	0.2%		11	Georgia	14	3.0%
29	Idaho	5	1.1%		11	Ohio	14	3.0%
9	Illinois	16	3.4%		13	Missouri	13	2.8%
6	Indiana	19	4.1%		14	Kentucky	11	2.4%
31	Iowa	4	0.9%		14	Tennessee	11	2.4%
31	Kansas	4	0.9%		14	Wisconsin	11	2.4%
14	Kentucky	11	2.4%		17	Alabama	10	2.2%
7	Louisiana	18	3.9%		17	Arkansas	10	2.2%
31	Maine	4	0.9%		17	Maryland	10	2.2%
17	Maryland	10	2.2%		17	North Carolina	10	2.2%
8	Massachusetts	17	3.7%		17	Oklahoma	10	2.2%
23	Michigan	8	1.7%		17	Virginia	10	2.2%
25	Minnesota	7	1.5%		23	Michigan	8	1.7%
31	Mississippi	4	0.9%		23	South Carolina	8	1.7%
13	Missouri	13	2.8%		25	Connecticut	7	1.5%
41	Montana	2	0.4%		25	Minnesota	7	1.5%
31	Nebraska	4	0.9%		27	Arizona	6	1.3%
37	Nevada	3	0.6%		27	Washington	6	1.3%
41	New Hampshire	2	0.4%		29	Colorado	5	1.1%
9	New Jersey	16	3.4%		29	Idaho	5	1.1%
41	New Mexico	2	0.4%		31	Iowa	4	0.9%
3	New York	29	6.2%		31	Kansas	4	0.9%
17	North Carolina	10	2.2%		31	Maine	4	0.9%
37	North Dakota	3	0.6%		31	Mississippi	4	0.9%
11	Ohio	14	3.0%		31	Nebraska	4	0.9%
17	Oklahoma	10	2.2%		31	West Virginia	4	0.9%
41	Oregon	2	0.4%		37	Delaware	3	0.6%
4	Pennsylvania	24	5.2%		37	Nevada	3	0.6%
41	Rhode Island	2	0.4%		37	North Dakota	3	0.6%
23	South Carolina	8	1.7%		37	Utah	3	0.6%
49	South Dakota	1	0.2%		41	Alaska	2	0.4%
14	Tennessee	11	2.4%		41	Montana	2	0.4%
1	Texas	32	6.9%		41	New Hampshire	2	0.4%
37	Utah	3	0.6%		41	New Mexico	2	0.4%
41	Vermont	2	0.4%		41	Oregon	2	0.4%
17	Virginia	10	2.2%		41	Rhode Island	2	0.4%
27	Washington	6	1.3%		41	Vermont	2	0.4%
31	West Virginia	4	0.9%		41	Wyoming	2	0.4%
14	Wisconsin	11	2.4%		49	Hawaii	1	0.2%
41	Wyoming	2	0.4%		49	South Dakota	1	0.2%
						District of Columbia	3	0.6%

Source: U.S. Department of Health and Human Services, Centers for Medicare and Medicaid Services
    OSCAR Database (January 10, 2005)
*Certified by CMS to participate in the Medicare/Medicaid programs. Excludes licensed facilities that do not accept federal funding and facilities managed by the Department of Veterans Affairs. National total does not include four certified psychiatric hospitals in U.S. territories.

Beds in Medicare and Medicaid Certified Psychiatric Hospitals in 2005

National Total = 54,722 Beds*

ALPHA ORDER

RANK	STATE	BEDS	% of USA
27	Alabama	661	1.2%
45	Alaska	169	0.3%
26	Arizona	768	1.4%
23	Arkansas	881	1.6%
8	California	2,195	4.0%
28	Colorado	561	1.0%
19	Connecticut	1,091	2.0%
40	Delaware	237	0.4%
4	Florida	2,679	4.9%
10	Georgia	1,568	2.9%
49	Hawaii	88	0.2%
42	Idaho	221	0.4%
9	Illinois	1,794	3.3%
17	Indiana	1,228	2.2%
35	Iowa	350	0.6%
28	Kansas	561	1.0%
15	Kentucky	1,291	2.4%
14	Louisiana	1,312	2.4%
32	Maine	403	0.7%
7	Maryland	2,282	4.2%
11	Massachusetts	1,509	2.8%
21	Michigan	1,059	1.9%
18	Minnesota	1,131	2.1%
37	Mississippi	296	0.5%
22	Missouri	954	1.7%
44	Montana	182	0.3%
36	Nebraska	347	0.6%
39	Nevada	268	0.5%
34	New Hampshire	356	0.6%
3	New Jersey	3,085	5.6%
47	New Mexico	151	0.3%
1	New York	6,425	11.7%
6	North Carolina	2,469	4.5%
41	North Dakota	229	0.4%
16	Ohio	1,237	2.3%
30	Oklahoma	540	1.0%
38	Oregon	281	0.5%
2	Pennsylvania	3,957	7.2%
46	Rhode Island	165	0.3%
25	South Carolina	822	1.5%
48	South Dakota	133	0.2%
20	Tennessee	1,084	2.0%
5	Texas	2,606	4.8%
33	Utah	391	0.7%
43	Vermont	203	0.4%
24	Virginia	860	1.6%
13	Washington	1,400	2.6%
31	West Virginia	463	0.8%
12	Wisconsin	1,419	2.6%
50	Wyoming	68	0.1%

RANK ORDER

RANK	STATE	BEDS	% of USA
1	New York	6,425	11.7%
2	Pennsylvania	3,957	7.2%
3	New Jersey	3,085	5.6%
4	Florida	2,679	4.9%
5	Texas	2,606	4.8%
6	North Carolina	2,469	4.5%
7	Maryland	2,282	4.2%
8	California	2,195	4.0%
9	Illinois	1,794	3.3%
10	Georgia	1,568	2.9%
11	Massachusetts	1,509	2.8%
12	Wisconsin	1,419	2.6%
13	Washington	1,400	2.6%
14	Louisiana	1,312	2.4%
15	Kentucky	1,291	2.4%
16	Ohio	1,237	2.3%
17	Indiana	1,228	2.2%
18	Minnesota	1,131	2.1%
19	Connecticut	1,091	2.0%
20	Tennessee	1,084	2.0%
21	Michigan	1,059	1.9%
22	Missouri	954	1.7%
23	Arkansas	881	1.6%
24	Virginia	860	1.6%
25	South Carolina	822	1.5%
26	Arizona	768	1.4%
27	Alabama	661	1.2%
28	Colorado	561	1.0%
28	Kansas	561	1.0%
30	Oklahoma	540	1.0%
31	West Virginia	463	0.8%
32	Maine	403	0.7%
33	Utah	391	0.7%
34	New Hampshire	356	0.6%
35	Iowa	350	0.6%
36	Nebraska	347	0.6%
37	Mississippi	296	0.5%
38	Oregon	281	0.5%
39	Nevada	268	0.5%
40	Delaware	237	0.4%
41	North Dakota	229	0.4%
42	Idaho	221	0.4%
43	Vermont	203	0.4%
44	Montana	182	0.3%
45	Alaska	169	0.3%
46	Rhode Island	165	0.3%
47	New Mexico	151	0.3%
48	South Dakota	133	0.2%
49	Hawaii	88	0.2%
50	Wyoming	68	0.1%
	District of Columbia	292	0.5%

Source: U.S. Department of Health and Human Services, Centers for Medicare and Medicaid Services
    OSCAR Database (January 10, 2005)

*Beds in hospitals certified by CMS to participate in the Medicare/Medicaid programs. Excludes licensed facilities that do not accept federal funding and facilities managed by the Department of Veterans Affairs. National total does not include 903 beds in U.S. territories.

Medicare and Medicaid Certified Community Mental Health Centers in 2005

National Total = 603 Centers*

ALPHA ORDER

RANK	STATE	CENTERS	% of USA
2	Alabama	65	10.8%
41	Alaska	0	0.0%
30	Arizona	3	0.5%
13	Arkansas	14	2.3%
8	California	20	3.3%
13	Colorado	14	2.3%
28	Connecticut	4	0.7%
41	Delaware	0	0.0%
1	Florida	115	19.1%
23	Georgia	7	1.2%
41	Hawaii	0	0.0%
41	Idaho	0	0.0%
18	Illinois	13	2.2%
21	Indiana	9	1.5%
26	Iowa	6	1.0%
11	Kansas	15	2.5%
19	Kentucky	12	2.0%
3	Louisiana	35	5.8%
41	Maine	0	0.0%
34	Maryland	2	0.3%
13	Massachusetts	14	2.3%
23	Michigan	7	1.2%
13	Minnesota	14	2.3%
27	Mississippi	5	0.8%
23	Missouri	7	1.2%
41	Montana	0	0.0%
39	Nebraska	1	0.2%
34	Nevada	2	0.3%
39	New Hampshire	1	0.2%
4	New Jersey	34	5.6%
11	New Mexico	15	2.5%
28	New York	4	0.7%
8	North Carolina	20	3.3%
41	North Dakota	0	0.0%
10	Ohio	16	2.7%
22	Oklahoma	8	1.3%
19	Oregon	12	2.0%
13	Pennsylvania	14	2.3%
41	Rhode Island	0	0.0%
30	South Carolina	3	0.5%
34	South Dakota	2	0.3%
7	Tennessee	21	3.5%
4	Texas	34	5.6%
34	Utah	2	0.3%
41	Vermont	0	0.0%
30	Virginia	3	0.5%
6	Washington	25	4.1%
34	West Virginia	2	0.3%
41	Wisconsin	0	0.0%
30	Wyoming	3	0.5%

RANK ORDER

RANK	STATE	CENTERS	% of USA
1	Florida	115	19.1%
2	Alabama	65	10.8%
3	Louisiana	35	5.8%
4	New Jersey	34	5.6%
4	Texas	34	5.6%
6	Washington	25	4.1%
7	Tennessee	21	3.5%
8	California	20	3.3%
8	North Carolina	20	3.3%
10	Ohio	16	2.7%
11	Kansas	15	2.5%
11	New Mexico	15	2.5%
13	Arkansas	14	2.3%
13	Colorado	14	2.3%
13	Massachusetts	14	2.3%
13	Minnesota	14	2.3%
13	Pennsylvania	14	2.3%
18	Illinois	13	2.2%
19	Kentucky	12	2.0%
19	Oregon	12	2.0%
21	Indiana	9	1.5%
22	Oklahoma	8	1.3%
23	Georgia	7	1.2%
23	Michigan	7	1.2%
23	Missouri	7	1.2%
26	Iowa	6	1.0%
27	Mississippi	5	0.8%
28	Connecticut	4	0.7%
28	New York	4	0.7%
30	Arizona	3	0.5%
30	South Carolina	3	0.5%
30	Virginia	3	0.5%
30	Wyoming	3	0.5%
34	Maryland	2	0.3%
34	Nevada	2	0.3%
34	South Dakota	2	0.3%
34	Utah	2	0.3%
34	West Virginia	2	0.3%
39	Nebraska	1	0.2%
39	New Hampshire	1	0.2%
41	Alaska	0	0.0%
41	Delaware	0	0.0%
41	Hawaii	0	0.0%
41	Idaho	0	0.0%
41	Maine	0	0.0%
41	Montana	0	0.0%
41	North Dakota	0	0.0%
41	Rhode Island	0	0.0%
41	Vermont	0	0.0%
41	Wisconsin	0	0.0%
	District of Columbia	0	0.0%

Source: U.S. Department of Health and Human Services, Centers for Medicare and Medicaid Services
  OSCAR Report 10 (January 10, 2005)
Certified by CMS to participate in the Medicare/Medicaid programs. Excludes licensed facilities that do not accept federal funding and facilities managed by the Department of Veterans Affairs. National total does not include nine certified mental health centers in U.S. territories.

Medicare and Medicaid Certified Outpatient Physical Therapy Facilities in 2005

National Total = 2,970 Facilities*

ALPHA ORDER

RANK ORDER

RANK	STATE	FACILITIES	% of USA		RANK	STATE	FACILITIES	% of USA
31	Alabama	26	0.9%		1	Florida	293	9.9%
36	Alaska	16	0.5%		2	Michigan	257	8.7%
29	Arizona	29	1.0%		3	Texas	221	7.4%
27	Arkansas	30	1.0%		4	California	198	6.7%
4	California	198	6.7%		5	Ohio	133	4.5%
22	Colorado	49	1.6%		6	Pennsylvania	128	4.3%
26	Connecticut	35	1.2%		7	Virginia	127	4.3%
36	Delaware	16	0.5%		8	Georgia	122	4.1%
1	Florida	293	9.9%		9	New Jersey	115	3.9%
8	Georgia	122	4.1%		10	Maryland	100	3.4%
41	Hawaii	8	0.3%		11	Illinois	95	3.2%
38	Idaho	15	0.5%		12	Tennessee	94	3.2%
11	Illinois	95	3.2%		13	Kentucky	81	2.7%
15	Indiana	60	2.0%		14	Missouri	61	2.1%
24	Iowa	41	1.4%		15	Indiana	60	2.0%
33	Kansas	21	0.7%		16	Louisiana	55	1.9%
13	Kentucky	81	2.7%		16	Mississippi	55	1.9%
16	Louisiana	55	1.9%		16	Wisconsin	55	1.9%
34	Maine	20	0.7%		19	South Carolina	54	1.8%
10	Maryland	100	3.4%		20	North Carolina	52	1.8%
40	Massachusetts	11	0.4%		21	Oklahoma	50	1.7%
2	Michigan	257	8.7%		22	Colorado	49	1.6%
23	Minnesota	47	1.6%		23	Minnesota	47	1.6%
16	Mississippi	55	1.9%		24	Iowa	41	1.4%
14	Missouri	61	2.1%		25	Washington	39	1.3%
41	Montana	8	0.3%		26	Connecticut	35	1.2%
41	Nebraska	8	0.3%		27	Arkansas	30	1.0%
32	Nevada	23	0.8%		27	New York	30	1.0%
39	New Hampshire	12	0.4%		29	Arizona	29	1.0%
9	New Jersey	115	3.9%		29	New Mexico	29	1.0%
29	New Mexico	29	1.0%		31	Alabama	26	0.9%
27	New York	30	1.0%		32	Nevada	23	0.8%
20	North Carolina	52	1.8%		33	Kansas	21	0.7%
48	North Dakota	3	0.1%		34	Maine	20	0.7%
5	Ohio	133	4.5%		35	Oregon	18	0.6%
21	Oklahoma	50	1.7%		36	Alaska	16	0.5%
35	Oregon	18	0.6%		36	Delaware	16	0.5%
6	Pennsylvania	128	4.3%		38	Idaho	15	0.5%
48	Rhode Island	3	0.1%		39	New Hampshire	12	0.4%
19	South Carolina	54	1.8%		40	Massachusetts	11	0.4%
46	South Dakota	5	0.2%		41	Hawaii	8	0.3%
12	Tennessee	94	3.2%		41	Montana	8	0.3%
3	Texas	221	7.4%		41	Nebraska	8	0.3%
45	Utah	6	0.2%		41	West Virginia	8	0.3%
50	Vermont	2	0.1%		45	Utah	6	0.2%
7	Virginia	127	4.3%		46	South Dakota	5	0.2%
25	Washington	39	1.3%		47	Wyoming	4	0.1%
41	West Virginia	8	0.3%		48	North Dakota	3	0.1%
16	Wisconsin	55	1.9%		48	Rhode Island	3	0.1%
47	Wyoming	4	0.1%		50	Vermont	2	0.1%
						District of Columbia	2	0.1%

Source: U.S. Department of Health and Human Services, Centers for Medicare and Medicaid Services
    OSCAR Report 10 (January 10, 2005)
*Certified by CMS to participate in the Medicare/Medicaid programs. Excludes licensed facilities that do not accept federal funding and facilities managed by the Department of Veterans Affairs. National total does not include four certified outpatient physical therapy facilities in U.S. territories.

Medicare and Medicaid Certified Rural Health Clinics in 2005

National Total = 3,535 Rural Health Clinics*

ALPHA ORDER

RANK ORDER

RANK	STATE	CLINICS	% of USA	RANK	STATE	CLINICS	% of USA
19	Alabama	66	1.9%	1	Texas	328	9.3%
42	Alaska	6	0.2%	2	Missouri	274	7.8%
39	Arizona	12	0.3%	3	California	241	6.8%
17	Arkansas	70	2.0%	4	Illinois	209	5.9%
3	California	241	6.8%	5	Kansas	177	5.0%
33	Colorado	37	1.0%	6	Michigan	158	4.5%
47	Connecticut	0	0.0%	7	Florida	154	4.4%
47	Delaware	0	0.0%	8	Mississippi	141	4.0%
7	Florida	154	4.4%	9	Iowa	133	3.8%
15	Georgia	93	2.6%	10	Kentucky	118	3.3%
44	Hawaii	1	0.0%	11	Washington	111	3.1%
28	Idaho	45	1.3%	12	North Carolina	103	2.9%
4	Illinois	209	5.9%	13	Nebraska	99	2.8%
25	Indiana	53	1.5%	14	South Carolina	95	2.7%
9	Iowa	133	3.8%	15	Georgia	93	2.6%
5	Kansas	177	5.0%	16	Minnesota	73	2.1%
10	Kentucky	118	3.3%	17	Arkansas	70	2.0%
21	Louisiana	61	1.7%	18	West Virginia	68	1.9%
27	Maine	46	1.3%	19	Alabama	66	1.9%
47	Maryland	0	0.0%	20	North Dakota	62	1.8%
44	Massachusetts	1	0.0%	21	Louisiana	61	1.7%
6	Michigan	158	4.5%	22	Wisconsin	58	1.6%
16	Minnesota	73	2.1%	23	Virginia	56	1.6%
8	Mississippi	141	4.0%	24	South Dakota	55	1.6%
2	Missouri	274	7.8%	25	Indiana	53	1.5%
29	Montana	42	1.2%	25	Oregon	53	1.5%
13	Nebraska	99	2.8%	27	Maine	46	1.3%
42	Nevada	6	0.2%	28	Idaho	45	1.3%
36	New Hampshire	17	0.5%	29	Montana	42	1.2%
47	New Jersey	0	0.0%	30	Pennsylvania	41	1.2%
39	New Mexico	12	0.3%	30	Tennessee	41	1.2%
41	New York	9	0.3%	32	Oklahoma	40	1.1%
12	North Carolina	103	2.9%	33	Colorado	37	1.0%
20	North Dakota	62	1.8%	34	Vermont	19	0.5%
36	Ohio	17	0.5%	34	Wyoming	19	0.5%
32	Oklahoma	40	1.1%	36	New Hampshire	17	0.5%
25	Oregon	53	1.5%	36	Ohio	17	0.5%
30	Pennsylvania	41	1.2%	38	Utah	14	0.4%
44	Rhode Island	1	0.0%	39	Arizona	12	0.3%
14	South Carolina	95	2.7%	39	New Mexico	12	0.3%
24	South Dakota	55	1.6%	41	New York	9	0.3%
30	Tennessee	41	1.2%	42	Alaska	6	0.2%
1	Texas	328	9.3%	42	Nevada	6	0.2%
38	Utah	14	0.4%	44	Hawaii	1	0.0%
34	Vermont	19	0.5%	44	Massachusetts	1	0.0%
23	Virginia	56	1.6%	44	Rhode Island	1	0.0%
11	Washington	111	3.1%	47	Connecticut	0	0.0%
18	West Virginia	68	1.9%	47	Delaware	0	0.0%
22	Wisconsin	58	1.6%	47	Maryland	0	0.0%
34	Wyoming	19	0.5%	47	New Jersey	0	0.0%
					District of Columbia	0	0.0%

*Source: U.S. Department of Health and Human Services, Centers for Medicare and Medicaid Services
OSCAR Report 10 (January 10, 2005)*
*Certified by CMS to participate in the Medicare/Medicaid programs. Excludes licensed facilities that do not accept federal funding and facilities managed by the Department of Veterans Affairs. There are no certified rural health centers in U.S. territories.

Medicare and Medicaid Certified Home Health Agencies in 2005

National Total = 7,607 Home Health Agencies*

ALPHA ORDER

RANK	STATE	AGENCIES	% of USA
18	Alabama	141	1.9%
47	Alaska	16	0.2%
29	Arizona	67	0.9%
14	Arkansas	173	2.3%
2	California	621	8.2%
21	Colorado	130	1.7%
26	Connecticut	84	1.1%
48	Delaware	15	0.2%
3	Florida	536	7.0%
25	Georgia	98	1.3%
49	Hawaii	14	0.2%
37	Idaho	49	0.6%
5	Illinois	328	4.3%
12	Indiana	185	2.4%
13	Iowa	181	2.4%
20	Kansas	135	1.8%
24	Kentucky	105	1.4%
8	Louisiana	225	3.0%
43	Maine	30	0.4%
39	Maryland	48	0.6%
23	Massachusetts	119	1.6%
7	Michigan	244	3.2%
9	Minnesota	213	2.8%
34	Mississippi	59	0.8%
17	Missouri	155	2.0%
41	Montana	40	0.5%
28	Nebraska	68	0.9%
36	Nevada	50	0.7%
42	New Hampshire	35	0.5%
35	New Jersey	52	0.7%
31	New Mexico	61	0.8%
11	New York	192	2.5%
15	North Carolina	169	2.2%
45	North Dakota	26	0.3%
4	Ohio	384	5.0%
10	Oklahoma	195	2.6%
32	Oregon	60	0.8%
6	Pennsylvania	292	3.8%
46	Rhode Island	22	0.3%
27	South Carolina	69	0.9%
40	South Dakota	46	0.6%
19	Tennessee	138	1.8%
1	Texas	1,219	16.0%
37	Utah	49	0.6%
50	Vermont	12	0.2%
16	Virginia	164	2.2%
32	Washington	60	0.8%
30	West Virginia	63	0.8%
22	Wisconsin	122	1.6%
43	Wyoming	30	0.4%

RANK ORDER

RANK	STATE	AGENCIES	% of USA
1	Texas	1,219	16.0%
2	California	621	8.2%
3	Florida	536	7.0%
4	Ohio	384	5.0%
5	Illinois	328	4.3%
6	Pennsylvania	292	3.8%
7	Michigan	244	3.2%
8	Louisiana	225	3.0%
9	Minnesota	213	2.8%
10	Oklahoma	195	2.6%
11	New York	192	2.5%
12	Indiana	185	2.4%
13	Iowa	181	2.4%
14	Arkansas	173	2.3%
15	North Carolina	169	2.2%
16	Virginia	164	2.2%
17	Missouri	155	2.0%
18	Alabama	141	1.9%
19	Tennessee	138	1.8%
20	Kansas	135	1.8%
21	Colorado	130	1.7%
22	Wisconsin	122	1.6%
23	Massachusetts	119	1.6%
24	Kentucky	105	1.4%
25	Georgia	98	1.3%
26	Connecticut	84	1.1%
27	South Carolina	69	0.9%
28	Nebraska	68	0.9%
29	Arizona	67	0.9%
30	West Virginia	63	0.8%
31	New Mexico	61	0.8%
32	Oregon	60	0.8%
32	Washington	60	0.8%
34	Mississippi	59	0.8%
35	New Jersey	52	0.7%
36	Nevada	50	0.7%
37	Idaho	49	0.6%
37	Utah	49	0.6%
39	Maryland	48	0.6%
40	South Dakota	46	0.6%
41	Montana	40	0.5%
42	New Hampshire	35	0.5%
43	Maine	30	0.4%
43	Wyoming	30	0.4%
45	North Dakota	26	0.3%
46	Rhode Island	22	0.3%
47	Alaska	16	0.2%
48	Delaware	15	0.2%
49	Hawaii	14	0.2%
50	Vermont	12	0.2%
	District of Columbia	18	0.2%

Source: U.S. Department of Health and Human Services, Centers for Medicare and Medicaid Services
    OSCAR Report 10 (January 10, 2005)

*Certified by CMS to participate in the Medicare/Medicaid programs. Excludes agencies that do not accept federal funding. National total does not include 51 certified home health agencies in U.S. territories. A home health agency provides health services to individuals in their homes for the purpose of promoting, maintaining or restoring health or maximizing the level of independence, while minimizing the effects of disability and illness.

Medicare and Medicaid Certified Hospices in 2005

National Total = 2,611 Hospices*

ALPHA ORDER

RANK	STATE	HOSPICES	% of USA
5	Alabama	106	4.1%
50	Alaska	3	0.1%
29	Arizona	39	1.5%
21	Arkansas	49	1.9%
2	California	175	6.7%
27	Colorado	41	1.6%
37	Connecticut	26	1.0%
49	Delaware	6	0.2%
28	Florida	40	1.5%
8	Georgia	91	3.5%
47	Hawaii	7	0.3%
35	Idaho	27	1.0%
6	Illinois	96	3.7%
11	Indiana	76	2.9%
15	Iowa	64	2.5%
22	Kansas	47	1.8%
35	Kentucky	27	1.0%
13	Louisiana	73	2.8%
41	Maine	18	0.7%
34	Maryland	28	1.1%
25	Massachusetts	44	1.7%
9	Michigan	87	3.3%
16	Minnesota	60	2.3%
14	Mississippi	69	2.6%
12	Missouri	75	2.9%
38	Montana	24	0.9%
33	Nebraska	30	1.1%
45	Nevada	11	0.4%
40	New Hampshire	19	0.7%
23	New Jersey	46	1.8%
29	New Mexico	39	1.5%
18	New York	54	2.1%
10	North Carolina	79	3.0%
43	North Dakota	15	0.6%
7	Ohio	92	3.5%
4	Oklahoma	124	4.7%
25	Oregon	44	1.7%
3	Pennsylvania	128	4.9%
47	Rhode Island	7	0.3%
24	South Carolina	45	1.7%
43	South Dakota	15	0.6%
19	Tennessee	51	2.0%
1	Texas	190	7.3%
31	Utah	36	1.4%
46	Vermont	10	0.4%
17	Virginia	58	2.2%
32	Washington	31	1.2%
39	West Virginia	20	0.8%
19	Wisconsin	51	2.0%
42	Wyoming	16	0.6%

RANK ORDER

RANK	STATE	HOSPICES	% of USA
1	Texas	190	7.3%
2	California	175	6.7%
3	Pennsylvania	128	4.9%
4	Oklahoma	124	4.7%
5	Alabama	106	4.1%
6	Illinois	96	3.7%
7	Ohio	92	3.5%
8	Georgia	91	3.5%
9	Michigan	87	3.3%
10	North Carolina	79	3.0%
11	Indiana	76	2.9%
12	Missouri	75	2.9%
13	Louisiana	73	2.8%
14	Mississippi	69	2.6%
15	Iowa	64	2.5%
16	Minnesota	60	2.3%
17	Virginia	58	2.2%
18	New York	54	2.1%
19	Tennessee	51	2.0%
19	Wisconsin	51	2.0%
21	Arkansas	49	1.9%
22	Kansas	47	1.8%
23	New Jersey	46	1.8%
24	South Carolina	45	1.7%
25	Massachusetts	44	1.7%
25	Oregon	44	1.7%
27	Colorado	41	1.6%
28	Florida	40	1.5%
29	Arizona	39	1.5%
29	New Mexico	39	1.5%
31	Utah	36	1.4%
32	Washington	31	1.2%
33	Nebraska	30	1.1%
34	Maryland	28	1.1%
35	Idaho	27	1.0%
35	Kentucky	27	1.0%
37	Connecticut	26	1.0%
38	Montana	24	0.9%
39	West Virginia	20	0.8%
40	New Hampshire	19	0.7%
41	Maine	18	0.7%
42	Wyoming	16	0.6%
43	North Dakota	15	0.6%
43	South Dakota	15	0.6%
45	Nevada	11	0.4%
46	Vermont	10	0.4%
47	Hawaii	7	0.3%
47	Rhode Island	7	0.3%
49	Delaware	6	0.2%
50	Alaska	3	0.1%
	District of Columbia	2	0.1%

Source: U.S. Department of Health and Human Services, Centers for Medicare and Medicaid Services
  OSCAR Report 10 (January 10, 2005)
*Certified by CMS to participate in the Medicare/Medicaid programs. Excludes licensed facilities that do not accept federal funding and facilities managed by the Department of Veterans Affairs. National total does not include 36 certified hospices in U.S. territories. An hospice provides specialized services for terminally ill people and their families.

218

Hospice Patients in Residential Facilities in 2005

National Total = 41,476 Patients*

ALPHA ORDER

RANK	STATE	PATIENTS	% of USA
23	Alabama	459	1.1%
50	Alaska	3	0.0%
24	Arizona	431	1.0%
30	Arkansas	308	0.7%
5	California	2,329	5.6%
19	Colorado	664	1.6%
31	Connecticut	244	0.6%
48	Delaware	8	0.0%
1	Florida	7,003	16.9%
9	Georgia	1,289	3.1%
39	Hawaii	51	0.1%
43	Idaho	47	0.1%
13	Illinois	965	2.3%
10	Indiana	1,097	2.6%
17	Iowa	721	1.7%
25	Kansas	425	1.0%
12	Kentucky	988	2.4%
28	Louisiana	346	0.8%
40	Maine	50	0.1%
32	Maryland	242	0.6%
18	Massachusetts	668	1.6%
7	Michigan	1,485	3.6%
20	Minnesota	610	1.5%
34	Mississippi	192	0.5%
8	Missouri	1,295	3.1%
42	Montana	48	0.1%
15	Nebraska	812	2.0%
35	Nevada	140	0.3%
44	New Hampshire	43	0.1%
22	New Jersey	481	1.2%
36	New Mexico	114	0.3%
11	New York	1,071	2.6%
14	North Carolina	874	2.1%
38	North Dakota	61	0.1%
4	Ohio	2,730	6.6%
6	Oklahoma	1,681	4.1%
16	Oregon	773	1.9%
3	Pennsylvania	4,328	10.4%
49	Rhode Island	6	0.0%
29	South Carolina	320	0.8%
47	South Dakota	17	0.0%
33	Tennessee	213	0.5%
2	Texas	4,408	10.6%
26	Utah	352	0.8%
45	Vermont	34	0.1%
41	Virginia	49	0.1%
27	Washington	351	0.8%
37	West Virginia	68	0.2%
21	Wisconsin	518	1.2%
46	Wyoming	18	0.0%

RANK ORDER

RANK	STATE	PATIENTS	% of USA
1	Florida	7,003	16.9%
2	Texas	4,408	10.6%
3	Pennsylvania	4,328	10.4%
4	Ohio	2,730	6.6%
5	California	2,329	5.6%
6	Oklahoma	1,681	4.1%
7	Michigan	1,485	3.6%
8	Missouri	1,295	3.1%
9	Georgia	1,289	3.1%
10	Indiana	1,097	2.6%
11	New York	1,071	2.6%
12	Kentucky	988	2.4%
13	Illinois	965	2.3%
14	North Carolina	874	2.1%
15	Nebraska	812	2.0%
16	Oregon	773	1.9%
17	Iowa	721	1.7%
18	Massachusetts	668	1.6%
19	Colorado	664	1.6%
20	Minnesota	610	1.5%
21	Wisconsin	518	1.2%
22	New Jersey	481	1.2%
23	Alabama	459	1.1%
24	Arizona	431	1.0%
25	Kansas	425	1.0%
26	Utah	352	0.8%
27	Washington	351	0.8%
28	Louisiana	346	0.8%
29	South Carolina	320	0.8%
30	Arkansas	308	0.7%
31	Connecticut	244	0.6%
32	Maryland	242	0.6%
33	Tennessee	213	0.5%
34	Mississippi	192	0.5%
35	Nevada	140	0.3%
36	New Mexico	114	0.3%
37	West Virginia	68	0.2%
38	North Dakota	61	0.1%
39	Hawaii	51	0.1%
40	Maine	50	0.1%
41	Virginia	49	0.1%
42	Montana	48	0.1%
43	Idaho	47	0.1%
44	New Hampshire	43	0.1%
45	Vermont	34	0.1%
46	Wyoming	18	0.0%
47	South Dakota	17	0.0%
48	Delaware	8	0.0%
49	Rhode Island	6	0.0%
50	Alaska	3	0.0%
	District of Columbia	46	0.1%

Source: U.S. Department of Health and Human Services, Centers for Medicare and Medicaid Services
    OSCAR Database (January 10, 2005)
*Patients in facilities certified by CMS to participate in the Medicare/Medicaid programs. Excludes licensed
facilities that do not accept federal funding and facilities managed by the Department of Veterans Affairs. National
total does not include 52 patients in U.S. territories. An hospice provides specialized services for terminally ill
people and their families.

Medicare and Medicaid Certified Nursing Care Facilities in 2005

National Total = 16,139 Nursing Care Facilities*

ALPHA ORDER

RANK	STATE	FACILITIES	% of USA
28	Alabama	228	1.4%
50	Alaska	14	0.1%
34	Arizona	134	0.8%
27	Arkansas	237	1.5%
1	California	1,311	8.1%
30	Colorado	215	1.3%
25	Connecticut	246	1.5%
47	Delaware	42	0.3%
6	Florida	690	4.3%
18	Georgia	362	2.2%
45	Hawaii	45	0.3%
43	Idaho	80	0.5%
4	Illinois	818	5.1%
9	Indiana	511	3.2%
11	Iowa	458	2.8%
16	Kansas	369	2.3%
22	Kentucky	295	1.8%
21	Louisiana	308	1.9%
36	Maine	117	0.7%
26	Maryland	241	1.5%
10	Massachusetts	475	2.9%
12	Michigan	430	2.7%
14	Minnesota	415	2.6%
31	Mississippi	205	1.3%
8	Missouri	524	3.2%
38	Montana	101	0.6%
29	Nebraska	227	1.4%
46	Nevada	43	0.3%
42	New Hampshire	81	0.5%
19	New Jersey	357	2.2%
43	New Mexico	80	0.5%
7	New York	661	4.1%
13	North Carolina	422	2.6%
41	North Dakota	83	0.5%
3	Ohio	980	6.1%
17	Oklahoma	365	2.3%
33	Oregon	138	0.9%
5	Pennsylvania	725	4.5%
39	Rhode Island	95	0.6%
32	South Carolina	177	1.1%
37	South Dakota	112	0.7%
20	Tennessee	333	2.1%
2	Texas	1,137	7.0%
40	Utah	90	0.6%
48	Vermont	41	0.3%
23	Virginia	280	1.7%
24	Washington	249	1.5%
35	West Virginia	133	0.8%
15	Wisconsin	400	2.5%
49	Wyoming	39	0.2%

RANK ORDER

RANK	STATE	FACILITIES	% of USA
1	California	1,311	8.1%
2	Texas	1,137	7.0%
3	Ohio	980	6.1%
4	Illinois	818	5.1%
5	Pennsylvania	725	4.5%
6	Florida	690	4.3%
7	New York	661	4.1%
8	Missouri	524	3.2%
9	Indiana	511	3.2%
10	Massachusetts	475	2.9%
11	Iowa	458	2.8%
12	Michigan	430	2.7%
13	North Carolina	422	2.6%
14	Minnesota	415	2.6%
15	Wisconsin	400	2.5%
16	Kansas	369	2.3%
17	Oklahoma	365	2.3%
18	Georgia	362	2.2%
19	New Jersey	357	2.2%
20	Tennessee	333	2.1%
21	Louisiana	308	1.9%
22	Kentucky	295	1.8%
23	Virginia	280	1.7%
24	Washington	249	1.5%
25	Connecticut	246	1.5%
26	Maryland	241	1.5%
27	Arkansas	237	1.5%
28	Alabama	228	1.4%
29	Nebraska	227	1.4%
30	Colorado	215	1.3%
31	Mississippi	205	1.3%
32	South Carolina	177	1.1%
33	Oregon	138	0.9%
34	Arizona	134	0.8%
35	West Virginia	133	0.8%
36	Maine	117	0.7%
37	South Dakota	112	0.7%
38	Montana	101	0.6%
39	Rhode Island	95	0.6%
40	Utah	90	0.6%
41	North Dakota	83	0.5%
42	New Hampshire	81	0.5%
43	Idaho	80	0.5%
43	New Mexico	80	0.5%
45	Hawaii	45	0.3%
46	Nevada	43	0.3%
47	Delaware	42	0.3%
48	Vermont	41	0.3%
49	Wyoming	39	0.2%
50	Alaska	14	0.1%
	District of Columbia	20	0.1%

*Source: U.S. Department of Health and Human Services, Centers for Medicare and Medicaid Services
OSCAR Database (January 10, 2005)*

Certified by CMS to participate in the Medicare/Medicaid programs. Excludes licensed facilities that do not accept federal funding and facilities managed by the Department of Veterans Affairs. National total does not include eight certified nursing facilities in U.S. territories.

Beds in Medicare and Medicaid Certified Nursing Care Facilities in 2005

National Total = 1,687,342 Beds*

ALPHA ORDER

RANK	STATE	BEDS	% of USA
24	Alabama	26,476	1.6%
50	Alaska	718	0.0%
32	Arizona	16,097	1.0%
27	Arkansas	23,829	1.4%
1	California	124,046	7.4%
29	Colorado	19,859	1.2%
22	Connecticut	30,280	1.8%
46	Delaware	4,320	0.3%
7	Florida	82,011	4.9%
14	Georgia	40,074	2.4%
47	Hawaii	4,026	0.2%
44	Idaho	6,188	0.4%
4	Illinois	98,660	5.8%
11	Indiana	48,041	2.8%
19	Iowa	33,393	2.0%
26	Kansas	24,281	1.4%
25	Kentucky	25,543	1.5%
16	Louisiana	37,859	2.2%
39	Maine	7,505	0.4%
23	Maryland	29,197	1.7%
8	Massachusetts	51,324	3.0%
12	Michigan	47,138	2.8%
17	Minnesota	37,715	2.2%
30	Mississippi	18,350	1.1%
10	Missouri	50,376	3.0%
40	Montana	7,447	0.4%
33	Nebraska	15,790	0.9%
45	Nevada	5,102	0.3%
37	New Hampshire	7,745	0.5%
9	New Jersey	50,605	3.0%
41	New Mexico	7,341	0.4%
2	New York	121,254	7.2%
13	North Carolina	42,942	2.5%
43	North Dakota	6,529	0.4%
5	Ohio	92,395	5.5%
20	Oklahoma	32,476	1.9%
34	Oregon	12,634	0.7%
6	Pennsylvania	89,271	5.3%
36	Rhode Island	9,368	0.6%
31	South Carolina	17,770	1.1%
42	South Dakota	7,253	0.4%
18	Tennessee	37,314	2.2%
3	Texas	115,181	6.8%
38	Utah	7,558	0.4%
48	Vermont	3,441	0.2%
21	Virginia	31,181	1.8%
28	Washington	22,565	1.3%
35	West Virginia	10,974	0.7%
15	Wisconsin	39,804	2.4%
49	Wyoming	3,061	0.2%

RANK ORDER

RANK	STATE	BEDS	% of USA
1	California	124,046	7.4%
2	New York	121,254	7.2%
3	Texas	115,181	6.8%
4	Illinois	98,660	5.8%
5	Ohio	92,395	5.5%
6	Pennsylvania	89,271	5.3%
7	Florida	82,011	4.9%
8	Massachusetts	51,324	3.0%
9	New Jersey	50,605	3.0%
10	Missouri	50,376	3.0%
11	Indiana	48,041	2.8%
12	Michigan	47,138	2.8%
13	North Carolina	42,942	2.5%
14	Georgia	40,074	2.4%
15	Wisconsin	39,804	2.4%
16	Louisiana	37,859	2.2%
17	Minnesota	37,715	2.2%
18	Tennessee	37,314	2.2%
19	Iowa	33,393	2.0%
20	Oklahoma	32,476	1.9%
21	Virginia	31,181	1.8%
22	Connecticut	30,280	1.8%
23	Maryland	29,197	1.7%
24	Alabama	26,476	1.6%
25	Kentucky	25,543	1.5%
26	Kansas	24,281	1.4%
27	Arkansas	23,829	1.4%
28	Washington	22,565	1.3%
29	Colorado	19,859	1.2%
30	Mississippi	18,350	1.1%
31	South Carolina	17,770	1.1%
32	Arizona	16,097	1.0%
33	Nebraska	15,790	0.9%
34	Oregon	12,634	0.7%
35	West Virginia	10,974	0.7%
36	Rhode Island	9,368	0.6%
37	New Hampshire	7,745	0.5%
38	Utah	7,558	0.4%
39	Maine	7,505	0.4%
40	Montana	7,447	0.4%
41	New Mexico	7,341	0.4%
42	South Dakota	7,253	0.4%
43	North Dakota	6,529	0.4%
44	Idaho	6,188	0.4%
45	Nevada	5,102	0.3%
46	Delaware	4,320	0.3%
47	Hawaii	4,026	0.2%
48	Vermont	3,441	0.2%
49	Wyoming	3,061	0.2%
50	Alaska	718	0.0%
	District of Columbia	3,035	0.2%

Source: U.S. Department of Health and Human Services, Centers for Medicare and Medicaid Services
    OSCAR Database (January 10, 2005)

*Beds in nursing care facilities certified by CMS to participate in the Medicare/Medicaid programs. National total does not include 349 beds in U.S. territories.

Rate of Beds in Medicare and Medicaid Certified Nursing Care Facilities in 2005

National Rate = 350 Beds per 1,000 Population 85 Years and Older*

ALPHA ORDER

RANK	STATE	RATE
27	Alabama	368
47	Alaska	211
48	Arizona	198
4	Arkansas	481
43	California	252
28	Colorado	363
19	Connecticut	408
31	Delaware	345
46	Florida	220
18	Georgia	411
50	Hawaii	172
40	Idaho	291
8	Illinois	465
5	Indiana	473
5	Iowa	473
10	Kansas	440
16	Kentucky	412
1	Louisiana	607
39	Maine	296
24	Maryland	375
21	Massachusetts	399
41	Michigan	290
23	Minnesota	394
14	Mississippi	417
3	Missouri	484
13	Montana	424
11	Nebraska	435
45	Nevada	230
24	New Hampshire	375
33	New Jersey	330
42	New Mexico	276
30	New York	351
29	North Carolina	361
20	North Dakota	404
7	Ohio	468
2	Oklahoma	547
49	Oregon	190
32	Pennsylvania	334
22	Rhode Island	397
37	South Carolina	303
15	South Dakota	416
12	Tennessee	425
9	Texas	450
37	Utah	303
36	Vermont	306
35	Virginia	312
44	Washington	231
34	West Virginia	327
26	Wisconsin	373
16	Wyoming	412

RANK ORDER

RANK	STATE	RATE
1	Louisiana	607
2	Oklahoma	547
3	Missouri	484
4	Arkansas	481
5	Indiana	473
5	Iowa	473
7	Ohio	468
8	Illinois	465
9	Texas	450
10	Kansas	440
11	Nebraska	435
12	Tennessee	425
13	Montana	424
14	Mississippi	417
15	South Dakota	416
16	Kentucky	412
16	Wyoming	412
18	Georgia	411
19	Connecticut	408
20	North Dakota	404
21	Massachusetts	399
22	Rhode Island	397
23	Minnesota	394
24	Maryland	375
24	New Hampshire	375
26	Wisconsin	373
27	Alabama	368
28	Colorado	363
29	North Carolina	361
30	New York	351
31	Delaware	345
32	Pennsylvania	334
33	New Jersey	330
34	West Virginia	327
35	Virginia	312
36	Vermont	306
37	South Carolina	303
37	Utah	303
39	Maine	296
40	Idaho	291
41	Michigan	290
42	New Mexico	276
43	California	252
44	Washington	231
45	Nevada	230
46	Florida	220
47	Alaska	211
48	Arizona	198
49	Oregon	190
50	Hawaii	172

| | District of Columbia | 321 |

Source: MQ Press using data from U.S. Dept of Health & Human Services, Centers for Medicare and Medicaid Services
OSCAR Database (January 10, 2005)
*Beds in nursing care facilities certified by CMS to participate in the Medicare/Medicaid programs. National rate does not include beds or population in U.S. territories. Calculated using 2003 Census population estimate.

Nursing Home Occupancy Rate in 2002

National Rate = 82.4% of Beds in Nursing Homes Occupied

RANK	STATE	RATE
10	Alabama	90.3
35	Alaska	79.4
35	Arizona	79.4
45	Arkansas	72.1
32	California	81.6
33	Colorado	80.3
6	Connecticut	91.9
28	Delaware	83.7
23	Florida	85.6
7	Georgia	91.2
2	Hawaii	93.6
43	Idaho	75.5
44	Illinois	74.7
42	Indiana	76.1
38	Iowa	77.8
37	Kansas	79.0
16	Kentucky	88.7
39	Louisiana	77.3
8	Maine	90.7
21	Maryland	86.8
14	Massachusetts	89.4
26	Michigan	84.3
4	Minnesota	92.2
17	Mississippi	88.2
49	Missouri	69.2
39	Montana	77.3
29	Nebraska	82.7
34	Nevada	79.9
10	New Hampshire	90.3
22	New Jersey	86.7
27	New Mexico	84.1
3	New York	93.0
18	North Carolina	88.0
1	North Dakota	94.1
41	Ohio	76.6
50	Oklahoma	68.4
48	Oregon	70.2
18	Pennsylvania	88.0
20	Rhode Island	87.9
15	South Carolina	89.2
5	South Dakota	92.1
13	Tennessee	89.5
47	Texas	70.3
45	Utah	72.1
9	Vermont	90.5
25	Virginia	84.5
30	Washington	82.5
12	West Virginia	90.2
24	Wisconsin	84.6
31	Wyoming	82.3

RANK	STATE	RATE
1	North Dakota	94.1
2	Hawaii	93.6
3	New York	93.0
4	Minnesota	92.2
5	South Dakota	92.1
6	Connecticut	91.9
7	Georgia	91.2
8	Maine	90.7
9	Vermont	90.5
10	Alabama	90.3
10	New Hampshire	90.3
12	West Virginia	90.2
13	Tennessee	89.5
14	Massachusetts	89.4
15	South Carolina	89.2
16	Kentucky	88.7
17	Mississippi	88.2
18	North Carolina	88.0
18	Pennsylvania	88.0
20	Rhode Island	87.9
21	Maryland	86.8
22	New Jersey	86.7
23	Florida	85.6
24	Wisconsin	84.6
25	Virginia	84.5
26	Michigan	84.3
27	New Mexico	84.1
28	Delaware	83.7
29	Nebraska	82.7
30	Washington	82.5
31	Wyoming	82.3
32	California	81.6
33	Colorado	80.3
34	Nevada	79.9
35	Alaska	79.4
35	Arizona	79.4
37	Kansas	79.0
38	Iowa	77.8
39	Louisiana	77.3
39	Montana	77.3
41	Ohio	76.6
42	Indiana	76.1
43	Idaho	75.5
44	Illinois	74.7
45	Arkansas	72.1
45	Utah	72.1
47	Texas	70.3
48	Oregon	70.2
49	Missouri	69.2
50	Oklahoma	68.4
	District of Columbia	90.5

Source: U.S. Department of Health and Human Services, Centers for Medicare and Medicaid Services
"Health, United States, 2004"

Nursing Home Resident Rate in 2002

National Rate = 317.5 Residents per 1,000 Population Age 85 and Older*

ALPHA ORDER

RANK	STATE	RATE
29	Alabama	331.8
45	Alaska	211.2
49	Arizona	169.1
17	Arkansas	371.3
42	California	226.0
32	Colorado	307.9
5	Connecticut	410.0
27	Delaware	333.5
47	Florida	196.4
16	Georgia	379.9
48	Hawaii	185.7
41	Idaho	242.6
11	Illinois	392.3
4	Indiana	416.9
3	Iowa	419.1
13	Kansas	391.7
18	Kentucky	371.1
1	Louisiana	483.5
38	Maine	279.5
24	Maryland	348.4
14	Massachusetts	385.8
39	Michigan	266.5
6	Minnesota	407.9
22	Mississippi	356.4
19	Missouri	367.4
23	Montana	351.0
9	Nebraska	396.4
46	Nevada	203.9
21	New Hampshire	356.6
35	New Jersey	299.5
40	New Mexico	243.5
26	New York	337.1
30	North Carolina	322.6
8	North Dakota	401.1
2	Ohio	422.6
15	Oklahoma	383.2
50	Oregon	143.2
31	Pennsylvania	318.4
10	Rhode Island	392.4
36	South Carolina	291.7
7	South Dakota	404.1
12	Tennessee	392.1
28	Texas	332.5
43	Utah	224.2
34	Vermont	304.5
37	Virginia	283.8
44	Washington	219.8
33	West Virginia	305.1
20	Wisconsin	359.6
25	Wyoming	346.2

RANK ORDER

RANK	STATE	RATE
1	Louisiana	483.5
2	Ohio	422.6
3	Iowa	419.1
4	Indiana	416.9
5	Connecticut	410.0
6	Minnesota	407.9
7	South Dakota	404.1
8	North Dakota	401.1
9	Nebraska	396.4
10	Rhode Island	392.4
11	Illinois	392.3
12	Tennessee	392.1
13	Kansas	391.7
14	Massachusetts	385.8
15	Oklahoma	383.2
16	Georgia	379.9
17	Arkansas	371.3
18	Kentucky	371.1
19	Missouri	367.4
20	Wisconsin	359.6
21	New Hampshire	356.6
22	Mississippi	356.4
23	Montana	351.0
24	Maryland	348.4
25	Wyoming	346.2
26	New York	337.1
27	Delaware	333.5
28	Texas	332.5
29	Alabama	331.8
30	North Carolina	322.6
31	Pennsylvania	318.4
32	Colorado	307.9
33	West Virginia	305.1
34	Vermont	304.5
35	New Jersey	299.5
36	South Carolina	291.7
37	Virginia	283.8
38	Maine	279.5
39	Michigan	266.5
40	New Mexico	243.5
41	Idaho	242.6
42	California	226.0
43	Utah	224.2
44	Washington	219.8
45	Alaska	211.2
46	Nevada	203.9
47	Florida	196.4
48	Hawaii	185.7
49	Arizona	169.1
50	Oregon	143.2

| | District of Columbia | 298.9 |

Source: U.S. Department of Health and Human Services, Centers for Medicare and Medicaid Services
    "Health, United States, 2004"
*Number of nursing home residents (all ages) per 1,000 resident population 85 years of age and over.

Nursing Home Population in 2002

National Total = 1,458,236

ALPHA ORDER

RANK	STATE	POPULATION	% of USA
23	Alabama	23,705	1.6%
50	Alaska	649	0.0%
33	Arizona	13,115	0.9%
28	Arkansas	18,179	1.2%
2	California	106,384	7.3%
29	Colorado	16,351	1.1%
19	Connecticut	28,734	2.0%
46	Delaware	3,942	0.3%
7	Florida	70,761	4.9%
16	Georgia	36,337	2.5%
47	Hawaii	3,780	0.3%
44	Idaho	4,780	0.3%
5	Illinois	81,147	5.6%
11	Indiana	40,988	2.8%
20	Iowa	28,720	2.0%
26	Kansas	21,117	1.4%
24	Kentucky	22,741	1.6%
18	Louisiana	29,674	2.0%
38	Maine	6,995	0.5%
22	Maryland	25,621	1.8%
8	Massachusetts	48,304	3.3%
10	Michigan	41,541	2.8%
13	Minnesota	37,374	2.6%
31	Mississippi	15,872	1.1%
12	Missouri	37,831	2.6%
42	Montana	5,815	0.4%
32	Nebraska	14,082	1.0%
45	Nevada	4,182	0.3%
37	New Hampshire	7,120	0.5%
9	New Jersey	44,605	3.1%
40	New Mexico	6,286	0.4%
1	New York	113,628	7.8%
14	North Carolina	37,278	2.6%
41	North Dakota	6,234	0.4%
6	Ohio	80,677	5.5%
25	Oklahoma	22,350	1.5%
35	Oregon	9,065	0.6%
4	Pennsylvania	82,411	5.7%
36	Rhode Island	8,910	0.6%
30	South Carolina	16,117	1.1%
39	South Dakota	6,878	0.5%
17	Tennessee	34,051	2.3%
3	Texas	84,980	5.8%
43	Utah	5,399	0.4%
48	Vermont	3,279	0.2%
21	Virginia	27,199	1.9%
27	Washington	20,461	1.4%
34	West Virginia	10,157	0.7%
15	Wisconsin	37,095	2.5%
49	Wyoming	2,518	0.2%

RANK ORDER

RANK	STATE	POPULATION	% of USA
1	New York	113,628	7.8%
2	California	106,384	7.3%
3	Texas	84,980	5.8%
4	Pennsylvania	82,411	5.7%
5	Illinois	81,147	5.6%
6	Ohio	80,677	5.5%
7	Florida	70,761	4.9%
8	Massachusetts	48,304	3.3%
9	New Jersey	44,605	3.1%
10	Michigan	41,541	2.8%
11	Indiana	40,988	2.8%
12	Missouri	37,831	2.6%
13	Minnesota	37,374	2.6%
14	North Carolina	37,278	2.6%
15	Wisconsin	37,095	2.5%
16	Georgia	36,337	2.5%
17	Tennessee	34,051	2.3%
18	Louisiana	29,674	2.0%
19	Connecticut	28,734	2.0%
20	Iowa	28,720	2.0%
21	Virginia	27,199	1.9%
22	Maryland	25,621	1.8%
23	Alabama	23,705	1.6%
24	Kentucky	22,741	1.6%
25	Oklahoma	22,350	1.5%
26	Kansas	21,117	1.4%
27	Washington	20,461	1.4%
28	Arkansas	18,179	1.2%
29	Colorado	16,351	1.1%
30	South Carolina	16,117	1.1%
31	Mississippi	15,872	1.1%
32	Nebraska	14,082	1.0%
33	Arizona	13,115	0.9%
34	West Virginia	10,157	0.7%
35	Oregon	9,065	0.6%
36	Rhode Island	8,910	0.6%
37	New Hampshire	7,120	0.5%
38	Maine	6,995	0.5%
39	South Dakota	6,878	0.5%
40	New Mexico	6,286	0.4%
41	North Dakota	6,234	0.4%
42	Montana	5,815	0.4%
43	Utah	5,399	0.4%
44	Idaho	4,780	0.3%
45	Nevada	4,182	0.3%
46	Delaware	3,942	0.3%
47	Hawaii	3,780	0.3%
48	Vermont	3,279	0.2%
49	Wyoming	2,518	0.2%
50	Alaska	649	0.0%
	District of Columbia	2,817	0.2%

Source: U.S. Department of Health and Human Services, Centers for Medicare and Medicaid Services
"Health, United States, 2004"

Health Care Establishments in 2002

National Total = 563,216 Establishments*

ALPHA ORDER

RANK	STATE	ESTABLISH'S	% of USA
27	Alabama	7,281	1.3%
48	Alaska	1,354	0.2%
19	Arizona	10,192	1.8%
32	Arkansas	4,967	0.9%
1	California	72,583	12.9%
21	Colorado	9,353	1.7%
26	Connecticut	7,567	1.3%
45	Delaware	1,556	0.3%
4	Florida	37,751	6.7%
10	Georgia	14,383	2.6%
41	Hawaii	2,644	0.5%
40	Idaho	2,756	0.5%
6	Illinois	22,665	4.0%
17	Indiana	10,604	1.9%
30	Iowa	5,470	1.0%
31	Kansas	5,321	0.9%
25	Kentucky	7,583	1.3%
23	Louisiana	8,481	1.5%
39	Maine	3,124	0.6%
15	Maryland	11,375	2.0%
12	Massachusetts	13,346	2.4%
9	Michigan	19,842	3.5%
22	Minnesota	9,244	1.6%
34	Mississippi	4,144	0.7%
16	Missouri	10,641	1.9%
44	Montana	2,123	0.4%
37	Nebraska	3,207	0.6%
35	Nevada	3,950	0.7%
43	New Hampshire	2,295	0.4%
8	New Jersey	19,851	3.5%
38	New Mexico	3,153	0.6%
2	New York	40,692	7.2%
11	North Carolina	13,672	2.4%
49	North Dakota	1,148	0.2%
7	Ohio	21,562	3.8%
28	Oklahoma	6,965	1.2%
24	Oregon	7,964	1.4%
5	Pennsylvania	26,209	4.7%
42	Rhode Island	2,395	0.4%
29	South Carolina	6,595	1.2%
46	South Dakota	1,477	0.3%
18	Tennessee	10,359	1.8%
3	Texas	38,777	6.9%
33	Utah	4,453	0.8%
47	Vermont	1,384	0.2%
14	Virginia	12,228	2.2%
13	Washington	12,308	2.2%
36	West Virginia	3,697	0.7%
20	Wisconsin	9,900	1.8%
50	Wyoming	1,118	0.2%

RANK ORDER

RANK	STATE	ESTABLISH'S	% of USA
1	California	72,583	12.9%
2	New York	40,692	7.2%
3	Texas	38,777	6.9%
4	Florida	37,751	6.7%
5	Pennsylvania	26,209	4.7%
6	Illinois	22,665	4.0%
7	Ohio	21,562	3.8%
8	New Jersey	19,851	3.5%
9	Michigan	19,842	3.5%
10	Georgia	14,383	2.6%
11	North Carolina	13,672	2.4%
12	Massachusetts	13,346	2.4%
13	Washington	12,308	2.2%
14	Virginia	12,228	2.2%
15	Maryland	11,375	2.0%
16	Missouri	10,641	1.9%
17	Indiana	10,604	1.9%
18	Tennessee	10,359	1.8%
19	Arizona	10,192	1.8%
20	Wisconsin	9,900	1.8%
21	Colorado	9,353	1.7%
22	Minnesota	9,244	1.6%
23	Louisiana	8,481	1.5%
24	Oregon	7,964	1.4%
25	Kentucky	7,583	1.3%
26	Connecticut	7,567	1.3%
27	Alabama	7,281	1.3%
28	Oklahoma	6,965	1.2%
29	South Carolina	6,595	1.2%
30	Iowa	5,470	1.0%
31	Kansas	5,321	0.9%
32	Arkansas	4,967	0.9%
33	Utah	4,453	0.8%
34	Mississippi	4,144	0.7%
35	Nevada	3,950	0.7%
36	West Virginia	3,697	0.7%
37	Nebraska	3,207	0.6%
38	New Mexico	3,153	0.6%
39	Maine	3,124	0.6%
40	Idaho	2,756	0.5%
41	Hawaii	2,644	0.5%
42	Rhode Island	2,395	0.4%
43	New Hampshire	2,295	0.4%
44	Montana	2,123	0.4%
45	Delaware	1,556	0.3%
46	South Dakota	1,477	0.3%
47	Vermont	1,384	0.2%
48	Alaska	1,354	0.2%
49	North Dakota	1,148	0.2%
50	Wyoming	1,118	0.2%
	District of Columbia	1,507	0.3%

Source: U.S. Bureau of the Census
"County Business Patterns 2002 (NAICS)" (http://censtats.census.gov/cbpnaic/cbpnaic.shtml)
*Includes establishments exempt from as well as subject to the federal income tax. Includes those establishments within the North American Industry Classification System (NAICS) classifications 621 (ambulatory health care services), 622 (hospitals) and 623 (nursing and residential care facilities).

IV. FINANCE

IV. FINANCE (Continued)

Average Medical Malpractice Payment in 2003

National Average = $294,814*

ALPHA ORDER

RANK	STATE	AVERAGE PAYMENT
5	Alabama	$389,028
21	Alaska	314,513
24	Arizona	301,293
7	Arkansas	378,643
46	California	176,986
36	Colorado	243,632
3	Connecticut	483,502
37	Delaware	238,781
19	Florida	315,272
9	Georgia	370,072
1	Hawaii	499,300
26	Idaho	276,723
2	Illinois	499,197
25	Indiana**	295,708
38	Iowa	237,750
44	Kansas**	185,452
40	Kentucky	214,632
45	Louisiana**	180,794
32	Maine	254,131
16	Maryland	331,070
4	Massachusetts	409,321
49	Michigan	134,405
15	Minnesota	331,746
27	Mississippi	273,715
33	Missouri	252,833
11	Montana	346,396
43	Nebraska**	192,058
8	Nevada	377,439
35	New Hampshire	248,806
17	New Jersey	326,101
47	New Mexico**	149,847
6	New York	387,228
14	North Carolina	331,776
42	North Dakota	195,812
12	Ohio	344,650
10	Oklahoma	347,800
20	Oregon	314,668
22	Pennsylvania**	306,538
13	Rhode Island	333,387
34	South Carolina**	250,062
30	South Dakota	259,597
28	Tennessee	269,737
39	Texas	229,314
50	Utah	125,099
48	Vermont	137,444
23	Virginia	306,413
29	Washington	269,730
18	West Virginia	322,646
31	Wisconsin**	257,536
41	Wyoming	203,155

RANK ORDER

RANK	STATE	AVERAGE PAYMENT
1	Hawaii	$499,300
2	Illinois	499,197
3	Connecticut	483,502
4	Massachusetts	409,321
5	Alabama	389,028
6	New York	387,228
7	Arkansas	378,643
8	Nevada	377,439
9	Georgia	370,072
10	Oklahoma	347,800
11	Montana	346,396
12	Ohio	344,650
13	Rhode Island	333,387
14	North Carolina	331,776
15	Minnesota	331,746
16	Maryland	331,070
17	New Jersey	326,101
18	West Virginia	322,646
19	Florida	315,272
20	Oregon	314,668
21	Alaska	314,513
22	Pennsylvania**	306,538
23	Virginia	306,413
24	Arizona	301,293
25	Indiana**	295,708
26	Idaho	276,723
27	Mississippi	273,715
28	Tennessee	269,737
29	Washington	269,730
30	South Dakota	259,597
31	Wisconsin**	257,536
32	Maine	254,131
33	Missouri	252,833
34	South Carolina**	250,062
35	New Hampshire	248,806
36	Colorado	243,632
37	Delaware	238,781
38	Iowa	237,750
39	Texas	229,314
40	Kentucky	214,632
41	Wyoming	203,155
42	North Dakota	195,812
43	Nebraska**	192,058
44	Kansas**	185,452
45	Louisiana**	180,794
46	California	176,986
47	New Mexico**	149,847
48	Vermont	137,444
49	Michigan	134,405
50	Utah	125,099
	District of Columbia	416,409

Source: U.S. Department of Health and Human Services, Bureau of Health Professions
   "National Practitioner Data Bank, 2003 Annual Report" (http://www.npdb-hipdb.com/annualrpt.html)
*National figure includes U.S. territories and U.S. Armed Forces locations overseas.
**The figures for these states have not been adjusted for payments by state compensation funds and other similar funds. Average payments for these states understate the actual average amounts received by claimants.

Percent of Private-Sector Establishments That Offer Health Insurance: 2002

National Percent = 57.2%

ALPHA ORDER				RANK ORDER		
RANK	STATE	PERCENT		RANK	STATE	PERCENT
11	Alabama	60.9		1	Hawaii	89.6
NA	Alaska*	NA		2	Ohio	67.4
34	Arizona	52.4		3	New Hampshire	67.0
NA	Arkansas*	NA		4	Pennsylvania	65.6
21	California	56.6		5	Michigan	63.3
18	Colorado	58.1		6	Massachusetts	62.8
7	Connecticut	62.4		7	Connecticut	62.4
22	Delaware	56.5		7	New Jersey	62.4
28	Florida	55.0		9	Nevada	61.7
29	Georgia	53.9		10	Maryland	61.0
1	Hawaii	89.6		11	Alabama	60.9
NA	Idaho*	NA		12	Wisconsin	60.0
16	Illinois	59.0		13	Indiana	59.4
13	Indiana	59.4		14	Kentucky	59.3
41	Iowa	46.9		15	Oregon	59.1
31	Kansas	53.6		16	Illinois	59.0
14	Kentucky	59.3		17	Virginia	58.9
29	Louisiana	53.9		18	Colorado	58.1
25	Maine	55.7		19	New York	57.1
10	Maryland	61.0		20	Washington	57.0
6	Massachusetts	62.8		21	California	56.6
5	Michigan	63.3		22	Delaware	56.5
22	Minnesota	56.5		22	Minnesota	56.5
37	Mississippi	48.5		24	Missouri	56.4
24	Missouri	56.4		25	Maine	55.7
41	Montana	46.9		26	Utah	55.3
43	Nebraska	43.6		27	West Virginia	55.2
9	Nevada	61.7		28	Florida	55.0
3	New Hampshire	67.0		29	Georgia	53.9
7	New Jersey	62.4		29	Louisiana	53.9
40	New Mexico	47.1		31	Kansas	53.6
19	New York	57.1		31	Tennessee	53.6
36	North Carolina	50.7		33	Oklahoma	52.5
NA	North Dakota*	NA		34	Arizona	52.4
2	Ohio	67.4		35	Texas	51.9
33	Oklahoma	52.5		36	North Carolina	50.7
15	Oregon	59.1		37	Mississippi	48.5
4	Pennsylvania	65.6		38	South Carolina	48.3
NA	Rhode Island*	NA		39	Wyoming	47.4
38	South Carolina	48.3		40	New Mexico	47.1
NA	South Dakota*	NA		41	Iowa	46.9
31	Tennessee	53.6		41	Montana	46.9
35	Texas	51.9		43	Nebraska	43.6
26	Utah	55.3		NA	Alaska*	NA
NA	Vermont*	NA		NA	Arkansas*	NA
17	Virginia	58.9		NA	Idaho*	NA
20	Washington	57.0		NA	North Dakota*	NA
27	West Virginia	55.2		NA	Rhode Island*	NA
12	Wisconsin	60.0		NA	South Dakota*	NA
39	Wyoming	47.4		NA	Vermont*	NA
					District of Columbia*	NA

Source: U.S. Department of Health and Human Services, Agency for Healthcare Research and Quality
   "Private-Sector Data by Firm Size and State" (Table II Series, Medical Expenditures Panel Survey, July 2004)
*Not shown separately. The figure for these states is 50.3 percent.

Percent of Private-Sector Establishments with Fewer Than 50 Employees That Offer Health Insurance: 2002
National Percent = 44.5%

ALPHA ORDER

RANK	STATE	PERCENT
14	Alabama	47.5
NA	Alaska*	NA
35	Arizona	36.4
NA	Arkansas*	NA
20	California	44.7
17	Colorado	45.8
6	Connecticut	52.5
26	Delaware	42.3
27	Florida	42.0
32	Georgia	38.2
1	Hawaii	86.1
NA	Idaho*	NA
12	Illinois	47.6
22	Indiana	44.2
38	Iowa	34.5
30	Kansas	39.7
24	Kentucky	43.0
29	Louisiana	40.2
21	Maine	44.6
11	Maryland	48.0
8	Massachusetts	51.9
5	Michigan	53.9
19	Minnesota	44.8
39	Mississippi	34.4
25	Missouri	42.5
33	Montana	37.5
42	Nebraska	32.1
9	Nevada	48.8
2	New Hampshire	57.9
7	New Jersey	52.3
40	New Mexico	33.8
12	New York	47.6
36	North Carolina	35.0
NA	North Dakota*	NA
4	Ohio	54.7
31	Oklahoma	39.5
15	Oregon	46.7
3	Pennsylvania	55.8
NA	Rhode Island*	NA
42	South Carolina	32.1
NA	South Dakota*	NA
41	Tennessee	33.3
37	Texas	34.8
22	Utah	44.2
NA	Vermont*	NA
16	Virginia	45.9
18	Washington	45.1
28	West Virginia	40.7
10	Wisconsin	48.2
34	Wyoming	36.7

RANK ORDER

RANK	STATE	PERCENT
1	Hawaii	86.1
2	New Hampshire	57.9
3	Pennsylvania	55.8
4	Ohio	54.7
5	Michigan	53.9
6	Connecticut	52.5
7	New Jersey	52.3
8	Massachusetts	51.9
9	Nevada	48.8
10	Wisconsin	48.2
11	Maryland	48.0
12	Illinois	47.6
12	New York	47.6
14	Alabama	47.5
15	Oregon	46.7
16	Virginia	45.9
17	Colorado	45.8
18	Washington	45.1
19	Minnesota	44.8
20	California	44.7
21	Maine	44.6
22	Indiana	44.2
22	Utah	44.2
24	Kentucky	43.0
25	Missouri	42.5
26	Delaware	42.3
27	Florida	42.0
28	West Virginia	40.7
29	Louisiana	40.2
30	Kansas	39.7
31	Oklahoma	39.5
32	Georgia	38.2
33	Montana	37.5
34	Wyoming	36.7
35	Arizona	36.4
36	North Carolina	35.0
37	Texas	34.8
38	Iowa	34.5
39	Mississippi	34.4
40	New Mexico	33.8
41	Tennessee	33.3
42	Nebraska	32.1
42	South Carolina	32.1
NA	Alaska*	NA
NA	Arkansas*	NA
NA	Idaho*	NA
NA	North Dakota*	NA
NA	Rhode Island*	NA
NA	South Dakota*	NA
NA	Vermont*	NA

District of Columbia*	NA

Source: U.S. Department of Health and Human Services, Agency for Healthcare Research and Quality
   "Private-Sector Data by Firm Size and State" (Table II Series, Medical Expenditures Panel Survey, July 2004)
*Not shown separately. The figure for these states is 37.6 percent.

Percent of Private-Sector Establishments with More Than 50 Employees That Offer Health Insurance: 2002
National Percent = 96.5%

ALPHA ORDER

RANK	STATE	PERCENT
1	Alabama	99.6
NA	Alaska*	NA
28	Arizona	95.7
NA	Arkansas*	NA
31	California	95.3
38	Colorado	93.9
3	Connecticut	99.0
42	Delaware	90.2
19	Florida	96.8
37	Georgia	94.0
2	Hawaii	99.3
NA	Idaho*	NA
9	Illinois	97.9
11	Indiana	97.6
36	Iowa	94.2
11	Kansas	97.6
22	Kentucky	96.6
32	Louisiana	95.2
3	Maine	99.0
6	Maryland	98.4
10	Massachusetts	97.8
21	Michigan	96.7
39	Minnesota	93.8
29	Mississippi	95.6
27	Missouri	95.8
41	Montana	92.2
33	Nebraska	94.7
24	Nevada	96.1
30	New Hampshire	95.4
18	New Jersey	97.1
43	New Mexico	86.5
8	New York	98.0
17	North Carolina	97.2
NA	North Dakota*	NA
14	Ohio	97.4
22	Oklahoma	96.6
11	Oregon	97.6
19	Pennsylvania	96.8
NA	Rhode Island*	NA
33	South Carolina	94.7
NA	South Dakota*	NA
15	Tennessee	97.3
24	Texas	96.1
40	Utah	92.5
NA	Vermont*	NA
5	Virginia	98.8
15	Washington	97.3
35	West Virginia	94.6
6	Wisconsin	98.4
26	Wyoming	95.9

RANK ORDER

RANK	STATE	PERCENT
1	Alabama	99.6
2	Hawaii	99.3
3	Connecticut	99.0
3	Maine	99.0
5	Virginia	98.8
6	Maryland	98.4
6	Wisconsin	98.4
8	New York	98.0
9	Illinois	97.9
10	Massachusetts	97.8
11	Indiana	97.6
11	Kansas	97.6
11	Oregon	97.6
14	Ohio	97.4
15	Tennessee	97.3
15	Washington	97.3
17	North Carolina	97.2
18	New Jersey	97.1
19	Florida	96.8
19	Pennsylvania	96.8
21	Michigan	96.7
22	Kentucky	96.6
22	Oklahoma	96.6
24	Nevada	96.1
24	Texas	96.1
26	Wyoming	95.9
27	Missouri	95.8
28	Arizona	95.7
29	Mississippi	95.6
30	New Hampshire	95.4
31	California	95.3
32	Louisiana	95.2
33	Nebraska	94.7
33	South Carolina	94.7
35	West Virginia	94.6
36	Iowa	94.2
37	Georgia	94.0
38	Colorado	93.9
39	Minnesota	93.8
40	Utah	92.5
41	Montana	92.2
42	Delaware	90.2
43	New Mexico	86.5
NA	Alaska*	NA
NA	Arkansas*	NA
NA	Idaho*	NA
NA	North Dakota*	NA
NA	Rhode Island*	NA
NA	South Dakota*	NA
NA	Vermont*	NA

District of Columbia*   NA

Source: U.S. Department of Health and Human Services, Agency for Healthcare Research and Quality
   "Private-Sector Data by Firm Size and State" (Table II Series, Medical Expenditures Panel Survey, July 2004)
Not shown separately. The figure for these states is 96.9 percent.

Average Annual Single Coverage Health Insurance Premium per Enrolled Employee in 2002
National Average = $3,189*

ALPHA ORDER

RANK	STATE	PREMIUM
37	Alabama	$2,945
NA	Alaska**	NA
33	Arizona	2,986
NA	Arkansas**	NA
39	California	2,936
13	Colorado	3,301
6	Connecticut	3,373
9	Delaware	3,332
18	Florida	3,258
30	Georgia	3,047
43	Hawaii	2,723
NA	Idaho**	NA
4	Illinois	3,458
19	Indiana	3,257
26	Iowa	3,124
40	Kansas	2,924
29	Kentucky	3,062
21	Louisiana	3,234
1	Maine	3,603
25	Maryland	3,164
8	Massachusetts	3,353
20	Michigan	3,250
14	Minnesota	3,293
36	Mississippi	2,962
32	Missouri	2,988
38	Montana	2,943
23	Nebraska	3,211
11	Nevada	3,315
17	New Hampshire	3,263
5	New Jersey	3,453
28	New Mexico	3,075
10	New York	3,326
24	North Carolina	3,167
NA	North Dakota**	NA
27	Ohio	3,087
22	Oklahoma	3,233
41	Oregon	2,909
12	Pennsylvania	3,311
NA	Rhode Island**	NA
42	South Carolina	2,898
NA	South Dakota**	NA
35	Tennessee	2,964
16	Texas	3,268
34	Utah	2,981
NA	Vermont**	NA
31	Virginia	3,010
15	Washington	3,287
7	West Virginia	3,371
2	Wisconsin	3,500
3	Wyoming	3,477

RANK ORDER

RANK	STATE	PREMIUM
1	Maine	$3,603
2	Wisconsin	3,500
3	Wyoming	3,477
4	Illinois	3,458
5	New Jersey	3,453
6	Connecticut	3,373
7	West Virginia	3,371
8	Massachusetts	3,353
9	Delaware	3,332
10	New York	3,326
11	Nevada	3,315
12	Pennsylvania	3,311
13	Colorado	3,301
14	Minnesota	3,293
15	Washington	3,287
16	Texas	3,268
17	New Hampshire	3,263
18	Florida	3,258
19	Indiana	3,257
20	Michigan	3,250
21	Louisiana	3,234
22	Oklahoma	3,233
23	Nebraska	3,211
24	North Carolina	3,167
25	Maryland	3,164
26	Iowa	3,124
27	Ohio	3,087
28	New Mexico	3,075
29	Kentucky	3,062
30	Georgia	3,047
31	Virginia	3,010
32	Missouri	2,988
33	Arizona	2,986
34	Utah	2,981
35	Tennessee	2,964
36	Mississippi	2,962
37	Alabama	2,945
38	Montana	2,943
39	California	2,936
40	Kansas	2,924
41	Oregon	2,909
42	South Carolina	2,898
43	Hawaii	2,723
NA	Alaska**	NA
NA	Arkansas**	NA
NA	Idaho**	NA
NA	North Dakota**	NA
NA	Rhode Island**	NA
NA	South Dakota**	NA
NA	Vermont**	NA
	District of Columbia**	NA

Source: U.S. Department of Health and Human Services, Agency for Healthcare Research and Quality
    "Private-Sector Data by Firm Size and State" (Table II Series, Medical Expenditures Panel Survey, July 2004)
*Enrolled employees at private-sector establishments that offer health insurance coverage.
**Not shown separately. The figure for these states is $3,255.

Average Annual Employee Contribution for Single Coverage
Health Insurance Coverage in 2002
National Average = $565*

ALPHA ORDER

RANK ORDER

RANK	STATE	PREMIUM	RANK	STATE	PREMIUM
15	Alabama	$620	1	Massachusetts	$708
NA	Alaska**	NA	2	Georgia	687
27	Arizona	547	3	Maine	684
NA	Arkansas**	NA	4	Oklahoma	680
38	California	446	5	Nebraska	678
20	Colorado	590	6	Maryland	670
15	Connecticut	620	7	Kentucky	669
36	Delaware	495	7	Minnesota	669
23	Florida	569	9	New Hampshire	665
2	Georgia	687	10	New York	648
43	Hawaii	257	11	Wisconsin	647
NA	Idaho**	NA	12	West Virginia	641
17	Illinois	615	13	Louisiana	622
18	Indiana	611	14	New Jersey	621
33	Iowa	505	15	Alabama	620
31	Kansas	524	15	Connecticut	620
7	Kentucky	669	17	Illinois	615
13	Louisiana	622	18	Indiana	611
3	Maine	684	19	Ohio	604
6	Maryland	670	20	Colorado	590
1	Massachusetts	708	21	Pennsylvania	580
34	Michigan	502	22	North Carolina	575
7	Minnesota	669	23	Florida	569
27	Mississippi	547	24	Tennessee	564
35	Missouri	496	25	Virginia	563
39	Montana	432	26	Utah	562
5	Nebraska	678	27	Arizona	547
40	Nevada	413	27	Mississippi	547
9	New Hampshire	665	29	New Mexico	536
14	New Jersey	621	30	Texas	530
29	New Mexico	536	31	Kansas	524
10	New York	648	32	South Carolina	517
22	North Carolina	575	33	Iowa	505
NA	North Dakota**	NA	34	Michigan	502
19	Ohio	604	35	Missouri	496
4	Oklahoma	680	36	Delaware	495
41	Oregon	350	37	Wyoming	487
21	Pennsylvania	580	38	California	446
NA	Rhode Island**	NA	39	Montana	432
32	South Carolina	517	40	Nevada	413
NA	South Dakota**	NA	41	Oregon	350
24	Tennessee	564	42	Washington	306
30	Texas	530	43	Hawaii	257
26	Utah	562	NA	Alaska**	NA
NA	Vermont**	NA	NA	Arkansas**	NA
25	Virginia	563	NA	Idaho**	NA
42	Washington	306	NA	North Dakota**	NA
12	West Virginia	641	NA	Rhode Island**	NA
11	Wisconsin	647	NA	South Dakota**	NA
37	Wyoming	487	NA	Vermont**	NA
				District of Columbia**	NA

Source: U.S. Department of Health and Human Services, Agency for Healthcare Research and Quality
    "Private-Sector Data by Firm Size and State" (Table II Series, Medical Expenditures Panel Survey, July 2004)
*Enrolled employees at private-sector establishments that offer health insurance coverage.
**Not shown separately. The figure for these states is $533.

Percent of Total Premiums for Single Coverage
Health Insurance Coverage Paid by Employees in 2002
National Average = 17.7%*

ALPHA ORDER

RANK	STATE	PERCENT
6	Alabama	21.0
NA	Alaska**	NA
22	Arizona	18.3
NA	Arkansas**	NA
36	California	15.2
25	Colorado	17.9
21	Connecticut	18.4
37	Delaware	14.9
30	Florida	17.4
1	Georgia	22.6
42	Hawaii	9.4
NA	Idaho**	NA
27	Illinois	17.8
17	Indiana	18.8
33	Iowa	16.2
25	Kansas	17.9
2	Kentucky	21.9
12	Louisiana	19.2
13	Maine	19.0
3	Maryland	21.2
4	Massachusetts	21.1
35	Michigan	15.4
9	Minnesota	20.3
19	Mississippi	18.5
32	Missouri	16.6
38	Montana	14.7
4	Nebraska	21.1
40	Nevada	12.5
8	New Hampshire	20.4
24	New Jersey	18.0
30	New Mexico	17.4
11	New York	19.5
23	North Carolina	18.2
NA	North Dakota**	NA
10	Ohio	19.6
6	Oklahoma	21.0
41	Oregon	12.0
29	Pennsylvania	17.5
NA	Rhode Island**	NA
27	South Carolina	17.8
NA	South Dakota**	NA
13	Tennessee	19.0
33	Texas	16.2
16	Utah	18.9
NA	Vermont**	NA
18	Virginia	18.7
43	Washington	9.3
13	West Virginia	19.0
19	Wisconsin	18.5
39	Wyoming	14.0

RANK ORDER

RANK	STATE	PERCENT
1	Georgia	22.6
2	Kentucky	21.9
3	Maryland	21.2
4	Massachusetts	21.1
4	Nebraska	21.1
6	Alabama	21.0
6	Oklahoma	21.0
8	New Hampshire	20.4
9	Minnesota	20.3
10	Ohio	19.6
11	New York	19.5
12	Louisiana	19.2
13	Maine	19.0
13	Tennessee	19.0
13	West Virginia	19.0
16	Utah	18.9
17	Indiana	18.8
18	Virginia	18.7
19	Mississippi	18.5
19	Wisconsin	18.5
21	Connecticut	18.4
22	Arizona	18.3
23	North Carolina	18.2
24	New Jersey	18.0
25	Colorado	17.9
25	Kansas	17.9
27	Illinois	17.8
27	South Carolina	17.8
29	Pennsylvania	17.5
30	Florida	17.4
30	New Mexico	17.4
32	Missouri	16.6
33	Iowa	16.2
33	Texas	16.2
35	Michigan	15.4
36	California	15.2
37	Delaware	14.9
38	Montana	14.7
39	Wyoming	14.0
40	Nevada	12.5
41	Oregon	12.0
42	Hawaii	9.4
43	Washington	9.3
NA	Alaska**	NA
NA	Arkansas**	NA
NA	Idaho**	NA
NA	North Dakota**	NA
NA	Rhode Island**	NA
NA	South Dakota**	NA
NA	Vermont**	NA

District of Columbia**   NA

Source: U.S. Department of Health and Human Services, Agency for Healthcare Research and Quality
  "Private-Sector Data by Firm Size and State" (Table II Series, Medical Expenditures Panel Survey, July 2004)
*Enrolled employees at private-sector establishments that offer health insurance coverage.
**Not shown separately. The figure for these states is 16.4 percent.

Average Annual Family Coverage Health Insurance Premium per Enrolled Employee in 2002
National Average = $8,469*

ALPHA ORDER

RANK	STATE	PREMIUM
41	Alabama	$7,574
NA	Alaska**	NA
33	Arizona	7,954
NA	Arkansas**	NA
21	California	8,380
17	Colorado	8,504
5	Connecticut	9,047
23	Delaware	8,370
11	Florida	8,748
34	Georgia	7,944
38	Hawaii	7,768
NA	Idaho**	NA
4	Illinois	9,067
26	Indiana	8,229
35	Iowa	7,873
25	Kansas	8,301
20	Kentucky	8,400
22	Louisiana	8,376
3	Maine	9,174
9	Maryland	8,809
10	Massachusetts	8,779
18	Michigan	8,452
7	Minnesota	8,899
42	Mississippi	7,525
36	Missouri	7,816
40	Montana	7,710
19	Nebraska	8,419
43	Nevada	7,378
1	New Hampshire	9,672
2	New Jersey	9,424
37	New Mexico	7,799
13	New York	8,691
31	North Carolina	8,025
NA	North Dakota**	NA
28	Ohio	8,163
16	Oklahoma	8,537
29	Oregon	8,141
27	Pennsylvania	8,217
NA	Rhode Island**	NA
32	South Carolina	8,024
NA	South Dakota**	NA
30	Tennessee	8,071
8	Texas	8,837
24	Utah	8,311
NA	Vermont**	NA
39	Virginia	7,755
14	Washington	8,642
6	West Virginia	8,941
12	Wisconsin	8,717
15	Wyoming	8,547

RANK ORDER

RANK	STATE	PREMIUM
1	New Hampshire	$9,672
2	New Jersey	9,424
3	Maine	9,174
4	Illinois	9,067
5	Connecticut	9,047
6	West Virginia	8,941
7	Minnesota	8,899
8	Texas	8,837
9	Maryland	8,809
10	Massachusetts	8,779
11	Florida	8,748
12	Wisconsin	8,717
13	New York	8,691
14	Washington	8,642
15	Wyoming	8,547
16	Oklahoma	8,537
17	Colorado	8,504
18	Michigan	8,452
19	Nebraska	8,419
20	Kentucky	8,400
21	California	8,380
22	Louisiana	8,376
23	Delaware	8,370
24	Utah	8,311
25	Kansas	8,301
26	Indiana	8,229
27	Pennsylvania	8,217
28	Ohio	8,163
29	Oregon	8,141
30	Tennessee	8,071
31	North Carolina	8,025
32	South Carolina	8,024
33	Arizona	7,954
34	Georgia	7,944
35	Iowa	7,873
36	Missouri	7,816
37	New Mexico	7,799
38	Hawaii	7,768
39	Virginia	7,755
40	Montana	7,710
41	Alabama	7,574
42	Mississippi	7,525
43	Nevada	7,378
NA	Alaska**	NA
NA	Arkansas**	NA
NA	Idaho**	NA
NA	North Dakota**	NA
NA	Rhode Island**	NA
NA	South Dakota**	NA
NA	Vermont**	NA
	District of Columbia**	NA

Source: U.S. Department of Health and Human Services, Agency for Healthcare Research and Quality
"Private-Sector Data by Firm Size and State" (Table II Series, Medical Expenditures Panel Survey, July 2004)
Enrolled employees at private-sector establishments that offer health insurance coverage.
**Not shown separately. The figure for these states is $8,403.*

Average Annual Employee Contribution for Family Coverage
Health Insurance Coverage in 2002
National Average = $1,987*

ALPHA ORDER

RANK	STATE	PREMIUM
11	Alabama	$2,164
NA	Alaska**	NA
12	Arizona	2,160
NA	Arkansas**	NA
21	California	1,996
15	Colorado	2,117
24	Connecticut	1,954
35	Delaware	1,735
10	Florida	2,178
8	Georgia	2,250
22	Hawaii	1,978
NA	Idaho**	NA
19	Illinois	2,016
42	Indiana	1,536
33	Iowa	1,781
29	Kansas	1,881
27	Kentucky	1,900
7	Louisiana	2,259
1	Maine	2,714
3	Maryland	2,583
17	Massachusetts	2,040
43	Michigan	1,361
18	Minnesota	2,033
34	Mississippi	1,777
26	Missouri	1,935
25	Montana	1,952
9	Nebraska	2,209
37	Nevada	1,694
5	New Hampshire	2,407
14	New Jersey	2,128
32	New Mexico	1,830
28	New York	1,886
16	North Carolina	2,110
NA	North Dakota**	NA
30	Ohio	1,841
2	Oklahoma	2,600
30	Oregon	1,841
39	Pennsylvania	1,656
NA	Rhode Island**	NA
13	South Carolina	2,155
NA	South Dakota**	NA
20	Tennessee	2,012
6	Texas	2,298
38	Utah	1,661
NA	Vermont**	NA
4	Virginia	2,447
40	Washington	1,623
36	West Virginia	1,710
41	Wisconsin	1,584
23	Wyoming	1,970

RANK ORDER

RANK	STATE	PREMIUM
1	Maine	$2,714
2	Oklahoma	2,600
3	Maryland	2,583
4	Virginia	2,447
5	New Hampshire	2,407
6	Texas	2,298
7	Louisiana	2,259
8	Georgia	2,250
9	Nebraska	2,209
10	Florida	2,178
11	Alabama	2,164
12	Arizona	2,160
13	South Carolina	2,155
14	New Jersey	2,128
15	Colorado	2,117
16	North Carolina	2,110
17	Massachusetts	2,040
18	Minnesota	2,033
19	Illinois	2,016
20	Tennessee	2,012
21	California	1,996
22	Hawaii	1,978
23	Wyoming	1,970
24	Connecticut	1,954
25	Montana	1,952
26	Missouri	1,935
27	Kentucky	1,900
28	New York	1,886
29	Kansas	1,881
30	Ohio	1,841
30	Oregon	1,841
32	New Mexico	1,830
33	Iowa	1,781
34	Mississippi	1,777
35	Delaware	1,735
36	West Virginia	1,710
37	Nevada	1,694
38	Utah	1,661
39	Pennsylvania	1,656
40	Washington	1,623
41	Wisconsin	1,584
42	Indiana	1,536
43	Michigan	1,361
NA	Alaska**	NA
NA	Arkansas**	NA
NA	Idaho**	NA
NA	North Dakota**	NA
NA	Rhode Island**	NA
NA	South Dakota**	NA
NA	Vermont**	NA
	District of Columbia**	NA

Source: U.S. Department of Health and Human Services, Agency for Healthcare Research and Quality
"Private-Sector Data by Firm Size and State" (Table II Series, Medical Expenditures Panel Survey, July 2004)
Enrolled employees at private-sector establishments that offer health insurance coverage.
**Not shown separately. The figure for these states is $2,112.*

Percent of Total Premiums for Family Coverage
Health Insurance Coverage Paid by Employees in 2002
National Average = 23.5%*

ALPHA ORDER

RANK ORDER

RANK	STATE	PERCENT	RANK	STATE	PERCENT
5	Alabama	28.6	1	Virginia	31.6
NA	Alaska**	NA	2	Oklahoma	30.5
7	Arizona	27.1	3	Maine	29.6
NA	Arkansas**	NA	4	Maryland	29.3
20	California	23.8	5	Alabama	28.6
15	Colorado	24.9	6	Georgia	28.3
35	Connecticut	21.6	7	Arizona	27.1
36	Delaware	20.7	8	Louisiana	27.0
15	Florida	24.9	9	South Carolina	26.9
6	Georgia	28.3	10	North Carolina	26.3
13	Hawaii	25.5	11	Nebraska	26.2
NA	Idaho**	NA	12	Texas	26.0
33	Illinois	22.2	13	Hawaii	25.5
41	Indiana	18.7	14	Montana	25.3
28	Iowa	22.6	15	Colorado	24.9
27	Kansas	22.7	15	Florida	24.9
28	Kentucky	22.6	15	New Hampshire	24.9
8	Louisiana	27.0	15	Tennessee	24.9
3	Maine	29.6	19	Missouri	24.8
4	Maryland	29.3	20	California	23.8
23	Massachusetts	23.2	21	Mississippi	23.6
43	Michigan	16.1	22	New Mexico	23.5
26	Minnesota	22.8	23	Massachusetts	23.2
21	Mississippi	23.6	24	Nevada	23.0
19	Missouri	24.8	24	Wyoming	23.0
14	Montana	25.3	26	Minnesota	22.8
11	Nebraska	26.2	27	Kansas	22.7
24	Nevada	23.0	28	Iowa	22.6
15	New Hampshire	24.9	28	Kentucky	22.6
28	New Jersey	22.6	28	New Jersey	22.6
22	New Mexico	23.5	28	Oregon	22.6
34	New York	21.7	32	Ohio	22.5
10	North Carolina	26.3	33	Illinois	22.2
NA	North Dakota**	NA	34	New York	21.7
32	Ohio	22.5	35	Connecticut	21.6
2	Oklahoma	30.5	36	Delaware	20.7
28	Oregon	22.6	37	Pennsylvania	20.2
37	Pennsylvania	20.2	38	Utah	20.0
NA	Rhode Island**	NA	39	West Virginia	19.1
9	South Carolina	26.9	40	Washington	18.8
NA	South Dakota**	NA	41	Indiana	18.7
15	Tennessee	24.9	42	Wisconsin	18.2
12	Texas	26.0	43	Michigan	16.1
38	Utah	20.0	NA	Alaska**	NA
NA	Vermont**	NA	NA	Arkansas**	NA
1	Virginia	31.6	NA	Idaho**	NA
40	Washington	18.8	NA	North Dakota**	NA
39	West Virginia	19.1	NA	Rhode Island**	NA
42	Wisconsin	18.2	NA	South Dakota**	NA
24	Wyoming	23.0	NA	Vermont**	NA
				District of Columbia**	NA

Source: U.S. Department of Health and Human Services, Agency for Healthcare Research and Quality
    "Private-Sector Data by Firm Size and State" (Table II Series, Medical Expenditures Panel Survey, July 2004)
Enrolled employees at private-sector establishments that offer health insurance coverage.
**Not shown separately. The figure for these states is 25.1 percent.*

236

Persons Not Covered by Health Insurance in 2003

National Total = 44,961,000 Uninsured

ALPHA ORDER

RANK	STATE	UNINSURED	% of USA
22	Alabama	629,000	1.4%
44	Alaska	122,000	0.3%
13	Arizona	951,000	2.1%
29	Arkansas	465,000	1.0%
1	California	6,499,000	14.5%
18	Colorado	772,000	1.7%
33	Connecticut	357,000	0.8%
46	Delaware	91,000	0.2%
3	Florida	3,071,000	6.8%
7	Georgia	1,409,000	3.1%
43	Hawaii	127,000	0.3%
38	Idaho	253,000	0.6%
5	Illinois	1,818,000	4.0%
16	Indiana	853,000	1.9%
34	Iowa	329,000	0.7%
37	Kansas	294,000	0.7%
27	Kentucky	574,000	1.3%
15	Louisiana	912,000	2.0%
41	Maine	133,000	0.3%
19	Maryland	762,000	1.7%
21	Massachusetts	682,000	1.5%
11	Michigan	1,080,000	2.4%
30	Minnesota	444,000	1.0%
28	Mississippi	511,000	1.1%
23	Missouri	620,000	1.4%
40	Montana	177,000	0.4%
39	Nebraska	195,000	0.4%
31	Nevada	426,000	0.9%
42	New Hampshire	131,000	0.3%
10	New Jersey	1,201,000	2.7%
32	New Mexico	414,000	0.9%
4	New York	2,866,000	6.4%
6	North Carolina	1,424,000	3.2%
49	North Dakota	69,000	0.2%
9	Ohio	1,362,000	3.0%
20	Oklahoma	701,000	1.6%
24	Oregon	613,000	1.4%
8	Pennsylvania	1,384,000	3.1%
45	Rhode Island	108,000	0.2%
26	South Carolina	584,000	1.3%
46	South Dakota	91,000	0.2%
17	Tennessee	778,000	1.7%
2	Texas	5,374,000	12.0%
35	Utah	298,000	0.7%
50	Vermont	58,000	0.1%
12	Virginia	962,000	2.1%
14	Washington	944,000	2.1%
36	West Virginia	296,000	0.7%
25	Wisconsin	593,000	1.3%
48	Wyoming	78,000	0.2%

RANK ORDER

RANK	STATE	UNINSURED	% of USA
1	California	6,499,000	14.5%
2	Texas	5,374,000	12.0%
3	Florida	3,071,000	6.8%
4	New York	2,866,000	6.4%
5	Illinois	1,818,000	4.0%
6	North Carolina	1,424,000	3.2%
7	Georgia	1,409,000	3.1%
8	Pennsylvania	1,384,000	3.1%
9	Ohio	1,362,000	3.0%
10	New Jersey	1,201,000	2.7%
11	Michigan	1,080,000	2.4%
12	Virginia	962,000	2.1%
13	Arizona	951,000	2.1%
14	Washington	944,000	2.1%
15	Louisiana	912,000	2.0%
16	Indiana	853,000	1.9%
17	Tennessee	778,000	1.7%
18	Colorado	772,000	1.7%
19	Maryland	762,000	1.7%
20	Oklahoma	701,000	1.6%
21	Massachusetts	682,000	1.5%
22	Alabama	629,000	1.4%
23	Missouri	620,000	1.4%
24	Oregon	613,000	1.4%
25	Wisconsin	593,000	1.3%
26	South Carolina	584,000	1.3%
27	Kentucky	574,000	1.3%
28	Mississippi	511,000	1.1%
29	Arkansas	465,000	1.0%
30	Minnesota	444,000	1.0%
31	Nevada	426,000	0.9%
32	New Mexico	414,000	0.9%
33	Connecticut	357,000	0.8%
34	Iowa	329,000	0.7%
35	Utah	298,000	0.7%
36	West Virginia	296,000	0.7%
37	Kansas	294,000	0.7%
38	Idaho	253,000	0.6%
39	Nebraska	195,000	0.4%
40	Montana	177,000	0.4%
41	Maine	133,000	0.3%
42	New Hampshire	131,000	0.3%
43	Hawaii	127,000	0.3%
44	Alaska	122,000	0.3%
45	Rhode Island	108,000	0.2%
46	Delaware	91,000	0.2%
46	South Dakota	91,000	0.2%
48	Wyoming	78,000	0.2%
49	North Dakota	69,000	0.2%
50	Vermont	58,000	0.1%
	District of Columbia	79,000	0.2%

Source: U.S. Bureau of the Census
"Health Insurance Coverage Status by State for All People: 2003"
(http://ferret.bls.census.gov/macro/032004/health/h06_000.htm)

Percent of Population Not Covered by Health Insurance in 2003

National Percent = 15.1% of Population*

RANK	STATE	PERCENT
25	Alabama	13.3
7	Alaska	17.8
10	Arizona	17.3
12	Arkansas	16.6
4	California	18.7
15	Colorado	16.3
40	Connecticut	10.4
42	Delaware	10.1
8	Florida	17.6
14	Georgia	16.4
43	Hawaii	9.9
9	Idaho	17.5
22	Illinois	14.0
29	Indiana	12.9
47	Iowa	9.5
35	Kansas	10.9
25	Kentucky	13.3
3	Louisiana	19.4
37	Maine	10.7
27	Maryland	13.2
46	Massachusetts	9.6
33	Michigan	11.0
50	Minnesota	8.2
11	Mississippi	17.0
35	Missouri	10.9
16	Montana	16.1
41	Nebraska	10.3
6	Nevada	18.3
43	New Hampshire	9.9
23	New Jersey	13.7
2	New Mexico	21.3
18	New York	15.5
16	North Carolina	16.1
39	North Dakota	10.5
32	Ohio	11.7
4	Oklahoma	18.7
19	Oregon	14.8
37	Pennsylvania	10.7
49	Rhode Island	9.3
28	South Carolina	13.1
33	South Dakota	11.0
31	Tennessee	11.8
1	Texas	24.6
24	Utah	13.6
43	Vermont	9.9
30	Virginia	12.5
21	Washington	14.3
19	West Virginia	14.8
47	Wisconsin	9.5
13	Wyoming	16.5

RANK	STATE	PERCENT
1	Texas	24.6
2	New Mexico	21.3
3	Louisiana	19.4
4	California	18.7
4	Oklahoma	18.7
6	Nevada	18.3
7	Alaska	17.8
8	Florida	17.6
9	Idaho	17.5
10	Arizona	17.3
11	Mississippi	17.0
12	Arkansas	16.6
13	Wyoming	16.5
14	Georgia	16.4
15	Colorado	16.3
16	Montana	16.1
16	North Carolina	16.1
18	New York	15.5
19	Oregon	14.8
19	West Virginia	14.8
21	Washington	14.3
22	Illinois	14.0
23	New Jersey	13.7
24	Utah	13.6
25	Alabama	13.3
25	Kentucky	13.3
27	Maryland	13.2
28	South Carolina	13.1
29	Indiana	12.9
30	Virginia	12.5
31	Tennessee	11.8
32	Ohio	11.7
33	Michigan	11.0
33	South Dakota	11.0
35	Kansas	10.9
35	Missouri	10.9
37	Maine	10.7
37	Pennsylvania	10.7
39	North Dakota	10.5
40	Connecticut	10.4
41	Nebraska	10.3
42	Delaware	10.1
43	Hawaii	9.9
43	New Hampshire	9.9
43	Vermont	9.9
46	Massachusetts	9.6
47	Iowa	9.5
47	Wisconsin	9.5
49	Rhode Island	9.3
50	Minnesota	8.2
	District of Columbia	13.3

Source: U.S. Bureau of the Census
"Income, Poverty and Health Insurance Covered in the United States: 2003"
(http://www.census.gov/hhes/hlthins/hlthin03/hi03t9.pdf)
*Three-year average for 2001 through 2003.

Numerical Change in Persons Uninsured: 1999 to 2003

National Change = 4,733,000 Increase

ALPHA ORDER

RANK	STATE	CHANGE
26	Alabama	46,000
37	Alaska	5,000
50	Arizona	(94,000)
19	Arkansas	85,000
49	California	(88,000)
17	Colorado	99,000
25	Connecticut	50,000
35	Delaware	14,000
6	Florida	230,000
7	Georgia	221,000
39	Hawaii	2,000
31	Idaho	27,000
12	Illinois	187,000
3	Indiana	297,000
16	Iowa	112,000
45	Kansas	(15,000)
22	Kentucky	66,000
46	Louisiana	(23,000)
41	Maine	(3,000)
11	Maryland	197,000
18	Massachusetts	98,000
24	Michigan	54,000
20	Minnesota	84,000
21	Mississippi	79,000
5	Missouri	246,000
33	Montana	18,000
32	Nebraska	25,000
27	Nevada	45,000
34	New Hampshire	16,000
10	New Jersey	202,000
47	New Mexico	(38,000)
48	New York	(65,000)
4	North Carolina	296,000
41	North Dakota	(3,000)
8	Ohio	218,000
13	Oklahoma	159,000
15	Oregon	133,000
2	Pennsylvania	395,000
28	Rhode Island	42,000
44	South Carolina	(9,000)
35	South Dakota	14,000
9	Tennessee	205,000
1	Texas	820,000
40	Utah	1,000
43	Vermont	(8,000)
23	Virginia	64,000
14	Washington	150,000
30	West Virginia	31,000
29	Wisconsin	41,000
38	Wyoming	4,000

RANK ORDER

RANK	STATE	CHANGE
1	Texas	820,000
2	Pennsylvania	395,000
3	Indiana	297,000
4	North Carolina	296,000
5	Missouri	246,000
6	Florida	230,000
7	Georgia	221,000
8	Ohio	218,000
9	Tennessee	205,000
10	New Jersey	202,000
11	Maryland	197,000
12	Illinois	187,000
13	Oklahoma	159,000
14	Washington	150,000
15	Oregon	133,000
16	Iowa	112,000
17	Colorado	99,000
18	Massachusetts	98,000
19	Arkansas	85,000
20	Minnesota	84,000
21	Mississippi	79,000
22	Kentucky	66,000
23	Virginia	64,000
24	Michigan	54,000
25	Connecticut	50,000
26	Alabama	46,000
27	Nevada	45,000
28	Rhode Island	42,000
29	Wisconsin	41,000
30	West Virginia	31,000
31	Idaho	27,000
32	Nebraska	25,000
33	Montana	18,000
34	New Hampshire	16,000
35	Delaware	14,000
35	South Dakota	14,000
37	Alaska	5,000
38	Wyoming	4,000
39	Hawaii	2,000
40	Utah	1,000
41	Maine	(3,000)
41	North Dakota	(3,000)
43	Vermont	(8,000)
44	South Carolina	(9,000)
45	Kansas	(15,000)
46	Louisiana	(23,000)
47	New Mexico	(38,000)
48	New York	(65,000)
49	California	(88,000)
50	Arizona	(94,000)

District of Columbia   2,000

Source: Morgan Quitno Press using data from U.S. Bureau of the Census
"Health Insurance Historical Table 4" (http://www.census.gov/hhes/hlthins/historic/hihistt4.html) and
"Health Insurance Coverage Status by State for All People: 2003"
(http://ferret.bls.census.gov/macro/032004/health/h06_000.htm)

Percent Change in Persons Uninsured: 1999 to 2003

National Percent Change = 11.8% Increase

ALPHA ORDER

RANK	STATE	PERCENT CHANGE
33	Alabama	7.9
38	Alaska	4.3
49	Arizona	(9.0)
12	Arkansas	22.4
41	California	(1.3)
23	Colorado	14.7
22	Connecticut	16.3
18	Delaware	18.2
32	Florida	8.1
16	Georgia	18.6
39	Hawaii	1.6
27	Idaho	11.9
30	Illinois	11.5
3	Indiana	53.4
4	Iowa	51.6
47	Kansas	(4.9)
26	Kentucky	13.0
45	Louisiana	(2.5)
43	Maine	(2.2)
7	Maryland	34.9
21	Massachusetts	16.8
37	Michigan	5.3
11	Minnesota	23.3
17	Mississippi	18.3
1	Missouri	65.8
31	Montana	11.3
23	Nebraska	14.7
28	Nevada	11.8
25	New Hampshire	13.9
13	New Jersey	20.2
48	New Mexico	(8.4)
43	New York	(2.2)
10	North Carolina	26.2
46	North Dakota	(4.2)
14	Ohio	19.1
8	Oklahoma	29.3
9	Oregon	27.7
5	Pennsylvania	39.9
2	Rhode Island	63.6
42	South Carolina	(1.5)
18	South Dakota	18.2
6	Tennessee	35.8
20	Texas	18.0
40	Utah	0.3
50	Vermont	(12.1)
35	Virginia	7.1
15	Washington	18.9
29	West Virginia	11.7
34	Wisconsin	7.4
36	Wyoming	5.4

RANK ORDER

RANK	STATE	PERCENT CHANGE
1	Missouri	65.8
2	Rhode Island	63.6
3	Indiana	53.4
4	Iowa	51.6
5	Pennsylvania	39.9
6	Tennessee	35.8
7	Maryland	34.9
8	Oklahoma	29.3
9	Oregon	27.7
10	North Carolina	26.2
11	Minnesota	23.3
12	Arkansas	22.4
13	New Jersey	20.2
14	Ohio	19.1
15	Washington	18.9
16	Georgia	18.6
17	Mississippi	18.3
18	Delaware	18.2
18	South Dakota	18.2
20	Texas	18.0
21	Massachusetts	16.8
22	Connecticut	16.3
23	Colorado	14.7
23	Nebraska	14.7
25	New Hampshire	13.9
26	Kentucky	13.0
27	Idaho	11.9
28	Nevada	11.8
29	West Virginia	11.7
30	Illinois	11.5
31	Montana	11.3
32	Florida	8.1
33	Alabama	7.9
34	Wisconsin	7.4
35	Virginia	7.1
36	Wyoming	5.4
37	Michigan	5.3
38	Alaska	4.3
39	Hawaii	1.6
40	Utah	0.3
41	California	(1.3)
42	South Carolina	(1.5)
43	Maine	(2.2)
43	New York	(2.2)
45	Louisiana	(2.5)
46	North Dakota	(4.2)
47	Kansas	(4.9)
48	New Mexico	(8.4)
49	Arizona	(9.0)
50	Vermont	(12.1)

District of Columbia   2.6

Source: Morgan Quitno Press using data from U.S. Bureau of the Census
"Health Insurance Historical Table 4" (http://www.census.gov/hhes/hlthins/historic/hihistt4.html) and
"Health Insurance Coverage Status by State for All People: 2003"
(http://ferret.bls.census.gov/macro/032004/health/h06_000.htm)

Change in Percent of Population Uninsured: 1999 to 2003

National Percent Change = 3.2% Decrease*

ALPHA ORDER

RANK	STATE	PERCENT CHANGE
43	Alabama	(13.1)
18	Alaska	(1.1)
50	Arizona	(25.1)
44	Arkansas	(13.5)
42	California	(11.0)
9	Colorado	6.5
34	Connecticut	(7.1)
48	Delaware	(19.8)
27	Florida	(4.3)
19	Georgia	(1.8)
6	Hawaii	7.6
21	Idaho	(2.2)
15	Illinois	2.9
3	Indiana	10.3
17	Iowa	(1.0)
22	Kansas	(3.5)
30	Kentucky	(5.7)
22	Louisiana	(3.5)
46	Maine	(16.4)
24	Maryland	(3.6)
39	Massachusetts	(10.3)
31	Michigan	(6.0)
28	Minnesota	(4.7)
37	Mississippi	(8.6)
5	Missouri	9.0
45	Montana	(14.8)
14	Nebraska	3.0
26	Nevada	(4.2)
35	New Hampshire	(7.5)
38	New Jersey	(8.7)
33	New Mexico	(6.6)
36	New York	(7.7)
7	North Carolina	7.3
49	North Dakota	(23.4)
4	Ohio	9.3
8	Oklahoma	6.9
9	Oregon	6.5
2	Pennsylvania	11.5
11	Rhode Island	4.5
47	South Carolina	(17.6)
41	South Dakota	(10.6)
25	Tennessee	(4.1)
13	Texas	3.4
16	Utah	0.0
20	Vermont	(2.0)
31	Virginia	(6.0)
1	Washington	14.4
39	West Virginia	(10.3)
29	Wisconsin	(5.0)
12	Wyoming	3.8

RANK ORDER

RANK	STATE	PERCENT CHANGE
1	Washington	14.4
2	Pennsylvania	11.5
3	Indiana	10.3
4	Ohio	9.3
5	Missouri	9.0
6	Hawaii	7.6
7	North Carolina	7.3
8	Oklahoma	6.9
9	Colorado	6.5
9	Oregon	6.5
11	Rhode Island	4.5
12	Wyoming	3.8
13	Texas	3.4
14	Nebraska	3.0
15	Illinois	2.9
16	Utah	0.0
17	Iowa	(1.0)
18	Alaska	(1.1)
19	Georgia	(1.8)
20	Vermont	(2.0)
21	Idaho	(2.2)
22	Kansas	(3.5)
22	Louisiana	(3.5)
24	Maryland	(3.6)
25	Tennessee	(4.1)
26	Nevada	(4.2)
27	Florida	(4.3)
28	Minnesota	(4.7)
29	Wisconsin	(5.0)
30	Kentucky	(5.7)
31	Michigan	(6.0)
31	Virginia	(6.0)
33	New Mexico	(6.6)
34	Connecticut	(7.1)
35	New Hampshire	(7.5)
36	New York	(7.7)
37	Mississippi	(8.6)
38	New Jersey	(8.7)
39	Massachusetts	(10.3)
39	West Virginia	(10.3)
41	South Dakota	(10.6)
42	California	(11.0)
43	Alabama	(13.1)
44	Arkansas	(13.5)
45	Montana	(14.8)
46	Maine	(16.4)
47	South Carolina	(17.6)
48	Delaware	(19.8)
49	North Dakota	(23.4)
50	Arizona	(25.1)

District of Columbia (15.3)

Source: Morgan Quitno Press using data from U.S. Bureau of the Census
"Health Insurance Historical Table 4" (http://www.census.gov/hhes/hlthins/historic/hihistt4.html) and
"Income, Poverty and Health Insurance Covered in the United States: 2003"
(http://www.census.gov/hhes/hlthins/hlthin03/hi03t9.pdf)
*Based on three-year averages for 2001 through 2003 and 1997 through 1999.

Percent of Children Not Covered by Health Insurance in 2003

National Percent = 11.4% of Children*

RANK	STATE	PERCENT
28	Alabama	8.7
15	Alaska	12.3
7	Arizona	14.6
20	Arkansas	10.5
13	California	12.5
8	Colorado	13.7
35	Connecticut	8.3
30	Delaware	8.5
5	Florida	15.5
8	Georgia	13.7
41	Hawaii	7.4
8	Idaho	13.7
22	Illinois	10.0
24	Indiana	9.0
29	Iowa	8.6
44	Kansas	6.4
20	Kentucky	10.5
6	Louisiana	15.2
46	Maine	6.0
37	Maryland	8.1
38	Massachusetts	7.9
47	Michigan	5.8
45	Minnesota	6.2
16	Mississippi	12.1
42	Missouri	7.3
3	Montana	17.7
43	Nebraska	7.0
4	Nevada	17.4
48	New Hampshire	5.5
18	New Jersey	11.0
12	New Mexico	13.2
23	New York	9.4
17	North Carolina	11.9
40	North Dakota	7.5
35	Ohio	8.3
2	Oklahoma	17.9
11	Oregon	13.5
31	Pennsylvania	8.4
49	Rhode Island	5.2
26	South Carolina	8.9
31	South Dakota	8.4
19	Tennessee	10.8
1	Texas	20.0
24	Utah	9.0
50	Vermont	3.9
26	Virginia	8.9
31	Washington	8.4
31	West Virginia	8.4
39	Wisconsin	7.7
13	Wyoming	12.5

RANK	STATE	PERCENT
1	Texas	20.0
2	Oklahoma	17.9
3	Montana	17.7
4	Nevada	17.4
5	Florida	15.5
6	Louisiana	15.2
7	Arizona	14.6
8	Colorado	13.7
8	Georgia	13.7
8	Idaho	13.7
11	Oregon	13.5
12	New Mexico	13.2
13	California	12.5
13	Wyoming	12.5
15	Alaska	12.3
16	Mississippi	12.1
17	North Carolina	11.9
18	New Jersey	11.0
19	Tennessee	10.8
20	Arkansas	10.5
20	Kentucky	10.5
22	Illinois	10.0
23	New York	9.4
24	Indiana	9.0
24	Utah	9.0
26	South Carolina	8.9
26	Virginia	8.9
28	Alabama	8.7
29	Iowa	8.6
30	Delaware	8.5
31	Pennsylvania	8.4
31	South Dakota	8.4
31	Washington	8.4
31	West Virginia	8.4
35	Connecticut	8.3
35	Ohio	8.3
37	Maryland	8.1
38	Massachusetts	7.9
39	Wisconsin	7.7
40	North Dakota	7.5
41	Hawaii	7.4
42	Missouri	7.3
43	Nebraska	7.0
44	Kansas	6.4
45	Minnesota	6.2
46	Maine	6.0
47	Michigan	5.8
48	New Hampshire	5.5
49	Rhode Island	5.2
50	Vermont	3.9

| | District of Columbia | 11.4 |

Source: U.S. Bureau of the Census
   "Health Insurance Coverage Status" (http://ferret.bls.census.gov/macro/032004/health/h05_000.htm)
*Children under 18 years old.

Persons Covered by Health Insurance in 2003

National Total = 243,320,000 Insured

ALPHA ORDER

RANK	STATE	INSURED	% of USA
22	Alabama	3,798,000	1.6%
49	Alaska	523,000	0.2%
21	Arizona	4,626,000	1.9%
33	Arkansas	2,206,000	0.9%
1	California	28,895,000	11.9%
23	Colorado	3,708,000	1.5%
27	Connecticut	3,065,000	1.3%
45	Delaware	729,000	0.3%
4	Florida	13,849,000	5.7%
10	Georgia	7,162,000	2.9%
41	Hawaii	1,126,000	0.5%
42	Idaho	1,107,000	0.5%
5	Illinois	10,810,000	4.4%
14	Indiana	5,296,000	2.2%
30	Iowa	2,593,000	1.1%
31	Kansas	2,389,000	1.0%
24	Kentucky	3,537,000	1.5%
25	Louisiana	3,517,000	1.4%
39	Maine	1,150,000	0.5%
19	Maryland	4,731,000	1.9%
13	Massachusetts	5,685,000	2.3%
8	Michigan	8,838,000	3.6%
20	Minnesota	4,633,000	1.9%
32	Mississippi	2,343,000	1.0%
17	Missouri	5,004,000	2.1%
44	Montana	739,000	0.3%
36	Nebraska	1,532,000	0.6%
35	Nevada	1,824,000	0.7%
40	New Hampshire	1,133,000	0.5%
9	New Jersey	7,378,000	3.0%
38	New Mexico	1,457,000	0.6%
3	New York	16,104,000	6.6%
11	North Carolina	6,829,000	2.8%
47	North Dakota	563,000	0.2%
7	Ohio	9,885,000	4.1%
29	Oklahoma	2,737,000	1.1%
28	Oregon	2,957,000	1.2%
6	Pennsylvania	10,771,000	4.4%
43	Rhode Island	946,000	0.4%
26	South Carolina	3,481,000	1.4%
46	South Dakota	659,000	0.3%
16	Tennessee	5,131,000	2.1%
2	Texas	16,484,000	6.8%
34	Utah	2,055,000	0.8%
48	Vermont	553,000	0.2%
12	Virginia	6,424,000	2.6%
15	Washington	5,147,000	2.1%
37	West Virginia	1,491,000	0.6%
18	Wisconsin	4,836,000	2.0%
50	Wyoming	411,000	0.2%

RANK ORDER

RANK	STATE	INSURED	% of USA
1	California	28,895,000	11.9%
2	Texas	16,484,000	6.8%
3	New York	16,104,000	6.6%
4	Florida	13,849,000	5.7%
5	Illinois	10,810,000	4.4%
6	Pennsylvania	10,771,000	4.4%
7	Ohio	9,885,000	4.1%
8	Michigan	8,838,000	3.6%
9	New Jersey	7,378,000	3.0%
10	Georgia	7,162,000	2.9%
11	North Carolina	6,829,000	2.8%
12	Virginia	6,424,000	2.6%
13	Massachusetts	5,685,000	2.3%
14	Indiana	5,296,000	2.2%
15	Washington	5,147,000	2.1%
16	Tennessee	5,131,000	2.1%
17	Missouri	5,004,000	2.1%
18	Wisconsin	4,836,000	2.0%
19	Maryland	4,731,000	1.9%
20	Minnesota	4,633,000	1.9%
21	Arizona	4,626,000	1.9%
22	Alabama	3,798,000	1.6%
23	Colorado	3,708,000	1.5%
24	Kentucky	3,537,000	1.5%
25	Louisiana	3,517,000	1.4%
26	South Carolina	3,481,000	1.4%
27	Connecticut	3,065,000	1.3%
28	Oregon	2,957,000	1.2%
29	Oklahoma	2,737,000	1.1%
30	Iowa	2,593,000	1.1%
31	Kansas	2,389,000	1.0%
32	Mississippi	2,343,000	1.0%
33	Arkansas	2,206,000	0.9%
34	Utah	2,055,000	0.8%
35	Nevada	1,824,000	0.7%
36	Nebraska	1,532,000	0.6%
37	West Virginia	1,491,000	0.6%
38	New Mexico	1,457,000	0.6%
39	Maine	1,150,000	0.5%
40	New Hampshire	1,133,000	0.5%
41	Hawaii	1,126,000	0.5%
42	Idaho	1,107,000	0.5%
43	Rhode Island	946,000	0.4%
44	Montana	739,000	0.3%
45	Delaware	729,000	0.3%
46	South Dakota	659,000	0.3%
47	North Dakota	563,000	0.2%
48	Vermont	553,000	0.2%
49	Alaska	523,000	0.2%
50	Wyoming	411,000	0.2%
	District of Columbia	475,000	0.2%

Source: U.S. Bureau of the Census
"Health Insurance Coverage Status by State for All People: 2003"
(http://ferret.bls.census.gov/macro/032004/health/h06_000.htm)

Percent of Population Covered by Health Insurance in 2003

National Percent = 84.9% of Population

ALPHA ORDER

RANK	STATE	PERCENT
25	Alabama	86.7
44	Alaska	82.2
41	Arizona	82.7
39	Arkansas	83.4
46	California	81.3
36	Colorado	83.7
11	Connecticut	89.6
9	Delaware	89.9
43	Florida	82.4
37	Georgia	83.6
6	Hawaii	90.1
42	Idaho	82.5
29	Illinois	86.0
22	Indiana	87.1
3	Iowa	90.5
15	Kansas	89.1
25	Kentucky	86.7
48	Louisiana	80.6
13	Maine	89.3
24	Maryland	86.8
5	Massachusetts	90.4
17	Michigan	89.0
1	Minnesota	91.8
40	Mississippi	83.0
15	Missouri	89.1
34	Montana	83.9
10	Nebraska	89.7
45	Nevada	81.7
6	New Hampshire	90.1
28	New Jersey	86.3
49	New Mexico	78.7
33	New York	84.5
34	North Carolina	83.9
12	North Dakota	89.5
19	Ohio	88.3
46	Oklahoma	81.3
31	Oregon	85.2
13	Pennsylvania	89.3
2	Rhode Island	90.7
23	South Carolina	86.9
17	South Dakota	89.0
20	Tennessee	88.2
50	Texas	75.4
27	Utah	86.4
6	Vermont	90.1
21	Virginia	87.5
30	Washington	85.7
31	West Virginia	85.2
3	Wisconsin	90.5
38	Wyoming	83.5

RANK ORDER

RANK	STATE	PERCENT
1	Minnesota	91.8
2	Rhode Island	90.7
3	Iowa	90.5
3	Wisconsin	90.5
5	Massachusetts	90.4
6	Hawaii	90.1
6	New Hampshire	90.1
6	Vermont	90.1
9	Delaware	89.9
10	Nebraska	89.7
11	Connecticut	89.6
12	North Dakota	89.5
13	Maine	89.3
13	Pennsylvania	89.3
15	Kansas	89.1
15	Missouri	89.1
17	Michigan	89.0
17	South Dakota	89.0
19	Ohio	88.3
20	Tennessee	88.2
21	Virginia	87.5
22	Indiana	87.1
23	South Carolina	86.9
24	Maryland	86.8
25	Alabama	86.7
25	Kentucky	86.7
27	Utah	86.4
28	New Jersey	86.3
29	Illinois	86.0
30	Washington	85.7
31	Oregon	85.2
31	West Virginia	85.2
33	New York	84.5
34	Montana	83.9
34	North Carolina	83.9
36	Colorado	83.7
37	Georgia	83.6
38	Wyoming	83.5
39	Arkansas	83.4
40	Mississippi	83.0
41	Arizona	82.7
42	Idaho	82.5
43	Florida	82.4
44	Alaska	82.2
45	Nevada	81.7
46	California	81.3
46	Oklahoma	81.3
48	Louisiana	80.6
49	New Mexico	78.7
50	Texas	75.4

	District of Columbia	86.7

Source: Morgan Quitno Press using data from U.S. Bureau of the Census
    "Income, Poverty and Health Insurance Covered in the United States: 2003"
    (http://www.census.gov/hhes/hlthins/hlthin03/hi03t9.pdf)
*Three-year average for 2001 through 2003.

Percent of Population Covered by Private Health Insurance in 2003

National Percent = 68.6% of Population*

ALPHA ORDER

RANK	STATE	PERCENT
33	Alabama	67.7
44	Alaska	61.5
40	Arizona	64.0
47	Arkansas	60.7
42	California	63.8
25	Colorado	69.8
8	Connecticut	75.8
10	Delaware	75.7
38	Florida	64.7
26	Georgia	69.5
19	Hawaii	74.0
35	Idaho	67.1
21	Illinois	73.2
20	Indiana	73.7
2	Iowa	79.3
11	Kansas	75.4
27	Kentucky	68.4
45	Louisiana	61.3
27	Maine	68.4
12	Maryland	75.2
17	Massachusetts	74.4
5	Michigan	76.2
1	Minnesota	81.0
48	Mississippi	59.4
14	Missouri	74.9
39	Montana	64.2
5	Nebraska	76.2
34	Nevada	67.5
2	New Hampshire	79.3
18	New Jersey	74.2
50	New Mexico	55.2
37	New York	66.4
41	North Carolina	63.9
7	North Dakota	76.0
15	Ohio	74.8
43	Oklahoma	62.1
29	Oregon	68.3
8	Pennsylvania	75.8
22	Rhode Island	72.7
29	South Carolina	68.3
16	South Dakota	74.6
36	Tennessee	66.6
49	Texas	57.9
4	Utah	77.8
24	Vermont	71.1
23	Virginia	71.8
29	Washington	68.3
46	West Virginia	60.9
12	Wisconsin	75.2
32	Wyoming	68.2

RANK ORDER

RANK	STATE	PERCENT
1	Minnesota	81.0
2	Iowa	79.3
2	New Hampshire	79.3
4	Utah	77.8
5	Michigan	76.2
5	Nebraska	76.2
7	North Dakota	76.0
8	Connecticut	75.8
8	Pennsylvania	75.8
10	Delaware	75.7
11	Kansas	75.4
12	Maryland	75.2
12	Wisconsin	75.2
14	Missouri	74.9
15	Ohio	74.8
16	South Dakota	74.6
17	Massachusetts	74.4
18	New Jersey	74.2
19	Hawaii	74.0
20	Indiana	73.7
21	Illinois	73.2
22	Rhode Island	72.7
23	Virginia	71.8
24	Vermont	71.1
25	Colorado	69.8
26	Georgia	69.5
27	Kentucky	68.4
27	Maine	68.4
29	Oregon	68.3
29	South Carolina	68.3
29	Washington	68.3
32	Wyoming	68.2
33	Alabama	67.7
34	Nevada	67.5
35	Idaho	67.1
36	Tennessee	66.6
37	New York	66.4
38	Florida	64.7
39	Montana	64.2
40	Arizona	64.0
41	North Carolina	63.9
42	California	63.8
43	Oklahoma	62.1
44	Alaska	61.5
45	Louisiana	61.3
46	West Virginia	60.9
47	Arkansas	60.7
48	Mississippi	59.4
49	Texas	57.9
50	New Mexico	55.2

| | District of Columbia | 64.6 |

Source: U.S. Bureau of the Census
"Health Insurance Coverage Status" (http://ferret.bls.census.gov/macro/032004/health/h05_000.htm)
*Private health insurance is coverage by a health plan provided through an employer or union or purchased by an individual from a private health insurance company.

Percent of Population Covered by
Employment-Based Health Insurance in 2003
National Percent = 60.4% of Population*

ALPHA ORDER

RANK	STATE	PERCENT
26	Alabama	60.5
38	Alaska	55.8
41	Arizona	54.8
48	Arkansas	51.1
39	California	55.5
24	Colorado	61.2
4	Connecticut	69.0
2	Delaware	70.5
43	Florida	54.2
20	Georgia	63.2
10	Hawaii	67.9
36	Idaho	57.3
18	Illinois	64.5
13	Indiana	65.7
14	Iowa	65.2
20	Kansas	63.2
28	Kentucky	59.8
45	Louisiana	52.8
33	Maine	58.1
9	Maryland	68.1
11	Massachusetts	66.0
4	Michigan	69.0
3	Minnesota	69.8
45	Mississippi	52.8
17	Missouri	64.6
49	Montana	49.9
23	Nebraska	61.4
25	Nevada	60.7
1	New Hampshire	73.3
8	New Jersey	68.3
50	New Mexico	48.9
28	New York	59.8
40	North Carolina	54.9
30	North Dakota	59.5
7	Ohio	68.4
44	Oklahoma	53.5
32	Oregon	58.7
16	Pennsylvania	64.9
15	Rhode Island	65.1
27	South Carolina	60.0
34	South Dakota	57.9
35	Tennessee	57.5
47	Texas	52.4
4	Utah	69.0
22	Vermont	62.2
19	Virginia	63.9
30	Washington	59.5
42	West Virginia	54.7
12	Wisconsin	65.8
37	Wyoming	56.3

RANK ORDER

RANK	STATE	PERCENT
1	New Hampshire	73.3
2	Delaware	70.5
3	Minnesota	69.8
4	Connecticut	69.0
4	Michigan	69.0
4	Utah	69.0
7	Ohio	68.4
8	New Jersey	68.3
9	Maryland	68.1
10	Hawaii	67.9
11	Massachusetts	66.0
12	Wisconsin	65.8
13	Indiana	65.7
14	Iowa	65.2
15	Rhode Island	65.1
16	Pennsylvania	64.9
17	Missouri	64.6
18	Illinois	64.5
19	Virginia	63.9
20	Georgia	63.2
20	Kansas	63.2
22	Vermont	62.2
23	Nebraska	61.4
24	Colorado	61.2
25	Nevada	60.7
26	Alabama	60.5
27	South Carolina	60.0
28	Kentucky	59.8
28	New York	59.8
30	North Dakota	59.5
30	Washington	59.5
32	Oregon	58.7
33	Maine	58.1
34	South Dakota	57.9
35	Tennessee	57.5
36	Idaho	57.3
37	Wyoming	56.3
38	Alaska	55.8
39	California	55.5
40	North Carolina	54.9
41	Arizona	54.8
42	West Virginia	54.7
43	Florida	54.2
44	Oklahoma	53.5
45	Louisiana	52.8
45	Mississippi	52.8
47	Texas	52.4
48	Arkansas	51.1
49	Montana	49.9
50	New Mexico	48.9
	District of Columbia	58.4

Source: U.S. Bureau of the Census
   "Health Insurance Coverage Status" (http://ferret.bls.census.gov/macro/032004/health/h05_000.htm)
*Employment-based health insurance is private insurance coverage offered through one's own employment or a relative's. It may be offered by an employer or by a union.

Percent of Population Covered by Direct Purchase Health Insurance in 2003

National Percent = 9.2% of Population*

ALPHA ORDER

RANK	STATE	PERCENT
32	Alabama	8.5
49	Alaska	5.9
30	Arizona	9.2
19	Arkansas	10.0
27	California	9.6
21	Colorado	9.8
38	Connecticut	7.7
47	Delaware	6.2
10	Florida	11.7
34	Georgia	7.9
34	Hawaii	7.9
9	Idaho	11.8
27	Illinois	9.6
17	Indiana	10.4
4	Iowa	15.2
7	Kansas	12.8
29	Kentucky	9.5
31	Louisiana	8.6
12	Maine	11.0
34	Maryland	7.9
33	Massachusetts	8.3
38	Michigan	7.7
8	Minnesota	12.5
37	Mississippi	7.8
16	Missouri	10.5
5	Montana	13.6
3	Nebraska	16.4
44	Nevada	7.1
44	New Hampshire	7.1
42	New Jersey	7.3
48	New Mexico	6.1
41	New York	7.4
13	North Carolina	10.8
1	North Dakota	17.2
46	Ohio	6.6
25	Oklahoma	9.7
14	Oregon	10.6
11	Pennsylvania	11.5
38	Rhode Island	7.7
21	South Carolina	9.8
2	South Dakota	16.9
25	Tennessee	9.7
50	Texas	5.7
21	Utah	9.8
20	Vermont	9.9
21	Virginia	9.8
14	Washington	10.6
42	West Virginia	7.3
18	Wisconsin	10.3
6	Wyoming	13.3

RANK ORDER

RANK	STATE	PERCENT
1	North Dakota	17.2
2	South Dakota	16.9
3	Nebraska	16.4
4	Iowa	15.2
5	Montana	13.6
6	Wyoming	13.3
7	Kansas	12.8
8	Minnesota	12.5
9	Idaho	11.8
10	Florida	11.7
11	Pennsylvania	11.5
12	Maine	11.0
13	North Carolina	10.8
14	Oregon	10.6
14	Washington	10.6
16	Missouri	10.5
17	Indiana	10.4
18	Wisconsin	10.3
19	Arkansas	10.0
20	Vermont	9.9
21	Colorado	9.8
21	South Carolina	9.8
21	Utah	9.8
21	Virginia	9.8
25	Oklahoma	9.7
25	Tennessee	9.7
27	California	9.6
27	Illinois	9.6
29	Kentucky	9.5
30	Arizona	9.2
31	Louisiana	8.6
32	Alabama	8.5
33	Massachusetts	8.3
34	Georgia	7.9
34	Hawaii	7.9
34	Maryland	7.9
37	Mississippi	7.8
38	Connecticut	7.7
38	Michigan	7.7
38	Rhode Island	7.7
41	New York	7.4
42	New Jersey	7.3
42	West Virginia	7.3
44	Nevada	7.1
44	New Hampshire	7.1
46	Ohio	6.6
47	Delaware	6.2
48	New Mexico	6.1
49	Alaska	5.9
50	Texas	5.7
	District of Columbia	7.4

Source: U.S. Bureau of the Census
   "Health Insurance Coverage Status" (http://ferret.bls.census.gov/macro/032004/health/h05_000.htm)
*Direct-purchase health insurance is private insurance coverage though a plan purchased by an individual from a private company.

Percent of Population Covered by Government Health Insurance in 2003

National Percent = 26.6% of Population*

ALPHA ORDER

RANK	STATE	PERCENT
18	Alabama	29.2
6	Alaska	33.5
13	Arizona	30.4
5	Arkansas	34.6
30	California	26.3
45	Colorado	21.5
31	Connecticut	25.8
29	Delaware	26.4
15	Florida	30.3
41	Georgia	23.4
11	Hawaii	30.5
35	Idaho	25.3
42	Illinois	22.9
43	Indiana	22.6
39	Iowa	24.3
28	Kansas	26.9
8	Kentucky	32.2
21	Louisiana	28.9
1	Maine	35.8
44	Maryland	21.8
36	Massachusetts	25.1
31	Michigan	25.8
47	Minnesota	21.1
4	Mississippi	34.9
22	Missouri	27.7
13	Montana	30.4
38	Nebraska	24.5
45	Nevada	21.5
48	New Hampshire	20.3
48	New Jersey	20.3
3	New Mexico	35.2
20	New York	29.0
16	North Carolina	29.4
22	North Dakota	27.7
40	Ohio	24.2
11	Oklahoma	30.5
33	Oregon	25.7
27	Pennsylvania	27.0
16	Rhode Island	29.4
9	South Carolina	31.2
24	South Dakota	27.6
10	Tennessee	30.6
37	Texas	24.8
50	Utah	19.5
7	Vermont	32.9
26	Virginia	27.4
25	Washington	27.5
1	West Virginia	35.8
34	Wisconsin	25.5
19	Wyoming	29.1

RANK ORDER

RANK	STATE	PERCENT
1	Maine	35.8
1	West Virginia	35.8
3	New Mexico	35.2
4	Mississippi	34.9
5	Arkansas	34.6
6	Alaska	33.5
7	Vermont	32.9
8	Kentucky	32.2
9	South Carolina	31.2
10	Tennessee	30.6
11	Hawaii	30.5
11	Oklahoma	30.5
13	Arizona	30.4
13	Montana	30.4
15	Florida	30.3
16	North Carolina	29.4
16	Rhode Island	29.4
18	Alabama	29.2
19	Wyoming	29.1
20	New York	29.0
21	Louisiana	28.9
22	Missouri	27.7
22	North Dakota	27.7
24	South Dakota	27.6
25	Washington	27.5
26	Virginia	27.4
27	Pennsylvania	27.0
28	Kansas	26.9
29	Delaware	26.4
30	California	26.3
31	Connecticut	25.8
31	Michigan	25.8
33	Oregon	25.7
34	Wisconsin	25.5
35	Idaho	25.3
36	Massachusetts	25.1
37	Texas	24.8
38	Nebraska	24.5
39	Iowa	24.3
40	Ohio	24.2
41	Georgia	23.4
42	Illinois	22.9
43	Indiana	22.6
44	Maryland	21.8
45	Colorado	21.5
45	Nevada	21.5
47	Minnesota	21.1
48	New Hampshire	20.3
48	New Jersey	20.3
50	Utah	19.5

	District of Columbia	30.5

Source: U.S. Bureau of the Census
   "Health Insurance Coverage Status" (http://ferret.bls.census.gov/macro/032004/health/h05_000.htm)
*Includes Medicaid, Medicare, State Children's Health Insurance Program (SCHIP) and military health care.

248

Percent of Population Covered by Military Health Care in 2003

National Percent = 3.5% of Population*

ALPHA ORDER

RANK	STATE	PERCENT
24	Alabama	4.1
1	Alaska	14.0
11	Arizona	6.3
7	Arkansas	7.0
36	California	2.7
13	Colorado	5.6
40	Connecticut	2.1
26	Delaware	3.9
19	Florida	4.7
32	Georgia	3.3
3	Hawaii	8.3
35	Idaho	3.0
45	Illinois	1.7
47	Indiana	1.5
36	Iowa	2.7
5	Kansas	7.6
12	Kentucky	6.0
21	Louisiana	4.4
23	Maine	4.2
29	Maryland	3.4
44	Massachusetts	1.8
48	Michigan	1.4
40	Minnesota	2.1
9	Mississippi	6.6
29	Missouri	3.4
6	Montana	7.4
17	Nebraska	4.8
25	Nevada	4.0
39	New Hampshire	2.4
48	New Jersey	1.4
17	New Mexico	4.8
50	New York	1.2
15	North Carolina	5.3
8	North Dakota	6.8
43	Ohio	2.0
10	Oklahoma	6.5
29	Oregon	3.4
40	Pennsylvania	2.1
38	Rhode Island	2.5
14	South Carolina	5.4
20	South Dakota	4.6
21	Tennessee	4.4
34	Texas	3.1
27	Utah	3.6
32	Vermont	3.3
2	Virginia	10.2
16	Washington	5.2
27	West Virginia	3.6
46	Wisconsin	1.6
4	Wyoming	7.8

RANK ORDER

RANK	STATE	PERCENT
1	Alaska	14.0
2	Virginia	10.2
3	Hawaii	8.3
4	Wyoming	7.8
5	Kansas	7.6
6	Montana	7.4
7	Arkansas	7.0
8	North Dakota	6.8
9	Mississippi	6.6
10	Oklahoma	6.5
11	Arizona	6.3
12	Kentucky	6.0
13	Colorado	5.6
14	South Carolina	5.4
15	North Carolina	5.3
16	Washington	5.2
17	Nebraska	4.8
17	New Mexico	4.8
19	Florida	4.7
20	South Dakota	4.6
21	Louisiana	4.4
21	Tennessee	4.4
23	Maine	4.2
24	Alabama	4.1
25	Nevada	4.0
26	Delaware	3.9
27	Utah	3.6
27	West Virginia	3.6
29	Maryland	3.4
29	Missouri	3.4
29	Oregon	3.4
32	Georgia	3.3
32	Vermont	3.3
34	Texas	3.1
35	Idaho	3.0
36	California	2.7
36	Iowa	2.7
38	Rhode Island	2.5
39	New Hampshire	2.4
40	Connecticut	2.1
40	Minnesota	2.1
40	Pennsylvania	2.1
43	Ohio	2.0
44	Massachusetts	1.8
45	Illinois	1.7
46	Wisconsin	1.6
47	Indiana	1.5
48	Michigan	1.4
48	New Jersey	1.4
50	New York	1.2

| | District of Columbia | 2.1 |

Source: U.S. Bureau of the Census
    "Health Insurance Coverage Status" (http://ferret.bls.census.gov/macro/032004/health/h05_000.htm)
*Includes CHAMPUS (Comprehensive Health and Medical Plan for Uniformed Services)/Tricare, Veterans and military health care.

Percent of Children Covered by Health Insurance in 2003

National Percent = 88.6% of Children*

ALPHA ORDER

RANK	STATE	PERCENT
23	Alabama	91.3
36	Alaska	87.7
44	Arizona	85.4
30	Arkansas	89.5
37	California	87.5
41	Colorado	86.3
15	Connecticut	91.7
21	Delaware	91.5
46	Florida	84.5
41	Georgia	86.3
10	Hawaii	92.6
41	Idaho	86.3
29	Illinois	90.0
26	Indiana	91.0
22	Iowa	91.4
7	Kansas	93.6
30	Kentucky	89.5
45	Louisiana	84.8
5	Maine	94.0
14	Maryland	91.9
13	Massachusetts	92.1
4	Michigan	94.2
6	Minnesota	93.8
35	Mississippi	87.9
9	Missouri	92.7
48	Montana	82.3
8	Nebraska	93.0
47	Nevada	82.6
3	New Hampshire	94.5
33	New Jersey	89.0
39	New Mexico	86.8
28	New York	90.6
34	North Carolina	88.1
11	North Dakota	92.5
15	Ohio	91.7
49	Oklahoma	82.1
40	Oregon	86.5
17	Pennsylvania	91.6
2	Rhode Island	94.8
24	South Carolina	91.1
17	South Dakota	91.6
32	Tennessee	89.2
50	Texas	80.0
26	Utah	91.0
1	Vermont	96.1
24	Virginia	91.1
17	Washington	91.6
17	West Virginia	91.6
12	Wisconsin	92.3
37	Wyoming	87.5

RANK ORDER

RANK	STATE	PERCENT
1	Vermont	96.1
2	Rhode Island	94.8
3	New Hampshire	94.5
4	Michigan	94.2
5	Maine	94.0
6	Minnesota	93.8
7	Kansas	93.6
8	Nebraska	93.0
9	Missouri	92.7
10	Hawaii	92.6
11	North Dakota	92.5
12	Wisconsin	92.3
13	Massachusetts	92.1
14	Maryland	91.9
15	Connecticut	91.7
15	Ohio	91.7
17	Pennsylvania	91.6
17	South Dakota	91.6
17	Washington	91.6
17	West Virginia	91.6
21	Delaware	91.5
22	Iowa	91.4
23	Alabama	91.3
24	South Carolina	91.1
24	Virginia	91.1
26	Indiana	91.0
26	Utah	91.0
28	New York	90.6
29	Illinois	90.0
30	Arkansas	89.5
30	Kentucky	89.5
32	Tennessee	89.2
33	New Jersey	89.0
34	North Carolina	88.1
35	Mississippi	87.9
36	Alaska	87.7
37	California	87.5
37	Wyoming	87.5
39	New Mexico	86.8
40	Oregon	86.5
41	Colorado	86.3
41	Georgia	86.3
41	Idaho	86.3
44	Arizona	85.4
45	Louisiana	84.8
46	Florida	84.5
47	Nevada	82.6
48	Montana	82.3
49	Oklahoma	82.1
50	Texas	80.0

	District of Columbia	88.6

Source: U.S. Bureau of the Census
   "Health Insurance Coverage Status" (http://ferret.bls.census.gov/macro/032004/health/h05_000.htm)
*Children under 18 covered by either private or government health insurance.

Percent of Children Covered by Private Health Insurance in 2003

National Percent = 65.9% of Children*

ALPHA ORDER

RANK	STATE	PERCENT
31	Alabama	65.3
42	Alaska	58.1
39	Arizona	60.7
44	Arkansas	56.4
40	California	60.5
24	Colorado	69.1
5	Connecticut	76.0
15	Delaware	73.4
37	Florida	61.7
33	Georgia	64.7
20	Hawaii	71.7
38	Idaho	61.1
19	Illinois	72.0
13	Indiana	74.1
4	Iowa	76.8
11	Kansas	74.3
34	Kentucky	63.9
45	Louisiana	55.3
30	Maine	65.6
9	Maryland	74.8
6	Massachusetts	75.4
8	Michigan	75.2
2	Minnesota	80.6
48	Mississippi	52.8
22	Missouri	71.3
46	Montana	55.1
18	Nebraska	73.2
26	Nevada	66.4
1	New Hampshire	81.4
7	New Jersey	75.3
50	New Mexico	47.7
32	New York	64.8
41	North Carolina	58.9
14	North Dakota	74.0
15	Ohio	73.4
46	Oklahoma	55.1
27	Oregon	66.2
10	Pennsylvania	74.4
12	Rhode Island	74.2
25	South Carolina	68.9
17	South Dakota	73.3
29	Tennessee	65.7
49	Texas	52.5
3	Utah	77.7
28	Vermont	65.8
23	Virginia	71.2
34	Washington	63.9
43	West Virginia	57.5
21	Wisconsin	71.6
36	Wyoming	62.7

RANK ORDER

RANK	STATE	PERCENT
1	New Hampshire	81.4
2	Minnesota	80.6
3	Utah	77.7
4	Iowa	76.8
5	Connecticut	76.0
6	Massachusetts	75.4
7	New Jersey	75.3
8	Michigan	75.2
9	Maryland	74.8
10	Pennsylvania	74.4
11	Kansas	74.3
12	Rhode Island	74.2
13	Indiana	74.1
14	North Dakota	74.0
15	Delaware	73.4
15	Ohio	73.4
17	South Dakota	73.3
18	Nebraska	73.2
19	Illinois	72.0
20	Hawaii	71.7
21	Wisconsin	71.6
22	Missouri	71.3
23	Virginia	71.2
24	Colorado	69.1
25	South Carolina	68.9
26	Nevada	66.4
27	Oregon	66.2
28	Vermont	65.8
29	Tennessee	65.7
30	Maine	65.6
31	Alabama	65.3
32	New York	64.8
33	Georgia	64.7
34	Kentucky	63.9
34	Washington	63.9
36	Wyoming	62.7
37	Florida	61.7
38	Idaho	61.1
39	Arizona	60.7
40	California	60.5
41	North Carolina	58.9
42	Alaska	58.1
43	West Virginia	57.5
44	Arkansas	56.4
45	Louisiana	55.3
46	Montana	55.1
46	Oklahoma	55.1
48	Mississippi	52.8
49	Texas	52.5
50	New Mexico	47.7

	District of Columbia	49.0

Source: U.S. Bureau of the Census
"Health Insurance Coverage Status" (http://ferret.bls.census.gov/macro/032004/health/h05_000.htm)
*Children under 18. Private health insurance is coverage by a health plan provided through an employer or union or purchased by an individual from a private health insurance company.

Percent of Children Covered by Employment-Based Health Insurance in 2003

National Percent = 61.2% of Children*

ALPHA ORDER

RANK	STATE	PERCENT
27	Alabama	61.3
41	Alaska	54.5
38	Arizona	55.1
44	Arkansas	52.1
40	California	54.7
24	Colorado	63.8
4	Connecticut	72.7
9	Delaware	70.1
37	Florida	55.5
30	Georgia	60.7
14	Hawaii	69.1
39	Idaho	54.8
20	Illinois	66.8
12	Indiana	69.5
15	Iowa	68.4
17	Kansas	67.7
34	Kentucky	59.0
48	Louisiana	49.0
32	Maine	60.0
8	Maryland	70.5
13	Massachusetts	69.4
5	Michigan	71.8
2	Minnesota	74.3
46	Mississippi	49.4
19	Missouri	67.2
49	Montana	48.6
23	Nebraska	65.4
31	Nevada	60.5
1	New Hampshire	78.8
3	New Jersey	73.2
50	New Mexico	45.6
27	New York	61.3
43	North Carolina	52.3
21	North Dakota	66.0
7	Ohio	70.7
45	Oklahoma	50.6
26	Oregon	61.5
10	Pennsylvania	70.0
10	Rhode Island	70.0
25	South Carolina	62.8
22	South Dakota	65.8
32	Tennessee	60.0
46	Texas	49.4
6	Utah	70.8
29	Vermont	61.1
18	Virginia	67.4
35	Washington	57.9
42	West Virginia	52.8
16	Wisconsin	67.9
36	Wyoming	56.4

RANK ORDER

RANK	STATE	PERCENT
1	New Hampshire	78.8
2	Minnesota	74.3
3	New Jersey	73.2
4	Connecticut	72.7
5	Michigan	71.8
6	Utah	70.8
7	Ohio	70.7
8	Maryland	70.5
9	Delaware	70.1
10	Pennsylvania	70.0
10	Rhode Island	70.0
12	Indiana	69.5
13	Massachusetts	69.4
14	Hawaii	69.1
15	Iowa	68.4
16	Wisconsin	67.9
17	Kansas	67.7
18	Virginia	67.4
19	Missouri	67.2
20	Illinois	66.8
21	North Dakota	66.0
22	South Dakota	65.8
23	Nebraska	65.4
24	Colorado	63.8
25	South Carolina	62.8
26	Oregon	61.5
27	Alabama	61.3
27	New York	61.3
29	Vermont	61.1
30	Georgia	60.7
31	Nevada	60.5
32	Maine	60.0
32	Tennessee	60.0
34	Kentucky	59.0
35	Washington	57.9
36	Wyoming	56.4
37	Florida	55.5
38	Arizona	55.1
39	Idaho	54.8
40	California	54.7
41	Alaska	54.5
42	West Virginia	52.8
43	North Carolina	52.3
44	Arkansas	52.1
45	Oklahoma	50.6
46	Mississippi	49.4
46	Texas	49.4
48	Louisiana	49.0
49	Montana	48.6
50	New Mexico	45.6
	District of Columbia	46.6

Source: U.S. Bureau of the Census
"Health Insurance Coverage Status" (http://ferret.bls.census.gov/macro/032004/health/h05_000.htm)
*Children under 18. Employment-based health insurance is private insurance coverage offered through one's own employment or a relative's. It may be offered by an employer or by a union.

Percent of Children Covered by Direct Purchase Health Insurance in 2003

National Percent = 5.3% of Children*

ALPHA ORDER

RANK	STATE	PERCENT
32	Alabama	4.5
35	Alaska	4.3
17	Arizona	6.1
30	Arkansas	4.6
13	California	6.8
16	Colorado	6.4
43	Connecticut	3.4
37	Delaware	4.0
12	Florida	6.9
20	Georgia	6.0
39	Hawaii	3.8
17	Idaho	6.1
15	Illinois	6.6
7	Indiana	7.2
2	Iowa	8.8
14	Kansas	6.7
36	Kentucky	4.1
22	Louisiana	5.9
26	Maine	5.1
29	Maryland	4.8
23	Massachusetts	5.7
43	Michigan	3.4
7	Minnesota	7.2
46	Mississippi	3.2
41	Missouri	3.7
17	Montana	6.1
1	Nebraska	9.1
24	Nevada	5.6
48	New Hampshire	2.8
47	New Jersey	2.9
50	New Mexico	2.2
37	New York	4.0
6	North Carolina	8.0
4	North Dakota	8.6
49	Ohio	2.6
32	Oklahoma	4.5
25	Oregon	5.4
34	Pennsylvania	4.4
41	Rhode Island	3.7
10	South Carolina	7.0
2	South Dakota	8.8
28	Tennessee	4.9
45	Texas	3.3
4	Utah	8.6
20	Vermont	6.0
27	Virginia	5.0
10	Washington	7.0
30	West Virginia	4.6
39	Wisconsin	3.8
9	Wyoming	7.1

RANK ORDER

RANK	STATE	PERCENT
1	Nebraska	9.1
2	Iowa	8.8
2	South Dakota	8.8
4	North Dakota	8.6
4	Utah	8.6
6	North Carolina	8.0
7	Indiana	7.2
7	Minnesota	7.2
9	Wyoming	7.1
10	South Carolina	7.0
10	Washington	7.0
12	Florida	6.9
13	California	6.8
14	Kansas	6.7
15	Illinois	6.6
16	Colorado	6.4
17	Arizona	6.1
17	Idaho	6.1
17	Montana	6.1
20	Georgia	6.0
20	Vermont	6.0
22	Louisiana	5.9
23	Massachusetts	5.7
24	Nevada	5.6
25	Oregon	5.4
26	Maine	5.1
27	Virginia	5.0
28	Tennessee	4.9
29	Maryland	4.8
30	Arkansas	4.6
30	West Virginia	4.6
32	Alabama	4.5
32	Oklahoma	4.5
34	Pennsylvania	4.4
35	Alaska	4.3
36	Kentucky	4.1
37	Delaware	4.0
37	New York	4.0
39	Hawaii	3.8
39	Wisconsin	3.8
41	Missouri	3.7
41	Rhode Island	3.7
43	Connecticut	3.4
43	Michigan	3.4
45	Texas	3.3
46	Mississippi	3.2
47	New Jersey	2.9
48	New Hampshire	2.8
49	Ohio	2.6
50	New Mexico	2.2

District of Columbia	1.9

Source: U.S. Bureau of the Census
    "Health Insurance Coverage Status" (http://ferret.bls.census.gov/macro/032004/health/h05_000.htm)
*Children under 18. Direct-purchase health insurance is private insurance coverage though a plan purchased by an individual from a private company.

Percent of Children Covered by Government Health Insurance in 2003

National Percent = 29.1% of Children*

<table>
<tr><td colspan="3">ALPHA ORDER</td><td colspan="3">RANK ORDER</td></tr>
<tr><th>RANK</th><th>STATE</th><th>PERCENT</th><th>RANK</th><th>STATE</th><th>PERCENT</th></tr>
<tr><td>19</td><td>Alabama</td><td>31.5</td><td>1</td><td>New Mexico</td><td>50.6</td></tr>
<tr><td>3</td><td>Alaska</td><td>44.4</td><td>2</td><td>Mississippi</td><td>45.8</td></tr>
<tr><td>22</td><td>Arizona</td><td>31.2</td><td>3</td><td>Alaska</td><td>44.4</td></tr>
<tr><td>4</td><td>Arkansas</td><td>42.6</td><td>4</td><td>Arkansas</td><td>42.6</td></tr>
<tr><td>17</td><td>California</td><td>32.0</td><td>5</td><td>Vermont</td><td>42.1</td></tr>
<tr><td>40</td><td>Colorado</td><td>22.5</td><td>6</td><td>West Virginia</td><td>40.9</td></tr>
<tr><td>44</td><td>Connecticut</td><td>21.2</td><td>7</td><td>Maine</td><td>39.1</td></tr>
<tr><td>25</td><td>Delaware</td><td>28.7</td><td>8</td><td>Washington</td><td>37.0</td></tr>
<tr><td>24</td><td>Florida</td><td>29.1</td><td>9</td><td>North Carolina</td><td>36.7</td></tr>
<tr><td>23</td><td>Georgia</td><td>29.4</td><td>10</td><td>Louisiana</td><td>35.7</td></tr>
<tr><td>19</td><td>Hawaii</td><td>31.5</td><td>11</td><td>Wyoming</td><td>35.4</td></tr>
<tr><td>21</td><td>Idaho</td><td>31.4</td><td>12</td><td>Oklahoma</td><td>33.6</td></tr>
<tr><td>39</td><td>Illinois</td><td>22.6</td><td>13</td><td>Montana</td><td>33.0</td></tr>
<tr><td>42</td><td>Indiana</td><td>22.4</td><td>14</td><td>South Carolina</td><td>32.5</td></tr>
<tr><td>48</td><td>Iowa</td><td>19.4</td><td>15</td><td>Texas</td><td>32.4</td></tr>
<tr><td>27</td><td>Kansas</td><td>28.4</td><td>16</td><td>New York</td><td>32.1</td></tr>
<tr><td>18</td><td>Kentucky</td><td>31.9</td><td>17</td><td>California</td><td>32.0</td></tr>
<tr><td>10</td><td>Louisiana</td><td>35.7</td><td>18</td><td>Kentucky</td><td>31.9</td></tr>
<tr><td>7</td><td>Maine</td><td>39.1</td><td>19</td><td>Alabama</td><td>31.5</td></tr>
<tr><td>40</td><td>Maryland</td><td>22.5</td><td>19</td><td>Hawaii</td><td>31.5</td></tr>
<tr><td>43</td><td>Massachusetts</td><td>22.1</td><td>21</td><td>Idaho</td><td>31.4</td></tr>
<tr><td>30</td><td>Michigan</td><td>28.2</td><td>22</td><td>Arizona</td><td>31.2</td></tr>
<tr><td>46</td><td>Minnesota</td><td>19.9</td><td>23</td><td>Georgia</td><td>29.4</td></tr>
<tr><td>2</td><td>Mississippi</td><td>45.8</td><td>24</td><td>Florida</td><td>29.1</td></tr>
<tr><td>27</td><td>Missouri</td><td>28.4</td><td>25</td><td>Delaware</td><td>28.7</td></tr>
<tr><td>13</td><td>Montana</td><td>33.0</td><td>25</td><td>Tennessee</td><td>28.7</td></tr>
<tr><td>34</td><td>Nebraska</td><td>26.5</td><td>27</td><td>Kansas</td><td>28.4</td></tr>
<tr><td>45</td><td>Nevada</td><td>20.0</td><td>27</td><td>Missouri</td><td>28.4</td></tr>
<tr><td>49</td><td>New Hampshire</td><td>18.8</td><td>27</td><td>Rhode Island</td><td>28.4</td></tr>
<tr><td>50</td><td>New Jersey</td><td>17.1</td><td>30</td><td>Michigan</td><td>28.2</td></tr>
<tr><td>1</td><td>New Mexico</td><td>50.6</td><td>31</td><td>North Dakota</td><td>27.2</td></tr>
<tr><td>16</td><td>New York</td><td>32.1</td><td>32</td><td>Wisconsin</td><td>27.1</td></tr>
<tr><td>9</td><td>North Carolina</td><td>36.7</td><td>33</td><td>Oregon</td><td>27.0</td></tr>
<tr><td>31</td><td>North Dakota</td><td>27.2</td><td>34</td><td>Nebraska</td><td>26.5</td></tr>
<tr><td>37</td><td>Ohio</td><td>25.3</td><td>34</td><td>South Dakota</td><td>26.5</td></tr>
<tr><td>12</td><td>Oklahoma</td><td>33.6</td><td>36</td><td>Virginia</td><td>26.2</td></tr>
<tr><td>33</td><td>Oregon</td><td>27.0</td><td>37</td><td>Ohio</td><td>25.3</td></tr>
<tr><td>38</td><td>Pennsylvania</td><td>24.0</td><td>38</td><td>Pennsylvania</td><td>24.0</td></tr>
<tr><td>27</td><td>Rhode Island</td><td>28.4</td><td>39</td><td>Illinois</td><td>22.6</td></tr>
<tr><td>14</td><td>South Carolina</td><td>32.5</td><td>40</td><td>Colorado</td><td>22.5</td></tr>
<tr><td>34</td><td>South Dakota</td><td>26.5</td><td>40</td><td>Maryland</td><td>22.5</td></tr>
<tr><td>25</td><td>Tennessee</td><td>28.7</td><td>42</td><td>Indiana</td><td>22.4</td></tr>
<tr><td>15</td><td>Texas</td><td>32.4</td><td>43</td><td>Massachusetts</td><td>22.1</td></tr>
<tr><td>47</td><td>Utah</td><td>19.6</td><td>44</td><td>Connecticut</td><td>21.2</td></tr>
<tr><td>5</td><td>Vermont</td><td>42.1</td><td>45</td><td>Nevada</td><td>20.0</td></tr>
<tr><td>36</td><td>Virginia</td><td>26.2</td><td>46</td><td>Minnesota</td><td>19.9</td></tr>
<tr><td>8</td><td>Washington</td><td>37.0</td><td>47</td><td>Utah</td><td>19.6</td></tr>
<tr><td>6</td><td>West Virginia</td><td>40.9</td><td>48</td><td>Iowa</td><td>19.4</td></tr>
<tr><td>32</td><td>Wisconsin</td><td>27.1</td><td>49</td><td>New Hampshire</td><td>18.8</td></tr>
<tr><td>11</td><td>Wyoming</td><td>35.4</td><td>50</td><td>New Jersey</td><td>17.1</td></tr>
<tr><td></td><td></td><td></td><td></td><td>District of Columbia</td><td>46.2</td></tr>
</table>

Source: U.S. Bureau of the Census
    "Health Insurance Coverage Status" (http://ferret.bls.census.gov/macro/032004/health/h05_000.htm)
*Children under 18. Includes Medicaid, Medicare, State Children's Health Insurance Program (SCHIP) and military health care.

Percent of Children Covered by Military Health Care in 2003

National Percent = 2.7% of Children*

ALPHA ORDER

RANK	STATE	PERCENT
31	Alabama	2.3
1	Alaska	16.6
17	Arizona	4.0
8	Arkansas	5.6
32	California	2.2
9	Colorado	5.5
41	Connecticut	1.6
16	Delaware	4.2
26	Florida	2.5
28	Georgia	2.4
2	Hawaii	9.8
44	Idaho	1.5
34	Illinois	2.0
46	Indiana	1.1
38	Iowa	1.7
4	Kansas	9.1
14	Kentucky	4.8
24	Louisiana	3.1
17	Maine	4.0
22	Maryland	3.3
45	Massachusetts	1.3
50	Michigan	0.8
35	Minnesota	1.8
6	Mississippi	6.5
28	Missouri	2.4
7	Montana	6.3
10	Nebraska	5.1
38	Nevada	1.7
41	New Hampshire	1.6
46	New Jersey	1.1
20	New Mexico	3.9
48	New York	0.9
12	North Carolina	5.0
4	North Dakota	9.1
38	Ohio	1.7
13	Oklahoma	4.9
35	Oregon	1.8
41	Pennsylvania	1.6
28	Rhode Island	2.4
17	South Carolina	4.0
26	South Dakota	2.5
20	Tennessee	3.9
35	Texas	1.8
22	Utah	3.3
24	Vermont	3.1
3	Virginia	9.4
10	Washington	5.1
33	West Virginia	2.1
48	Wisconsin	0.9
14	Wyoming	4.8

RANK ORDER

RANK	STATE	PERCENT
1	Alaska	16.6
2	Hawaii	9.8
3	Virginia	9.4
4	Kansas	9.1
4	North Dakota	9.1
6	Mississippi	6.5
7	Montana	6.3
8	Arkansas	5.6
9	Colorado	5.5
10	Nebraska	5.1
10	Washington	5.1
12	North Carolina	5.0
13	Oklahoma	4.9
14	Kentucky	4.8
14	Wyoming	4.8
16	Delaware	4.2
17	Arizona	4.0
17	Maine	4.0
17	South Carolina	4.0
20	New Mexico	3.9
20	Tennessee	3.9
22	Maryland	3.3
22	Utah	3.3
24	Louisiana	3.1
24	Vermont	3.1
26	Florida	2.5
26	South Dakota	2.5
28	Georgia	2.4
28	Missouri	2.4
28	Rhode Island	2.4
31	Alabama	2.3
32	California	2.2
33	West Virginia	2.1
34	Illinois	2.0
35	Minnesota	1.8
35	Oregon	1.8
35	Texas	1.8
38	Iowa	1.7
38	Nevada	1.7
38	Ohio	1.7
41	Connecticut	1.6
41	New Hampshire	1.6
41	Pennsylvania	1.6
44	Idaho	1.5
45	Massachusetts	1.3
46	Indiana	1.1
46	New Jersey	1.1
48	New York	0.9
48	Wisconsin	0.9
50	Michigan	0.8

District of Columbia	1.5

Source: U.S. Bureau of the Census
   "Health Insurance Coverage Status" (http://ferret.bls.census.gov/macro/032004/health/h05_000.htm)
Children under 18. Includes CHAMPUS (Comprehensive Health and Medical Plan for Uniformed Services)/Tricare,
Veterans and military health care.

Percent of Children Covered by Medicaid in 2003

National Percent = 26.4% of Children*

ALPHA ORDER

RANK	STATE	PERCENT
18	Alabama	28.6
12	Alaska	29.9
21	Arizona	27.2
4	Arkansas	39.0
14	California	29.8
48	Colorado	16.8
41	Connecticut	19.5
30	Delaware	24.7
23	Florida	26.9
24	Georgia	26.7
34	Hawaii	22.3
14	Idaho	29.8
37	Illinois	20.7
36	Indiana	21.3
47	Iowa	17.1
39	Kansas	19.6
20	Kentucky	27.6
8	Louisiana	32.1
6	Maine	35.4
39	Maryland	19.6
37	Massachusetts	20.7
22	Michigan	27.0
44	Minnesota	17.9
2	Mississippi	39.2
25	Missouri	26.6
16	Montana	29.7
35	Nebraska	21.5
43	Nevada	18.5
45	New Hampshire	17.4
49	New Jersey	16.5
1	New Mexico	46.0
9	New York	31.3
11	North Carolina	30.3
42	North Dakota	19.1
32	Ohio	23.4
17	Oklahoma	28.9
28	Oregon	25.3
33	Pennsylvania	22.5
26	Rhode Island	26.2
19	South Carolina	28.5
31	South Dakota	23.9
28	Tennessee	25.3
10	Texas	30.7
50	Utah	16.1
2	Vermont	39.2
46	Virginia	17.2
7	Washington	32.4
5	West Virginia	38.7
27	Wisconsin	26.0
12	Wyoming	29.9

RANK ORDER

RANK	STATE	PERCENT
1	New Mexico	46.0
2	Mississippi	39.2
2	Vermont	39.2
4	Arkansas	39.0
5	West Virginia	38.7
6	Maine	35.4
7	Washington	32.4
8	Louisiana	32.1
9	New York	31.3
10	Texas	30.7
11	North Carolina	30.3
12	Alaska	29.9
12	Wyoming	29.9
14	California	29.8
14	Idaho	29.8
16	Montana	29.7
17	Oklahoma	28.9
18	Alabama	28.6
19	South Carolina	28.5
20	Kentucky	27.6
21	Arizona	27.2
22	Michigan	27.0
23	Florida	26.9
24	Georgia	26.7
25	Missouri	26.6
26	Rhode Island	26.2
27	Wisconsin	26.0
28	Oregon	25.3
28	Tennessee	25.3
30	Delaware	24.7
31	South Dakota	23.9
32	Ohio	23.4
33	Pennsylvania	22.5
34	Hawaii	22.3
35	Nebraska	21.5
36	Indiana	21.3
37	Illinois	20.7
37	Massachusetts	20.7
39	Kansas	19.6
39	Maryland	19.6
41	Connecticut	19.5
42	North Dakota	19.1
43	Nevada	18.5
44	Minnesota	17.9
45	New Hampshire	17.4
46	Virginia	17.2
47	Iowa	17.1
48	Colorado	16.8
49	New Jersey	16.5
50	Utah	16.1
	District of Columbia	44.5

Source: U.S. Bureau of the Census
    "Health Insurance Coverage Status" (http://ferret.bls.census.gov/macro/032004/health/h05_000.htm)
*Children under 18 years old. Medicaid is a form of government insurance.

State Children's Health Insurance Program (SCHIP) Enrollment in 2003

National Total = 5,874,259 Children*

ALPHA ORDER

RANK	STATE	CHILDREN	% of USA
20	Alabama	78,554	1.3%
35	Alaska	22,934	0.4%
18	Arizona	90,468	1.5%
NA	Arkansas**	NA	NA
1	California	955,152	16.3%
23	Colorado	74,144	1.3%
36	Connecticut	20,971	0.4%
42	Delaware	9,903	0.2%
4	Florida	443,177	7.5%
5	Georgia	251,711	4.3%
41	Hawaii	12,022	0.2%
38	Idaho	16,877	0.3%
10	Illinois	135,609	2.3%
24	Indiana	73,762	1.3%
31	Iowa	37,060	0.6%
27	Kansas	45,662	0.8%
15	Kentucky	94,053	1.6%
14	Louisiana	104,908	1.8%
33	Maine	29,474	0.5%
11	Maryland	130,161	2.2%
12	Massachusetts	128,790	2.2%
21	Michigan	77,467	1.3%
NA	Minnesota**	NA	NA
22	Mississippi	75,010	1.3%
8	Missouri	150,954	2.6%
39	Montana	13,084	0.2%
28	Nebraska	45,490	0.8%
26	Nevada	47,183	0.8%
43	New Hampshire	9,893	0.2%
13	New Jersey	119,272	2.0%
37	New Mexico	18,841	0.3%
2	New York	795,111	13.5%
9	North Carolina	150,444	2.6%
47	North Dakota	4,953	0.1%
6	Ohio	207,854	3.5%
16	Oklahoma	91,914	1.6%
29	Oregon	44,752	0.8%
7	Pennsylvania	160,015	2.7%
34	Rhode Island	24,505	0.4%
17	South Carolina	90,764	1.5%
40	South Dakota	12,288	0.2%
NA	Tennessee**	NA	NA
3	Texas	726,428	12.4%
30	Utah	37,766	0.6%
45	Vermont	6,467	0.1%
19	Virginia	83,716	1.4%
44	Washington	9,571	0.2%
32	West Virginia	35,320	0.6%
25	Wisconsin	68,641	1.2%
46	Wyoming	5,241	0.1%

RANK ORDER

RANK	STATE	CHILDREN	% of USA
1	California	955,152	16.3%
2	New York	795,111	13.5%
3	Texas	726,428	12.4%
4	Florida	443,177	7.5%
5	Georgia	251,711	4.3%
6	Ohio	207,854	3.5%
7	Pennsylvania	160,015	2.7%
8	Missouri	150,954	2.6%
9	North Carolina	150,444	2.6%
10	Illinois	135,609	2.3%
11	Maryland	130,161	2.2%
12	Massachusetts	128,790	2.2%
13	New Jersey	119,272	2.0%
14	Louisiana	104,908	1.8%
15	Kentucky	94,053	1.6%
16	Oklahoma	91,914	1.6%
17	South Carolina	90,764	1.5%
18	Arizona	90,468	1.5%
19	Virginia	83,716	1.4%
20	Alabama	78,554	1.3%
21	Michigan	77,467	1.3%
22	Mississippi	75,010	1.3%
23	Colorado	74,144	1.3%
24	Indiana	73,762	1.3%
25	Wisconsin	68,641	1.2%
26	Nevada	47,183	0.8%
27	Kansas	45,662	0.8%
28	Nebraska	45,490	0.8%
29	Oregon	44,752	0.8%
30	Utah	37,766	0.6%
31	Iowa	37,060	0.6%
32	West Virginia	35,320	0.6%
33	Maine	29,474	0.5%
34	Rhode Island	24,505	0.4%
35	Alaska	22,934	0.4%
36	Connecticut	20,971	0.4%
37	New Mexico	18,841	0.3%
38	Idaho	16,877	0.3%
39	Montana	13,084	0.2%
40	South Dakota	12,288	0.2%
41	Hawaii	12,022	0.2%
42	Delaware	9,903	0.2%
43	New Hampshire	9,893	0.2%
44	Washington	9,571	0.2%
45	Vermont	6,467	0.1%
46	Wyoming	5,241	0.1%
47	North Dakota	4,953	0.1%
NA	Arkansas**	NA	NA
NA	Minnesota**	NA	NA
NA	Tennessee**	NA	NA
	District of Columbia	5,875	0.1%

Source: U.S. Department of Health and Human Services, Centers for Medicare and Medicaid Services
    "Children's Health Insurance Program" (http://www.cms.hhs.gov/schip/enrollment/schip03r.pdf)
Revised figures for fiscal year 2003. The State Children's Health Insurance Program (SCHIP) was created in 1997 to help states expand health insurance to children whose families earn too much to qualify for Medicaid, yet not enough to afford private health insurance.
**Not reported.

Percent Change in State Children's Health Insurance
Program (SCHIP) Enrollment: 2002 to 2003
National Percent Change = 9.7% Increase*

ALPHA ORDER

RANK	STATE	PERCENT CHANGE
47	Alabama	(5.8)
34	Alaska	2.8
44	Arizona	(2.4)
NA	Arkansas**	NA
22	California	10.9
3	Colorado	43.1
35	Connecticut	2.3
36	Delaware	1.9
13	Florida	20.4
16	Georgia	13.9
4	Hawaii	41.9
39	Idaho	(0.1)
2	Illinois	99.3
20	Indiana	11.4
29	Iowa	7.4
18	Kansas	11.8
41	Kentucky	(0.6)
5	Louisiana	40.5
7	Maine	30.5
32	Maryland	4.0
27	Massachusetts	7.6
26	Michigan	7.8
NA	Minnesota**	NA
14	Mississippi	15.7
38	Missouri	0.3
46	Montana	(5.7)
1	Nebraska	180.3
10	Nevada	24.6
12	New Hampshire	21.6
36	New Jersey	1.9
45	New Mexico	(5.5)
42	New York	(1.5)
9	North Carolina	25.0
21	North Dakota	11.0
17	Ohio	13.6
25	Oklahoma	8.8
31	Oregon	4.1
27	Pennsylvania	7.6
8	Rhode Island	25.6
6	South Carolina	36.3
23	South Dakota	9.4
NA	Tennessee**	NA
39	Texas	(0.1)
19	Utah	11.7
30	Vermont	4.9
11	Virginia	23.2
24	Washington	9.3
43	West Virginia	(1.7)
15	Wisconsin	14.7
33	Wyoming	3.6

RANK ORDER

RANK	STATE	PERCENT CHANGE
1	Nebraska	180.3
2	Illinois	99.3
3	Colorado	43.1
4	Hawaii	41.9
5	Louisiana	40.5
6	South Carolina	36.3
7	Maine	30.5
8	Rhode Island	25.6
9	North Carolina	25.0
10	Nevada	24.6
11	Virginia	23.2
12	New Hampshire	21.6
13	Florida	20.4
14	Mississippi	15.7
15	Wisconsin	14.7
16	Georgia	13.9
17	Ohio	13.6
18	Kansas	11.8
19	Utah	11.7
20	Indiana	11.4
21	North Dakota	11.0
22	California	10.9
23	South Dakota	9.4
24	Washington	9.3
25	Oklahoma	8.8
26	Michigan	7.8
27	Massachusetts	7.6
27	Pennsylvania	7.6
29	Iowa	7.4
30	Vermont	4.9
31	Oregon	4.1
32	Maryland	4.0
33	Wyoming	3.6
34	Alaska	2.8
35	Connecticut	2.3
36	Delaware	1.9
36	New Jersey	1.9
38	Missouri	0.3
39	Idaho	(0.1)
39	Texas	(0.1)
41	Kentucky	(0.6)
42	New York	(1.5)
43	West Virginia	(1.7)
44	Arizona	(2.4)
45	New Mexico	(5.5)
46	Montana	(5.7)
47	Alabama	(5.8)
NA	Arkansas**	NA
NA	Minnesota**	NA
NA	Tennessee**	NA

District of Columbia   16.1

Source: MQ Press using data from U.S. Dept of Health & Human Services, Centers for Medicare and Medicaid Services "Children's Health Insurance Program" (http://www.cms.hhs.gov/schip/enrollment/schip03r.pdf)
*Revised figures for fiscal year 2003. The State Children's Health Insurance Program (SCHIP) was created in 1997 to help states expand health insurance to children whose families earn too much to qualify for Medicaid, yet not enough to afford private health insurance.
**Not available.

Percent of Children Enrolled in State Children's Health Insurance Program (SCHIP) in 2003
National Percent = 8.1% of Children 17 Years and Younger*

ALPHA ORDER

RANK	STATE	PERCENT
22	Alabama	7.1
2	Alaska	12.2
27	Arizona	6.0
NA	Arkansas**	NA
10	California	10.2
24	Colorado	6.5
46	Connecticut	2.5
34	Delaware	5.0
4	Florida	11.4
5	Georgia	11.0
41	Hawaii	4.1
37	Idaho	4.6
40	Illinois	4.2
37	Indiana	4.6
30	Iowa	5.4
23	Kansas	6.7
13	Kentucky	9.5
16	Louisiana	9.0
9	Maine	10.3
13	Maryland	9.5
18	Massachusetts	8.7
45	Michigan	3.1
NA	Minnesota**	NA
12	Mississippi	9.9
6	Missouri	10.8
26	Montana	6.1
8	Nebraska	10.4
19	Nevada	8.2
44	New Hampshire	3.3
29	New Jersey	5.6
42	New Mexico	3.8
1	New York	17.7
21	North Carolina	7.3
43	North Dakota	3.4
20	Ohio	7.4
7	Oklahoma	10.5
31	Oregon	5.3
28	Pennsylvania	5.7
11	Rhode Island	10.1
17	South Carolina	8.9
25	South Dakota	6.4
NA	Tennessee**	NA
3	Texas	11.7
33	Utah	5.1
35	Vermont	4.8
36	Virginia	4.7
47	Washington	0.6
15	West Virginia	9.1
32	Wisconsin	5.2
39	Wyoming	4.4

RANK ORDER

RANK	STATE	PERCENT
1	New York	17.7
2	Alaska	12.2
3	Texas	11.7
4	Florida	11.4
5	Georgia	11.0
6	Missouri	10.8
7	Oklahoma	10.5
8	Nebraska	10.4
9	Maine	10.3
10	California	10.2
11	Rhode Island	10.1
12	Mississippi	9.9
13	Kentucky	9.5
13	Maryland	9.5
15	West Virginia	9.1
16	Louisiana	9.0
17	South Carolina	8.9
18	Massachusetts	8.7
19	Nevada	8.2
20	Ohio	7.4
21	North Carolina	7.3
22	Alabama	7.1
23	Kansas	6.7
24	Colorado	6.5
25	South Dakota	6.4
26	Montana	6.1
27	Arizona	6.0
28	Pennsylvania	5.7
29	New Jersey	5.6
30	Iowa	5.4
31	Oregon	5.3
32	Wisconsin	5.2
33	Utah	5.1
34	Delaware	5.0
35	Vermont	4.8
36	Virginia	4.7
37	Idaho	4.6
37	Indiana	4.6
39	Wyoming	4.4
40	Illinois	4.2
41	Hawaii	4.1
42	New Mexico	3.8
43	North Dakota	3.4
44	New Hampshire	3.3
45	Michigan	3.1
46	Connecticut	2.5
47	Washington	0.6
NA	Arkansas**	NA
NA	Minnesota**	NA
NA	Tennessee**	NA
	District of Columbia	5.5

Source: MQ Press using data from U.S. Dept of Health & Human Services, Centers for Medicare and Medicaid Services "Children's Health Insurance Program" (http://www.cms.hhs.gov/schip/enrollment/schip03r.pdf)
*Revised figures for fiscal year 2003. The State Children's Health Insurance Program (SCHIP) was created in 1997 to help states expand health insurance to children whose families earn too much to qualify for Medicaid, yet not enough to afford private health insurance. Calculated using 2003 Census estimates for 17 and younger.
**Not available.

State Children's Health Insurance Program (SCHIP) Allotments in 2004

National Total = $3,142,125,000*

ALPHA ORDER

RANK ORDER

RANK	STATE	ALLOTMENTS	% of USA
16	Alabama	$54,679,333	1.7%
45	Alaska	7,156,891	0.2%
10	Arizona	87,023,654	2.8%
29	Arkansas	35,073,372	1.1%
1	California	533,990,797	17.0%
20	Colorado	44,865,429	1.4%
33	Connecticut	27,975,129	0.9%
43	Delaware	7,817,461	0.2%
4	Florida	193,614,837	6.2%
6	Georgia	103,892,954	3.3%
40	Hawaii	9,647,963	0.3%
37	Idaho	16,958,002	0.5%
5	Illinois	120,969,643	3.8%
17	Indiana	54,026,680	1.7%
35	Iowa	19,703,423	0.6%
34	Kansas	23,541,920	0.7%
25	Kentucky	39,286,749	1.3%
12	Louisiana	64,523,178	2.1%
41	Maine	9,474,540	0.3%
28	Maryland	36,121,348	1.1%
19	Massachusetts	46,201,047	1.5%
9	Michigan	89,138,280	2.8%
32	Minnesota	30,626,504	1.0%
27	Mississippi	36,897,326	1.2%
24	Missouri	41,923,481	1.3%
39	Montana	10,193,881	0.3%
38	Nebraska	13,872,884	0.4%
31	Nevada	31,163,957	1.0%
42	New Hampshire	8,013,366	0.3%
13	New Jersey	64,389,677	2.0%
30	New Mexico	32,788,606	1.0%
3	New York	216,455,790	6.9%
11	North Carolina	85,753,907	2.7%
47	North Dakota	5,436,695	0.2%
7	Ohio	103,803,316	3.3%
21	Oklahoma	44,621,756	1.4%
26	Oregon	38,056,795	1.2%
8	Pennsylvania	98,747,809	3.1%
44	Rhode Island	7,379,988	0.2%
23	South Carolina	43,355,057	1.4%
46	South Dakota	5,790,144	0.2%
14	Tennessee	57,957,983	1.8%
2	Texas	330,851,106	10.5%
49	Utah	3,813,156	0.1%
49	Vermont	3,813,156	0.1%
15	Virginia	55,714,814	1.8%
18	Washington	50,326,484	1.6%
36	West Virginia	18,760,354	0.6%
22	Wisconsin	43,504,958	1.4%
48	Wyoming	4,952,110	0.2%

RANK	STATE	ALLOTMENTS	% of USA
1	California	$533,990,797	17.0%
2	Texas	330,851,106	10.5%
3	New York	216,455,790	6.9%
4	Florida	193,614,837	6.2%
5	Illinois	120,969,643	3.8%
6	Georgia	103,892,954	3.3%
7	Ohio	103,803,316	3.3%
8	Pennsylvania	98,747,809	3.1%
9	Michigan	89,138,280	2.8%
10	Arizona	87,023,654	2.8%
11	North Carolina	85,753,907	2.7%
12	Louisiana	64,523,178	2.1%
13	New Jersey	64,389,677	2.0%
14	Tennessee	57,957,983	1.8%
15	Virginia	55,714,814	1.8%
16	Alabama	54,679,333	1.7%
17	Indiana	54,026,680	1.7%
18	Washington	50,326,484	1.6%
19	Massachusetts	46,201,047	1.5%
20	Colorado	44,865,429	1.4%
21	Oklahoma	44,621,756	1.4%
22	Wisconsin	43,504,958	1.4%
23	South Carolina	43,355,057	1.4%
24	Missouri	41,923,481	1.3%
25	Kentucky	39,286,749	1.3%
26	Oregon	38,056,795	1.2%
27	Mississippi	36,897,326	1.2%
28	Maryland	36,121,348	1.1%
29	Arkansas	35,073,372	1.1%
30	New Mexico	32,788,606	1.0%
31	Nevada	31,163,957	1.0%
32	Minnesota	30,626,504	1.0%
33	Connecticut	27,975,129	0.9%
34	Kansas	23,541,920	0.7%
35	Iowa	19,703,423	0.6%
36	West Virginia	18,760,354	0.6%
37	Idaho	16,958,002	0.5%
38	Nebraska	13,872,884	0.4%
39	Montana	10,193,881	0.3%
40	Hawaii	9,647,963	0.3%
41	Maine	9,474,540	0.3%
42	New Hampshire	8,013,366	0.3%
43	Delaware	7,817,461	0.2%
44	Rhode Island	7,379,988	0.2%
45	Alaska	7,156,891	0.2%
46	South Dakota	5,790,144	0.2%
47	North Dakota	5,436,695	0.2%
48	Wyoming	4,952,110	0.2%
49	Utah	3,813,156	0.1%
49	Vermont	3,813,156	0.1%
	District of Columbia	7,198,952	0.2%

Source: U.S. Department of Health and Human Services, Centers for Medicare and Medicaid Services
  "SCHIP Allotments" (http://www.cms.gov/schip/regulations/allotments/)
For fiscal year 2004. Allotments are distributed based on the number of low-income children and health care cost factors in each state. States have three years to spend their SCHIP allotments. SCHIP was created in 1997 to help states expand health insurance to children whose families earn too much to qualify for Medicaid, yet not enough to afford private health insurance. Total does not include $33,075,000 in allotments to U.S. territories.

Per Capita State Children's Health Insurance Program (SCHIP) Allotments in 2004
National Per Capita = $10.70*

ALPHA ORDER

RANK	STATE	PER CAPITA
11	Alabama	$12.07
16	Alaska	10.92
2	Arizona	15.15
7	Arkansas	12.74
3	California	14.88
23	Colorado	9.75
33	Connecticut	7.98
26	Delaware	9.41
14	Florida	11.13
12	Georgia	11.77
37	Hawaii	7.64
10	Idaho	12.17
24	Illinois	9.51
29	Indiana	8.66
45	Iowa	6.67
30	Kansas	8.61
25	Kentucky	9.48
5	Louisiana	14.29
43	Maine	7.19
46	Maryland	6.50
42	Massachusetts	7.20
28	Michigan	8.81
49	Minnesota	6.00
8	Mississippi	12.71
41	Missouri	7.29
15	Montana	11.00
35	Nebraska	7.94
6	Nevada	13.35
47	New Hampshire	6.17
40	New Jersey	7.40
1	New Mexico	17.23
13	New York	11.26
20	North Carolina	10.04
31	North Dakota	8.57
27	Ohio	9.06
9	Oklahoma	12.66
17	Oregon	10.59
34	Pennsylvania	7.96
44	Rhode Island	6.83
18	South Carolina	10.33
38	South Dakota	7.51
21	Tennessee	9.82
4	Texas	14.71
50	Utah	1.60
48	Vermont	6.14
39	Virginia	7.47
32	Washington	8.11
18	West Virginia	10.33
36	Wisconsin	7.90
22	Wyoming	9.78

RANK ORDER

RANK	STATE	PER CAPITA
1	New Mexico	$17.23
2	Arizona	15.15
3	California	14.88
4	Texas	14.71
5	Louisiana	14.29
6	Nevada	13.35
7	Arkansas	12.74
8	Mississippi	12.71
9	Oklahoma	12.66
10	Idaho	12.17
11	Alabama	12.07
12	Georgia	11.77
13	New York	11.26
14	Florida	11.13
15	Montana	11.00
16	Alaska	10.92
17	Oregon	10.59
18	South Carolina	10.33
18	West Virginia	10.33
20	North Carolina	10.04
21	Tennessee	9.82
22	Wyoming	9.78
23	Colorado	9.75
24	Illinois	9.51
25	Kentucky	9.48
26	Delaware	9.41
27	Ohio	9.06
28	Michigan	8.81
29	Indiana	8.66
30	Kansas	8.61
31	North Dakota	8.57
32	Washington	8.11
33	Connecticut	7.98
34	Pennsylvania	7.96
35	Nebraska	7.94
36	Wisconsin	7.90
37	Hawaii	7.64
38	South Dakota	7.51
39	Virginia	7.47
40	New Jersey	7.40
41	Missouri	7.29
42	Massachusetts	7.20
43	Maine	7.19
44	Rhode Island	6.83
45	Iowa	6.67
46	Maryland	6.50
47	New Hampshire	6.17
48	Vermont	6.14
49	Minnesota	6.00
50	Utah	1.60

District of Columbia   13.01

Source: Morgan Quitno Press using data from U.S. Dept of HHS, Centers for Medicare and Medicaid Services
    "SCHIP Allotments" (http://www.cms.gov/schip/regulations/allotments/)
*For fiscal year 2004. Allotments are distributed based on the number of low-income children and health care cost factors in each state. States have three years to spend their SCHIP allotments. SCHIP was created in 1997 to help states expand health insurance to children whose families earn too much to qualify for Medicaid, yet not enough to afford private health insurance. National per capita does not include allotments to U.S. territories.

Expenditures for State Children's Health Insurance Program (SCHIP) in 2002

National Total = $5,313,023,149*

ALPHA ORDER

RANK	STATE	EXPENDITURES	% of USA
20	Alabama	$69,331,278	1.3%
33	Alaska	29,943,737	0.6%
8	Arizona	167,950,645	3.2%
50	Arkansas	1,909,978	0.0%
2	California	688,375,800	13.0%
27	Colorado	47,971,251	0.9%
34	Connecticut	24,873,938	0.5%
48	Delaware	4,015,741	0.1%
4	Florida	388,478,373	7.3%
10	Georgia	148,512,336	2.8%
44	Hawaii	5,616,974	0.1%
37	Idaho	18,002,709	0.3%
23	Illinois	55,864,061	1.1%
18	Indiana	82,261,316	1.5%
28	Iowa	38,817,621	0.7%
26	Kansas	49,811,709	0.9%
15	Kentucky	91,103,213	1.7%
19	Louisiana	82,164,345	1.5%
35	Maine	23,234,195	0.4%
6	Maryland	183,381,755	3.5%
14	Massachusetts	92,672,672	1.7%
22	Michigan	56,974,700	1.1%
13	Minnesota	99,513,047	1.9%
17	Mississippi	83,755,754	1.6%
16	Missouri	85,492,822	1.6%
40	Montana	14,935,804	0.3%
39	Nebraska	16,623,206	0.3%
32	Nevada	31,433,945	0.6%
43	New Hampshire	6,025,576	0.1%
5	New Jersey	388,473,026	7.3%
38	New Mexico	17,125,552	0.3%
3	New York	571,634,828	10.8%
11	North Carolina	117,820,812	2.2%
46	North Dakota	4,847,508	0.1%
7	Ohio	181,349,593	3.4%
29	Oklahoma	38,023,894	0.7%
36	Oregon	22,796,830	0.4%
9	Pennsylvania	152,372,663	2.9%
25	Rhode Island	51,641,583	1.0%
24	South Carolina	52,894,359	1.0%
42	South Dakota	11,370,254	0.2%
45	Tennessee	5,358,112	0.1%
1	Texas	742,802,504	14.0%
30	Utah	32,706,432	0.6%
49	Vermont	3,443,510	0.1%
21	Virginia	60,183,556	1.1%
41	Washington	12,319,513	0.2%
31	West Virginia	32,521,009	0.6%
12	Wisconsin	113,060,766	2.1%
47	Wyoming	4,304,677	0.1%

RANK ORDER

RANK	STATE	EXPENDITURES	% of USA
1	Texas	$742,802,504	14.0%
2	California	688,375,800	13.0%
3	New York	571,634,828	10.8%
4	Florida	388,478,373	7.3%
5	New Jersey	388,473,026	7.3%
6	Maryland	183,381,755	3.5%
7	Ohio	181,349,593	3.4%
8	Arizona	167,950,645	3.2%
9	Pennsylvania	152,372,663	2.9%
10	Georgia	148,512,336	2.8%
11	North Carolina	117,820,812	2.2%
12	Wisconsin	113,060,766	2.1%
13	Minnesota	99,513,047	1.9%
14	Massachusetts	92,672,672	1.7%
15	Kentucky	91,103,213	1.7%
16	Missouri	85,492,822	1.6%
17	Mississippi	83,755,754	1.6%
18	Indiana	82,261,316	1.5%
19	Louisiana	82,164,345	1.5%
20	Alabama	69,331,278	1.3%
21	Virginia	60,183,556	1.1%
22	Michigan	56,974,700	1.1%
23	Illinois	55,864,061	1.1%
24	South Carolina	52,894,359	1.0%
25	Rhode Island	51,641,583	1.0%
26	Kansas	49,811,709	0.9%
27	Colorado	47,971,251	0.9%
28	Iowa	38,817,621	0.7%
29	Oklahoma	38,023,894	0.7%
30	Utah	32,706,432	0.6%
31	West Virginia	32,521,009	0.6%
32	Nevada	31,433,945	0.6%
33	Alaska	29,943,737	0.6%
34	Connecticut	24,873,938	0.5%
35	Maine	23,234,195	0.4%
36	Oregon	22,796,830	0.4%
37	Idaho	18,002,709	0.3%
38	New Mexico	17,125,552	0.3%
39	Nebraska	16,623,206	0.3%
40	Montana	14,935,804	0.3%
41	Washington	12,319,513	0.2%
42	South Dakota	11,370,254	0.2%
43	New Hampshire	6,025,576	0.1%
44	Hawaii	5,616,974	0.1%
45	Tennessee	5,358,112	0.1%
46	North Dakota	4,847,508	0.1%
47	Wyoming	4,304,677	0.1%
48	Delaware	4,015,741	0.1%
49	Vermont	3,443,510	0.1%
50	Arkansas	1,909,978	0.0%
	District of Columbia	6,923,667	0.1%

Source: U.S. Department of Health and Human Services, Centers for Medicare and Medicaid Services "Statement of Expenditures for the SCHIP Program" (CMS-21 Report)

*Federal and state expenditures for fiscal year 2002. National total does not include $105,040,084 spent in U.S. territories. The State Children's Health Insurance Program (SCHIP) was created in 1997 to help states expand health insurance to children whose families earn too much to qualify for Medicaid, yet not enough to afford private health insurance. Includes administrative expenditures.

Per Capita Expenditures for State Children's
Health Insurance Program (SCHIP) in 2002
National Per Capita = $18.45*

ALPHA ORDER

RANK	STATE	PER CAPITA
21	Alabama	$15.47
2	Alaska	46.73
6	Arizona	30.88
50	Arkansas	0.71
13	California	19.67
34	Colorado	10.66
40	Connecticut	7.19
44	Delaware	4.98
9	Florida	23.29
18	Georgia	17.39
46	Hawaii	4.55
28	Idaho	13.40
47	Illinois	4.44
29	Indiana	13.36
30	Iowa	13.23
14	Kansas	18.36
10	Kentucky	22.27
15	Louisiana	18.35
17	Maine	17.90
5	Maryland	33.70
25	Massachusetts	14.45
42	Michigan	5.67
12	Minnesota	19.80
8	Mississippi	29.21
22	Missouri	15.05
19	Montana	16.40
35	Nebraska	9.63
24	Nevada	14.50
45	New Hampshire	4.72
3	New Jersey	45.29
36	New Mexico	9.23
7	New York	29.85
26	North Carolina	14.17
39	North Dakota	7.65
20	Ohio	15.89
33	Oklahoma	10.90
41	Oregon	6.47
32	Pennsylvania	12.36
1	Rhode Island	48.31
31	South Carolina	12.88
23	South Dakota	14.95
49	Tennessee	0.93
4	Texas	34.19
27	Utah	14.10
43	Vermont	5.59
38	Virginia	8.27
48	Washington	2.03
16	West Virginia	18.01
11	Wisconsin	20.78
37	Wyoming	8.62

RANK ORDER

RANK	STATE	PER CAPITA
1	Rhode Island	$48.31
2	Alaska	46.73
3	New Jersey	45.29
4	Texas	34.19
5	Maryland	33.70
6	Arizona	30.88
7	New York	29.85
8	Mississippi	29.21
9	Florida	23.29
10	Kentucky	22.27
11	Wisconsin	20.78
12	Minnesota	19.80
13	California	19.67
14	Kansas	18.36
15	Louisiana	18.35
16	West Virginia	18.01
17	Maine	17.90
18	Georgia	17.39
19	Montana	16.40
20	Ohio	15.89
21	Alabama	15.47
22	Missouri	15.05
23	South Dakota	14.95
24	Nevada	14.50
25	Massachusetts	14.45
26	North Carolina	14.17
27	Utah	14.10
28	Idaho	13.40
29	Indiana	13.36
30	Iowa	13.23
31	South Carolina	12.88
32	Pennsylvania	12.36
33	Oklahoma	10.90
34	Colorado	10.66
35	Nebraska	9.63
36	New Mexico	9.23
37	Wyoming	8.62
38	Virginia	8.27
39	North Dakota	7.65
40	Connecticut	7.19
41	Oregon	6.47
42	Michigan	5.67
43	Vermont	5.59
44	Delaware	4.98
45	New Hampshire	4.72
46	Hawaii	4.55
47	Illinois	4.44
48	Washington	2.03
49	Tennessee	0.93
50	Arkansas	0.71
	District of Columbia	12.26

Source: MQ Press using data from U.S. Dept of Health & Human Services, Centers for Medicare and Medicaid Services
"Statement of Expenditures for the SCHIP Program" (CMS-21 Report)
*Federal and state expenditures for fiscal year 2002. National figure does not include expenditures in U.S.
territories. The State Children's Health Insurance Program (SCHIP) was created in 1997 to help states expand
health insurance to children whose families earn too much to qualify for Medicaid, yet not enough to afford private
health insurance. Includes administrative expenditures.

Expenditures per State Children's Health Insurance Program (SCHIP)
Participant in 2002
National Per Participant = $992*

ALPHA ORDER

ALPHA ORDER | | | RANK ORDER | |

RANK	STATE	PER PARTICIPANT	RANK	STATE	PER PARTICIPANT
33	Alabama	$832	1	New Jersey	$3,319
7	Alaska	1,342	2	Rhode Island	2,646
4	Arizona	1,812	3	Wisconsin	1,889
23	Arkansas	999	4	Arizona	1,812
36	California	799	5	Maryland	1,465
28	Colorado	926	6	Washington	1,407
11	Connecticut	1,213	7	Alaska	1,342
49	Delaware	413	8	Mississippi	1,292
17	Florida	1,055	9	Indiana	1,242
42	Georgia	672	10	Kansas	1,220
43	Hawaii	663	11	Connecticut	1,213
16	Idaho	1,066	12	Iowa	1,125
35	Illinois	821	13	Louisiana	1,101
9	Indiana	1,242	14	North Dakota	1,086
12	Iowa	1,125	15	Montana	1,076
10	Kansas	1,220	16	Idaho	1,066
27	Kentucky	963	17	Florida	1,055
13	Louisiana	1,101	18	Maine	1,029
18	Maine	1,029	19	Pennsylvania	1,025
5	Maryland	1,465	20	Nebraska	1,024
39	Massachusetts	774	21	Texas	1,021
38	Michigan	793	22	South Dakota	1,012
NA	Minnesota**	NA	23	Arkansas	999
8	Mississippi	1,292	24	Ohio	991
44	Missouri	568	25	North Carolina	979
15	Montana	1,076	26	Utah	967
20	Nebraska	1,024	27	Kentucky	963
34	Nevada	830	28	Colorado	926
40	New Hampshire	740	29	West Virginia	905
1	New Jersey	3,319	30	Virginia	885
31	New Mexico	859	31	New Mexico	859
41	New York	708	32	Wyoming	851
25	North Carolina	979	33	Alabama	832
14	North Dakota	1,086	34	Nevada	830
24	Ohio	991	35	Illinois	821
48	Oklahoma	450	36	California	799
46	Oregon	530	37	South Carolina	794
19	Pennsylvania	1,025	38	Michigan	793
2	Rhode Island	2,646	39	Massachusetts	774
37	South Carolina	794	40	New Hampshire	740
22	South Dakota	1,012	41	New York	708
47	Tennessee	524	42	Georgia	672
21	Texas	1,021	43	Hawaii	663
26	Utah	967	44	Missouri	568
45	Vermont	559	45	Vermont	559
30	Virginia	885	46	Oregon	530
6	Washington	1,407	47	Tennessee	524
29	West Virginia	905	48	Oklahoma	450
3	Wisconsin	1,889	49	Delaware	413
32	Wyoming	851	NA	Minnesota**	NA
				District of Columbia	1,368

Source: MQ Press using data from U.S. Dept of Health & Human Services, Centers for Medicare and Medicaid Services
   "Statement of Expenditures for the SCHIP Program" (CMS-21 Report)
*Federal and state expenditures for fiscal year 2002. National figure does not include expenditures in U.S.
territories. The State Children's Health Insurance Program (SCHIP) was created in 1997 to help states expand
health insurance to children whose families earn too much to qualify for Medicaid, yet not enough to afford private
health insurance. Includes administrative expenditures. **Not available.

Health Maintenance Organizations (HMOs) in 2004

National Total = 408 HMOs*

ALPHA ORDER

RANK ORDER

RANK	STATE	HMOs	% of USA		RANK	STATE	HMOs	% of USA
37	Alabama	3	0.7%		1	California	30	7.4%
50	Alaska	0	0.0%		2	Michigan	24	5.9%
21	Arizona	7	1.7%		3	New York	23	5.6%
37	Arkansas	3	0.7%		4	Florida	21	5.1%
1	California	30	7.4%		5	Ohio	18	4.4%
12	Colorado	11	2.7%		5	Texas	18	4.4%
21	Connecticut	7	1.7%		5	Wisconsin	18	4.4%
28	Delaware	4	1.0%		8	Missouri	17	4.2%
4	Florida	21	5.1%		9	Illinois	14	3.4%
15	Georgia	9	2.2%		9	Pennsylvania	14	3.4%
43	Hawaii	2	0.5%		11	New Jersey	12	2.9%
37	Idaho	3	0.7%		12	Colorado	11	2.7%
9	Illinois	14	3.4%		12	Indiana	11	2.7%
12	Indiana	11	2.7%		14	Virginia	10	2.5%
28	Iowa	4	1.0%		15	Georgia	9	2.2%
28	Kansas	4	1.0%		15	Massachusetts	9	2.2%
25	Kentucky	6	1.5%		15	Tennessee	9	2.2%
21	Louisiana	7	1.7%		18	Maryland	8	2.0%
28	Maine	4	1.0%		18	Minnesota	8	2.0%
18	Maryland	8	2.0%		18	North Carolina	8	2.0%
15	Massachusetts	9	2.2%		21	Arizona	7	1.7%
2	Michigan	24	5.9%		21	Connecticut	7	1.7%
18	Minnesota	8	2.0%		21	Louisiana	7	1.7%
43	Mississippi	2	0.5%		21	Utah	7	1.7%
8	Missouri	17	4.2%		25	Kentucky	6	1.5%
43	Montana	2	0.5%		25	Nevada	6	1.5%
28	Nebraska	4	1.0%		27	Oregon	5	1.2%
25	Nevada	6	1.5%		28	Delaware	4	1.0%
37	New Hampshire	3	0.7%		28	Iowa	4	1.0%
11	New Jersey	12	2.9%		28	Kansas	4	1.0%
28	New Mexico	4	1.0%		28	Maine	4	1.0%
3	New York	23	5.6%		28	Nebraska	4	1.0%
18	North Carolina	8	2.0%		28	New Mexico	4	1.0%
48	North Dakota	1	0.2%		28	Oklahoma	4	1.0%
5	Ohio	18	4.4%		28	South Carolina	4	1.0%
28	Oklahoma	4	1.0%		28	Washington	4	1.0%
27	Oregon	5	1.2%		37	Alabama	3	0.7%
9	Pennsylvania	14	3.4%		37	Arkansas	3	0.7%
37	Rhode Island	3	0.7%		37	Idaho	3	0.7%
28	South Carolina	4	1.0%		37	New Hampshire	3	0.7%
37	South Dakota	3	0.7%		37	Rhode Island	3	0.7%
15	Tennessee	9	2.2%		37	South Dakota	3	0.7%
5	Texas	18	4.4%		43	Hawaii	2	0.5%
21	Utah	7	1.7%		43	Mississippi	2	0.5%
43	Vermont	2	0.5%		43	Montana	2	0.5%
14	Virginia	10	2.5%		43	Vermont	2	0.5%
28	Washington	4	1.0%		43	West Virginia	2	0.5%
43	West Virginia	2	0.5%		48	North Dakota	1	0.2%
5	Wisconsin	18	4.4%		48	Wyoming	1	0.2%
48	Wyoming	1	0.2%		50	Alaska	0	0.0%
						District of Columbia	5	1.2%

Source: InterStudy Publications (St. Paul, MN)
    "Managed Care Industry Report, Fall 2004"
As of January 1, 2004. Total does not include one HMO in Guam and three in Puerto Rico. Health plans are allocated to states based upon their primary service areas. This means each plan is counted once. However, many plans serve more than one state.

Enrollees in Health Maintenance Organizations (HMOs) in 2004

National Total = 67,240,805 Enrollees*

ALPHA ORDER

RANK ORDER

RANK	STATE	ENROLLEES	% of USA		RANK	STATE	ENROLLEES	% of USA
41	Alabama	128,203	0.2%		1	California	17,021,620	25.3%
50	Alaska	0	0.0%		2	New York	5,742,910	8.5%
20	Arizona	1,112,341	1.7%		3	Florida	4,224,656	6.3%
39	Arkansas	145,102	0.2%		4	Pennsylvania	3,856,232	5.7%
1	California	17,021,620	25.3%		5	Michigan	2,743,714	4.1%
17	Colorado	1,244,058	1.9%		6	Massachusetts	2,405,343	3.6%
14	Connecticut	1,361,558	2.0%		7	Texas	2,353,838	3.5%
42	Delaware	120,103	0.2%		8	New Jersey	2,135,705	3.2%
3	Florida	4,224,656	6.3%		9	Ohio	2,059,376	3.1%
18	Georgia	1,192,886	1.8%		10	Maryland**	1,698,300	2.5%
30	Hawaii	373,407	0.6%		11	Illinois	1,624,940	2.4%
46	Idaho	39,359	0.1%		12	Missouri	1,564,063	2.3%
11	Illinois	1,624,940	2.4%		13	Wisconsin	1,556,039	2.3%
25	Indiana	702,230	1.0%		14	Connecticut	1,361,558	2.0%
32	Iowa	294,932	0.4%		15	Virginia**	1,343,197	2.0%
38	Kansas	175,264	0.3%		16	Minnesota	1,334,830	2.0%
19	Kentucky	1,163,792	1.7%		17	Colorado	1,244,058	1.9%
29	Louisiana	523,974	0.8%		18	Georgia	1,192,886	1.8%
35	Maine	258,937	0.4%		19	Kentucky	1,163,792	1.7%
10	Maryland**	1,698,300	2.5%		20	Arizona	1,112,341	1.7%
6	Massachusetts	2,405,343	3.6%		21	North Carolina	835,980	1.2%
5	Michigan	2,743,714	4.1%		22	Washington	785,615	1.2%
16	Minnesota	1,334,830	2.0%		23	Oregon	777,625	1.2%
47	Mississippi	11,814	0.0%		24	Tennessee	749,035	1.1%
12	Missouri	1,564,063	2.3%		25	Indiana	702,230	1.0%
43	Montana	85,556	0.1%		26	Utah	597,684	0.9%
40	Nebraska	130,107	0.2%		27	New Mexico	576,506	0.9%
28	Nevada	537,814	0.8%		28	Nevada	537,814	0.8%
33	New Hampshire	284,494	0.4%		29	Louisiana	523,974	0.8%
8	New Jersey	2,135,705	3.2%		30	Hawaii	373,407	0.6%
27	New Mexico	576,506	0.9%		31	Rhode Island	340,407	0.5%
2	New York	5,742,910	8.5%		32	Iowa	294,932	0.4%
21	North Carolina	835,980	1.2%		33	New Hampshire	284,494	0.4%
49	North Dakota	2,101	0.0%		34	Oklahoma	277,454	0.4%
9	Ohio	2,059,376	3.1%		35	Maine	258,937	0.4%
34	Oklahoma	277,454	0.4%		36	South Carolina	253,428	0.4%
23	Oregon	777,625	1.2%		37	West Virginia**	179,455	0.3%
4	Pennsylvania	3,856,232	5.7%		38	Kansas	175,264	0.3%
31	Rhode Island	340,407	0.5%		39	Arkansas	145,102	0.2%
36	South Carolina	253,428	0.4%		40	Nebraska	130,107	0.2%
44	South Dakota	82,083	0.1%		41	Alabama	128,203	0.2%
24	Tennessee	749,035	1.1%		42	Delaware	120,103	0.2%
7	Texas	2,353,838	3.5%		43	Montana	85,556	0.1%
26	Utah	597,684	0.9%		44	South Dakota	82,083	0.1%
45	Vermont	59,483	0.1%		45	Vermont	59,483	0.1%
15	Virginia**	1,343,197	2.0%		46	Idaho	39,359	0.1%
22	Washington	785,615	1.2%		47	Mississippi	11,814	0.0%
37	West Virginia**	179,455	0.3%		48	Wyoming	11,000	0.0%
13	Wisconsin	1,556,039	2.3%		49	North Dakota	2,101	0.0%
48	Wyoming	11,000	0.0%		50	Alaska	0	0.0%
						District of Columbia	162,255	0.2%

Source: InterStudy Publications (St. Paul, MN)
    "Managed Care Industry Report, Fall 2004"

*As of January 1, 2004. Total does not include 1,567,257 enrollees in U.S. territories.
**Maryland, Virginia and West Virginia include partial enrollment from five HMOs serving the Washington, DC metropolitan area.

Percent Change in Enrollees in Health Maintenance Organizations (HMOs): 2003 to 2004
National Percent Change = 4.1% Decrease*

ALPHA ORDER

RANK	STATE	PERCENT CHANGE
46	Alabama	(24.9)
NA	Alaska**	NA
26	Arizona	(4.2)
45	Arkansas	(24.5)
13	California	0.0
35	Colorado	(8.9)
6	Connecticut	4.2
21	Delaware	(2.7)
19	Florida	(2.6)
7	Georgia	3.6
13	Hawaii	0.0
8	Idaho	3.0
37	Illinois	(12.3)
25	Indiana	(4.0)
4	Iowa	5.8
44	Kansas	(16.8)
35	Kentucky	(8.9)
27	Louisiana	(4.3)
29	Maine	(5.3)
10	Maryland	1.7
23	Massachusetts	(3.4)
5	Michigan	5.0
24	Minnesota	(3.7)
49	Mississippi	(50.6)
42	Missouri	(14.5)
1	Montana	81.7
40	Nebraska	(14.3)
2	Nevada	17.3
39	New Hampshire	(14.0)
32	New Jersey	(8.0)
9	New Mexico	2.6
31	New York	(7.5)
38	North Carolina	(13.2)
30	North Dakota	(6.2)
22	Ohio	(3.0)
48	Oklahoma	(42.9)
34	Oregon	(8.7)
16	Pennsylvania	(1.4)
12	Rhode Island	0.5
28	South Carolina	(4.8)
11	South Dakota	1.6
47	Tennessee	(28.4)
43	Texas	(15.6)
15	Utah	(0.3)
19	Vermont	(2.6)
3	Virginia	11.7
41	Washington	(14.4)
18	West Virginia	(1.8)
17	Wisconsin	(1.6)
33	Wyoming	(8.3)

RANK ORDER

RANK	STATE	PERCENT CHANGE
1	Montana	81.7
2	Nevada	17.3
3	Virginia	11.7
4	Iowa	5.8
5	Michigan	5.0
6	Connecticut	4.2
7	Georgia	3.6
8	Idaho	3.0
9	New Mexico	2.6
10	Maryland	1.7
11	South Dakota	1.6
12	Rhode Island	0.5
13	California	0.0
13	Hawaii	0.0
15	Utah	(0.3)
16	Pennsylvania	(1.4)
17	Wisconsin	(1.6)
18	West Virginia	(1.8)
19	Florida	(2.6)
19	Vermont	(2.6)
21	Delaware	(2.7)
22	Ohio	(3.0)
23	Massachusetts	(3.4)
24	Minnesota	(3.7)
25	Indiana	(4.0)
26	Arizona	(4.2)
27	Louisiana	(4.3)
28	South Carolina	(4.8)
29	Maine	(5.3)
30	North Dakota	(6.2)
31	New York	(7.5)
32	New Jersey	(8.0)
33	Wyoming	(8.3)
34	Oregon	(8.7)
35	Colorado	(8.9)
35	Kentucky	(8.9)
37	Illinois	(12.3)
38	North Carolina	(13.2)
39	New Hampshire	(14.0)
40	Nebraska	(14.3)
41	Washington	(14.4)
42	Missouri	(14.5)
43	Texas	(15.6)
44	Kansas	(16.8)
45	Arkansas	(24.5)
46	Alabama	(24.9)
47	Tennessee	(28.4)
48	Oklahoma	(42.9)
49	Mississippi	(50.6)
NA	Alaska**	NA

District of Columbia 2.2

Source: InterStudy Publications (St. Paul, MN)
   "Managed Care Industry Report, Fall 2004"
*As of January 1, 2004. National rate does not include enrollees in U.S. territories.
**Not applicable.

Percent of Population Enrolled in Health Maintenance Organizations (HMOs) in 2004
National Percent = 22.9% Enrolled in HMOs*

ALPHA ORDER

RANK	STATE	PERCENT
45	Alabama	2.8
50	Alaska	0.0
23	Arizona	19.4
44	Arkansas	5.3
1	California	47.4
14	Colorado	27.0
2	Connecticut	38.9
26	Delaware	14.5
18	Florida	24.3
27	Georgia	13.5
9	Hawaii	29.6
45	Idaho	2.8
28	Illinois	12.8
32	Indiana	11.3
35	Iowa	10.0
42	Kansas	6.4
11	Kentucky	28.1
31	Louisiana	11.6
22	Maine	19.7
6	Maryland	30.6
3	Massachusetts	37.5
13	Michigan	27.1
15	Minnesota	26.2
48	Mississippi	0.4
12	Missouri	27.2
39	Montana	9.2
41	Nebraska	7.4
19	Nevada	23.0
20	New Hampshire	21.9
17	New Jersey	24.6
7	New Mexico	30.3
8	New York	29.9
37	North Carolina	9.8
49	North Dakota	0.3
24	Ohio	18.0
40	Oklahoma	7.9
21	Oregon	21.6
5	Pennsylvania	31.1
4	Rhode Island	31.5
43	South Carolina	6.0
33	South Dakota	10.6
29	Tennessee	12.7
34	Texas	10.5
16	Utah	25.0
38	Vermont	9.6
24	Virginia	18.0
29	Washington	12.7
36	West Virginia	9.9
10	Wisconsin	28.2
47	Wyoming	2.2

RANK ORDER

RANK	STATE	PERCENT
1	California	47.4
2	Connecticut	38.9
3	Massachusetts	37.5
4	Rhode Island	31.5
5	Pennsylvania	31.1
6	Maryland	30.6
7	New Mexico	30.3
8	New York	29.9
9	Hawaii	29.6
10	Wisconsin	28.2
11	Kentucky	28.1
12	Missouri	27.2
13	Michigan	27.1
14	Colorado	27.0
15	Minnesota	26.2
16	Utah	25.0
17	New Jersey	24.6
18	Florida	24.3
19	Nevada	23.0
20	New Hampshire	21.9
21	Oregon	21.6
22	Maine	19.7
23	Arizona	19.4
24	Ohio	18.0
24	Virginia	18.0
26	Delaware	14.5
27	Georgia	13.5
28	Illinois	12.8
29	Tennessee	12.7
29	Washington	12.7
31	Louisiana	11.6
32	Indiana	11.3
33	South Dakota	10.6
34	Texas	10.5
35	Iowa	10.0
36	West Virginia	9.9
37	North Carolina	9.8
38	Vermont	9.6
39	Montana	9.2
40	Oklahoma	7.9
41	Nebraska	7.4
42	Kansas	6.4
43	South Carolina	6.0
44	Arkansas	5.3
45	Alabama	2.8
45	Idaho	2.8
47	Wyoming	2.2
48	Mississippi	0.4
49	North Dakota	0.3
50	Alaska	0.0

| | District of Columbia | 29.3 |

Source: Morgan Quitno Press using data from InterStudy Publications (St. Paul, MN)
    "Managed Care Industry Report, Fall 2004"

*As of January 1, 2004. Calculated using Census 2004 population estimates. National percent does not include enrollees or population in U.S. territories.

Percent of Insured Population Enrolled in
Health Maintenance Organizations (HMOs) in 2004
National Percent = 27.6% of Insured are Enrolled in HMOs*

ALPHA ORDER

RANK	STATE	PERCENT
46	Alabama	3.4
50	Alaska	0.0
22	Arizona	24.0
44	Arkansas	6.6
1	California	58.9
9	Colorado	33.6
2	Connecticut	44.4
27	Delaware	16.5
15	Florida	30.5
26	Georgia	16.7
10	Hawaii	33.2
45	Idaho	3.6
29	Illinois	15.0
33	Indiana	13.3
38	Iowa	11.4
42	Kansas	7.3
11	Kentucky	32.9
30	Louisiana	14.9
23	Maine	22.5
6	Maryland	35.9
3	Massachusetts	42.3
14	Michigan	31.0
19	Minnesota	28.8
48	Mississippi	0.5
13	Missouri	31.3
37	Montana	11.6
41	Nebraska	8.5
16	Nevada	29.5
21	New Hampshire	25.1
18	New Jersey	28.9
4	New Mexico	39.6
8	New York	35.7
35	North Carolina	12.2
49	North Dakota	0.4
25	Ohio	20.8
40	Oklahoma	10.1
20	Oregon	26.3
7	Pennsylvania	35.8
5	Rhode Island	36.0
42	South Carolina	7.3
34	South Dakota	12.5
31	Tennessee	14.6
32	Texas	14.3
17	Utah	29.1
39	Vermont	10.8
24	Virginia	20.9
28	Washington	15.3
36	West Virginia	12.0
12	Wisconsin	32.2
47	Wyoming	2.7

RANK ORDER

RANK	STATE	PERCENT
1	California	58.9
2	Connecticut	44.4
3	Massachusetts	42.3
4	New Mexico	39.6
5	Rhode Island	36.0
6	Maryland	35.9
7	Pennsylvania	35.8
8	New York	35.7
9	Colorado	33.6
10	Hawaii	33.2
11	Kentucky	32.9
12	Wisconsin	32.2
13	Missouri	31.3
14	Michigan	31.0
15	Florida	30.5
16	Nevada	29.5
17	Utah	29.1
18	New Jersey	28.9
19	Minnesota	28.8
20	Oregon	26.3
21	New Hampshire	25.1
22	Arizona	24.0
23	Maine	22.5
24	Virginia	20.9
25	Ohio	20.8
26	Georgia	16.7
27	Delaware	16.5
28	Washington	15.3
29	Illinois	15.0
30	Louisiana	14.9
31	Tennessee	14.6
32	Texas	14.3
33	Indiana	13.3
34	South Dakota	12.5
35	North Carolina	12.2
36	West Virginia	12.0
37	Montana	11.6
38	Iowa	11.4
39	Vermont	10.8
40	Oklahoma	10.1
41	Nebraska	8.5
42	Kansas	7.3
42	South Carolina	7.3
44	Arkansas	6.6
45	Idaho	3.6
46	Alabama	3.4
47	Wyoming	2.7
48	Mississippi	0.5
49	North Dakota	0.4
50	Alaska	0.0
	District of Columbia	34.2

Source: Morgan Quitno Press using data from InterStudy Publications (St. Paul, MN)
  "Managed Care Industry Report, Fall 2004"
As of January 1, 2004. Calculated using estimated number of insured as of 2003 from the U.S. Census Bureau.

Medicare Enrollees in 2003

National Total = 41,086,981 Enrollees*

ALPHA ORDER

ALPHA ORDER

RANK ORDER

RANK	STATE	ENROLLEES	% of USA	RANK	STATE	ENROLLEES	% of USA
20	Alabama	719,246	1.8%	1	California	4,078,426	9.9%
50	Alaska	47,749	0.1%	2	Florida	2,920,971	7.1%
19	Arizona	728,885	1.8%	3	New York	2,763,299	6.7%
31	Arkansas	452,676	1.1%	4	Texas	2,390,053	5.8%
1	California	4,078,426	9.9%	5	Pennsylvania	2,110,470	5.1%
29	Colorado	493,454	1.2%	6	Ohio	1,727,096	4.2%
26	Connecticut	522,403	1.3%	7	Illinois	1,661,454	4.0%
46	Delaware	119,302	0.3%	8	Michigan	1,444,987	3.5%
2	Florida	2,920,971	7.1%	9	New Jersey	1,219,935	3.0%
11	Georgia	973,794	2.4%	10	North Carolina	1,205,466	2.9%
42	Hawaii	174,633	0.4%	11	Georgia	973,794	2.4%
41	Idaho	177,700	0.4%	12	Massachusetts	965,943	2.4%
7	Illinois	1,661,454	4.0%	13	Virginia	946,470	2.3%
15	Indiana	877,954	2.1%	14	Missouri	884,449	2.2%
30	Iowa	482,340	1.2%	15	Indiana	877,954	2.1%
33	Kansas	394,206	1.0%	16	Tennessee	871,938	2.1%
23	Kentucky	648,400	1.6%	17	Wisconsin	803,678	2.0%
24	Louisiana	620,196	1.5%	18	Washington	775,358	1.9%
38	Maine	226,696	0.6%	19	Arizona	728,885	1.8%
22	Maryland	674,448	1.6%	20	Alabama	719,246	1.8%
12	Massachusetts	965,943	2.4%	21	Minnesota	676,156	1.6%
8	Michigan	1,444,987	3.5%	22	Maryland	674,448	1.6%
21	Minnesota	676,156	1.6%	23	Kentucky	648,400	1.6%
32	Mississippi	436,677	1.1%	24	Louisiana	620,196	1.5%
14	Missouri	884,449	2.2%	25	South Carolina	606,323	1.5%
44	Montana	142,457	0.3%	26	Connecticut	522,403	1.3%
36	Nebraska	257,171	0.6%	27	Oklahoma	521,286	1.3%
35	Nevada	273,724	0.7%	28	Oregon	513,253	1.2%
40	New Hampshire	179,564	0.4%	29	Colorado	493,454	1.2%
9	New Jersey	1,219,935	3.0%	30	Iowa	482,340	1.2%
37	New Mexico	250,113	0.6%	31	Arkansas	452,676	1.1%
3	New York	2,763,299	6.7%	32	Mississippi	436,677	1.1%
10	North Carolina	1,205,466	2.9%	33	Kansas	394,206	1.0%
47	North Dakota	103,220	0.3%	34	West Virginia	347,459	0.8%
6	Ohio	1,727,096	4.2%	35	Nevada	273,724	0.7%
27	Oklahoma	521,286	1.3%	36	Nebraska	257,171	0.6%
28	Oregon	513,253	1.2%	37	New Mexico	250,113	0.6%
5	Pennsylvania	2,110,470	5.1%	38	Maine	226,696	0.6%
43	Rhode Island	172,474	0.4%	39	Utah	220,221	0.5%
25	South Carolina	606,323	1.5%	40	New Hampshire	179,564	0.4%
45	South Dakota	121,777	0.3%	41	Idaho	177,700	0.4%
16	Tennessee	871,938	2.1%	42	Hawaii	174,633	0.4%
4	Texas	2,390,053	5.8%	43	Rhode Island	172,474	0.4%
39	Utah	220,221	0.5%	44	Montana	142,457	0.3%
48	Vermont	92,724	0.2%	45	South Dakota	121,777	0.3%
13	Virginia	946,470	2.3%	46	Delaware	119,302	0.3%
18	Washington	775,358	1.9%	47	North Dakota	103,220	0.3%
34	West Virginia	347,459	0.8%	48	Vermont	92,724	0.2%
17	Wisconsin	803,678	2.0%	49	Wyoming	68,590	0.2%
49	Wyoming	68,590	0.2%	50	Alaska	47,749	0.1%
					District of Columbia	73,794	0.2%

*Source: U.S. Department of Health and Human Services, Centers for Medicare and Medicaid Services
"Medicare Enrollment" (http://www.cms.hhs.gov/statistics/enrollment/st03all.asp)*
*As of July 2003. Includes aged and disabled enrollees. Total includes 574,799 enrollees in Puerto Rico and 351,124 enrollees in other outlying areas, foreign countries or whose address is unknown.

Percent Change in Medicare Enrollees: 2002 to 2003

National Percent Change = 1.5% Increase

ALPHA ORDER

RANK	STATE	PERCENT CHANGE
17	Alabama	1.9
2	Alaska	4.3
3	Arizona	2.9
28	Arkansas	1.5
23	California	1.7
15	Colorado	2.0
40	Connecticut	0.8
5	Delaware	2.5
25	Florida	1.6
9	Georgia	2.3
15	Hawaii	2.0
4	Idaho	2.8
38	Illinois	0.9
28	Indiana	1.5
42	Iowa	0.6
42	Kansas	0.6
20	Kentucky	1.8
31	Louisiana	1.4
23	Maine	1.7
25	Maryland	1.6
48	Massachusetts	0.3
32	Michigan	1.3
32	Minnesota	1.3
20	Mississippi	1.8
35	Missouri	1.2
25	Montana	1.6
46	Nebraska	0.5
1	Nevada	4.7
12	New Hampshire	2.1
42	New Jersey	0.6
5	New Mexico	2.5
42	New York	0.6
9	North Carolina	2.3
50	North Dakota	0.0
40	Ohio	0.8
32	Oklahoma	1.3
17	Oregon	1.9
46	Pennsylvania	0.5
49	Rhode Island	0.2
8	South Carolina	2.4
38	South Dakota	0.9
17	Tennessee	1.9
11	Texas	2.2
5	Utah	2.5
28	Vermont	1.5
12	Virginia	2.1
12	Washington	2.1
35	West Virginia	1.2
35	Wisconsin	1.2
20	Wyoming	1.8

RANK ORDER

RANK	STATE	PERCENT CHANGE
1	Nevada	4.7
2	Alaska	4.3
3	Arizona	2.9
4	Idaho	2.8
5	Delaware	2.5
5	New Mexico	2.5
5	Utah	2.5
8	South Carolina	2.4
9	Georgia	2.3
9	North Carolina	2.3
11	Texas	2.2
12	New Hampshire	2.1
12	Virginia	2.1
12	Washington	2.1
15	Colorado	2.0
15	Hawaii	2.0
17	Alabama	1.9
17	Oregon	1.9
17	Tennessee	1.9
20	Kentucky	1.8
20	Mississippi	1.8
20	Wyoming	1.8
23	California	1.7
23	Maine	1.7
25	Florida	1.6
25	Maryland	1.6
25	Montana	1.6
28	Arkansas	1.5
28	Indiana	1.5
28	Vermont	1.5
31	Louisiana	1.4
32	Michigan	1.3
32	Minnesota	1.3
32	Oklahoma	1.3
35	Missouri	1.2
35	West Virginia	1.2
35	Wisconsin	1.2
38	Illinois	0.9
38	South Dakota	0.9
40	Connecticut	0.8
40	Ohio	0.8
42	Iowa	0.6
42	Kansas	0.6
42	New Jersey	0.6
42	New York	0.6
46	Nebraska	0.5
46	Pennsylvania	0.5
48	Massachusetts	0.3
49	Rhode Island	0.2
50	North Dakota	0.0

District of Columbia   (0.5)

Source: MQ Press using data from U.S. Dept of Health & Human Services, Centers for Medicare and Medicaid Services
"Medicare Enrollment" (http://www.cms.hhs.gov/statistics/enrollment/st03all.asp)
*As of July. Includes aged and disabled enrollees. National rate includes enrollees in Puerto Rico and other
outlying areas, foreign countries or whose address is unknown.

Percent of Population Enrolled in Medicare in 2003

National Percent = 13.8% of Population*

ALPHA ORDER

RANK	STATE	PERCENT
8	Alabama	16.0
50	Alaska	7.4
38	Arizona	13.1
5	Arkansas	16.6
45	California	11.5
47	Colorado	10.9
16	Connecticut	15.0
23	Delaware	14.6
3	Florida	17.2
46	Georgia	11.2
32	Hawaii	14.0
40	Idaho	13.0
38	Illinois	13.1
30	Indiana	14.2
6	Iowa	16.4
25	Kansas	14.5
11	Kentucky	15.7
34	Louisiana	13.8
2	Maine	17.3
43	Maryland	12.2
16	Massachusetts	15.0
28	Michigan	14.3
36	Minnesota	13.4
14	Mississippi	15.1
12	Missouri	15.5
12	Montana	15.5
21	Nebraska	14.8
43	Nevada	12.2
33	New Hampshire	13.9
31	New Jersey	14.1
37	New Mexico	13.3
26	New York	14.4
28	North Carolina	14.3
7	North Dakota	16.3
14	Ohio	15.1
19	Oklahoma	14.9
26	Oregon	14.4
4	Pennsylvania	17.1
8	Rhode Island	16.0
23	South Carolina	14.6
10	South Dakota	15.9
19	Tennessee	14.9
48	Texas	10.8
49	Utah	9.4
16	Vermont	15.0
41	Virginia	12.9
42	Washington	12.6
1	West Virginia	19.2
22	Wisconsin	14.7
35	Wyoming	13.7

RANK ORDER

RANK	STATE	PERCENT
1	West Virginia	19.2
2	Maine	17.3
3	Florida	17.2
4	Pennsylvania	17.1
5	Arkansas	16.6
6	Iowa	16.4
7	North Dakota	16.3
8	Alabama	16.0
8	Rhode Island	16.0
10	South Dakota	15.9
11	Kentucky	15.7
12	Missouri	15.5
12	Montana	15.5
14	Mississippi	15.1
14	Ohio	15.1
16	Connecticut	15.0
16	Massachusetts	15.0
16	Vermont	15.0
19	Oklahoma	14.9
19	Tennessee	14.9
21	Nebraska	14.8
22	Wisconsin	14.7
23	Delaware	14.6
23	South Carolina	14.6
25	Kansas	14.5
26	New York	14.4
26	Oregon	14.4
28	Michigan	14.3
28	North Carolina	14.3
30	Indiana	14.2
31	New Jersey	14.1
32	Hawaii	14.0
33	New Hampshire	13.9
34	Louisiana	13.8
35	Wyoming	13.7
36	Minnesota	13.4
37	New Mexico	13.3
38	Arizona	13.1
38	Illinois	13.1
40	Idaho	13.0
41	Virginia	12.9
42	Washington	12.6
43	Maryland	12.2
43	Nevada	12.2
45	California	11.5
46	Georgia	11.2
47	Colorado	10.9
48	Texas	10.8
49	Utah	9.4
50	Alaska	7.4

District of Columbia — 13.2

Source: MQ Press using data from U.S. Dept of Health & Human Services, Centers for Medicare and Medicaid Services "Medicare Enrollment" (http://www.cms.hhs.gov/statistics/enrollment/st03all.asp)

*For fiscal year 2003. Includes aged and disabled enrollees. National rate includes only residents of the 50 states and the District of Columbia.

Medicare Managed Care Enrollees in 2005

National Total = 5,438,359 Enrollees*

ALPHA ORDER					RANK ORDER			
RANK	STATE	ENROLLEES	% of USA		RANK	STATE	ENROLLEES	% of USA
22	Alabama	57,837	1.1%		1	California	1,363,771	25.1%
42	Alaska	0	0.0%		2	Florida	570,074	10.5%
6	Arizona	203,321	3.7%		3	New York	517,389	9.5%
42	Arkansas	0	0.0%		4	Pennsylvania	510,708	9.4%
1	California	1,363,771	25.1%		5	Ohio	231,659	4.3%
10	Colorado	136,540	2.5%		6	Arizona	203,321	3.7%
27	Connecticut	28,241	0.5%		7	Texas	189,511	3.5%
42	Delaware	0	0.0%		8	Oregon	186,326	3.4%
2	Florida	570,074	10.5%		9	Massachusetts	161,400	3.0%
31	Georgia	16,941	0.3%		10	Colorado	136,540	2.5%
20	Hawaii	59,495	1.1%		11	Missouri	134,613	2.5%
33	Idaho	16,483	0.3%		12	Washington	124,922	2.3%
16	Illinois	81,505	1.5%		13	Minnesota	100,835	1.9%
30	Indiana	17,377	0.3%		14	New Jersey	90,775	1.7%
35	Iowa	6,876	0.1%		15	Nevada	84,131	1.5%
41	Kansas	300	0.0%		16	Illinois	81,505	1.5%
29	Kentucky	18,159	0.3%		17	Tennessee	75,263	1.4%
18	Louisiana	68,685	1.3%		18	Louisiana	68,685	1.3%
42	Maine	0	0.0%		19	North Carolina	60,075	1.1%
23	Maryland	41,668	0.8%		20	Hawaii	59,495	1.1%
9	Massachusetts	161,400	3.0%		21	Rhode Island	58,077	1.1%
28	Michigan	20,166	0.4%		22	Alabama	57,837	1.1%
13	Minnesota	100,835	1.9%		23	Maryland	41,668	0.8%
42	Mississippi	0	0.0%		24	New Mexico	41,321	0.8%
11	Missouri	134,613	2.5%		25	Oklahoma	40,492	0.7%
42	Montana	0	0.0%		26	Wisconsin	37,389	0.7%
34	Nebraska	10,348	0.2%		27	Connecticut	28,241	0.5%
15	Nevada	84,131	1.5%		28	Michigan	20,166	0.4%
38	New Hampshire	1,088	0.0%		29	Kentucky	18,159	0.3%
14	New Jersey	90,775	1.7%		30	Indiana	17,377	0.3%
24	New Mexico	41,321	0.8%		31	Georgia	16,941	0.3%
3	New York	517,389	9.5%		32	Utah	16,545	0.3%
19	North Carolina	60,075	1.1%		33	Idaho	16,483	0.3%
39	North Dakota	611	0.0%		34	Nebraska	10,348	0.2%
5	Ohio	231,659	4.3%		35	Iowa	6,876	0.1%
25	Oklahoma	40,492	0.7%		36	West Virginia	6,183	0.1%
8	Oregon	186,326	3.4%		37	Virginia	2,742	0.1%
4	Pennsylvania	510,708	9.4%		38	New Hampshire	1,088	0.0%
21	Rhode Island	58,077	1.1%		39	North Dakota	611	0.0%
40	South Carolina	312	0.0%		40	South Carolina	312	0.0%
42	South Dakota	0	0.0%		41	Kansas	300	0.0%
17	Tennessee	75,263	1.4%		42	Alaska	0	0.0%
7	Texas	189,511	3.5%		42	Arkansas	0	0.0%
32	Utah	16,545	0.3%		42	Delaware	0	0.0%
42	Vermont	0	0.0%		42	Maine	0	0.0%
37	Virginia	2,742	0.1%		42	Mississippi	0	0.0%
12	Washington	124,922	2.3%		42	Montana	0	0.0%
36	West Virginia	6,183	0.1%		42	South Dakota	0	0.0%
26	Wisconsin	37,389	0.7%		42	Vermont	0	0.0%
42	Wyoming	0	0.0%		42	Wyoming	0	0.0%
						District of Columbia	0	0.0%

Source: U.S. Department of Health and Human Services, Centers for Medicare and Medicaid Services
   "Medicare Managed Care Report" (http://www.cms.hhs.gov/healthplans/statistics/mmcc/mmcc012005.pdf)
*As of January 2005. Includes M + C, Cost, Health Care Prepayment Plans (HCPP) and other demo plans. National total includes 48,205 enrollees in the United Mine Workers' plan not shown separately by state.

Percent of Medicare Enrollees in Managed Care Programs in 2005

National Percent = 14% of Medicare Enrollees*

ALPHA ORDER

RANK	STATE	PERCENT
20	Alabama	8
39	Alaska	0
6	Arizona	29
39	Arkansas	0
3	California	34
6	Colorado	29
26	Connecticut	5
39	Delaware	0
9	Florida	19
32	Georgia	2
2	Hawaii	35
18	Idaho	9
26	Illinois	5
32	Indiana	2
35	Iowa	1
39	Kansas	0
31	Kentucky	3
17	Louisiana	11
39	Maine	0
25	Maryland	7
11	Massachusetts	17
35	Michigan	1
14	Minnesota	15
39	Mississippi	0
14	Missouri	15
39	Montana	0
29	Nebraska	4
4	Nevada	33
35	New Hampshire	1
20	New Jersey	8
11	New Mexico	17
9	New York	19
26	North Carolina	5
35	North Dakota	1
16	Ohio	13
20	Oklahoma	8
1	Oregon	38
8	Pennsylvania	24
4	Rhode Island	33
39	South Carolina	0
39	South Dakota	0
18	Tennessee	9
20	Texas	8
20	Utah	8
39	Vermont	0
39	Virginia	0
11	Washington	17
32	West Virginia	2
29	Wisconsin	4
39	Wyoming	0

RANK ORDER

RANK	STATE	PERCENT
1	Oregon	38
2	Hawaii	35
3	California	34
4	Nevada	33
4	Rhode Island	33
6	Arizona	29
6	Colorado	29
8	Pennsylvania	24
9	Florida	19
9	New York	19
11	Massachusetts	17
11	New Mexico	17
11	Washington	17
14	Minnesota	15
14	Missouri	15
16	Ohio	13
17	Louisiana	11
18	Idaho	9
18	Tennessee	9
20	Alabama	8
20	New Jersey	8
20	Oklahoma	8
20	Texas	8
20	Utah	8
25	Maryland	7
26	Connecticut	5
26	Illinois	5
26	North Carolina	5
29	Nebraska	4
29	Wisconsin	4
31	Kentucky	3
32	Georgia	2
32	Indiana	2
32	West Virginia	2
35	Iowa	1
35	Michigan	1
35	New Hampshire	1
35	North Dakota	1
39	Alaska	0
39	Arkansas	0
39	Delaware	0
39	Kansas	0
39	Maine	0
39	Mississippi	0
39	Montana	0
39	South Carolina	0
39	South Dakota	0
39	Vermont	0
39	Virginia	0
39	Wyoming	0
	District of Columbia	0

Source: U.S. Department of Health and Human Services, Centers for Medicare and Medicaid Services
"Medicare Managed Care Report" (http://www.cms.hhs.gov/healthplans/statistics/mmcc/mmcc012005.pdf)
*As of January 2005. Includes M + C, Cost, Health Care Prepayment Plans (HCPP) and other demo plans. National figure includes enrollees in the United Mine Workers' plan not shown separately by state.

Medicare Physicians in 2003

National Total = 914,303 Physicians*

ALPHA ORDER

RANK	STATE	PHYSICIANS	% of USA
28	Alabama	10,389	1.1%
49	Alaska	2,161	0.2%
23	Arizona	14,289	1.6%
31	Arkansas	8,762	1.0%
1	California	90,222	9.9%
22	Colorado	14,835	1.6%
29	Connecticut	10,064	1.1%
48	Delaware	2,689	0.3%
4	Florida	51,245	5.6%
12	Georgia	22,944	2.5%
41	Hawaii**	4,540	0.5%
27	Idaho	10,402	1.1%
42	Illinois	3,687	0.4%
8	Indiana	35,555	3.9%
18	Iowa	17,543	1.9%
30	Kansas	8,971	1.0%
24	Kentucky	12,473	1.4%
21	Louisiana	15,668	1.7%
6	Maine	37,314	4.1%
14	Maryland	21,154	2.3%
34	Massachusetts	6,350	0.7%
9	Michigan	32,264	3.5%
20	Minnesota	15,872	1.7%
15	Mississippi	19,600	2.1%
35	Missouri	6,289	0.7%
44	Montana	3,367	0.4%
11	Nebraska	25,715	2.8%
46	Nevada	2,875	0.3%
38	New Hampshire	5,809	0.6%
37	New Jersey	5,853	0.6%
10	New Mexico	32,038	3.5%
39	New York	4,951	0.5%
40	North Carolina	4,925	0.5%
2	North Dakota	74,194	8.1%
7	Ohio	37,111	4.1%
32	Oklahoma	8,445	0.9%
25	Oregon	11,834	1.3%
5	Pennsylvania	45,990	5.0%
43	Rhode Island	3,430	0.4%
26	South Carolina	11,577	1.3%
47	South Dakota	2,709	0.3%
16	Tennessee	19,309	2.1%
3	Texas	52,595	5.8%
33	Utah	6,566	0.7%
19	Vermont	17,204	1.9%
45	Virginia	3,029	0.3%
13	Washington	21,302	2.3%
17	West Virginia	19,198	2.1%
36	Wisconsin	5,914	0.6%
50	Wyoming	1,635	0.2%

RANK ORDER

RANK	STATE	PHYSICIANS	% of USA
1	California	90,222	9.9%
2	North Dakota	74,194	8.1%
3	Texas	52,595	5.8%
4	Florida	51,245	5.6%
5	Pennsylvania	45,990	5.0%
6	Maine	37,314	4.1%
7	Ohio	37,111	4.1%
8	Indiana	35,555	3.9%
9	Michigan	32,264	3.5%
10	New Mexico	32,038	3.5%
11	Nebraska	25,715	2.8%
12	Georgia	22,944	2.5%
13	Washington	21,302	2.3%
14	Maryland	21,154	2.3%
15	Mississippi	19,600	2.1%
16	Tennessee	19,309	2.1%
17	West Virginia	19,198	2.1%
18	Iowa	17,543	1.9%
19	Vermont	17,204	1.9%
20	Minnesota	15,872	1.7%
21	Louisiana	15,668	1.7%
22	Colorado	14,835	1.6%
23	Arizona	14,289	1.6%
24	Kentucky	12,473	1.4%
25	Oregon	11,834	1.3%
26	South Carolina	11,577	1.3%
27	Idaho	10,402	1.1%
28	Alabama	10,389	1.1%
29	Connecticut	10,064	1.1%
30	Kansas	8,971	1.0%
31	Arkansas	8,762	1.0%
32	Oklahoma	8,445	0.9%
33	Utah	6,566	0.7%
34	Massachusetts	6,350	0.7%
35	Missouri	6,289	0.7%
36	Wisconsin	5,914	0.6%
37	New Jersey	5,853	0.6%
38	New Hampshire	5,809	0.6%
39	New York	4,951	0.5%
40	North Carolina	4,925	0.5%
41	Hawaii**	4,540	0.5%
42	Illinois	3,687	0.4%
43	Rhode Island	3,430	0.4%
44	Montana	3,367	0.4%
45	Virginia	3,029	0.3%
46	Nevada	2,875	0.3%
47	South Dakota	2,709	0.3%
48	Delaware	2,689	0.3%
49	Alaska	2,161	0.2%
50	Wyoming	1,635	0.2%
	District of Columbia	4,546	0.5%

Source: U.S. Department of Health and Human Services, Centers for Medicare and Medicaid Services
"2003 Data Compendium" (http://www.cms.gov/researchers/pubs/datacompendium/)
*Medicare Part B. "Physicians" include MD, DO, DDM, DDS, DPM, OD and CH. National total includes 6,891
physicians in Puerto Rico and the Virgin Islands.*
**Physicians for Guam are included in Hawaii's total.*

Percent of Physicians Participating in Medicare in 2003

National Percent = 91.5% of Physicians Participate in Medicare*

ALPHA ORDER

RANK	STATE	PERCENT
4	Alabama	96.4
45	Alaska	87.2
35	Arizona	91.1
7	Arkansas	95.9
40	California	89.5
39	Colorado	90.0
25	Connecticut	93.4
32	Delaware	92.4
31	Florida	92.5
38	Georgia	90.4
15	Hawaii	94.7
47	Idaho	84.0
25	Illinois	93.4
44	Indiana	87.4
16	Iowa	94.6
11	Kansas	95.4
20	Kentucky	94.0
32	Louisiana	92.4
13	Maine	94.8
19	Maryland	94.3
6	Massachusetts	96.0
1	Michigan	97.3
49	Minnesota	80.6
46	Mississippi	86.1
20	Missouri	94.0
36	Montana	90.9
16	Nebraska	94.6
10	Nevada	95.6
20	New Hampshire	94.0
42	New Jersey	88.9
28	New Mexico	93.3
48	New York	82.3
34	North Carolina	91.9
1	North Dakota	97.3
9	Ohio	95.7
18	Oklahoma	94.4
25	Oregon	93.4
4	Pennsylvania	96.4
50	Rhode Island	77.2
29	South Carolina	92.8
37	South Dakota	90.6
30	Tennessee	92.6
41	Texas	89.4
3	Utah	97.0
23	Vermont	93.8
24	Virginia	93.7
8	Washington	95.8
13	West Virginia	94.8
12	Wisconsin	95.0
43	Wyoming	88.0

RANK ORDER

RANK	STATE	PERCENT
1	Michigan	97.3
1	North Dakota	97.3
3	Utah	97.0
4	Alabama	96.4
4	Pennsylvania	96.4
6	Massachusetts	96.0
7	Arkansas	95.9
8	Washington	95.8
9	Ohio	95.7
10	Nevada	95.6
11	Kansas	95.4
12	Wisconsin	95.0
13	Maine	94.8
13	West Virginia	94.8
15	Hawaii	94.7
16	Iowa	94.6
16	Nebraska	94.6
18	Oklahoma	94.4
19	Maryland	94.3
20	Kentucky	94.0
20	Missouri	94.0
20	New Hampshire	94.0
23	Vermont	93.8
24	Virginia	93.7
25	Connecticut	93.4
25	Illinois	93.4
25	Oregon	93.4
28	New Mexico	93.3
29	South Carolina	92.8
30	Tennessee	92.6
31	Florida	92.5
32	Delaware	92.4
32	Louisiana	92.4
34	North Carolina	91.9
35	Arizona	91.1
36	Montana	90.9
37	South Dakota	90.6
38	Georgia	90.4
39	Colorado	90.0
40	California	89.5
41	Texas	89.4
42	New Jersey	88.9
43	Wyoming	88.0
44	Indiana	87.4
45	Alaska	87.2
46	Mississippi	86.1
47	Idaho	84.0
48	New York	82.3
49	Minnesota	80.6
50	Rhode Island	77.2
	District of Columbia	91.3

Source: U.S. Department of Health and Human Services, Centers for Medicare and Medicaid Services
    "2003 Data Compendium" (http://www.cms.gov/researchers/pubs/datacompendium/)
*As of January 1, 2003. Refers to Medicare Part B. Physicians include MDs, DOs, limited license practitioners and non-physician practitioners.

Medicare Benefit Payments in 2001

National Total = $236,492,552,000*

ALPHA ORDER

RANK	STATE	BENEFITS	% of USA
18	Alabama	$4,270,957,000	1.8%
50	Alaska	169,288,000	0.1%
23	Arizona	3,322,292,000	1.4%
28	Arkansas	2,420,406,000	1.0%
1	California	24,858,719,000	10.5%
27	Colorado	2,698,488,000	1.1%
26	Connecticut	3,117,052,000	1.3%
47	Delaware	500,000,000	0.2%
2	Florida	21,580,488,000	9.1%
17	Georgia	4,397,178,000	1.9%
42	Hawaii	717,998,000	0.3%
41	Idaho	741,441,000	0.3%
7	Illinois	8,001,947,000	3.4%
13	Indiana	4,999,250,000	2.1%
34	Iowa	1,632,032,000	0.7%
31	Kansas	2,141,312,000	0.9%
21	Kentucky	3,640,057,000	1.5%
14	Louisiana	4,902,926,000	2.1%
40	Maine	875,798,000	0.4%
16	Maryland	4,611,432,000	1.9%
11	Massachusetts	5,963,041,000	2.5%
8	Michigan	7,012,604,000	3.0%
25	Minnesota	3,136,907,000	1.3%
32	Mississippi	2,140,391,000	0.9%
15	Missouri	4,755,402,000	2.0%
44	Montana	663,416,000	0.3%
35	Nebraska	1,366,977,000	0.6%
36	Nevada	1,272,774,000	0.5%
43	New Hampshire	714,188,000	0.3%
9	New Jersey	6,885,642,000	2.9%
39	New Mexico	879,540,000	0.4%
3	New York	20,436,630,000	8.6%
10	North Carolina	6,797,677,000	2.9%
46	North Dakota	562,654,000	0.2%
6	Ohio	10,685,164,000	4.5%
29	Oklahoma	2,343,403,000	1.0%
30	Oregon	2,181,557,000	0.9%
5	Pennsylvania	15,141,847,000	6.4%
37	Rhode Island	1,146,888,000	0.5%
22	South Carolina	3,356,574,000	1.4%
45	South Dakota	622,092,000	0.3%
12	Tennessee	5,545,549,000	2.3%
4	Texas	16,336,061,000	6.9%
38	Utah	1,077,334,000	0.5%
48	Vermont	361,871,000	0.2%
20	Virginia	3,897,031,000	1.6%
24	Washington	3,209,406,000	1.4%
33	West Virginia	1,822,039,000	0.8%
19	Wisconsin	3,961,455,000	1.7%
49	Wyoming	281,639,000	0.1%

RANK ORDER

RANK	STATE	BENEFITS	% of USA
1	California	$24,858,719,000	10.5%
2	Florida	21,580,488,000	9.1%
3	New York	20,436,630,000	8.6%
4	Texas	16,336,061,000	6.9%
5	Pennsylvania	15,141,847,000	6.4%
6	Ohio	10,685,164,000	4.5%
7	Illinois	8,001,947,000	3.4%
8	Michigan	7,012,604,000	3.0%
9	New Jersey	6,885,642,000	2.9%
10	North Carolina	6,797,677,000	2.9%
11	Massachusetts	5,963,041,000	2.5%
12	Tennessee	5,545,549,000	2.3%
13	Indiana	4,999,250,000	2.1%
14	Louisiana	4,902,926,000	2.1%
15	Missouri	4,755,402,000	2.0%
16	Maryland	4,611,432,000	1.9%
17	Georgia	4,397,178,000	1.9%
18	Alabama	4,270,957,000	1.8%
19	Wisconsin	3,961,455,000	1.7%
20	Virginia	3,897,031,000	1.6%
21	Kentucky	3,640,057,000	1.5%
22	South Carolina	3,356,574,000	1.4%
23	Arizona	3,322,292,000	1.4%
24	Washington	3,209,406,000	1.4%
25	Minnesota	3,136,907,000	1.3%
26	Connecticut	3,117,052,000	1.3%
27	Colorado	2,698,488,000	1.1%
28	Arkansas	2,420,406,000	1.0%
29	Oklahoma	2,343,403,000	1.0%
30	Oregon	2,181,557,000	0.9%
31	Kansas	2,141,312,000	0.9%
32	Mississippi	2,140,391,000	0.9%
33	West Virginia	1,822,039,000	0.8%
34	Iowa	1,632,032,000	0.7%
35	Nebraska	1,366,977,000	0.6%
36	Nevada	1,272,774,000	0.5%
37	Rhode Island	1,146,888,000	0.5%
38	Utah	1,077,334,000	0.5%
39	New Mexico	879,540,000	0.4%
40	Maine	875,798,000	0.4%
41	Idaho	741,441,000	0.3%
42	Hawaii	717,998,000	0.3%
43	New Hampshire	714,188,000	0.3%
44	Montana	663,416,000	0.3%
45	South Dakota	622,092,000	0.3%
46	North Dakota	562,654,000	0.2%
47	Delaware	500,000,000	0.2%
48	Vermont	361,871,000	0.2%
49	Wyoming	281,639,000	0.1%
50	Alaska	169,288,000	0.1%
	District of Columbia	792,265,000	0.3%

Source: U.S. Department of Health and Human Services, Centers for Medicare and Medicaid Services
   "Medicare Estimated Benefit Payments by State" (www.cms.gov/statistics/feeforservice/BenefitPayments01.pdf)
*For fiscal year 2001. Includes payments to aged and disabled enrollees. Total includes $1,454,823,000 in
payments to enrollees in Puerto Rico and $88,652,000 to enrollees in "other outlying areas."

Per Capita Medicare Benefit Payments in 2001

National Per Capita = $823*

ALPHA ORDER

RANK	STATE	PER CAPITA
8	Alabama	$956
50	Alaska	267
36	Arizona	626
12	Arkansas	898
28	California	718
37	Colorado	609
11	Connecticut	908
34	Delaware	628
1	Florida	1,318
47	Georgia	523
40	Hawaii	585
43	Idaho	561
32	Illinois	639
20	Indiana	816
44	Iowa	557
23	Kansas	792
13	Kentucky	895
3	Louisiana	1,097
30	Maine	682
15	Maryland	856
10	Massachusetts	932
29	Michigan	701
33	Minnesota	629
25	Mississippi	748
16	Missouri	844
26	Montana	733
22	Nebraska	795
38	Nevada	607
42	New Hampshire	567
21	New Jersey	809
48	New Mexico	480
5	New York	1,071
17	North Carolina	828
14	North Dakota	884
9	Ohio	938
31	Oklahoma	675
34	Oregon	628
2	Pennsylvania	1,231
4	Rhode Island	1,082
18	South Carolina	826
19	South Dakota	820
7	Tennessee	965
24	Texas	764
49	Utah	473
39	Vermont	590
45	Virginia	541
46	Washington	535
6	West Virginia	1,012
26	Wisconsin	733
41	Wyoming	570

RANK ORDER

RANK	STATE	PER CAPITA
1	Florida	$1,318
2	Pennsylvania	1,231
3	Louisiana	1,097
4	Rhode Island	1,082
5	New York	1,071
6	West Virginia	1,012
7	Tennessee	965
8	Alabama	956
9	Ohio	938
10	Massachusetts	932
11	Connecticut	908
12	Arkansas	898
13	Kentucky	895
14	North Dakota	884
15	Maryland	856
16	Missouri	844
17	North Carolina	828
18	South Carolina	826
19	South Dakota	820
20	Indiana	816
21	New Jersey	809
22	Nebraska	795
23	Kansas	792
24	Texas	764
25	Mississippi	748
26	Montana	733
26	Wisconsin	733
28	California	718
29	Michigan	701
30	Maine	682
31	Oklahoma	675
32	Illinois	639
33	Minnesota	629
34	Delaware	628
34	Oregon	628
36	Arizona	626
37	Colorado	609
38	Nevada	607
39	Vermont	590
40	Hawaii	585
41	Wyoming	570
42	New Hampshire	567
43	Idaho	561
44	Iowa	557
45	Virginia	541
46	Washington	535
47	Georgia	523
48	New Mexico	480
49	Utah	473
50	Alaska	267

District of Columbia   1,381

Source: MQ Press using data from U.S. Dept of Health & Human Services, Centers for Medicare and Medicaid Services "Medicare Estimated Benefit Payments by State" (www.cms.gov/statistics/feeforservice/BenefitPayments01.pdf)
*For fiscal year 2001. Includes aged and disabled enrollees. National rate does not include payments or enrollees in Puerto Rico and in "other outlying areas." Payments are based on the state of the provider or plan. Thus data showing payments per capita should be viewed as estimates and interpreted with caution.

Percent Change in Medicare Benefit Payments: 1997 to 2001

National Percent Change = 14.2% Increase*

ALPHA ORDER

RANK	STATE	PERCENT CHANGE
22	Alabama	19.2
37	Alaska	4.1
39	Arizona	3.5
10	Arkansas	27.0
30	California	12.5
17	Colorado	21.8
40	Connecticut	1.1
34	Delaware	6.1
15	Florida	23.1
48	Georgia	(6.9)
32	Hawaii	9.5
6	Idaho	31.2
45	Illinois	(3.7)
16	Indiana	22.5
47	Iowa	(6.1)
11	Kansas	26.6
12	Kentucky	26.0
27	Louisiana	14.4
43	Maine	(0.4)
2	Maryland	34.1
49	Massachusetts	(7.6)
46	Michigan	(5.2)
26	Minnesota	14.8
44	Mississippi	(3.3)
38	Missouri	3.8
3	Montana	33.8
5	Nebraska	32.8
29	Nevada	13.3
42	New Hampshire	0.1
36	New Jersey	4.8
41	New Mexico	0.7
14	New York	24.2
3	North Carolina	33.8
21	North Dakota	20.1
13	Ohio	24.9
50	Oklahoma	(12.5)
25	Oregon	15.6
18	Pennsylvania	21.7
24	Rhode Island	16.0
1	South Carolina	41.8
8	South Dakota	30.6
23	Tennessee	17.5
27	Texas	14.4
19	Utah	21.5
31	Vermont	10.3
33	Virginia	7.2
35	Washington	5.8
20	West Virginia	21.2
9	Wisconsin	27.4
7	Wyoming	30.7

RANK ORDER

RANK	STATE	PERCENT CHANGE
1	South Carolina	41.8
2	Maryland	34.1
3	Montana	33.8
3	North Carolina	33.8
5	Nebraska	32.8
6	Idaho	31.2
7	Wyoming	30.7
8	South Dakota	30.6
9	Wisconsin	27.4
10	Arkansas	27.0
11	Kansas	26.6
12	Kentucky	26.0
13	Ohio	24.9
14	New York	24.2
15	Florida	23.1
16	Indiana	22.5
17	Colorado	21.8
18	Pennsylvania	21.7
19	Utah	21.5
20	West Virginia	21.2
21	North Dakota	20.1
22	Alabama	19.2
23	Tennessee	17.5
24	Rhode Island	16.0
25	Oregon	15.6
26	Minnesota	14.8
27	Louisiana	14.4
27	Texas	14.4
29	Nevada	13.3
30	California	12.5
31	Vermont	10.3
32	Hawaii	9.5
33	Virginia	7.2
34	Delaware	6.1
35	Washington	5.8
36	New Jersey	4.8
37	Alaska	4.1
38	Missouri	3.8
39	Arizona	3.5
40	Connecticut	1.1
41	New Mexico	0.7
42	New Hampshire	0.1
43	Maine	(0.4)
44	Mississippi	(3.3)
45	Illinois	(3.7)
46	Michigan	(5.2)
47	Iowa	(6.1)
48	Georgia	(6.9)
49	Massachusetts	(7.6)
50	Oklahoma	(12.5)

District of Columbia   (37.3)

Source: Morgan Quitno Press using data from U.S. Department of HHS, Centers for Medicare and Medicaid Services
"Medicare Estimated Benefit Payments by State" (www.cms.gov/statistics/feeforservice/BenefitPayments01.pdf)
*For fiscal years 1997 and 2001. Includes payments to aged and disabled enrollees. Total includes payments to
enrollees in Puerto Rico and to enrollees in "other outlying areas."

Medicare Payments per Enrollee in 2001

National Rate = $6,003*

ALPHA ORDER

RANK	STATE	PER ENROLLEE
12	Alabama	$6,144
48	Alaska	3,864
33	Arizona	4,811
21	Arkansas	5,478
9	California	6,285
19	Colorado	5,674
13	Connecticut	6,037
40	Delaware	4,387
2	Florida	7,603
36	Georgia	4,713
43	Hawaii	4,266
39	Idaho	4,399
32	Illinois	4,879
15	Indiana	5,826
50	Iowa	3,414
22	Kansas	5,475
17	Kentucky	5,781
1	Louisiana	8,099
47	Maine	3,993
6	Maryland	7,045
11	Massachusetts	6,202
31	Michigan	4,959
35	Minnesota	4,750
29	Mississippi	5,055
20	Missouri	5,486
34	Montana	4,798
24	Nebraska	5,367
28	Nevada	5,080
45	New Hampshire	4,135
18	New Jersey	5,702
49	New Mexico	3,689
3	New York	7,489
14	North Carolina	5,886
23	North Dakota	5,456
10	Ohio	6,266
37	Oklahoma	4,590
38	Oregon	4,401
4	Pennsylvania	7,226
7	Rhode Island	6,675
16	South Carolina	5,791
26	South Dakota	5,183
8	Tennessee	6,584
5	Texas	7,104
27	Utah	5,120
46	Vermont	4,019
42	Virginia	4,285
41	Washington	4,303
25	West Virginia	5,361
30	Wisconsin	5,031
44	Wyoming	4,239

RANK ORDER

RANK	STATE	PER ENROLLEE
1	Louisiana	$8,099
2	Florida	7,603
3	New York	7,489
4	Pennsylvania	7,226
5	Texas	7,104
6	Maryland	7,045
7	Rhode Island	6,675
8	Tennessee	6,584
9	California	6,285
10	Ohio	6,266
11	Massachusetts	6,202
12	Alabama	6,144
13	Connecticut	6,037
14	North Carolina	5,886
15	Indiana	5,826
16	South Carolina	5,791
17	Kentucky	5,781
18	New Jersey	5,702
19	Colorado	5,674
20	Missouri	5,486
21	Arkansas	5,478
22	Kansas	5,475
23	North Dakota	5,456
24	Nebraska	5,367
25	West Virginia	5,361
26	South Dakota	5,183
27	Utah	5,120
28	Nevada	5,080
29	Mississippi	5,055
30	Wisconsin	5,031
31	Michigan	4,959
32	Illinois	4,879
33	Arizona	4,811
34	Montana	4,798
35	Minnesota	4,750
36	Georgia	4,713
37	Oklahoma	4,590
38	Oregon	4,401
39	Idaho	4,399
40	Delaware	4,387
41	Washington	4,303
42	Virginia	4,285
43	Hawaii	4,266
44	Wyoming	4,239
45	New Hampshire	4,135
46	Vermont	4,019
47	Maine	3,993
48	Alaska	3,864
49	New Mexico	3,689
50	Iowa	3,414

| | District of Columbia | 10,606 |

Source: MQ Press using data from U.S. Dept of Health & Human Services, Centers for Medicare and Medicaid Services
"Medicare Estimated Benefit Payments by State" (www.cms.gov/statistics/feeforservice/BenefitPayments01.pdf)
*For fiscal year 2001. Includes aged and disabled enrollees. National rate does not include payments or enrollees
in Puerto Rico and in "other outlying areas." Payments are based on the state of the provider or plan. Thus data
showing payments per beneficiary should be viewed as estimates and interpreted with caution.

Percent Change in Medicare Benefit Payments per Enrollee: 1997 to 2001

National Percent Change = 11.1% Increase*

ALPHA ORDER

RANK ORDER

RANK	STATE	PERCENT CHANGE		RANK	STATE	PERCENT CHANGE
22	Alabama	13.2		1	Nebraska	30.7
48	Alaska	(12.6)		2	South Carolina	30.4
40	Arizona	(5.3)		3	Montana	28.6
9	Arkansas	23.4		4	South Dakota	28.1
29	California	6.0		5	Maryland	26.5
21	Colorado	13.3		6	Kansas	25.1
36	Connecticut	(0.6)		7	Wisconsin	24.6
37	Delaware	(1.9)		8	North Carolina	24.2
19	Florida	17.3		9	Arkansas	23.4
49	Georgia	(13.6)		10	Wyoming	23.2
32	Hawaii	1.5		11	Ohio	23.0
12	Idaho	21.0		12	Idaho	21.0
39	Illinois	(4.9)		12	New York	21.0
17	Indiana	18.9		14	Pennsylvania	20.7
43	Iowa	(6.6)		15	Kentucky	20.3
6	Kansas	25.1		16	North Dakota	19.9
15	Kentucky	20.3		17	Indiana	18.9
24	Louisiana	11.6		18	West Virginia	18.4
41	Maine	(5.5)		19	Florida	17.3
5	Maryland	26.5		20	Rhode Island	14.1
47	Massachusetts	(9.2)		21	Colorado	13.3
46	Michigan	(8.3)		22	Alabama	13.2
25	Minnesota	11.0		23	Utah	12.6
45	Mississippi	(7.2)		24	Louisiana	11.6
33	Missouri	1.0		25	Minnesota	11.0
3	Montana	28.6		26	Oregon	10.9
1	Nebraska	30.7		27	Tennessee	10.7
38	Nevada	(4.1)		28	Texas	7.2
42	New Hampshire	(6.3)		29	California	6.0
31	New Jersey	2.4		30	Vermont	4.9
44	New Mexico	(6.7)		31	New Jersey	2.4
12	New York	21.0		32	Hawaii	1.5
8	North Carolina	24.2		33	Missouri	1.0
16	North Dakota	19.9		34	Washington	0.3
11	Ohio	23.0		35	Virginia	(0.2)
50	Oklahoma	(15.1)		36	Connecticut	(0.6)
26	Oregon	10.9		37	Delaware	(1.9)
14	Pennsylvania	20.7		38	Nevada	(4.1)
20	Rhode Island	14.1		39	Illinois	(4.9)
2	South Carolina	30.4		40	Arizona	(5.3)
4	South Dakota	28.1		41	Maine	(5.5)
27	Tennessee	10.7		42	New Hampshire	(6.3)
28	Texas	7.2		43	Iowa	(6.6)
23	Utah	12.6		44	New Mexico	(6.7)
30	Vermont	4.9		45	Mississippi	(7.2)
35	Virginia	(0.2)		46	Michigan	(8.3)
34	Washington	0.3		47	Massachusetts	(9.2)
18	West Virginia	18.4		48	Alaska	(12.6)
7	Wisconsin	24.6		49	Georgia	(13.6)
10	Wyoming	23.2		50	Oklahoma	(15.1)
					District of Columbia	(36.1)

Source: Morgan Quitno Press using data from U.S. Department of HHS, Centers for Medicare and Medicaid Services
"Medicare Estimated Benefit Payments by State" (www.cms.gov/statistics/feeforservice/BenefitPayments01.pdf)
*For fiscal years 1997 and 2001. Includes payments to aged and disabled enrollees. Total includes payments to enrollees in Puerto Rico and to enrollees in "other outlying areas."

Medicaid Enrollment in 2003

National Total = 42,740,719 Enrollees*

ALPHA ORDER

RANK	STATE	ENROLLEES	% of USA
19	Alabama	760,527	1.8%
45	Alaska	95,335	0.2%
15	Arizona	901,655	2.1%
26	Arkansas	557,074	1.3%
1	California	6,272,109	14.7%
32	Colorado	330,499	0.8%
30	Connecticut	405,064	0.9%
44	Delaware	121,676	0.3%
4	Florida	2,214,058	5.2%
8	Georgia	1,448,645	3.4%
39	Hawaii	179,522	0.4%
42	Idaho	156,935	0.4%
5	Illinois	1,580,944	3.7%
22	Indiana	707,168	1.7%
34	Iowa	266,737	0.6%
36	Kansas	246,186	0.6%
24	Kentucky	663,002	1.6%
17	Louisiana	861,846	2.0%
35	Maine	249,738	0.6%
23	Maryland	681,096	1.6%
14	Massachusetts	915,114	2.1%
9	Michigan	1,322,261	3.1%
27	Minnesota	552,779	1.3%
21	Mississippi	720,304	1.7%
13	Missouri	950,694	2.2%
48	Montana	80,378	0.2%
37	Nebraska	197,378	0.5%
41	Nevada	164,033	0.4%
47	New Hampshire	91,261	0.2%
18	New Jersey	782,309	1.8%
31	New Mexico	404,497	0.9%
2	New York	3,645,834	8.5%
11	North Carolina	1,074,616	2.5%
50	North Dakota	53,806	0.1%
6	Ohio	1,515,712	3.5%
28	Oklahoma	498,031	1.2%
29	Oregon	425,627	1.0%
7	Pennsylvania	1,492,095	3.5%
40	Rhode Island	178,543	0.4%
16	South Carolina	862,175	2.0%
46	South Dakota	93,208	0.2%
10	Tennessee	1,304,794	3.1%
3	Texas	2,559,248	6.0%
38	Utah	187,823	0.4%
43	Vermont	131,051	0.3%
25	Virginia	583,999	1.4%
12	Washington	1,059,865	2.5%
33	West Virginia	296,220	0.7%
20	Wisconsin	739,431	1.7%
49	Wyoming	56,209	0.1%

RANK ORDER

RANK	STATE	ENROLLEES	% of USA
1	California	6,272,109	14.7%
2	New York	3,645,834	8.5%
3	Texas	2,559,248	6.0%
4	Florida	2,214,058	5.2%
5	Illinois	1,580,944	3.7%
6	Ohio	1,515,712	3.5%
7	Pennsylvania	1,492,095	3.5%
8	Georgia	1,448,645	3.4%
9	Michigan	1,322,261	3.1%
10	Tennessee	1,304,794	3.1%
11	North Carolina	1,074,616	2.5%
12	Washington	1,059,865	2.5%
13	Missouri	950,694	2.2%
14	Massachusetts	915,114	2.1%
15	Arizona	901,655	2.1%
16	South Carolina	862,175	2.0%
17	Louisiana	861,846	2.0%
18	New Jersey	782,309	1.8%
19	Alabama	760,527	1.8%
20	Wisconsin	739,431	1.7%
21	Mississippi	720,304	1.7%
22	Indiana	707,168	1.7%
23	Maryland	681,096	1.6%
24	Kentucky	663,002	1.6%
25	Virginia	583,999	1.4%
26	Arkansas	557,074	1.3%
27	Minnesota	552,779	1.3%
28	Oklahoma	498,031	1.2%
29	Oregon	425,627	1.0%
30	Connecticut	405,064	0.9%
31	New Mexico	404,497	0.9%
32	Colorado	330,499	0.8%
33	West Virginia	296,220	0.7%
34	Iowa	266,737	0.6%
35	Maine	249,738	0.6%
36	Kansas	246,186	0.6%
37	Nebraska	197,378	0.5%
38	Utah	187,823	0.4%
39	Hawaii	179,522	0.4%
40	Rhode Island	178,543	0.4%
41	Nevada	164,033	0.4%
42	Idaho	156,935	0.4%
43	Vermont	131,051	0.3%
44	Delaware	121,676	0.3%
45	Alaska	95,335	0.2%
46	South Dakota	93,208	0.2%
47	New Hampshire	91,261	0.2%
48	Montana	80,378	0.2%
49	Wyoming	56,209	0.1%
50	North Dakota	53,806	0.1%
	District of Columbia	128,185	0.3%

Source: U.S. Department of Health and Human Services, Centers for Medicare and Medicaid Services
   "Medicaid Managed Care State Enrollment" (http://www.cms.hhs.gov/medicaid/managedcare/mcsten03.pdf)
As of June 30, 2003.   National total includes 973,423 Medicaid enrollees in Puerto Rico and the Virgin Islands.

Percent of Population Enrolled in Medicaid in 2003

National Percent = 14.4% of Population*

<table>
<tr><td colspan="3">ALPHA ORDER</td><td colspan="3">RANK ORDER</td></tr>
<tr><td>RANK</td><td>STATE</td><td>PERCENT</td><td>RANK</td><td>STATE</td><td>PERCENT</td></tr>
<tr><td>12</td><td>Alabama</td><td>16.9</td><td>1</td><td>Mississippi</td><td>25.0</td></tr>
<tr><td>20</td><td>Alaska</td><td>14.7</td><td>2</td><td>Tennessee</td><td>22.3</td></tr>
<tr><td>17</td><td>Arizona</td><td>16.2</td><td>3</td><td>New Mexico</td><td>21.5</td></tr>
<tr><td>6</td><td>Arkansas</td><td>20.4</td><td>4</td><td>Vermont</td><td>21.2</td></tr>
<tr><td>10</td><td>California</td><td>17.7</td><td>5</td><td>South Carolina</td><td>20.8</td></tr>
<tr><td>48</td><td>Colorado</td><td>7.3</td><td>6</td><td>Arkansas</td><td>20.4</td></tr>
<tr><td>34</td><td>Connecticut</td><td>11.6</td><td>7</td><td>Louisiana</td><td>19.2</td></tr>
<tr><td>19</td><td>Delaware</td><td>14.9</td><td>8</td><td>Maine</td><td>19.1</td></tr>
<tr><td>27</td><td>Florida</td><td>13.0</td><td>9</td><td>New York</td><td>19.0</td></tr>
<tr><td>13</td><td>Georgia</td><td>16.7</td><td>10</td><td>California</td><td>17.7</td></tr>
<tr><td>21</td><td>Hawaii</td><td>14.4</td><td>11</td><td>Washington</td><td>17.3</td></tr>
<tr><td>36</td><td>Idaho</td><td>11.5</td><td>12</td><td>Alabama</td><td>16.9</td></tr>
<tr><td>29</td><td>Illinois</td><td>12.5</td><td>13</td><td>Georgia</td><td>16.7</td></tr>
<tr><td>37</td><td>Indiana</td><td>11.4</td><td>14</td><td>Missouri</td><td>16.6</td></tr>
<tr><td>41</td><td>Iowa</td><td>9.1</td><td>14</td><td>Rhode Island</td><td>16.6</td></tr>
<tr><td>43</td><td>Kansas</td><td>9.0</td><td>16</td><td>West Virginia</td><td>16.4</td></tr>
<tr><td>18</td><td>Kentucky</td><td>16.1</td><td>17</td><td>Arizona</td><td>16.2</td></tr>
<tr><td>7</td><td>Louisiana</td><td>19.2</td><td>18</td><td>Kentucky</td><td>16.1</td></tr>
<tr><td>8</td><td>Maine</td><td>19.1</td><td>19</td><td>Delaware</td><td>14.9</td></tr>
<tr><td>30</td><td>Maryland</td><td>12.4</td><td>20</td><td>Alaska</td><td>14.7</td></tr>
<tr><td>22</td><td>Massachusetts</td><td>14.3</td><td>21</td><td>Hawaii</td><td>14.4</td></tr>
<tr><td>26</td><td>Michigan</td><td>13.1</td><td>22</td><td>Massachusetts</td><td>14.3</td></tr>
<tr><td>40</td><td>Minnesota</td><td>10.9</td><td>23</td><td>Oklahoma</td><td>14.2</td></tr>
<tr><td>1</td><td>Mississippi</td><td>25.0</td><td>24</td><td>Wisconsin</td><td>13.5</td></tr>
<tr><td>14</td><td>Missouri</td><td>16.6</td><td>25</td><td>Ohio</td><td>13.3</td></tr>
<tr><td>44</td><td>Montana</td><td>8.8</td><td>26</td><td>Michigan</td><td>13.1</td></tr>
<tr><td>37</td><td>Nebraska</td><td>11.4</td><td>27</td><td>Florida</td><td>13.0</td></tr>
<tr><td>48</td><td>Nevada</td><td>7.3</td><td>28</td><td>North Carolina</td><td>12.8</td></tr>
<tr><td>50</td><td>New Hampshire</td><td>7.1</td><td>29</td><td>Illinois</td><td>12.5</td></tr>
<tr><td>41</td><td>New Jersey</td><td>9.1</td><td>30</td><td>Maryland</td><td>12.4</td></tr>
<tr><td>3</td><td>New Mexico</td><td>21.5</td><td>31</td><td>South Dakota</td><td>12.2</td></tr>
<tr><td>9</td><td>New York</td><td>19.0</td><td>32</td><td>Pennsylvania</td><td>12.1</td></tr>
<tr><td>28</td><td>North Carolina</td><td>12.8</td><td>33</td><td>Oregon</td><td>11.9</td></tr>
<tr><td>45</td><td>North Dakota</td><td>8.5</td><td>34</td><td>Connecticut</td><td>11.6</td></tr>
<tr><td>25</td><td>Ohio</td><td>13.3</td><td>34</td><td>Texas</td><td>11.6</td></tr>
<tr><td>23</td><td>Oklahoma</td><td>14.2</td><td>36</td><td>Idaho</td><td>11.5</td></tr>
<tr><td>33</td><td>Oregon</td><td>11.9</td><td>37</td><td>Indiana</td><td>11.4</td></tr>
<tr><td>32</td><td>Pennsylvania</td><td>12.1</td><td>37</td><td>Nebraska</td><td>11.4</td></tr>
<tr><td>14</td><td>Rhode Island</td><td>16.6</td><td>39</td><td>Wyoming</td><td>11.2</td></tr>
<tr><td>5</td><td>South Carolina</td><td>20.8</td><td>40</td><td>Minnesota</td><td>10.9</td></tr>
<tr><td>31</td><td>South Dakota</td><td>12.2</td><td>41</td><td>Iowa</td><td>9.1</td></tr>
<tr><td>2</td><td>Tennessee</td><td>22.3</td><td>41</td><td>New Jersey</td><td>9.1</td></tr>
<tr><td>34</td><td>Texas</td><td>11.6</td><td>43</td><td>Kansas</td><td>9.0</td></tr>
<tr><td>46</td><td>Utah</td><td>8.0</td><td>44</td><td>Montana</td><td>8.8</td></tr>
<tr><td>4</td><td>Vermont</td><td>21.2</td><td>45</td><td>North Dakota</td><td>8.5</td></tr>
<tr><td>47</td><td>Virginia</td><td>7.9</td><td>46</td><td>Utah</td><td>8.0</td></tr>
<tr><td>11</td><td>Washington</td><td>17.3</td><td>47</td><td>Virginia</td><td>7.9</td></tr>
<tr><td>16</td><td>West Virginia</td><td>16.4</td><td>48</td><td>Colorado</td><td>7.3</td></tr>
<tr><td>24</td><td>Wisconsin</td><td>13.5</td><td>48</td><td>Nevada</td><td>7.3</td></tr>
<tr><td>39</td><td>Wyoming</td><td>11.2</td><td>50</td><td>New Hampshire</td><td>7.1</td></tr>
<tr><td></td><td></td><td></td><td></td><td>District of Columbia</td><td>23.0</td></tr>
</table>

Source: MQ Press using data from U.S. Dept of Health & Human Services, Centers for Medicare and Medicaid Services
"Medicaid Managed Care State Enrollment" (http://www.cms.hhs.gov/medicaid/managedcare/mcsten03.pdf)
*As of June 30, 2003. National percent does not include recipients or population in U.S. territories.

Medicaid Managed Care Enrollment in 2003

National Total = 25,262,873 Enrollees*

ALPHA ORDER

RANK	STATE	ENROLLEES	% of USA
20	Alabama	404,797	1.6%
48	Alaska	0	0.0%
10	Arizona	808,506	3.2%
21	Arkansas	374,067	1.5%
1	California	3,258,787	12.9%
28	Colorado	262,263	1.0%
26	Connecticut	294,331	1.2%
41	Delaware	86,709	0.3%
3	Florida	1,354,025	5.4%
6	Georgia	1,212,639	4.8%
35	Hawaii	141,399	0.6%
39	Idaho	101,257	0.4%
37	Illinois	137,682	0.5%
16	Indiana	502,401	2.0%
30	Iowa	243,954	1.0%
36	Kansas	141,119	0.6%
12	Kentucky	611,878	2.4%
15	Louisiana	505,434	2.0%
33	Maine	148,151	0.6%
17	Maryland	466,688	1.8%
13	Massachusetts	572,835	2.3%
4	Michigan	1,314,810	5.2%
22	Minnesota	362,349	1.4%
48	Mississippi	0	0.0%
19	Missouri	425,161	1.7%
45	Montana	55,372	0.2%
34	Nebraska	142,377	0.6%
43	Nevada	74,923	0.3%
47	New Hampshire	13,407	0.1%
14	New Jersey	525,864	2.1%
29	New Mexico	261,015	1.0%
2	New York	1,914,794	7.6%
11	North Carolina	749,152	3.0%
46	North Dakota	35,515	0.1%
18	Ohio	436,146	1.7%
24	Oklahoma	338,859	1.3%
25	Oregon	330,874	1.3%
7	Pennsylvania	1,192,031	4.7%
38	Rhode Island	119,257	0.5%
44	South Carolina	71,195	0.3%
40	South Dakota	90,733	0.4%
5	Tennessee	1,304,794	5.2%
8	Texas	1,065,945	4.2%
31	Utah	162,364	0.6%
42	Vermont	85,751	0.3%
27	Virginia	262,961	1.0%
9	Washington	854,861	3.4%
32	West Virginia	151,515	0.6%
23	Wisconsin	349,246	1.4%
48	Wyoming	0	0.0%

RANK ORDER

RANK	STATE	ENROLLEES	% of USA
1	California	3,258,787	12.9%
2	New York	1,914,794	7.6%
3	Florida	1,354,025	5.4%
4	Michigan	1,314,810	5.2%
5	Tennessee	1,304,794	5.2%
6	Georgia	1,212,639	4.8%
7	Pennsylvania	1,192,031	4.7%
8	Texas	1,065,945	4.2%
9	Washington	854,861	3.4%
10	Arizona	808,506	3.2%
11	North Carolina	749,152	3.0%
12	Kentucky	611,878	2.4%
13	Massachusetts	572,835	2.3%
14	New Jersey	525,864	2.1%
15	Louisiana	505,434	2.0%
16	Indiana	502,401	2.0%
17	Maryland	466,688	1.8%
18	Ohio	436,146	1.7%
19	Missouri	425,161	1.7%
20	Alabama	404,797	1.6%
21	Arkansas	374,067	1.5%
22	Minnesota	362,349	1.4%
23	Wisconsin	349,246	1.4%
24	Oklahoma	338,859	1.3%
25	Oregon	330,874	1.3%
26	Connecticut	294,331	1.2%
27	Virginia	262,961	1.0%
28	Colorado	262,263	1.0%
29	New Mexico	261,015	1.0%
30	Iowa	243,954	1.0%
31	Utah	162,364	0.6%
32	West Virginia	151,515	0.6%
33	Maine	148,151	0.6%
34	Nebraska	142,377	0.6%
35	Hawaii	141,399	0.6%
36	Kansas	141,119	0.6%
37	Illinois	137,682	0.5%
38	Rhode Island	119,257	0.5%
39	Idaho	101,257	0.4%
40	South Dakota	90,733	0.4%
41	Delaware	86,709	0.3%
42	Vermont	85,751	0.3%
43	Nevada	74,923	0.3%
44	South Carolina	71,195	0.3%
45	Montana	55,372	0.2%
46	North Dakota	35,515	0.1%
47	New Hampshire	13,407	0.1%
48	Alaska	0	0.0%
48	Mississippi	0	0.0%
48	Wyoming	0	0.0%
	District of Columbia	85,370	0.3%

Source: U.S. Department of Health and Human Services, Centers for Medicare and Medicaid Services
"Medicaid Managed Care State Enrollment" (http://www.cms.hhs.gov/medicaid/managedcare/mcsten03.pdf)
*As of June 30, 2003. Enrollment in state health care reform programs that expand eligibility beyond traditional Medicaid standards. National total includes 857,310 Medicaid managed care enrollees in Puerto Rico.

Percent of Medicaid Enrollees in Managed Care in 2003

National Percent = 59.1% of Medicaid Enrollees*

ALPHA ORDER

RANK ORDER

RANK	STATE	PERCENT
35	Alabama	53.2
48	Alaska	0.0
6	Arizona	89.7
22	Arkansas	67.2
37	California	52.0
11	Colorado	79.4
14	Connecticut	72.7
16	Delaware	71.3
31	Florida	61.2
8	Georgia	83.7
12	Hawaii	78.8
28	Idaho	64.5
46	Illinois	8.7
17	Indiana	71.0
5	Iowa	91.5
34	Kansas	57.3
4	Kentucky	92.3
33	Louisiana	58.7
32	Maine	59.3
20	Maryland	68.5
30	Massachusetts	62.6
2	Michigan	99.4
26	Minnesota	65.6
48	Mississippi	0.0
42	Missouri	44.7
19	Montana	68.9
15	Nebraska	72.1
40	Nevada	45.7
45	New Hampshire	14.7
22	New Jersey	67.2
28	New Mexico	64.5
36	New York	52.5
18	North Carolina	69.7
25	North Dakota	66.0
44	Ohio	28.8
21	Oklahoma	68.0
13	Oregon	77.7
10	Pennsylvania	79.9
24	Rhode Island	66.8
47	South Carolina	8.3
3	South Dakota	97.3
1	Tennessee	100.0
43	Texas	41.7
7	Utah	86.5
27	Vermont	65.4
41	Virginia	45.0
9	Washington	80.7
38	West Virginia	51.2
39	Wisconsin	47.2
48	Wyoming	0.0

RANK	STATE	PERCENT
1	Tennessee	100.0
2	Michigan	99.4
3	South Dakota	97.3
4	Kentucky	92.3
5	Iowa	91.5
6	Arizona	89.7
7	Utah	86.5
8	Georgia	83.7
9	Washington	80.7
10	Pennsylvania	79.9
11	Colorado	79.4
12	Hawaii	78.8
13	Oregon	77.7
14	Connecticut	72.7
15	Nebraska	72.1
16	Delaware	71.3
17	Indiana	71.0
18	North Carolina	69.7
19	Montana	68.9
20	Maryland	68.5
21	Oklahoma	68.0
22	Arkansas	67.2
22	New Jersey	67.2
24	Rhode Island	66.8
25	North Dakota	66.0
26	Minnesota	65.6
27	Vermont	65.4
28	Idaho	64.5
28	New Mexico	64.5
30	Massachusetts	62.6
31	Florida	61.2
32	Maine	59.3
33	Louisiana	58.7
34	Kansas	57.3
35	Alabama	53.2
36	New York	52.5
37	California	52.0
38	West Virginia	51.2
39	Wisconsin	47.2
40	Nevada	45.7
41	Virginia	45.0
42	Missouri	44.7
43	Texas	41.7
44	Ohio	28.8
45	New Hampshire	14.7
46	Illinois	8.7
47	South Carolina	8.3
48	Alaska	0.0
48	Mississippi	0.0
48	Wyoming	0.0

District of Columbia   66.6

Source: U.S. Department of Health and Human Services, Centers for Medicare and Medicaid Services
"Medicaid Managed Care State Enrollment" (http://www.cms.hhs.gov/medicaid/managedcare/mcsten03.pdf)
As of June 30, 2003. Enrollment in state health care reform programs that expand eligibility beyond traditional Medicaid standards. National percent includes Medicaid enrollees in Puerto Rico and the Virgin Islands.

Medicaid Expenditures in 2002

National Total = $246,283,943,000*

RANK	STATE	EXPENDITURES	% of USA
26	Alabama	$3,093,271,000	1.3%
44	Alaska	685,773,000	0.3%
23	Arizona	3,541,599,000	1.4%
32	Arkansas	2,237,818,000	0.9%
2	California	26,890,541,000	10.9%
30	Colorado	2,323,069,000	0.9%
24	Connecticut	3,456,339,000	1.4%
46	Delaware	634,046,000	0.3%
5	Florida	9,871,508,000	4.0%
12	Georgia	6,241,211,000	2.5%
43	Hawaii	740,007,000	0.3%
42	Idaho	773,535,000	0.3%
7	Illinois	8,809,060,000	3.6%
17	Indiana	4,448,318,000	1.8%
28	Iowa	2,575,146,000	1.0%
33	Kansas	1,836,717,000	0.7%
21	Kentucky	3,763,204,000	1.5%
16	Louisiana	4,885,972,000	2.0%
36	Maine	1,430,109,000	0.6%
22	Maryland	3,613,476,000	1.5%
8	Massachusetts	8,063,005,000	3.3%
10	Michigan	7,562,053,000	3.1%
18	Minnesota	4,414,511,000	1.8%
27	Mississippi	2,877,014,000	1.2%
14	Missouri	5,360,608,000	2.2%
47	Montana	571,456,000	0.2%
38	Nebraska	1,339,132,000	0.5%
41	Nevada	808,198,000	0.3%
39	New Hampshire	1,016,095,000	0.4%
9	New Jersey	7,745,878,000	3.1%
34	New Mexico	1,776,812,000	0.7%
1	New York	36,295,107,000	14.7%
11	North Carolina	6,723,599,000	2.7%
49	North Dakota	461,402,000	0.2%
6	Ohio	9,658,041,000	3.9%
31	Oklahoma	2,260,404,000	0.9%
29	Oregon	2,571,561,000	1.0%
4	Pennsylvania	12,130,925,000	4.9%
37	Rhode Island	1,358,501,000	0.6%
25	South Carolina	3,292,901,000	1.3%
48	South Dakota	549,884,000	0.2%
13	Tennessee	5,787,079,000	2.3%
3	Texas	13,523,486,000	5.5%
40	Utah	984,161,000	0.4%
45	Vermont	660,732,000	0.3%
20	Virginia	3,812,166,000	1.5%
15	Washington	5,168,512,000	2.1%
35	West Virginia	1,584,166,000	0.6%
19	Wisconsin	4,193,175,000	1.7%
50	Wyoming	274,565,000	0.1%

RANK	STATE	EXPENDITURES	% of USA
1	New York	$36,295,107,000	14.7%
2	California	26,890,541,000	10.9%
3	Texas	13,523,486,000	5.5%
4	Pennsylvania	12,130,925,000	4.9%
5	Florida	9,871,508,000	4.0%
6	Ohio	9,658,041,000	3.9%
7	Illinois	8,809,060,000	3.6%
8	Massachusetts	8,063,005,000	3.3%
9	New Jersey	7,745,878,000	3.1%
10	Michigan	7,562,053,000	3.1%
11	North Carolina	6,723,599,000	2.7%
12	Georgia	6,241,211,000	2.5%
13	Tennessee	5,787,079,000	2.3%
14	Missouri	5,360,608,000	2.2%
15	Washington	5,168,512,000	2.1%
16	Louisiana	4,885,972,000	2.0%
17	Indiana	4,448,318,000	1.8%
18	Minnesota	4,414,511,000	1.8%
19	Wisconsin	4,193,175,000	1.7%
20	Virginia	3,812,166,000	1.5%
21	Kentucky	3,763,204,000	1.5%
22	Maryland	3,613,476,000	1.5%
23	Arizona	3,541,599,000	1.4%
24	Connecticut	3,456,339,000	1.4%
25	South Carolina	3,292,901,000	1.3%
26	Alabama	3,093,271,000	1.3%
27	Mississippi	2,877,014,000	1.2%
28	Iowa	2,575,146,000	1.0%
29	Oregon	2,571,561,000	1.0%
30	Colorado	2,323,069,000	0.9%
31	Oklahoma	2,260,404,000	0.9%
32	Arkansas	2,237,818,000	0.9%
33	Kansas	1,836,717,000	0.7%
34	New Mexico	1,776,812,000	0.7%
35	West Virginia	1,584,166,000	0.6%
36	Maine	1,430,109,000	0.6%
37	Rhode Island	1,358,501,000	0.6%
38	Nebraska	1,339,132,000	0.5%
39	New Hampshire	1,016,095,000	0.4%
40	Utah	984,161,000	0.4%
41	Nevada	808,198,000	0.3%
42	Idaho	773,535,000	0.3%
43	Hawaii	740,007,000	0.3%
44	Alaska	685,773,000	0.3%
45	Vermont	660,732,000	0.3%
46	Delaware	634,046,000	0.3%
47	Montana	571,456,000	0.2%
48	South Dakota	549,884,000	0.2%
49	North Dakota	461,402,000	0.2%
50	Wyoming	274,565,000	0.1%
	District of Columbia	1,021,773,000	0.4%

Source: U.S. Department of Health and Human Services, Centers for Medicare and Medicaid Services
    "Medicaid Financial Statistics Tables (CMS-64 Report)"
*For fiscal year 2002. National total includes $586,322,000 in expenditures in U.S. territories. Includes Medical Assistance Payments and Administrative Costs.

Per Capita Medicaid Expenditures in 2002

National Per Capita = $852*

ALPHA ORDER

RANK ORDER

RANK	STATE	PER CAPITA	RANK	STATE	PER CAPITA
36	Alabama	$689	1	New York	$1,895
7	Alaska	1,065	2	Rhode Island	1,270
39	Arizona	649	3	Massachusetts	1,254
21	Arkansas	826	4	Maine	1,105
28	California	766	5	Louisiana	1,090
48	Colorado	515	6	Vermont	1,072
9	Connecticut	999	7	Alaska	1,065
25	Delaware	785	8	Mississippi	1,002
44	Florida	591	9	Connecticut	999
31	Georgia	729	10	Tennessee	998
43	Hawaii	594	11	Pennsylvania	983
45	Idaho	577	12	New Mexico	958
35	Illinois	699	13	Missouri	945
34	Indiana	722	14	Kentucky	919
18	Iowa	877	15	New Jersey	902
37	Kansas	676	16	Minnesota	879
14	Kentucky	919	16	West Virginia	879
5	Louisiana	1,090	18	Iowa	877
4	Maine	1,105	19	Washington	852
38	Maryland	662	20	Ohio	846
3	Massachusetts	1,254	21	Arkansas	826
29	Michigan	752	22	North Carolina	808
16	Minnesota	879	23	South Carolina	802
8	Mississippi	1,002	24	New Hampshire	797
13	Missouri	945	25	Delaware	785
41	Montana	628	26	Nebraska	774
26	Nebraska	774	27	Wisconsin	771
50	Nevada	372	28	California	766
24	New Hampshire	797	29	Michigan	752
15	New Jersey	902	30	Oregon	730
12	New Mexico	958	31	Georgia	729
1	New York	1,895	32	North Dakota	728
22	North Carolina	808	33	South Dakota	723
32	North Dakota	728	34	Indiana	722
20	Ohio	846	35	Illinois	699
40	Oklahoma	647	36	Alabama	689
30	Oregon	730	37	Kansas	676
11	Pennsylvania	983	38	Maryland	662
2	Rhode Island	1,270	39	Arizona	649
23	South Carolina	802	40	Oklahoma	647
33	South Dakota	723	41	Montana	628
10	Tennessee	998	42	Texas	621
42	Texas	621	43	Hawaii	594
49	Utah	425	44	Florida	591
6	Vermont	1,072	45	Idaho	577
47	Virginia	523	46	Wyoming	551
19	Washington	852	47	Virginia	523
16	West Virginia	879	48	Colorado	515
27	Wisconsin	771	49	Utah	425
46	Wyoming	551	50	Nevada	372

District of Columbia 1,790

Source: MQ Press using data from U.S. Dept of Health & Human Services, Centers for Medicare and Medicaid Services
"Medicaid Financial Statistics Tables (CMS-64 Report)"
*For fiscal year 2002. National figure does not include expenditures or enrollees in U.S. territories. Includes Medical Assistance Payments and Administrative Costs.

Percent Change in Medicaid Expenditures: 1998 to 2002

National Percent Change = 45.8% Increase*

ALPHA ORDER

RANK	STATE	PERCENT CHANGE
45	Alabama	33.1
3	Alaska	89.0
2	Arizona	90.3
14	Arkansas	59.1
26	California	46.7
34	Colorado	44.8
49	Connecticut	22.1
21	Delaware	53.1
18	Florida	55.1
5	Georgia	79.0
48	Hawaii	26.3
4	Idaho	88.8
43	Illinois	35.2
8	Indiana	72.6
1	Iowa	91.2
10	Kansas	68.1
33	Kentucky	45.0
20	Louisiana	53.9
46	Maine	32.6
38	Maryland	40.2
26	Massachusetts	46.7
47	Michigan	31.8
25	Minnesota	47.7
7	Mississippi	73.8
12	Missouri	63.3
28	Montana	46.3
15	Nebraska	58.3
16	Nevada	57.6
42	New Hampshire	36.8
36	New Jersey	42.5
6	New Mexico	76.0
44	New York	33.2
24	North Carolina	47.8
39	North Dakota	39.6
32	Ohio	45.1
9	Oklahoma	68.6
23	Oregon	50.5
35	Pennsylvania	42.6
37	Rhode Island	41.5
29	South Carolina	45.7
19	South Dakota	54.7
30	Tennessee	45.6
41	Texas	38.3
31	Utah	45.4
11	Vermont	66.3
13	Virginia	62.7
17	Washington	55.9
50	West Virginia	16.5
22	Wisconsin	52.0
40	Wyoming	39.1

RANK ORDER

RANK	STATE	PERCENT CHANGE
1	Iowa	91.2
2	Arizona	90.3
3	Alaska	89.0
4	Idaho	88.8
5	Georgia	79.0
6	New Mexico	76.0
7	Mississippi	73.8
8	Indiana	72.6
9	Oklahoma	68.6
10	Kansas	68.1
11	Vermont	66.3
12	Missouri	63.3
13	Virginia	62.7
14	Arkansas	59.1
15	Nebraska	58.3
16	Nevada	57.6
17	Washington	55.9
18	Florida	55.1
19	South Dakota	54.7
20	Louisiana	53.9
21	Delaware	53.1
22	Wisconsin	52.0
23	Oregon	50.5
24	North Carolina	47.8
25	Minnesota	47.7
26	California	46.7
26	Massachusetts	46.7
28	Montana	46.3
29	South Carolina	45.7
30	Tennessee	45.6
31	Utah	45.4
32	Ohio	45.1
33	Kentucky	45.0
34	Colorado	44.8
35	Pennsylvania	42.6
36	New Jersey	42.5
37	Rhode Island	41.5
38	Maryland	40.2
39	North Dakota	39.6
40	Wyoming	39.1
41	Texas	38.3
42	New Hampshire	36.8
43	Illinois	35.2
44	New York	33.2
45	Alabama	33.1
46	Maine	32.6
47	Michigan	31.8
48	Hawaii	26.3
49	Connecticut	22.1
50	West Virginia	16.5

District of Columbia	18.1

Source: MQ Press using data from U.S. Dept of Health & Human Services, Centers for Medicare and Medicaid Services "Medicaid Financial Statistics Tables (CMS-64 Report)"

For fiscal years 2002 and 1998. National figure includes expenditures in U.S. territories. Figures do not include administrative costs.

Medicaid Expenditures per Enrollee in 2002

National Rate = $5,985 per Enrollee*

ALPHA ORDER

RANK	STATE	PER ENROLLEE
49	Alabama	$4,204
12	Alaska	7,479
46	Arizona	4,310
48	Arkansas	4,247
45	California	4,344
14	Colorado	7,418
5	Connecticut	8,972
35	Delaware	5,079
41	Florida	4,679
40	Georgia	4,717
50	Hawaii	4,168
34	Idaho	5,110
33	Illinois	5,195
16	Indiana	6,478
4	Iowa	9,716
10	Kansas	7,789
22	Kentucky	6,229
26	Louisiana	5,859
17	Maine	6,464
32	Maryland	5,452
7	Massachusetts	8,379
19	Michigan	6,347
9	Minnesota	7,934
43	Mississippi	4,421
27	Missouri	5,763
13	Montana	7,472
20	Nebraska	6,325
38	Nevada	4,916
1	New Hampshire	11,286
3	New Jersey	10,197
42	New Mexico	4,564
2	New York	10,710
18	North Carolina	6,391
6	North Dakota	8,720
21	Ohio	6,251
39	Oklahoma	4,887
25	Oregon	6,015
8	Pennsylvania	8,316
11	Rhode Island	7,741
47	South Carolina	4,268
24	South Dakota	6,058
44	Tennessee	4,371
29	Texas	5,605
27	Utah	5,763
37	Vermont	4,987
15	Virginia	7,187
31	Washington	5,462
30	West Virginia	5,499
23	Wisconsin	6,199
36	Wyoming	5,024

RANK ORDER

RANK	STATE	PER ENROLLEE
1	New Hampshire	$11,286
2	New York	10,710
3	New Jersey	10,197
4	Iowa	9,716
5	Connecticut	8,972
6	North Dakota	8,720
7	Massachusetts	8,379
8	Pennsylvania	8,316
9	Minnesota	7,934
10	Kansas	7,789
11	Rhode Island	7,741
12	Alaska	7,479
13	Montana	7,472
14	Colorado	7,418
15	Virginia	7,187
16	Indiana	6,478
17	Maine	6,464
18	North Carolina	6,391
19	Michigan	6,347
20	Nebraska	6,325
21	Ohio	6,251
22	Kentucky	6,229
23	Wisconsin	6,199
24	South Dakota	6,058
25	Oregon	6,015
26	Louisiana	5,859
27	Missouri	5,763
27	Utah	5,763
29	Texas	5,605
30	West Virginia	5,499
31	Washington	5,462
32	Maryland	5,452
33	Illinois	5,195
34	Idaho	5,110
35	Delaware	5,079
36	Wyoming	5,024
37	Vermont	4,987
38	Nevada	4,916
39	Oklahoma	4,887
40	Georgia	4,717
41	Florida	4,679
42	New Mexico	4,564
43	Mississippi	4,421
44	Tennessee	4,371
45	California	4,344
46	Arizona	4,310
47	South Carolina	4,268
48	Arkansas	4,247
49	Alabama	4,204
50	Hawaii	4,168
	District of Columbia	7,931

Source: MQ Press using data from U.S. Dept of Health & Human Services, Centers for Medicare and Medicaid Services
"Medicaid Financial Statistics Tables (CMS-64 Report)"
*For fiscal year 2002. National figure includes expenditures and enrollees in U.S. territories. Includes Medical
Assistance Payments and Administrative Costs.

Percent Change in Expenditures per Medicaid Enrollee: 1998 to 2002

National Percent Change = 10.2% Increase*

ALPHA ORDER

RANK	STATE	PERCENT CHANGE
45	Alabama	(7.5)
9	Alaska	25.5
39	Arizona	(0.8)
34	Arkansas	5.6
17	California	17.0
38	Colorado	(0.4)
40	Connecticut	(1.9)
37	Delaware	(0.3)
31	Florida	5.9
11	Georgia	22.9
21	Hawaii	14.0
41	Idaho	(3.0)
35	Illinois	3.6
23	Indiana	12.6
2	Iowa	49.8
15	Kansas	21.0
13	Kentucky	22.8
29	Louisiana	7.3
44	Maine	(3.7)
36	Maryland	0.5
6	Massachusetts	31.1
16	Michigan	17.9
27	Minnesota	11.0
32	Mississippi	5.8
24	Missouri	12.5
8	Montana	26.4
14	Nebraska	22.0
50	Nevada	(17.3)
22	New Hampshire	13.7
18	New Jersey	15.4
11	New Mexico	22.9
49	New York	(12.5)
20	North Carolina	14.1
26	North Dakota	11.9
43	Ohio	(3.6)
10	Oklahoma	25.1
5	Oregon	32.1
7	Pennsylvania	28.5
42	Rhode Island	(3.2)
46	South Carolina	(10.9)
25	South Dakota	12.2
3	Tennessee	41.7
32	Texas	5.8
30	Utah	6.5
4	Vermont	38.3
1	Virginia	50.8
19	Washington	15.3
28	West Virginia	9.3
47	Wisconsin	(11.3)
47	Wyoming	(11.3)

RANK ORDER

RANK	STATE	PERCENT CHANGE
1	Virginia	50.8
2	Iowa	49.8
3	Tennessee	41.7
4	Vermont	38.3
5	Oregon	32.1
6	Massachusetts	31.1
7	Pennsylvania	28.5
8	Montana	26.4
9	Alaska	25.5
10	Oklahoma	25.1
11	Georgia	22.9
11	New Mexico	22.9
13	Kentucky	22.8
14	Nebraska	22.0
15	Kansas	21.0
16	Michigan	17.9
17	California	17.0
18	New Jersey	15.4
19	Washington	15.3
20	North Carolina	14.1
21	Hawaii	14.0
22	New Hampshire	13.7
23	Indiana	12.6
24	Missouri	12.5
25	South Dakota	12.2
26	North Dakota	11.9
27	Minnesota	11.0
28	West Virginia	9.3
29	Louisiana	7.3
30	Utah	6.5
31	Florida	5.9
32	Mississippi	5.8
32	Texas	5.8
34	Arkansas	5.6
35	Illinois	3.6
36	Maryland	0.5
37	Delaware	(0.3)
38	Colorado	(0.4)
39	Arizona	(0.8)
40	Connecticut	(1.9)
41	Idaho	(3.0)
42	Rhode Island	(3.2)
43	Ohio	(3.6)
44	Maine	(3.7)
45	Alabama	(7.5)
46	South Carolina	(10.9)
47	Wisconsin	(11.3)
47	Wyoming	(11.3)
49	New York	(12.5)
50	Nevada	(17.3)

District of Columbia   6.1

Source: MQ Press using data from U.S. Dept of Health & Human Services, Centers for Medicare and Medicaid Services "Medicaid Financial Statistics Tables (CMS-64 Report)"
*For fiscal years 2002 and 1998. National figure includes expenditures and enrollees in U.S. territories. Figures do not include administrative costs.

Federal Medicaid Matching Fund Rate for 2005

National Average = 72.62% of States' Funds Matched by Federal Government*

ALPHA ORDER

RANK	STATE	RATE
8	Alabama	79.58
33	Alaska	70.31
14	Arizona	77.22
2	Arkansas	82.33
39	California	65.00
39	Colorado	65.00
39	Connecticut	65.00
38	Delaware	65.27
29	Florida	71.23
25	Georgia	72.31
30	Hawaii	70.93
9	Idaho	79.43
39	Illinois	65.00
20	Indiana	73.95
19	Iowa	74.49
23	Kansas	72.71
12	Kentucky	78.72
7	Louisiana	79.73
16	Maine	75.42
39	Maryland	65.00
39	Massachusetts	65.00
34	Michigan	69.70
39	Minnesota	65.00
1	Mississippi	83.96
21	Missouri	72.81
6	Montana	80.33
28	Nebraska	71.75
35	Nevada	69.13
39	New Hampshire	65.00
39	New Jersey	65.00
4	New Mexico	82.01
39	New York	65.00
18	North Carolina	74.54
13	North Dakota	77.24
27	Ohio	71.78
10	Oklahoma	79.13
22	Oregon	72.78
37	Pennsylvania	67.69
36	Rhode Island	68.77
11	South Carolina	78.92
15	South Dakota	76.22
17	Tennessee	75.37
24	Texas	72.61
5	Utah	80.50
26	Vermont	72.08
39	Virginia	65.00
39	Washington	65.00
3	West Virginia	82.26
31	Wisconsin	70.82
32	Wyoming	70.53

RANK ORDER

RANK	STATE	RATE
1	Mississippi	83.96
2	Arkansas	82.33
3	West Virginia	82.26
4	New Mexico	82.01
5	Utah	80.50
6	Montana	80.33
7	Louisiana	79.73
8	Alabama	79.58
9	Idaho	79.43
10	Oklahoma	79.13
11	South Carolina	78.92
12	Kentucky	78.72
13	North Dakota	77.24
14	Arizona	77.22
15	South Dakota	76.22
16	Maine	75.42
17	Tennessee	75.37
18	North Carolina	74.54
19	Iowa	74.49
20	Indiana	73.95
21	Missouri	72.81
22	Oregon	72.78
23	Kansas	72.71
24	Texas	72.61
25	Georgia	72.31
26	Vermont	72.08
27	Ohio	71.78
28	Nebraska	71.75
29	Florida	71.23
30	Hawaii	70.93
31	Wisconsin	70.82
32	Wyoming	70.53
33	Alaska	70.31
34	Michigan	69.70
35	Nevada	69.13
36	Rhode Island	68.77
37	Pennsylvania	67.69
38	Delaware	65.27
39	California	65.00
39	Colorado	65.00
39	Connecticut	65.00
39	Illinois	65.00
39	Maryland	65.00
39	Massachusetts	65.00
39	Minnesota	65.00
39	New Hampshire	65.00
39	New Jersey	65.00
39	New York	65.00
39	Virginia	65.00
39	Washington	65.00
	District of Columbia	79.00

Source: U.S. Department of Health and Human Services, Centers for Medicare and Medicaid Services
"Enhanced Federal Medical Assistance Percentages" (http://aspe.os.dhhs.gov/health/fmap05.htm)
*For fiscal year 2005. These are "enhanced" matching rates established by the Children's Health Insurance
Program, signed into law in August 1997. Sixty-five percent is the minimum. National average is a simple average of
the 51 individual rates and is not weighted for population or funds.

Ryan White CARE Act Funding in 2002

National Total = $1,776,693,108*

ALPHA ORDER

RANK ORDER

RANK	STATE	FUNDING	% of USA		RANK	STATE	FUNDING	% of USA
22	Alabama	$18,231,999	1.0%		1	New York	$324,557,906	18.3%
42	Alaska	2,088,958	0.1%		2	California	256,736,116	14.5%
20	Arizona	20,092,282	1.1%		3	Florida	192,878,364	10.9%
32	Arkansas	5,960,095	0.3%		4	Texas	127,712,408	7.2%
2	California	256,736,116	14.5%		5	New Jersey	86,828,754	4.9%
23	Colorado	17,046,608	1.0%		6	Pennsylvania	72,371,827	4.1%
12	Connecticut	29,568,818	1.7%		7	Illinois	64,274,543	3.6%
33	Delaware	5,553,429	0.3%		8	Georgia	59,713,150	3.4%
3	Florida	192,878,364	10.9%		9	Maryland	51,049,588	2.9%
8	Georgia	59,713,150	3.4%		10	Massachusetts	48,845,635	2.7%
39	Hawaii	3,179,231	0.2%		11	Louisiana	34,763,202	2.0%
45	Idaho	1,661,432	0.1%		12	Connecticut	29,568,818	1.7%
7	Illinois	64,274,543	3.6%		13	Virginia	29,347,675	1.7%
26	Indiana	10,721,722	0.6%		14	Michigan	27,213,618	1.5%
38	Iowa	3,422,491	0.2%		15	North Carolina	25,416,151	1.4%
37	Kansas	3,827,934	0.2%		16	South Carolina	23,361,278	1.3%
28	Kentucky	9,374,329	0.5%		17	Missouri	22,735,983	1.3%
11	Louisiana	34,763,202	2.0%		18	Ohio	22,190,441	1.2%
43	Maine	1,985,769	0.1%		19	Washington	21,780,359	1.2%
9	Maryland	51,049,588	2.9%		20	Arizona	20,092,282	1.1%
10	Massachusetts	48,845,635	2.7%		21	Tennessee	19,417,971	1.1%
14	Michigan	27,213,618	1.5%		22	Alabama	18,231,999	1.0%
30	Minnesota	8,262,242	0.5%		23	Colorado	17,046,608	1.0%
24	Mississippi	12,504,167	0.7%		24	Mississippi	12,504,167	0.7%
17	Missouri	22,735,983	1.3%		25	Nevada	11,698,447	0.7%
46	Montana	1,373,270	0.1%		26	Indiana	10,721,722	0.6%
41	Nebraska	2,429,384	0.1%		27	Oregon	10,387,710	0.6%
25	Nevada	11,698,447	0.7%		28	Kentucky	9,374,329	0.5%
44	New Hampshire	1,868,740	0.1%		29	Oklahoma	8,523,718	0.5%
5	New Jersey	86,828,754	4.9%		30	Minnesota	8,262,242	0.5%
34	New Mexico	5,432,896	0.3%		31	Wisconsin	8,009,633	0.5%
1	New York	324,557,906	18.3%		32	Arkansas	5,960,095	0.3%
15	North Carolina	25,416,151	1.4%		33	Delaware	5,553,429	0.3%
50	North Dakota	288,717	0.0%		34	New Mexico	5,432,896	0.3%
18	Ohio	22,190,441	1.2%		35	Rhode Island	4,724,711	0.3%
29	Oklahoma	8,523,718	0.5%		36	Utah	3,893,056	0.2%
27	Oregon	10,387,710	0.6%		37	Kansas	3,827,934	0.2%
6	Pennsylvania	72,371,827	4.1%		38	Iowa	3,422,491	0.2%
35	Rhode Island	4,724,711	0.3%		39	Hawaii	3,179,231	0.2%
16	South Carolina	23,361,278	1.3%		40	West Virginia	2,683,120	0.2%
48	South Dakota	772,293	0.0%		41	Nebraska	2,429,384	0.1%
21	Tennessee	19,417,971	1.1%		42	Alaska	2,088,958	0.1%
4	Texas	127,712,408	7.2%		43	Maine	1,985,769	0.1%
36	Utah	3,893,056	0.2%		44	New Hampshire	1,868,740	0.1%
47	Vermont	1,306,601	0.1%		45	Idaho	1,661,432	0.1%
13	Virginia	29,347,675	1.7%		46	Montana	1,373,270	0.1%
19	Washington	21,780,359	1.2%		47	Vermont	1,306,601	0.1%
40	West Virginia	2,683,120	0.2%		48	South Dakota	772,293	0.0%
31	Wisconsin	8,009,633	0.5%		49	Wyoming	390,041	0.0%
49	Wyoming	390,041	0.0%		50	North Dakota	288,717	0.0%
						District of Columbia	48,234,296	2.7%

Source: U.S. Department of Health and Human Services, Health Resources and Services Admin., HIV/AIDS Bureau (http://hab.hrsa.gov)
*The Ryan White CARE Act was established in 1990 to provide health care and support services to medically underserved individuals and families affected by HIV/AIDS. It is named after Ryan White, an Indiana teenager who worked to educate the nation about AIDS-related discrimination. He died in 1990.

Per Capita Ryan White CARE Act Funding in 2002

National Per Capita = $6.17*

ALPHA ORDER

RANK	STATE	PER CAPITA
18	Alabama	$4.07
25	Alaska	3.26
22	Arizona	3.69
33	Arkansas	2.20
8	California	7.34
21	Colorado	3.79
5	Connecticut	8.55
10	Delaware	6.89
2	Florida	11.56
9	Georgia	6.99
30	Hawaii	2.58
46	Idaho	1.24
15	Illinois	5.11
36	Indiana	1.74
47	Iowa	1.17
44	Kansas	1.41
32	Kentucky	2.29
6	Louisiana	7.76
39	Maine	1.53
4	Maryland	9.38
7	Massachusetts	7.62
29	Michigan	2.71
38	Minnesota	1.64
17	Mississippi	4.36
20	Missouri	4.00
40	Montana	1.51
44	Nebraska	1.41
14	Nevada	5.40
43	New Hampshire	1.46
3	New Jersey	10.12
28	New Mexico	2.93
1	New York	16.95
26	North Carolina	3.06
50	North Dakota	0.46
35	Ohio	1.94
31	Oklahoma	2.44
27	Oregon	2.95
12	Pennsylvania	5.87
16	Rhode Island	4.42
13	South Carolina	5.69
48	South Dakota	1.02
24	Tennessee	3.35
11	Texas	5.88
37	Utah	1.68
34	Vermont	2.12
19	Virginia	4.03
23	Washington	3.59
41	West Virginia	1.49
42	Wisconsin	1.47
49	Wyoming	0.78

RANK ORDER

RANK	STATE	PER CAPITA
1	New York	$16.95
2	Florida	11.56
3	New Jersey	10.12
4	Maryland	9.38
5	Connecticut	8.55
6	Louisiana	7.76
7	Massachusetts	7.62
8	California	7.34
9	Georgia	6.99
10	Delaware	6.89
11	Texas	5.88
12	Pennsylvania	5.87
13	South Carolina	5.69
14	Nevada	5.40
15	Illinois	5.11
16	Rhode Island	4.42
17	Mississippi	4.36
18	Alabama	4.07
19	Virginia	4.03
20	Missouri	4.00
21	Colorado	3.79
22	Arizona	3.69
23	Washington	3.59
24	Tennessee	3.35
25	Alaska	3.26
26	North Carolina	3.06
27	Oregon	2.95
28	New Mexico	2.93
29	Michigan	2.71
30	Hawaii	2.58
31	Oklahoma	2.44
32	Kentucky	2.29
33	Arkansas	2.20
34	Vermont	2.12
35	Ohio	1.94
36	Indiana	1.74
37	Utah	1.68
38	Minnesota	1.64
39	Maine	1.53
40	Montana	1.51
41	West Virginia	1.49
42	Wisconsin	1.47
43	New Hampshire	1.46
44	Kansas	1.41
44	Nebraska	1.41
46	Idaho	1.24
47	Iowa	1.17
48	South Dakota	1.02
49	Wyoming	0.78
50	North Dakota	0.46
	District of Columbia	85.42

Source: Morgan Quitno Press using data from U.S. Department of Health and Human Services, Health Resources and Services Admin., HIV/AIDS Bureau (http://hab.hrsa.gov)
*The Ryan White CARE Act was established in 1990 to provide health care and support services to medically underserved individuals and families affected by HIV/AIDS. It is named after Ryan White, an Indiana teenager who worked to educate the nation about AIDS-related discrimination. He died in 1990.

State and Local Government Expenditures for Hospitals in 2002

National Total = $87,247,337,000*

ALPHA ORDER

RANK	STATE	EXPENDITURES	% of USA
7	Alabama	$3,099,637,000	3.6%
44	Alaska	96,212,000	0.1%
34	Arizona	469,395,000	0.5%
31	Arkansas	626,078,000	0.7%
1	California	11,147,510,000	12.8%
26	Colorado	1,080,688,000	1.2%
23	Connecticut	1,379,290,000	1.6%
47	Delaware	68,578,000	0.1%
4	Florida	4,306,698,000	4.9%
6	Georgia	3,498,875,000	4.0%
41	Hawaii	184,789,000	0.2%
37	Idaho	445,773,000	0.5%
12	Illinois	2,209,318,000	2.5%
13	Indiana	2,201,067,000	2.5%
21	Iowa	1,452,361,000	1.7%
32	Kansas	624,755,000	0.7%
29	Kentucky	717,087,000	0.8%
8	Louisiana	3,066,062,000	3.5%
42	Maine	116,256,000	0.1%
39	Maryland	400,821,000	0.5%
25	Massachusetts	1,178,524,000	1.4%
16	Michigan	2,069,991,000	2.4%
24	Minnesota	1,180,564,000	1.4%
18	Mississippi	1,865,839,000	2.1%
19	Missouri	1,730,692,000	2.0%
45	Montana	87,915,000	0.1%
35	Nebraska	468,136,000	0.5%
30	Nevada	665,836,000	0.8%
48	New Hampshire	45,807,000	0.1%
20	New Jersey	1,496,652,000	1.7%
36	New Mexico	460,797,000	0.5%
2	New York	9,189,139,000	10.5%
5	North Carolina	4,088,445,000	4.7%
49	North Dakota	44,424,000	0.1%
9	Ohio	2,373,885,000	2.7%
28	Oklahoma	834,967,000	1.0%
22	Oregon	1,424,243,000	1.6%
15	Pennsylvania	2,148,955,000	2.5%
43	Rhode Island	114,204,000	0.1%
10	South Carolina	2,364,115,000	2.7%
46	South Dakota	75,162,000	0.1%
11	Tennessee	2,261,897,000	2.6%
3	Texas	7,418,558,000	8.5%
33	Utah	529,725,000	0.6%
50	Vermont	9,485,000	0.0%
17	Virginia	2,048,955,000	2.3%
14	Washington	2,161,826,000	2.5%
40	West Virginia	285,092,000	0.3%
27	Wisconsin	851,907,000	1.0%
38	Wyoming	403,430,000	0.5%

RANK ORDER

RANK	STATE	EXPENDITURES	% of USA
1	California	$11,147,510,000	12.8%
2	New York	9,189,139,000	10.5%
3	Texas	7,418,558,000	8.5%
4	Florida	4,306,698,000	4.9%
5	North Carolina	4,088,445,000	4.7%
6	Georgia	3,498,875,000	4.0%
7	Alabama	3,099,637,000	3.6%
8	Louisiana	3,066,062,000	3.5%
9	Ohio	2,373,885,000	2.7%
10	South Carolina	2,364,115,000	2.7%
11	Tennessee	2,261,897,000	2.6%
12	Illinois	2,209,318,000	2.5%
13	Indiana	2,201,067,000	2.5%
14	Washington	2,161,826,000	2.5%
15	Pennsylvania	2,148,955,000	2.5%
16	Michigan	2,069,991,000	2.4%
17	Virginia	2,048,955,000	2.3%
18	Mississippi	1,865,839,000	2.1%
19	Missouri	1,730,692,000	2.0%
20	New Jersey	1,496,652,000	1.7%
21	Iowa	1,452,361,000	1.7%
22	Oregon	1,424,243,000	1.6%
23	Connecticut	1,379,290,000	1.6%
24	Minnesota	1,180,564,000	1.4%
25	Massachusetts	1,178,524,000	1.4%
26	Colorado	1,080,688,000	1.2%
27	Wisconsin	851,907,000	1.0%
28	Oklahoma	834,967,000	1.0%
29	Kentucky	717,087,000	0.8%
30	Nevada	665,836,000	0.8%
31	Arkansas	626,078,000	0.7%
32	Kansas	624,755,000	0.7%
33	Utah	529,725,000	0.6%
34	Arizona	469,395,000	0.5%
35	Nebraska	468,136,000	0.5%
36	New Mexico	460,797,000	0.5%
37	Idaho	445,773,000	0.5%
38	Wyoming	403,430,000	0.5%
39	Maryland	400,821,000	0.5%
40	West Virginia	285,092,000	0.3%
41	Hawaii	184,789,000	0.2%
42	Maine	116,256,000	0.1%
43	Rhode Island	114,204,000	0.1%
44	Alaska	96,212,000	0.1%
45	Montana	87,915,000	0.1%
46	South Dakota	75,162,000	0.1%
47	Delaware	68,578,000	0.1%
48	New Hampshire	45,807,000	0.1%
49	North Dakota	44,424,000	0.1%
50	Vermont	9,485,000	0.0%
	District of Columbia	176,920,000	0.2%

Source: U.S. Bureau of the Census, Governments Division
   "State and Local Government Finances: 2002 Census" (http://www.census.gov/govs/www/estimate02.html)
*Financing, construction, acquisition, maintenance or operation of hospital facilities, provision of hospital care and support of public or private hospitals.

Per Capita State and Local Government Expenditures for Hospitals in 2002

National Per Capita = $303*

ALPHA ORDER

RANK	STATE	PER CAPITA
2	Alabama	$692
39	Alaska	150
45	Arizona	86
27	Arkansas	231
17	California	319
24	Colorado	240
11	Connecticut	399
46	Delaware	85
22	Florida	258
9	Georgia	410
39	Hawaii	150
16	Idaho	332
33	Illinois	176
13	Indiana	357
6	Iowa	495
28	Kansas	230
34	Kentucky	175
3	Louisiana	685
44	Maine	90
47	Maryland	74
32	Massachusetts	184
31	Michigan	206
26	Minnesota	235
4	Mississippi	651
19	Missouri	305
43	Montana	97
21	Nebraska	271
18	Nevada	307
49	New Hampshire	36
35	New Jersey	174
23	New Mexico	248
8	New York	480
7	North Carolina	492
48	North Dakota	70
30	Ohio	208
25	Oklahoma	239
10	Oregon	404
35	Pennsylvania	174
41	Rhode Island	107
5	South Carolina	576
42	South Dakota	99
12	Tennessee	391
15	Texas	342
29	Utah	228
50	Vermont	15
20	Virginia	282
14	Washington	356
37	West Virginia	158
38	Wisconsin	157
1	Wyoming	808

RANK ORDER

RANK	STATE	PER CAPITA
1	Wyoming	$808
2	Alabama	692
3	Louisiana	685
4	Mississippi	651
5	South Carolina	576
6	Iowa	495
7	North Carolina	492
8	New York	480
9	Georgia	410
10	Oregon	404
11	Connecticut	399
12	Tennessee	391
13	Indiana	357
14	Washington	356
15	Texas	342
16	Idaho	332
17	California	319
18	Nevada	307
19	Missouri	305
20	Virginia	282
21	Nebraska	271
22	Florida	258
23	New Mexico	248
24	Colorado	240
25	Oklahoma	239
26	Minnesota	235
27	Arkansas	231
28	Kansas	230
29	Utah	228
30	Ohio	208
31	Michigan	206
32	Massachusetts	184
33	Illinois	176
34	Kentucky	175
35	New Jersey	174
35	Pennsylvania	174
37	West Virginia	158
38	Wisconsin	157
39	Alaska	150
39	Hawaii	150
41	Rhode Island	107
42	South Dakota	99
43	Montana	97
44	Maine	90
45	Arizona	86
46	Delaware	85
47	Maryland	74
48	North Dakota	70
49	New Hampshire	36
50	Vermont	15

District of Columbia 313

Source: Morgan Quitno Press using data from U.S. Bureau of the Census, Governments Division
"State and Local Government Finances: 2002 Census" (http://www.census.gov/govs/www/estimate02.html)
*Financing, construction, acquisition, maintenance or operation of hospital facilities, provision of hospital care and support of public or private hospitals.

Percent of State and Local Government Expenditures
Used for Hospitals in 2002
National Percent = 5.0%*

RANK	STATE	PERCENT
1	Alabama	12.6
47	Alaska	1.1
40	Arizona	1.9
21	Arkansas	4.8
23	California	4.7
27	Colorado	4.0
15	Connecticut	5.7
45	Delaware	1.3
20	Florida	4.9
8	Georgia	7.8
39	Hawaii	2.2
11	Idaho	6.6
33	Illinois	3.0
10	Indiana	6.7
7	Iowa	8.5
25	Kansas	4.2
32	Kentucky	3.3
1	Louisiana	12.6
44	Maine	1.5
45	Maryland	1.3
36	Massachusetts	2.8
30	Michigan	3.4
30	Minnesota	3.4
3	Mississippi	12.1
14	Missouri	6.0
42	Montana	1.7
21	Nebraska	4.8
15	Nevada	5.7
49	New Hampshire	0.7
36	New Jersey	2.8
27	New Mexico	4.0
15	New York	5.7
6	North Carolina	9.2
47	North Dakota	1.1
29	Ohio	3.5
24	Oklahoma	4.6
13	Oregon	6.2
34	Pennsylvania	2.9
42	Rhode Island	1.7
5	South Carolina	9.9
40	South Dakota	1.9
8	Tennessee	7.8
11	Texas	6.6
26	Utah	4.1
50	Vermont	0.2
19	Virginia	5.2
18	Washington	5.6
34	West Virginia	2.9
38	Wisconsin	2.5
4	Wyoming	10.5

RANK	STATE	PERCENT
1	Alabama	12.6
1	Louisiana	12.6
3	Mississippi	12.1
4	Wyoming	10.5
5	South Carolina	9.9
6	North Carolina	9.2
7	Iowa	8.5
8	Georgia	7.8
8	Tennessee	7.8
10	Indiana	6.7
11	Idaho	6.6
11	Texas	6.6
13	Oregon	6.2
14	Missouri	6.0
15	Connecticut	5.7
15	Nevada	5.7
15	New York	5.7
18	Washington	5.6
19	Virginia	5.2
20	Florida	4.9
21	Arkansas	4.8
21	Nebraska	4.8
23	California	4.7
24	Oklahoma	4.6
25	Kansas	4.2
26	Utah	4.1
27	Colorado	4.0
27	New Mexico	4.0
29	Ohio	3.5
30	Michigan	3.4
30	Minnesota	3.4
32	Kentucky	3.3
33	Illinois	3.0
34	Pennsylvania	2.9
34	West Virginia	2.9
36	Massachusetts	2.8
36	New Jersey	2.8
38	Wisconsin	2.5
39	Hawaii	2.2
40	Arizona	1.9
40	South Dakota	1.9
42	Montana	1.7
42	Rhode Island	1.7
44	Maine	1.5
45	Delaware	1.3
45	Maryland	1.3
47	Alaska	1.1
47	North Dakota	1.1
49	New Hampshire	0.7
50	Vermont	0.2

District of Columbia	2.9

Source: Morgan Quitno Press using data from U.S. Bureau of the Census, Governments Division
"State and Local Government Finances: 2002 Census" (http://www.census.gov/govs/www/estimate02.html)
As a percent of direct general expenditures. Financing, construction, acquisition, maintenance or operation of hospital facilities, provision of hospital care and support of public or private hospitals.

State and Local Government Expenditures for Health Programs in 2002

National Total = $59,132,241,000*

ALPHA ORDER

RANK	STATE	EXPENDITURES	% of USA
18	Alabama	$982,547,000	1.7%
43	Alaska	166,727,000	0.3%
23	Arizona	739,853,000	1.3%
37	Arkansas	289,169,000	0.5%
1	California	9,813,693,000	16.6%
19	Colorado	959,754,000	1.6%
29	Connecticut	523,784,000	0.9%
39	Delaware	258,062,000	0.4%
4	Florida	3,184,348,000	5.4%
12	Georgia	1,333,214,000	2.3%
31	Hawaii	466,935,000	0.8%
44	Idaho	159,685,000	0.3%
7	Illinois	2,989,614,000	5.1%
26	Indiana	675,081,000	1.1%
32	Iowa	433,367,000	0.7%
27	Kansas	606,145,000	1.0%
24	Kentucky	728,385,000	1.2%
28	Louisiana	555,215,000	0.9%
33	Maine	383,724,000	0.6%
16	Maryland	1,089,312,000	1.8%
10	Massachusetts	1,995,701,000	3.4%
3	Michigan	3,276,613,000	5.5%
20	Minnesota	784,524,000	1.3%
38	Mississippi	274,402,000	0.5%
25	Missouri	702,516,000	1.2%
36	Montana	290,174,000	0.5%
45	Nebraska	138,569,000	0.2%
40	Nevada	256,822,000	0.4%
46	New Hampshire	137,748,000	0.2%
13	New Jersey	1,239,632,000	2.1%
34	New Mexico	368,268,000	0.6%
2	New York	3,819,062,000	6.5%
9	North Carolina	1,998,981,000	3.4%
50	North Dakota	59,264,000	0.1%
5	Ohio	3,079,714,000	5.2%
30	Oklahoma	470,344,000	0.8%
22	Oregon	769,376,000	1.3%
6	Pennsylvania	3,003,948,000	5.1%
42	Rhode Island	184,603,000	0.3%
21	South Carolina	779,193,000	1.3%
48	South Dakota	95,543,000	0.2%
17	Tennessee	1,038,348,000	1.8%
8	Texas	2,685,724,000	4.5%
35	Utah	328,753,000	0.6%
49	Vermont	78,036,000	0.1%
15	Virginia	1,134,990,000	1.9%
11	Washington	1,851,162,000	3.1%
41	West Virginia	231,148,000	0.4%
14	Wisconsin	1,229,637,000	2.1%
47	Wyoming	112,886,000	0.2%

RANK ORDER

RANK	STATE	EXPENDITURES	% of USA
1	California	$9,813,693,000	16.6%
2	New York	3,819,062,000	6.5%
3	Michigan	3,276,613,000	5.5%
4	Florida	3,184,348,000	5.4%
5	Ohio	3,079,714,000	5.2%
6	Pennsylvania	3,003,948,000	5.1%
7	Illinois	2,989,614,000	5.1%
8	Texas	2,685,724,000	4.5%
9	North Carolina	1,998,981,000	3.4%
10	Massachusetts	1,995,701,000	3.4%
11	Washington	1,851,162,000	3.1%
12	Georgia	1,333,214,000	2.3%
13	New Jersey	1,239,632,000	2.1%
14	Wisconsin	1,229,637,000	2.1%
15	Virginia	1,134,990,000	1.9%
16	Maryland	1,089,312,000	1.8%
17	Tennessee	1,038,348,000	1.8%
18	Alabama	982,547,000	1.7%
19	Colorado	959,754,000	1.6%
20	Minnesota	784,524,000	1.3%
21	South Carolina	779,193,000	1.3%
22	Oregon	769,376,000	1.3%
23	Arizona	739,853,000	1.3%
24	Kentucky	728,385,000	1.2%
25	Missouri	702,516,000	1.2%
26	Indiana	675,081,000	1.1%
27	Kansas	606,145,000	1.0%
28	Louisiana	555,215,000	0.9%
29	Connecticut	523,784,000	0.9%
30	Oklahoma	470,344,000	0.8%
31	Hawaii	466,935,000	0.8%
32	Iowa	433,367,000	0.7%
33	Maine	383,724,000	0.6%
34	New Mexico	368,268,000	0.6%
35	Utah	328,753,000	0.6%
36	Montana	290,174,000	0.5%
37	Arkansas	289,169,000	0.5%
38	Mississippi	274,402,000	0.5%
39	Delaware	258,062,000	0.4%
40	Nevada	256,822,000	0.4%
41	West Virginia	231,148,000	0.4%
42	Rhode Island	184,603,000	0.3%
43	Alaska	166,727,000	0.3%
44	Idaho	159,685,000	0.3%
45	Nebraska	138,569,000	0.2%
46	New Hampshire	137,748,000	0.2%
47	Wyoming	112,886,000	0.2%
48	South Dakota	95,543,000	0.2%
49	Vermont	78,036,000	0.1%
50	North Dakota	59,264,000	0.1%
	District of Columbia	377,946,000	0.6%

Source: U.S. Bureau of the Census, Governments Division
   "State and Local Government Finances: 2002 Census" (http://www.census.gov/govs/www/estimate02.html)
*Includes outpatient health services other than hospital care, research and education, categorical health programs,
treatment and immunization clinics, nursing and environmental health activities. Includes capital expenditures.

Per Capita State and Local Government Expenditures for Health Programs in 2002
National Per Capita = $205*

ALPHA ORDER

RANK	STATE	PER CAPITA
17	Alabama	$219
10	Alaska	260
35	Arizona	136
47	Arkansas	107
8	California	280
19	Colorado	213
31	Connecticut	151
3	Delaware	320
23	Florida	191
28	Georgia	156
1	Hawaii	378
43	Idaho	119
13	Illinois	238
45	Indiana	110
32	Iowa	148
16	Kansas	223
26	Kentucky	178
40	Louisiana	124
7	Maine	296
20	Maryland	200
5	Massachusetts	311
2	Michigan	326
28	Minnesota	156
48	Mississippi	96
40	Missouri	124
4	Montana	319
50	Nebraska	80
44	Nevada	118
46	New Hampshire	108
33	New Jersey	145
21	New Mexico	199
21	New York	199
12	North Carolina	240
49	North Dakota	94
9	Ohio	270
36	Oklahoma	135
18	Oregon	218
11	Pennsylvania	244
27	Rhode Island	173
24	South Carolina	190
39	South Dakota	126
25	Tennessee	179
40	Texas	124
34	Utah	142
38	Vermont	127
28	Virginia	156
6	Washington	305
37	West Virginia	128
14	Wisconsin	226
14	Wyoming	226

RANK ORDER

RANK	STATE	PER CAPITA
1	Hawaii	$378
2	Michigan	326
3	Delaware	320
4	Montana	319
5	Massachusetts	311
6	Washington	305
7	Maine	296
8	California	280
9	Ohio	270
10	Alaska	260
11	Pennsylvania	244
12	North Carolina	240
13	Illinois	238
14	Wisconsin	226
14	Wyoming	226
16	Kansas	223
17	Alabama	219
18	Oregon	218
19	Colorado	213
20	Maryland	200
21	New Mexico	199
21	New York	199
23	Florida	191
24	South Carolina	190
25	Tennessee	179
26	Kentucky	178
27	Rhode Island	173
28	Georgia	156
28	Minnesota	156
28	Virginia	156
31	Connecticut	151
32	Iowa	148
33	New Jersey	145
34	Utah	142
35	Arizona	136
36	Oklahoma	135
37	West Virginia	128
38	Vermont	127
39	South Dakota	126
40	Louisiana	124
40	Missouri	124
40	Texas	124
43	Idaho	119
44	Nevada	118
45	Indiana	110
46	New Hampshire	108
47	Arkansas	107
48	Mississippi	96
49	North Dakota	94
50	Nebraska	80

District of Columbia   669

Source: Morgan Quitno Press using data from U.S. Bureau of the Census, Governments Division
"State and Local Government Finances: 2002 Census" (http://www.census.gov/govs/www/estimate02.html)
*Includes outpatient health services other than hospital care, research and education, categorical health programs, treatment and immunization clinics, nursing and environmental health activities. Includes capital expenditures.

Percent of State and Local Government Expenditures
Used for Health Programs in 2002
National Percent = 3.4%*

ALPHA ORDER

RANK	STATE	PERCENT
13	Alabama	4.0
47	Alaska	2.0
25	Arizona	2.9
40	Arkansas	2.2
10	California	4.2
18	Colorado	3.5
40	Connecticut	2.2
4	Delaware	4.8
15	Florida	3.7
24	Georgia	3.0
2	Hawaii	5.6
36	Idaho	2.3
13	Illinois	4.0
45	Indiana	2.1
31	Iowa	2.5
11	Kansas	4.1
19	Kentucky	3.4
36	Louisiana	2.3
4	Maine	4.8
19	Maryland	3.4
7	Massachusetts	4.7
3	Michigan	5.4
40	Minnesota	2.2
48	Mississippi	1.8
33	Missouri	2.4
1	Montana	5.7
50	Nebraska	1.4
40	Nevada	2.2
40	New Hampshire	2.2
36	New Jersey	2.3
23	New Mexico	3.2
33	New York	2.4
9	North Carolina	4.5
49	North Dakota	1.5
8	Ohio	4.6
29	Oklahoma	2.6
21	Oregon	3.3
11	Pennsylvania	4.1
28	Rhode Island	2.7
21	South Carolina	3.3
31	South Dakota	2.5
16	Tennessee	3.6
33	Texas	2.4
29	Utah	2.6
45	Vermont	2.1
25	Virginia	2.9
4	Washington	4.8
36	West Virginia	2.3
16	Wisconsin	3.6
25	Wyoming	2.9

RANK ORDER

RANK	STATE	PERCENT
1	Montana	5.7
2	Hawaii	5.6
3	Michigan	5.4
4	Delaware	4.8
4	Maine	4.8
4	Washington	4.8
7	Massachusetts	4.7
8	Ohio	4.6
9	North Carolina	4.5
10	California	4.2
11	Kansas	4.1
11	Pennsylvania	4.1
13	Alabama	4.0
13	Illinois	4.0
15	Florida	3.7
16	Tennessee	3.6
16	Wisconsin	3.6
18	Colorado	3.5
19	Kentucky	3.4
19	Maryland	3.4
21	Oregon	3.3
21	South Carolina	3.3
23	New Mexico	3.2
24	Georgia	3.0
25	Arizona	2.9
25	Virginia	2.9
25	Wyoming	2.9
28	Rhode Island	2.7
29	Oklahoma	2.6
29	Utah	2.6
31	Iowa	2.5
31	South Dakota	2.5
33	Missouri	2.4
33	New York	2.4
33	Texas	2.4
36	Idaho	2.3
36	Louisiana	2.3
36	New Jersey	2.3
36	West Virginia	2.3
40	Arkansas	2.2
40	Connecticut	2.2
40	Minnesota	2.2
40	Nevada	2.2
40	New Hampshire	2.2
45	Indiana	2.1
45	Vermont	2.1
47	Alaska	2.0
48	Mississippi	1.8
49	North Dakota	1.5
50	Nebraska	1.4

District of Columbia 6.1

Source: Morgan Quitno Press using data from U.S. Bureau of the Census, Governments Division
   "State and Local Government Finances: 2002 Census" (http://www.census.gov/govs/www/estimate02.html)
*As a percent of direct general expenditures. Includes outpatient health services other than hospital care, research
and education, categorical health programs, treatment and immunization clinics, nursing and environmental health
activities. Includes capital expenditures.

Estimated Tobacco Settlement Revenues in FY 2005

National Total = $7,055,000,000*

ALPHA ORDER

RANK	STATE	REVENUE	% of USA
25	Alabama	$96,100,000	1.4%
49	Alaska	20,300,000	0.3%
26	Arizona	87,600,000	1.2%
34	Arkansas	49,200,000	0.7%
1	California	759,000,000	10.8%
27	Colorado	81,500,000	1.2%
23	Connecticut	110,400,000	1.6%
45	Delaware	23,500,000	0.3%
4	Florida	380,300,000	5.4%
12	Georgia	146,000,000	2.1%
39	Hawaii	35,800,000	0.5%
47	Idaho	21,600,000	0.3%
7	Illinois	276,800,000	3.9%
21	Indiana	121,300,000	1.7%
32	Iowa	51,700,000	0.7%
33	Kansas	49,600,000	0.7%
24	Kentucky	104,700,000	1.5%
17	Louisiana	134,100,000	1.9%
35	Maine	45,800,000	0.6%
16	Maryland	134,400,000	1.9%
9	Massachusetts	240,200,000	3.4%
8	Michigan	258,800,000	3.7%
11	Minnesota	179,600,000	2.5%
22	Mississippi	117,500,000	1.7%
15	Missouri	135,300,000	1.9%
43	Montana	25,300,000	0.4%
41	Nebraska	35,400,000	0.5%
38	Nevada	36,300,000	0.5%
37	New Hampshire	39,600,000	0.6%
10	New Jersey	230,000,000	3.3%
40	New Mexico	35,500,000	0.5%
2	New York	758,900,000	10.8%
14	North Carolina	138,700,000	2.0%
46	North Dakota	21,800,000	0.3%
6	Ohio	299,600,000	4.2%
30	Oklahoma	61,600,000	0.9%
29	Oregon	68,200,000	1.0%
5	Pennsylvania	341,800,000	4.8%
36	Rhode Island	42,800,000	0.6%
28	South Carolina	70,000,000	1.0%
48	South Dakota	20,800,000	0.3%
13	Tennessee	145,200,000	2.1%
3	Texas	501,300,000	7.1%
42	Utah	26,500,000	0.4%
44	Vermont	24,500,000	0.3%
20	Virginia	121,600,000	1.7%
19	Washington	122,100,000	1.7%
31	West Virginia	52,700,000	0.7%
18	Wisconsin	123,200,000	1.7%
50	Wyoming	14,800,000	0.2%

RANK ORDER

RANK	STATE	REVENUE	% of USA
1	California	$759,000,000	10.8%
2	New York	758,900,000	10.8%
3	Texas	501,300,000	7.1%
4	Florida	380,300,000	5.4%
5	Pennsylvania	341,800,000	4.8%
6	Ohio	299,600,000	4.2%
7	Illinois	276,800,000	3.9%
8	Michigan	258,800,000	3.7%
9	Massachusetts	240,200,000	3.4%
10	New Jersey	230,000,000	3.3%
11	Minnesota	179,600,000	2.5%
12	Georgia	146,000,000	2.1%
13	Tennessee	145,200,000	2.1%
14	North Carolina	138,700,000	2.0%
15	Missouri	135,300,000	1.9%
16	Maryland	134,400,000	1.9%
17	Louisiana	134,100,000	1.9%
18	Wisconsin	123,200,000	1.7%
19	Washington	122,100,000	1.7%
20	Virginia	121,600,000	1.7%
21	Indiana	121,300,000	1.7%
22	Mississippi	117,500,000	1.7%
23	Connecticut	110,400,000	1.6%
24	Kentucky	104,700,000	1.5%
25	Alabama	96,100,000	1.4%
26	Arizona	87,600,000	1.2%
27	Colorado	81,500,000	1.2%
28	South Carolina	70,000,000	1.0%
29	Oregon	68,200,000	1.0%
30	Oklahoma	61,600,000	0.9%
31	West Virginia	52,700,000	0.7%
32	Iowa	51,700,000	0.7%
33	Kansas	49,600,000	0.7%
34	Arkansas	49,200,000	0.7%
35	Maine	45,800,000	0.6%
36	Rhode Island	42,800,000	0.6%
37	New Hampshire	39,600,000	0.6%
38	Nevada	36,300,000	0.5%
39	Hawaii	35,800,000	0.5%
40	New Mexico	35,500,000	0.5%
41	Nebraska	35,400,000	0.5%
42	Utah	26,500,000	0.4%
43	Montana	25,300,000	0.4%
44	Vermont	24,500,000	0.3%
45	Delaware	23,500,000	0.3%
46	North Dakota	21,800,000	0.3%
47	Idaho	21,600,000	0.3%
48	South Dakota	20,800,000	0.3%
49	Alaska	20,300,000	0.3%
50	Wyoming	14,800,000	0.2%
	District of Columbia	36,100,000	0.5%

Source: Campaign for Tobacco-Free Kids
    "A Broken Promise to Our Children" (http://tobaccofreekids.org/reports/settlements/)
*For fiscal year 2005. Settlement originally reached in November 1998 and called for an estimated 25 years of payments.

Personal Health Care Expenditures in 1998

National Total = $1,016,129,000,000*

ALPHA ORDER

RANK	STATE	EXPENDITURES	% of USA
22	Alabama	$15,611,000,000	1.5%
48	Alaska	2,085,000,000	0.2%
24	Arizona	15,010,000,000	1.5%
33	Arkansas	8,532,000,000	0.8%
1	California	112,848,000,000	11.1%
26	Colorado	13,552,000,000	1.3%
23	Connecticut	15,336,000,000	1.5%
44	Delaware	3,070,000,000	0.3%
4	Florida	60,306,000,000	5.9%
11	Georgia	27,213,000,000	2.7%
41	Hawaii	4,579,000,000	0.5%
43	Idaho	3,419,000,000	0.3%
6	Illinois	44,170,000,000	4.3%
15	Indiana	21,221,000,000	2.1%
30	Iowa	10,192,000,000	1.0%
31	Kansas	9,309,000,000	0.9%
25	Kentucky	14,471,000,000	1.4%
21	Louisiana	16,434,000,000	1.6%
39	Maine	4,895,000,000	0.5%
19	Maryland	19,507,000,000	1.9%
10	Massachusetts	30,198,000,000	3.0%
8	Michigan	35,256,000,000	3.5%
17	Minnesota	19,989,000,000	2.0%
32	Mississippi	9,034,000,000	0.9%
16	Missouri	21,150,000,000	2.1%
45	Montana	2,855,000,000	0.3%
35	Nebraska	6,109,000,000	0.6%
37	Nevada	5,581,000,000	0.5%
40	New Hampshire	4,610,000,000	0.5%
9	New Jersey	32,772,000,000	3.2%
38	New Mexico	5,364,000,000	0.5%
2	New York	85,156,000,000	8.4%
12	North Carolina	26,853,000,000	2.6%
47	North Dakota	2,669,000,000	0.3%
7	Ohio	41,798,000,000	4.1%
29	Oklahoma	10,897,000,000	1.1%
28	Oregon	10,950,000,000	1.1%
5	Pennsylvania	50,760,000,000	5.0%
42	Rhode Island	4,400,000,000	0.4%
27	South Carolina	13,006,000,000	1.3%
46	South Dakota	2,774,000,000	0.3%
14	Tennessee	21,798,000,000	2.1%
3	Texas	68,385,000,000	6.7%
36	Utah	5,933,000,000	0.6%
49	Vermont	2,052,000,000	0.2%
13	Virginia	22,158,000,000	2.2%
20	Washington	19,331,000,000	1.9%
34	West Virginia	7,015,000,000	0.7%
18	Wisconsin	19,806,000,000	1.9%
50	Wyoming	1,398,000,000	0.1%

RANK ORDER

RANK	STATE	EXPENDITURES	% of USA
1	California	$112,848,000,000	11.1%
2	New York	85,156,000,000	8.4%
3	Texas	68,385,000,000	6.7%
4	Florida	60,306,000,000	5.9%
5	Pennsylvania	50,760,000,000	5.0%
6	Illinois	44,170,000,000	4.3%
7	Ohio	41,798,000,000	4.1%
8	Michigan	35,256,000,000	3.5%
9	New Jersey	32,772,000,000	3.2%
10	Massachusetts	30,198,000,000	3.0%
11	Georgia	27,213,000,000	2.7%
12	North Carolina	26,853,000,000	2.6%
13	Virginia	22,158,000,000	2.2%
14	Tennessee	21,798,000,000	2.1%
15	Indiana	21,221,000,000	2.1%
16	Missouri	21,150,000,000	2.1%
17	Minnesota	19,989,000,000	2.0%
18	Wisconsin	19,806,000,000	1.9%
19	Maryland	19,507,000,000	1.9%
20	Washington	19,331,000,000	1.9%
21	Louisiana	16,434,000,000	1.6%
22	Alabama	15,611,000,000	1.5%
23	Connecticut	15,336,000,000	1.5%
24	Arizona	15,010,000,000	1.5%
25	Kentucky	14,471,000,000	1.4%
26	Colorado	13,552,000,000	1.3%
27	South Carolina	13,006,000,000	1.3%
28	Oregon	10,950,000,000	1.1%
29	Oklahoma	10,897,000,000	1.1%
30	Iowa	10,192,000,000	1.0%
31	Kansas	9,309,000,000	0.9%
32	Mississippi	9,034,000,000	0.9%
33	Arkansas	8,532,000,000	0.8%
34	West Virginia	7,015,000,000	0.7%
35	Nebraska	6,109,000,000	0.6%
36	Utah	5,933,000,000	0.6%
37	Nevada	5,581,000,000	0.5%
38	New Mexico	5,364,000,000	0.5%
39	Maine	4,895,000,000	0.5%
40	New Hampshire	4,610,000,000	0.5%
41	Hawaii	4,579,000,000	0.5%
42	Rhode Island	4,400,000,000	0.4%
43	Idaho	3,419,000,000	0.3%
44	Delaware	3,070,000,000	0.3%
45	Montana	2,855,000,000	0.3%
46	South Dakota	2,774,000,000	0.3%
47	North Dakota	2,669,000,000	0.3%
48	Alaska	2,085,000,000	0.2%
49	Vermont	2,052,000,000	0.2%
50	Wyoming	1,398,000,000	0.1%
	District of Columbia	4,312,000,000	0.4%

Source: U.S. Department of Health and Human Services, Centers for Medicare and Medicaid Services
"State Health Care Expenditures" (http://www.cms.hhs.gov/statistics/nhe/)
*By state of provider. Includes hospital care, physician services, dental services, home health care, drugs, vision products, nursing home care and other personal health care services and products. Revised figures.

Health Care Expenditures as a Percent of Gross State Product in 1998

National Percent = 11.6% of Total Gross State Product*

ALPHA ORDER

RANK	STATE	PERCENT
8	Alabama	14.2
49	Alaska	8.5
32	Arizona	11.3
9	Arkansas	13.9
43	California	10.0
45	Colorado	9.7
36	Connecticut	10.7
47	Delaware	9.4
5	Florida	14.5
36	Georgia	10.7
30	Hawaii	11.6
35	Idaho	11.0
40	Illinois	10.4
25	Indiana	12.0
21	Iowa	12.3
23	Kansas	12.1
12	Kentucky	13.4
12	Louisiana	13.4
3	Maine	15.2
27	Maryland	11.9
20	Massachusetts	12.5
25	Michigan	12.0
21	Minnesota	12.3
4	Mississippi	14.6
16	Missouri	12.9
6	Montana	14.3
27	Nebraska	11.9
48	Nevada	8.7
31	New Hampshire	11.4
41	New Jersey	10.3
33	New Mexico	11.1
29	New York	11.8
33	North Carolina	11.1
2	North Dakota	15.7
23	Ohio	12.1
15	Oklahoma	13.3
39	Oregon	10.6
9	Pennsylvania	13.9
6	Rhode Island	14.3
17	South Carolina	12.8
11	South Dakota	13.5
12	Tennessee	13.4
36	Texas	10.7
43	Utah	10.0
18	Vermont	12.6
45	Virginia	9.7
42	Washington	10.1
1	West Virginia	18.0
18	Wisconsin	12.6
49	Wyoming	8.5

RANK ORDER

RANK	STATE	PERCENT
1	West Virginia	18.0
2	North Dakota	15.7
3	Maine	15.2
4	Mississippi	14.6
5	Florida	14.5
6	Montana	14.3
6	Rhode Island	14.3
8	Alabama	14.2
9	Arkansas	13.9
9	Pennsylvania	13.9
11	South Dakota	13.5
12	Kentucky	13.4
12	Louisiana	13.4
12	Tennessee	13.4
15	Oklahoma	13.3
16	Missouri	12.9
17	South Carolina	12.8
18	Vermont	12.6
18	Wisconsin	12.6
20	Massachusetts	12.5
21	Iowa	12.3
21	Minnesota	12.3
23	Kansas	12.1
23	Ohio	12.1
25	Indiana	12.0
25	Michigan	12.0
27	Maryland	11.9
27	Nebraska	11.9
29	New York	11.8
30	Hawaii	11.6
31	New Hampshire	11.4
32	Arizona	11.3
33	New Mexico	11.1
33	North Carolina	11.1
35	Idaho	11.0
36	Connecticut	10.7
36	Georgia	10.7
36	Texas	10.7
39	Oregon	10.6
40	Illinois	10.4
41	New Jersey	10.3
42	Washington	10.1
43	California	10.0
43	Utah	10.0
45	Colorado	9.7
45	Virginia	9.7
47	Delaware	9.4
48	Nevada	8.7
49	Alaska	8.5
49	Wyoming	8.5
	District of Columbia	8.3

Source: MQ Press using data from U.S. Dept of Health & Human Services, Centers for Medicare and Medicaid Services "State Health Care Expenditures" (http://www.cms.hhs.gov/statistics/nhe/)
*By state of provider. Includes hospital care, physician services, dental services, home health care, drugs, vision products, nursing home care and other personal health care services and products. Revised figures.

Per Capita Personal Health Care Expenditures in 1998

National Per Capita = $3,760*

ALPHA ORDER

RANK	STATE	PER CAPITA
27	Alabama	$3,588
37	Alaska	3,389
45	Arizona	3,216
39	Arkansas	3,361
34	California	3,453
35	Colorado	3,414
3	Connecticut	4,686
8	Delaware	4,126
10	Florida	4,045
28	Georgia	3,564
16	Hawaii	3,846
50	Idaho	2,778
24	Illinois	3,660
25	Indiana	3,592
29	Iowa	3,562
31	Kansas	3,528
22	Kentucky	3,678
20	Louisiana	3,767
12	Maine	3,924
17	Maryland	3,802
1	Massachusetts	4,915
26	Michigan	3,590
5	Minnesota	4,229
41	Mississippi	3,283
13	Missouri	3,890
44	Montana	3,246
22	Nebraska	3,678
46	Nevada	3,201
14	New Hampshire	3,888
9	New Jersey	4,048
47	New Mexico	3,094
2	New York	4,689
30	North Carolina	3,559
7	North Dakota	4,185
21	Ohio	3,719
43	Oklahoma	3,263
40	Oregon	3,336
5	Pennsylvania	4,229
4	Rhode Island	4,455
38	South Carolina	3,387
18	South Dakota	3,796
11	Tennessee	4,012
33	Texas	3,469
49	Utah	2,824
32	Vermont	3,475
42	Virginia	3,264
36	Washington	3,399
15	West Virginia	3,872
19	Wisconsin	3,793
48	Wyoming	2,912

RANK ORDER

RANK	STATE	PER CAPITA
1	Massachusetts	$4,915
2	New York	4,689
3	Connecticut	4,686
4	Rhode Island	4,455
5	Minnesota	4,229
5	Pennsylvania	4,229
7	North Dakota	4,185
8	Delaware	4,126
9	New Jersey	4,048
10	Florida	4,045
11	Tennessee	4,012
12	Maine	3,924
13	Missouri	3,890
14	New Hampshire	3,888
15	West Virginia	3,872
16	Hawaii	3,846
17	Maryland	3,802
18	South Dakota	3,796
19	Wisconsin	3,793
20	Louisiana	3,767
21	Ohio	3,719
22	Kentucky	3,678
22	Nebraska	3,678
24	Illinois	3,660
25	Indiana	3,592
26	Michigan	3,590
27	Alabama	3,588
28	Georgia	3,564
29	Iowa	3,562
30	North Carolina	3,559
31	Kansas	3,528
32	Vermont	3,475
33	Texas	3,469
34	California	3,453
35	Colorado	3,414
36	Washington	3,399
37	Alaska	3,389
38	South Carolina	3,387
39	Arkansas	3,361
40	Oregon	3,336
41	Mississippi	3,283
42	Virginia	3,264
43	Oklahoma	3,263
44	Montana	3,246
45	Arizona	3,216
46	Nevada	3,201
47	New Mexico	3,094
48	Wyoming	2,912
49	Utah	2,824
50	Idaho	2,778

| | District of Columbia | 8,270 |

Source: MQ Press using data from U.S. Dept of Health & Human Services, Centers for Medicare and Medicaid Services
"State Health Care Expenditures" (http://www.cms.hhs.gov/statistics/nhe/)
*By state of provider. Per capita calculated using resident population. These figures may be skewed due to residents crossing state borders for care. Includes hospital care, physician services, dental services, home health care, drugs, vision products, nursing home care and other personal health care services and products. Revised figures

Expenditures for Hospital Care in 1998

National Total = $379,834,000,000*

ALPHA ORDER

RANK	STATE	EXPENDITURES	% of USA
22	Alabama	$6,169,000,000	1.6%
48	Alaska	909,000,000	0.2%
25	Arizona	5,199,000,000	1.4%
33	Arkansas	3,394,000,000	0.9%
1	California	37,717,000,000	9.9%
27	Colorado	4,729,000,000	1.2%
26	Connecticut	4,798,000,000	1.3%
47	Delaware	1,142,000,000	0.3%
4	Florida	20,313,000,000	5.3%
12	Georgia	10,381,000,000	2.7%
40	Hawaii	1,697,000,000	0.4%
44	Idaho	1,266,000,000	0.3%
6	Illinois	17,856,000,000	4.7%
15	Indiana	8,474,000,000	2.2%
29	Iowa	4,077,000,000	1.1%
32	Kansas	3,498,000,000	0.9%
23	Kentucky	5,783,000,000	1.5%
19	Louisiana	7,070,000,000	1.9%
39	Maine	1,818,000,000	0.5%
17	Maryland	7,178,000,000	1.9%
9	Massachusetts	11,464,000,000	3.0%
8	Michigan	14,246,000,000	3.8%
21	Minnesota	6,209,000,000	1.6%
30	Mississippi	4,000,000,000	1.1%
13	Missouri	9,063,000,000	2.4%
45	Montana	1,245,000,000	0.3%
35	Nebraska	2,611,000,000	0.7%
38	Nevada	1,843,000,000	0.5%
42	New Hampshire	1,510,000,000	0.4%
10	New Jersey	11,260,000,000	3.0%
36	New Mexico	2,336,000,000	0.6%
2	New York	31,990,000,000	8.4%
11	North Carolina	10,513,000,000	2.8%
43	North Dakota	1,271,000,000	0.3%
7	Ohio	15,985,000,000	4.2%
28	Oklahoma	4,127,000,000	1.1%
31	Oregon	3,652,000,000	1.0%
5	Pennsylvania	19,634,000,000	5.2%
41	Rhode Island	1,591,000,000	0.4%
24	South Carolina	5,399,000,000	1.4%
46	South Dakota	1,200,000,000	0.3%
16	Tennessee	8,049,000,000	2.1%
3	Texas	25,952,000,000	6.8%
37	Utah	2,261,000,000	0.6%
49	Vermont	698,000,000	0.2%
14	Virginia	8,585,000,000	2.3%
20	Washington	6,415,000,000	1.7%
34	West Virginia	2,932,000,000	0.8%
18	Wisconsin	7,108,000,000	1.9%
50	Wyoming	573,000,000	0.2%

RANK ORDER

RANK	STATE	EXPENDITURES	% of USA
1	California	$37,717,000,000	9.9%
2	New York	31,990,000,000	8.4%
3	Texas	25,952,000,000	6.8%
4	Florida	20,313,000,000	5.3%
5	Pennsylvania	19,634,000,000	5.2%
6	Illinois	17,856,000,000	4.7%
7	Ohio	15,985,000,000	4.2%
8	Michigan	14,246,000,000	3.8%
9	Massachusetts	11,464,000,000	3.0%
10	New Jersey	11,260,000,000	3.0%
11	North Carolina	10,513,000,000	2.8%
12	Georgia	10,381,000,000	2.7%
13	Missouri	9,063,000,000	2.4%
14	Virginia	8,585,000,000	2.3%
15	Indiana	8,474,000,000	2.2%
16	Tennessee	8,049,000,000	2.1%
17	Maryland	7,178,000,000	1.9%
18	Wisconsin	7,108,000,000	1.9%
19	Louisiana	7,070,000,000	1.9%
20	Washington	6,415,000,000	1.7%
21	Minnesota	6,209,000,000	1.6%
22	Alabama	6,169,000,000	1.6%
23	Kentucky	5,783,000,000	1.5%
24	South Carolina	5,399,000,000	1.4%
25	Arizona	5,199,000,000	1.4%
26	Connecticut	4,798,000,000	1.3%
27	Colorado	4,729,000,000	1.2%
28	Oklahoma	4,127,000,000	1.1%
29	Iowa	4,077,000,000	1.1%
30	Mississippi	4,000,000,000	1.1%
31	Oregon	3,652,000,000	1.0%
32	Kansas	3,498,000,000	0.9%
33	Arkansas	3,394,000,000	0.9%
34	West Virginia	2,932,000,000	0.8%
35	Nebraska	2,611,000,000	0.7%
36	New Mexico	2,336,000,000	0.6%
37	Utah	2,261,000,000	0.6%
38	Nevada	1,843,000,000	0.5%
39	Maine	1,818,000,000	0.5%
40	Hawaii	1,697,000,000	0.4%
41	Rhode Island	1,591,000,000	0.4%
42	New Hampshire	1,510,000,000	0.4%
43	North Dakota	1,271,000,000	0.3%
44	Idaho	1,266,000,000	0.3%
45	Montana	1,245,000,000	0.3%
46	South Dakota	1,200,000,000	0.3%
47	Delaware	1,142,000,000	0.3%
48	Alaska	909,000,000	0.2%
49	Vermont	698,000,000	0.2%
50	Wyoming	573,000,000	0.2%
	District of Columbia	2,644,000,000	0.7%

*Source: U.S. Department of Health and Human Services, Centers for Medicare and Medicaid Services
"State Health Care Expenditures" (http://www.cms.hhs.gov/statistics/nhe/)*
By state of provider. Revised figures

Percent of Total Personal Health Care Expenditures
Spent on Hospital Care in 1998
National Percent = 37.4%*

ALPHA ORDER

RANK	STATE	PERCENT
19	Alabama	39.5
3	Alaska	43.6
40	Arizona	34.6
18	Arkansas	39.8
44	California	33.4
39	Colorado	34.9
49	Connecticut	31.3
31	Delaware	37.2
43	Florida	33.7
24	Georgia	38.1
32	Hawaii	37.1
34	Idaho	37.0
13	Illinois	40.4
17	Indiana	39.9
15	Iowa	40.0
29	Kansas	37.6
15	Kentucky	40.0
7	Louisiana	43.0
32	Maine	37.1
36	Maryland	36.8
26	Massachusetts	38.0
13	Michigan	40.4
50	Minnesota	31.1
2	Mississippi	44.3
8	Missouri	42.9
3	Montana	43.6
9	Nebraska	42.7
47	Nevada	33.0
48	New Hampshire	32.8
41	New Jersey	34.4
5	New Mexico	43.5
29	New York	37.6
20	North Carolina	39.2
1	North Dakota	47.6
23	Ohio	38.2
27	Oklahoma	37.9
44	Oregon	33.4
21	Pennsylvania	38.7
37	Rhode Island	36.2
11	South Carolina	41.5
6	South Dakota	43.3
35	Tennessee	36.9
27	Texas	37.9
24	Utah	38.1
42	Vermont	34.0
21	Virginia	38.7
46	Washington	33.2
10	West Virginia	41.8
38	Wisconsin	35.9
12	Wyoming	41.0

RANK ORDER

RANK	STATE	PERCENT
1	North Dakota	47.6
2	Mississippi	44.3
3	Alaska	43.6
3	Montana	43.6
5	New Mexico	43.5
6	South Dakota	43.3
7	Louisiana	43.0
8	Missouri	42.9
9	Nebraska	42.7
10	West Virginia	41.8
11	South Carolina	41.5
12	Wyoming	41.0
13	Illinois	40.4
13	Michigan	40.4
15	Iowa	40.0
15	Kentucky	40.0
17	Indiana	39.9
18	Arkansas	39.8
19	Alabama	39.5
20	North Carolina	39.2
21	Pennsylvania	38.7
21	Virginia	38.7
23	Ohio	38.2
24	Georgia	38.1
24	Utah	38.1
26	Massachusetts	38.0
27	Oklahoma	37.9
27	Texas	37.9
29	Kansas	37.6
29	New York	37.6
31	Delaware	37.2
32	Hawaii	37.1
32	Maine	37.1
34	Idaho	37.0
35	Tennessee	36.9
36	Maryland	36.8
37	Rhode Island	36.2
38	Wisconsin	35.9
39	Colorado	34.9
40	Arizona	34.6
41	New Jersey	34.4
42	Vermont	34.0
43	Florida	33.7
44	California	33.4
44	Oregon	33.4
46	Washington	33.2
47	Nevada	33.0
48	New Hampshire	32.8
49	Connecticut	31.3
50	Minnesota	31.1

| | District of Columbia | 61.3 |

Source: MQ Press using data from U.S. Dept of Health & Human Services, Centers for Medicare and Medicaid Services
"State Health Care Expenditures" (http://www.cms.hhs.gov/statistics/nhe/)
*By state of provider. Revised figures.

Per Capita Expenditures for Hospital Care in 1998

National Per Capita = $1,406*

ALPHA ORDER

RANK	STATE	PER CAPITA
24	Alabama	$1,418
14	Alaska	1,478
46	Arizona	1,114
34	Arkansas	1,337
44	California	1,154
42	Colorado	1,191
16	Connecticut	1,466
11	Delaware	1,535
30	Florida	1,363
32	Georgia	1,359
21	Hawaii	1,425
50	Idaho	1,028
13	Illinois	1,479
20	Indiana	1,434
21	Iowa	1,425
35	Kansas	1,326
15	Kentucky	1,470
7	Louisiana	1,621
17	Maine	1,457
27	Maryland	1,399
2	Massachusetts	1,866
19	Michigan	1,451
37	Minnesota	1,314
18	Mississippi	1,454
4	Missouri	1,667
25	Montana	1,416
10	Nebraska	1,572
49	Nevada	1,057
38	New Hampshire	1,273
29	New Jersey	1,391
33	New Mexico	1,348
3	New York	1,762
28	North Carolina	1,393
1	North Dakota	1,993
23	Ohio	1,422
40	Oklahoma	1,236
47	Oregon	1,113
6	Pennsylvania	1,636
9	Rhode Island	1,611
26	South Carolina	1,406
5	South Dakota	1,642
12	Tennessee	1,482
36	Texas	1,317
48	Utah	1,076
43	Vermont	1,182
39	Virginia	1,265
45	Washington	1,128
8	West Virginia	1,618
31	Wisconsin	1,361
41	Wyoming	1,194

RANK ORDER

RANK	STATE	PER CAPITA
1	North Dakota	$1,993
2	Massachusetts	1,866
3	New York	1,762
4	Missouri	1,667
5	South Dakota	1,642
6	Pennsylvania	1,636
7	Louisiana	1,621
8	West Virginia	1,618
9	Rhode Island	1,611
10	Nebraska	1,572
11	Delaware	1,535
12	Tennessee	1,482
13	Illinois	1,479
14	Alaska	1,478
15	Kentucky	1,470
16	Connecticut	1,466
17	Maine	1,457
18	Mississippi	1,454
19	Michigan	1,451
20	Indiana	1,434
21	Hawaii	1,425
21	Iowa	1,425
23	Ohio	1,422
24	Alabama	1,418
25	Montana	1,416
26	South Carolina	1,406
27	Maryland	1,399
28	North Carolina	1,393
29	New Jersey	1,391
30	Florida	1,363
31	Wisconsin	1,361
32	Georgia	1,359
33	New Mexico	1,348
34	Arkansas	1,337
35	Kansas	1,326
36	Texas	1,317
37	Minnesota	1,314
38	New Hampshire	1,273
39	Virginia	1,265
40	Oklahoma	1,236
41	Wyoming	1,194
42	Colorado	1,191
43	Vermont	1,182
44	California	1,154
45	Washington	1,128
46	Arizona	1,114
47	Oregon	1,113
48	Utah	1,076
49	Nevada	1,057
50	Idaho	1,028

| | District of Columbia | 5,071 |

Source: MQ Press using data from U.S. Dept of Health & Human Services, Centers for Medicare and Medicaid Services "State Health Care Expenditures" (http://www.cms.hhs.gov/statistics/nhe/)
*By state of provider. Per capita calculated using resident population. These figures may be skewed due to residents crossing state borders for care. Revised figures.

Expenditures for Physician and Other Professional Services in 1998

National Total = $296,102,000,000*

ALPHA ORDER

RANK	STATE	EXPENDITURES	% of USA
22	Alabama	$4,609,000,000	1.6%
48	Alaska	568,000,000	0.2%
21	Arizona	5,135,000,000	1.7%
32	Arkansas	2,225,000,000	0.8%
1	California	44,239,000,000	14.9%
23	Colorado	4,314,000,000	1.5%
24	Connecticut	4,292,000,000	1.4%
44	Delaware	792,000,000	0.3%
4	Florida	18,985,000,000	6.4%
10	Georgia	8,510,000,000	2.9%
37	Hawaii	1,594,000,000	0.5%
43	Idaho	935,000,000	0.3%
6	Illinois	11,975,000,000	4.0%
19	Indiana	5,613,000,000	1.9%
31	Iowa	2,457,000,000	0.8%
30	Kansas	2,538,000,000	0.9%
26	Kentucky	3,785,000,000	1.3%
25	Louisiana	4,249,000,000	1.4%
41	Maine	1,219,000,000	0.4%
16	Maryland	5,978,000,000	2.0%
11	Massachusetts	8,322,000,000	2.8%
9	Michigan	9,186,000,000	3.1%
12	Minnesota	7,183,000,000	2.4%
33	Mississippi	2,212,000,000	0.7%
20	Missouri	5,310,000,000	1.8%
46	Montana	695,000,000	0.2%
40	Nebraska	1,367,000,000	0.5%
34	Nevada	1,918,000,000	0.6%
39	New Hampshire	1,405,000,000	0.5%
8	New Jersey	9,506,000,000	3.2%
38	New Mexico	1,415,000,000	0.5%
2	New York	20,103,000,000	6.8%
13	North Carolina	7,106,000,000	2.4%
47	North Dakota	612,000,000	0.2%
7	Ohio	11,024,000,000	3.7%
29	Oklahoma	2,978,000,000	1.0%
27	Oregon	3,285,000,000	1.1%
5	Pennsylvania	13,434,000,000	4.5%
42	Rhode Island	1,095,000,000	0.4%
28	South Carolina	3,254,000,000	1.1%
45	South Dakota	747,000,000	0.3%
14	Tennessee	6,719,000,000	2.3%
3	Texas	20,071,000,000	6.8%
36	Utah	1,648,000,000	0.6%
49	Vermont	563,000,000	0.2%
15	Virginia	6,265,000,000	2.1%
17	Washington	5,908,000,000	2.0%
35	West Virginia	1,793,000,000	0.6%
18	Wisconsin	5,844,000,000	2.0%
50	Wyoming	343,000,000	0.1%

RANK ORDER

RANK	STATE	EXPENDITURES	% of USA
1	California	$44,239,000,000	14.9%
2	New York	20,103,000,000	6.8%
3	Texas	20,071,000,000	6.8%
4	Florida	18,985,000,000	6.4%
5	Pennsylvania	13,434,000,000	4.5%
6	Illinois	11,975,000,000	4.0%
7	Ohio	11,024,000,000	3.7%
8	New Jersey	9,506,000,000	3.2%
9	Michigan	9,186,000,000	3.1%
10	Georgia	8,510,000,000	2.9%
11	Massachusetts	8,322,000,000	2.8%
12	Minnesota	7,183,000,000	2.4%
13	North Carolina	7,106,000,000	2.4%
14	Tennessee	6,719,000,000	2.3%
15	Virginia	6,265,000,000	2.1%
16	Maryland	5,978,000,000	2.0%
17	Washington	5,908,000,000	2.0%
18	Wisconsin	5,844,000,000	2.0%
19	Indiana	5,613,000,000	1.9%
20	Missouri	5,310,000,000	1.8%
21	Arizona	5,135,000,000	1.7%
22	Alabama	4,609,000,000	1.6%
23	Colorado	4,314,000,000	1.5%
24	Connecticut	4,292,000,000	1.4%
25	Louisiana	4,249,000,000	1.4%
26	Kentucky	3,785,000,000	1.3%
27	Oregon	3,285,000,000	1.1%
28	South Carolina	3,254,000,000	1.1%
29	Oklahoma	2,978,000,000	1.0%
30	Kansas	2,538,000,000	0.9%
31	Iowa	2,457,000,000	0.8%
32	Arkansas	2,225,000,000	0.8%
33	Mississippi	2,212,000,000	0.7%
34	Nevada	1,918,000,000	0.6%
35	West Virginia	1,793,000,000	0.6%
36	Utah	1,648,000,000	0.6%
37	Hawaii	1,594,000,000	0.5%
38	New Mexico	1,415,000,000	0.5%
39	New Hampshire	1,405,000,000	0.5%
40	Nebraska	1,367,000,000	0.5%
41	Maine	1,219,000,000	0.4%
42	Rhode Island	1,095,000,000	0.4%
43	Idaho	935,000,000	0.3%
44	Delaware	792,000,000	0.3%
45	South Dakota	747,000,000	0.3%
46	Montana	695,000,000	0.2%
47	North Dakota	612,000,000	0.2%
48	Alaska	568,000,000	0.2%
49	Vermont	563,000,000	0.2%
50	Wyoming	343,000,000	0.1%
	District of Columbia	781,000,000	0.3%

Source: U.S. Department of Health and Human Services, Centers for Medicare and Medicaid Services
   "State Health Care Expenditures" (http://www.cms.hhs.gov/statistics/nhe/)
By state of provider. Includes "other professional services" previously listed as a separate category. These include services of licensed professionals such as chiropractors, optometrists, podiatrists and independently practicing nurses. Also includes specialty clinics, independently billing laboratories and Medicare ambulance services. Revised figures.

Percent of Total Personal Health Care Expenditures
Spent on Physician and Other Professional Services in 1998
National Percent = 29.1%*

ALPHA ORDER

RANK	STATE	PERCENT
14	Alabama	29.5
26	Alaska	27.2
5	Arizona	34.2
35	Arkansas	26.1
1	California	39.2
6	Colorado	31.8
19	Connecticut	28.0
38	Delaware	25.8
7	Florida	31.5
8	Georgia	31.3
3	Hawaii	34.8
23	Idaho	27.3
27	Illinois	27.1
29	Indiana	26.5
47	Iowa	24.1
23	Kansas	27.3
34	Kentucky	26.2
37	Louisiana	25.9
42	Maine	24.9
10	Maryland	30.6
21	Massachusetts	27.6
35	Michigan	26.1
2	Minnesota	35.9
44	Mississippi	24.5
40	Missouri	25.1
46	Montana	24.3
50	Nebraska	22.4
4	Nevada	34.4
12	New Hampshire	30.5
17	New Jersey	29.0
32	New Mexico	26.4
48	New York	23.6
29	North Carolina	26.5
49	North Dakota	22.9
32	Ohio	26.4
23	Oklahoma	27.3
13	Oregon	30.0
29	Pennsylvania	26.5
42	Rhode Island	24.9
41	South Carolina	25.0
28	South Dakota	26.9
9	Tennessee	30.8
16	Texas	29.4
20	Utah	27.8
22	Vermont	27.4
18	Virginia	28.3
10	Washington	30.6
39	West Virginia	25.6
14	Wisconsin	29.5
44	Wyoming	24.5

RANK ORDER

RANK	STATE	PERCENT
1	California	39.2
2	Minnesota	35.9
3	Hawaii	34.8
4	Nevada	34.4
5	Arizona	34.2
6	Colorado	31.8
7	Florida	31.5
8	Georgia	31.3
9	Tennessee	30.8
10	Maryland	30.6
10	Washington	30.6
12	New Hampshire	30.5
13	Oregon	30.0
14	Alabama	29.5
14	Wisconsin	29.5
16	Texas	29.4
17	New Jersey	29.0
18	Virginia	28.3
19	Connecticut	28.0
20	Utah	27.8
21	Massachusetts	27.6
22	Vermont	27.4
23	Idaho	27.3
23	Kansas	27.3
23	Oklahoma	27.3
26	Alaska	27.2
27	Illinois	27.1
28	South Dakota	26.9
29	Indiana	26.5
29	North Carolina	26.5
29	Pennsylvania	26.5
32	New Mexico	26.4
32	Ohio	26.4
34	Kentucky	26.2
35	Arkansas	26.1
35	Michigan	26.1
37	Louisiana	25.9
38	Delaware	25.8
39	West Virginia	25.6
40	Missouri	25.1
41	South Carolina	25.0
42	Maine	24.9
42	Rhode Island	24.9
44	Mississippi	24.5
44	Wyoming	24.5
46	Montana	24.3
47	Iowa	24.1
48	New York	23.6
49	North Dakota	22.9
50	Nebraska	22.4

District of Columbia   18.1

*Source: MQ Press using data from U.S. Dept of Health & Human Services, Centers for Medicare and Medicaid Services
"State Health Care Expenditures" (http://www.cms.hhs.gov/statistics/nhe/)*

By state of provider. Includes "other professional services" previously listed as a separate category. These include services of licensed professionals such as chiropractors, optometrists, podiatrists and independently practicing nurses. Also includes specialty clinics, independently billing laboratories and Medicare ambulance services. Revised figures.

Per Capita Expenditures for Physician and Other Professional Services in 1998

National Per Capita = $1,096*

ALPHA ORDER

RANK ORDER

RANK	STATE	PER CAPITA
20	Alabama	$1,059
38	Alaska	923
16	Arizona	1,100
41	Arkansas	877
2	California	1,354
18	Colorado	1,087
5	Connecticut	1,312
19	Delaware	1,064
6	Florida	1,273
13	Georgia	1,114
4	Hawaii	1,339
49	Idaho	760
25	Illinois	992
35	Indiana	950
42	Iowa	859
31	Kansas	962
31	Kentucky	962
30	Louisiana	974
28	Maine	977
10	Maryland	1,165
2	Massachusetts	1,354
37	Michigan	935
1	Minnesota	1,520
46	Mississippi	804
28	Missouri	977
47	Montana	790
44	Nebraska	823
16	Nevada	1,100
8	New Hampshire	1,185
9	New Jersey	1,174
45	New Mexico	816
15	New York	1,107
36	North Carolina	942
33	North Dakota	960
27	Ohio	981
40	Oklahoma	892
24	Oregon	1,001
11	Pennsylvania	1,119
14	Rhode Island	1,109
43	South Carolina	847
22	South Dakota	1,022
7	Tennessee	1,237
23	Texas	1,018
48	Utah	785
34	Vermont	953
38	Virginia	923
21	Washington	1,039
26	West Virginia	990
11	Wisconsin	1,119
50	Wyoming	715

RANK	STATE	PER CAPITA
1	Minnesota	$1,520
2	California	1,354
2	Massachusetts	1,354
4	Hawaii	1,339
5	Connecticut	1,312
6	Florida	1,273
7	Tennessee	1,237
8	New Hampshire	1,185
9	New Jersey	1,174
10	Maryland	1,165
11	Pennsylvania	1,119
11	Wisconsin	1,119
13	Georgia	1,114
14	Rhode Island	1,109
15	New York	1,107
16	Arizona	1,100
16	Nevada	1,100
18	Colorado	1,087
19	Delaware	1,064
20	Alabama	1,059
21	Washington	1,039
22	South Dakota	1,022
23	Texas	1,018
24	Oregon	1,001
25	Illinois	992
26	West Virginia	990
27	Ohio	981
28	Maine	977
28	Missouri	977
30	Louisiana	974
31	Kansas	962
31	Kentucky	962
33	North Dakota	960
34	Vermont	953
35	Indiana	950
36	North Carolina	942
37	Michigan	935
38	Alaska	923
38	Virginia	923
40	Oklahoma	892
41	Arkansas	877
42	Iowa	859
43	South Carolina	847
44	Nebraska	823
45	New Mexico	816
46	Mississippi	804
47	Montana	790
48	Utah	785
49	Idaho	760
50	Wyoming	715

District of Columbia 1,498

Source: MQ Press using data from U.S. Dept of Health & Human Services, Centers for Medicare and Medicaid Services "State Health Care Expenditures" (http://www.cms.hhs.gov/statistics/nhe/)

*By state of provider. Per capita calculated using resident population. These figures may be skewed due to residents crossing state borders for care. Includes "other professional services" previously listed as a separate category. Services include licensed professionals such as chiropractors, optometrists, podiatrists and independently practicing nurses. Revised figures.

Expenditures for Drugs and
Other Medical Non-Durables in 1998
National Total = $121,906,000,000*

ALPHA ORDER

RANK	STATE	EXPENDITURES	% of USA
21	Alabama	$2,049,000,000	1.7%
49	Alaska	221,000,000	0.2%
20	Arizona	2,066,000,000	1.7%
32	Arkansas	1,177,000,000	1.0%
1	California	11,604,000,000	9.5%
27	Colorado	1,546,000,000	1.3%
26	Connecticut	1,705,000,000	1.4%
44	Delaware	390,000,000	0.3%
4	Florida	8,226,000,000	6.7%
11	Georgia	3,367,000,000	2.8%
41	Hawaii	514,000,000	0.4%
43	Idaho	474,000,000	0.4%
6	Illinois	5,174,000,000	4.2%
15	Indiana	2,649,000,000	2.2%
31	Iowa	1,219,000,000	1.0%
33	Kansas	1,087,000,000	0.9%
24	Kentucky	1,966,000,000	1.6%
23	Louisiana	1,992,000,000	1.6%
39	Maine	559,000,000	0.5%
18	Maryland	2,304,000,000	1.9%
13	Massachusetts	2,882,000,000	2.4%
8	Michigan	4,884,000,000	4.0%
22	Minnesota	2,004,000,000	1.6%
30	Mississippi	1,222,000,000	1.0%
16	Missouri	2,403,000,000	2.0%
45	Montana	349,000,000	0.3%
37	Nebraska	791,000,000	0.6%
36	Nevada	825,000,000	0.7%
40	New Hampshire	539,000,000	0.4%
9	New Jersey	4,564,000,000	3.7%
38	New Mexico	630,000,000	0.5%
2	New York	8,940,000,000	7.3%
10	North Carolina	3,411,000,000	2.8%
47	North Dakota	250,000,000	0.2%
7	Ohio	5,027,000,000	4.1%
28	Oklahoma	1,418,000,000	1.2%
29	Oregon	1,386,000,000	1.1%
5	Pennsylvania	6,162,000,000	5.1%
42	Rhode Island	505,000,000	0.4%
25	South Carolina	1,721,000,000	1.4%
46	South Dakota	268,000,000	0.2%
14	Tennessee	2,751,000,000	2.3%
3	Texas	8,672,000,000	7.1%
35	Utah	828,000,000	0.7%
48	Vermont	237,000,000	0.2%
12	Virginia	2,947,000,000	2.4%
17	Washington	2,365,000,000	1.9%
34	West Virginia	949,000,000	0.8%
19	Wisconsin	2,269,000,000	1.9%
50	Wyoming	178,000,000	0.1%

RANK ORDER

RANK	STATE	EXPENDITURES	% of USA
1	California	$11,604,000,000	9.5%
2	New York	8,940,000,000	7.3%
3	Texas	8,672,000,000	7.1%
4	Florida	8,226,000,000	6.7%
5	Pennsylvania	6,162,000,000	5.1%
6	Illinois	5,174,000,000	4.2%
7	Ohio	5,027,000,000	4.1%
8	Michigan	4,884,000,000	4.0%
9	New Jersey	4,564,000,000	3.7%
10	North Carolina	3,411,000,000	2.8%
11	Georgia	3,367,000,000	2.8%
12	Virginia	2,947,000,000	2.4%
13	Massachusetts	2,882,000,000	2.4%
14	Tennessee	2,751,000,000	2.3%
15	Indiana	2,649,000,000	2.2%
16	Missouri	2,403,000,000	2.0%
17	Washington	2,365,000,000	1.9%
18	Maryland	2,304,000,000	1.9%
19	Wisconsin	2,269,000,000	1.9%
20	Arizona	2,066,000,000	1.7%
21	Alabama	2,049,000,000	1.7%
22	Minnesota	2,004,000,000	1.6%
23	Louisiana	1,992,000,000	1.6%
24	Kentucky	1,966,000,000	1.6%
25	South Carolina	1,721,000,000	1.4%
26	Connecticut	1,705,000,000	1.4%
27	Colorado	1,546,000,000	1.3%
28	Oklahoma	1,418,000,000	1.2%
29	Oregon	1,386,000,000	1.1%
30	Mississippi	1,222,000,000	1.0%
31	Iowa	1,219,000,000	1.0%
32	Arkansas	1,177,000,000	1.0%
33	Kansas	1,087,000,000	0.9%
34	West Virginia	949,000,000	0.8%
35	Utah	828,000,000	0.7%
36	Nevada	825,000,000	0.7%
37	Nebraska	791,000,000	0.6%
38	New Mexico	630,000,000	0.5%
39	Maine	559,000,000	0.5%
40	New Hampshire	539,000,000	0.4%
41	Hawaii	514,000,000	0.4%
42	Rhode Island	505,000,000	0.4%
43	Idaho	474,000,000	0.4%
44	Delaware	390,000,000	0.3%
45	Montana	349,000,000	0.3%
46	South Dakota	268,000,000	0.2%
47	North Dakota	250,000,000	0.2%
48	Vermont	237,000,000	0.2%
49	Alaska	221,000,000	0.2%
50	Wyoming	178,000,000	0.1%
	District of Columbia	239,000,000	0.2%

Source: U.S. Department of Health and Human Services, Centers for Medicare and Medicaid Services
"State Health Care Expenditures" (http://www.cms.hhs.gov/statistics/nhe/)
*Purchases in retail outlets. By state of outlet. Includes prescription drugs, over-the-counter drugs and sundries.
Revised figures.

Percent of Total Personal Health Care Expenditures Spent on Drugs and Other Medical Non-Durables in 1998
National Percent = 12.0%*

ALPHA ORDER

RANK	STATE	PERCENT
14	Alabama	13.1
44	Alaska	10.6
6	Arizona	13.8
6	Arkansas	13.8
46	California	10.3
39	Colorado	11.4
43	Connecticut	11.1
17	Delaware	12.7
8	Florida	13.6
24	Georgia	12.4
42	Hawaii	11.2
3	Idaho	13.9
32	Illinois	11.7
23	Indiana	12.5
29	Iowa	12.0
32	Kansas	11.7
8	Kentucky	13.6
27	Louisiana	12.1
39	Maine	11.4
31	Maryland	11.8
49	Massachusetts	9.5
3	Michigan	13.9
47	Minnesota	10.0
10	Mississippi	13.5
39	Missouri	11.4
25	Montana	12.2
16	Nebraska	12.9
1	Nevada	14.8
32	New Hampshire	11.7
3	New Jersey	13.9
32	New Mexico	11.7
45	New York	10.5
17	North Carolina	12.7
50	North Dakota	9.4
29	Ohio	12.0
15	Oklahoma	13.0
17	Oregon	12.7
27	Pennsylvania	12.1
36	Rhode Island	11.5
13	South Carolina	13.2
48	South Dakota	9.7
22	Tennessee	12.6
17	Texas	12.7
2	Utah	14.0
36	Vermont	11.5
12	Virginia	13.3
25	Washington	12.2
10	West Virginia	13.5
36	Wisconsin	11.5
17	Wyoming	12.7

RANK ORDER

RANK	STATE	PERCENT
1	Nevada	14.8
2	Utah	14.0
3	Idaho	13.9
3	Michigan	13.9
3	New Jersey	13.9
6	Arizona	13.8
6	Arkansas	13.8
8	Florida	13.6
8	Kentucky	13.6
10	Mississippi	13.5
10	West Virginia	13.5
12	Virginia	13.3
13	South Carolina	13.2
14	Alabama	13.1
15	Oklahoma	13.0
16	Nebraska	12.9
17	Delaware	12.7
17	North Carolina	12.7
17	Oregon	12.7
17	Texas	12.7
17	Wyoming	12.7
22	Tennessee	12.6
23	Indiana	12.5
24	Georgia	12.4
25	Montana	12.2
25	Washington	12.2
27	Louisiana	12.1
27	Pennsylvania	12.1
29	Iowa	12.0
29	Ohio	12.0
31	Maryland	11.8
32	Illinois	11.7
32	Kansas	11.7
32	New Hampshire	11.7
32	New Mexico	11.7
36	Rhode Island	11.5
36	Vermont	11.5
36	Wisconsin	11.5
39	Colorado	11.4
39	Maine	11.4
39	Missouri	11.4
42	Hawaii	11.2
43	Connecticut	11.1
44	Alaska	10.6
45	New York	10.5
46	California	10.3
47	Minnesota	10.0
48	South Dakota	9.7
49	Massachusetts	9.5
50	North Dakota	9.4

District of Columbia 5.5

Source: MQ Press using data from U.S. Dept of Health & Human Services, Centers for Medicare and Medicaid Services
  "State Health Care Expenditures" (http://www.cms.hhs.gov/statistics/nhe/)
*Purchases in retail outlets. By state of outlet. Includes prescription drugs, over-the-counter drugs and sundries.
Revised figures.

Per Capita Expenditures for Drugs and
Other Medical Non-Durables in 1998
National Per Capita = $451*

RANK	STATE	PER CAPITA
14	Alabama	$471
49	Alaska	359
26	Arizona	443
16	Arkansas	464
50	California	355
44	Colorado	390
5	Connecticut	521
3	Delaware	524
2	Florida	552
28	Georgia	441
32	Hawaii	432
45	Idaho	385
33	Illinois	429
21	Indiana	448
34	Iowa	426
39	Kansas	412
9	Kentucky	500
17	Louisiana	457
21	Maine	448
20	Maryland	449
15	Massachusetts	469
10	Michigan	497
36	Minnesota	424
25	Mississippi	444
27	Missouri	442
41	Montana	397
12	Nebraska	476
13	Nevada	473
18	New Hampshire	455
1	New Jersey	564
48	New Mexico	363
11	New York	492
19	North Carolina	452
43	North Dakota	392
24	Ohio	447
35	Oklahoma	425
37	Oregon	422
6	Pennsylvania	513
7	Rhode Island	511
21	South Carolina	448
47	South Dakota	367
8	Tennessee	506
29	Texas	440
42	Utah	394
40	Vermont	401
30	Virginia	434
38	Washington	416
3	West Virginia	524
30	Wisconsin	434
46	Wyoming	371

RANK	STATE	PER CAPITA
1	New Jersey	$564
2	Florida	552
3	Delaware	524
3	West Virginia	524
5	Connecticut	521
6	Pennsylvania	513
7	Rhode Island	511
8	Tennessee	506
9	Kentucky	500
10	Michigan	497
11	New York	492
12	Nebraska	476
13	Nevada	473
14	Alabama	471
15	Massachusetts	469
16	Arkansas	464
17	Louisiana	457
18	New Hampshire	455
19	North Carolina	452
20	Maryland	449
21	Indiana	448
21	Maine	448
21	South Carolina	448
24	Ohio	447
25	Mississippi	444
26	Arizona	443
27	Missouri	442
28	Georgia	441
29	Texas	440
30	Virginia	434
30	Wisconsin	434
32	Hawaii	432
33	Illinois	429
34	Iowa	426
35	Oklahoma	425
36	Minnesota	424
37	Oregon	422
38	Washington	416
39	Kansas	412
40	Vermont	401
41	Montana	397
42	Utah	394
43	North Dakota	392
44	Colorado	390
45	Idaho	385
46	Wyoming	371
47	South Dakota	367
48	New Mexico	363
49	Alaska	359
50	California	355
	District of Columbia	458

*Source: MQ Press using data from U.S. Dept of Health & Human Services, Centers for Medicare and Medicaid Services
"State Health Care Expenditures" (http://www.cms.hhs.gov/statistics/nhe)*
**Purchases in retail outlets. By state of outlet. Includes prescription drugs, over-the-counter drugs and sundries.
Per capita calculated using resident population. These figures may be skewed due to residents crossing state
borders to make purchases. Revised figures.*

Expenditures for Prescription Drugs in 1998

National Total = $90,648,000,000*

ALPHA ORDER

RANK	STATE	EXPENDITURES	% of USA
21	Alabama	$1,552,000,000	1.7%
49	Alaska	133,000,000	0.1%
24	Arizona	1,397,000,000	1.5%
32	Arkansas	903,000,000	1.0%
1	California	7,537,000,000	8.3%
28	Colorado	970,000,000	1.1%
25	Connecticut	1,354,000,000	1.5%
44	Delaware	300,000,000	0.3%
3	Florida	6,204,000,000	6.8%
11	Georgia	2,460,000,000	2.7%
43	Hawaii	311,000,000	0.3%
42	Idaho	334,000,000	0.4%
6	Illinois	3,964,000,000	4.4%
15	Indiana	2,058,000,000	2.3%
30	Iowa	945,000,000	1.0%
33	Kansas	854,000,000	0.9%
20	Kentucky	1,564,000,000	1.7%
22	Louisiana	1,507,000,000	1.7%
38	Maine	456,000,000	0.5%
18	Maryland	1,678,000,000	1.9%
12	Massachusetts	2,172,000,000	2.4%
8	Michigan	3,885,000,000	4.3%
23	Minnesota	1,491,000,000	1.6%
29	Mississippi	962,000,000	1.1%
16	Missouri	1,814,000,000	2.0%
45	Montana	234,000,000	0.3%
35	Nebraska	626,000,000	0.7%
37	Nevada	478,000,000	0.5%
41	New Hampshire	391,000,000	0.4%
9	New Jersey	3,545,000,000	3.9%
39	New Mexico	402,000,000	0.4%
2	New York	7,122,000,000	7.9%
10	North Carolina	2,566,000,000	2.8%
47	North Dakota	192,000,000	0.2%
7	Ohio	3,898,000,000	4.3%
27	Oklahoma	1,056,000,000	1.2%
31	Oregon	918,000,000	1.0%
5	Pennsylvania	5,035,000,000	5.6%
40	Rhode Island	400,000,000	0.4%
26	South Carolina	1,315,000,000	1.5%
46	South Dakota	201,000,000	0.2%
14	Tennessee	2,129,000,000	2.3%
4	Texas	6,023,000,000	6.6%
36	Utah	564,000,000	0.6%
48	Vermont	183,000,000	0.2%
13	Virginia	2,130,000,000	2.3%
19	Washington	1,603,000,000	1.8%
34	West Virginia	776,000,000	0.9%
17	Wisconsin	1,745,000,000	1.9%
49	Wyoming	133,000,000	0.1%

RANK ORDER

RANK	STATE	EXPENDITURES	% of USA
1	California	$7,537,000,000	8.3%
2	New York	7,122,000,000	7.9%
3	Florida	6,204,000,000	6.8%
4	Texas	6,023,000,000	6.6%
5	Pennsylvania	5,035,000,000	5.6%
6	Illinois	3,964,000,000	4.4%
7	Ohio	3,898,000,000	4.3%
8	Michigan	3,885,000,000	4.3%
9	New Jersey	3,545,000,000	3.9%
10	North Carolina	2,566,000,000	2.8%
11	Georgia	2,460,000,000	2.7%
12	Massachusetts	2,172,000,000	2.4%
13	Virginia	2,130,000,000	2.3%
14	Tennessee	2,129,000,000	2.3%
15	Indiana	2,058,000,000	2.3%
16	Missouri	1,814,000,000	2.0%
17	Wisconsin	1,745,000,000	1.9%
18	Maryland	1,678,000,000	1.9%
19	Washington	1,603,000,000	1.8%
20	Kentucky	1,564,000,000	1.7%
21	Alabama	1,552,000,000	1.7%
22	Louisiana	1,507,000,000	1.7%
23	Minnesota	1,491,000,000	1.6%
24	Arizona	1,397,000,000	1.5%
25	Connecticut	1,354,000,000	1.5%
26	South Carolina	1,315,000,000	1.5%
27	Oklahoma	1,056,000,000	1.2%
28	Colorado	970,000,000	1.1%
29	Mississippi	962,000,000	1.1%
30	Iowa	945,000,000	1.0%
31	Oregon	918,000,000	1.0%
32	Arkansas	903,000,000	1.0%
33	Kansas	854,000,000	0.9%
34	West Virginia	776,000,000	0.9%
35	Nebraska	626,000,000	0.7%
36	Utah	564,000,000	0.6%
37	Nevada	478,000,000	0.5%
38	Maine	456,000,000	0.5%
39	New Mexico	402,000,000	0.4%
40	Rhode Island	400,000,000	0.4%
41	New Hampshire	391,000,000	0.4%
42	Idaho	334,000,000	0.4%
43	Hawaii	311,000,000	0.3%
44	Delaware	300,000,000	0.3%
45	Montana	234,000,000	0.3%
46	South Dakota	201,000,000	0.2%
47	North Dakota	192,000,000	0.2%
48	Vermont	183,000,000	0.2%
49	Alaska	133,000,000	0.1%
49	Wyoming	133,000,000	0.1%
	District of Columbia	180,000,000	0.2%

Source: U.S. Department of Health and Human Services, Centers for Medicare and Medicaid Services
   "State Health Care Expenditures" (http://www.cms.hhs.gov/statistics/nhe/)
*Purchases in retail outlets. By state of outlet. Revised figures.

Percent of Total Personal Health Care Expenditures
Spent on Prescription Drugs in 1998
National Percent = 8.9%*

ALPHA ORDER

RANK	STATE	PERCENT
10	Alabama	9.9
50	Alaska	6.4
21	Arizona	9.3
5	Arkansas	10.6
49	California	6.7
44	Colorado	7.2
31	Connecticut	8.8
12	Delaware	9.8
7	Florida	10.3
28	Georgia	9.0
48	Hawaii	6.8
12	Idaho	9.8
28	Illinois	9.0
15	Indiana	9.7
21	Iowa	9.3
25	Kansas	9.2
3	Kentucky	10.8
25	Louisiana	9.2
21	Maine	9.3
34	Maryland	8.6
44	Massachusetts	7.2
2	Michigan	11.0
42	Minnesota	7.5
5	Mississippi	10.6
34	Missouri	8.6
41	Montana	8.2
8	Nebraska	10.2
34	Nevada	8.6
37	New Hampshire	8.5
3	New Jersey	10.8
42	New Mexico	7.5
38	New York	8.4
17	North Carolina	9.6
44	North Dakota	7.2
21	Ohio	9.3
15	Oklahoma	9.7
38	Oregon	8.4
10	Pennsylvania	9.9
27	Rhode Island	9.1
9	South Carolina	10.1
44	South Dakota	7.2
12	Tennessee	9.8
31	Texas	8.8
19	Utah	9.5
30	Vermont	8.9
17	Virginia	9.6
40	Washington	8.3
1	West Virginia	11.1
31	Wisconsin	8.8
19	Wyoming	9.5

RANK ORDER

RANK	STATE	PERCENT
1	West Virginia	11.1
2	Michigan	11.0
3	Kentucky	10.8
3	New Jersey	10.8
5	Arkansas	10.6
5	Mississippi	10.6
7	Florida	10.3
8	Nebraska	10.2
9	South Carolina	10.1
10	Alabama	9.9
10	Pennsylvania	9.9
12	Delaware	9.8
12	Idaho	9.8
12	Tennessee	9.8
15	Indiana	9.7
15	Oklahoma	9.7
17	North Carolina	9.6
17	Virginia	9.6
19	Utah	9.5
19	Wyoming	9.5
21	Arizona	9.3
21	Iowa	9.3
21	Maine	9.3
21	Ohio	9.3
25	Kansas	9.2
25	Louisiana	9.2
27	Rhode Island	9.1
28	Georgia	9.0
28	Illinois	9.0
30	Vermont	8.9
31	Connecticut	8.8
31	Texas	8.8
31	Wisconsin	8.8
34	Maryland	8.6
34	Missouri	8.6
34	Nevada	8.6
37	New Hampshire	8.5
38	New York	8.4
38	Oregon	8.4
40	Washington	8.3
41	Montana	8.2
42	Minnesota	7.5
42	New Mexico	7.5
44	Colorado	7.2
44	Massachusetts	7.2
44	North Dakota	7.2
44	South Dakota	7.2
48	Hawaii	6.8
49	California	6.7
50	Alaska	6.4

District of Columbia   4.2

Source: MQ Press using data from U.S. Dept of Health & Human Services, Centers for Medicare and Medicaid Services
"State Health Care Expenditures" (http://www.cms.hhs.gov/statistics/nhe/)
*Purchases in retail outlets. By state of outlet. Revised figures.

Per Capita Expenditures for Prescription Drugs in 1998

National Per Capita = $335*

ALPHA ORDER				RANK ORDER		
RANK	STATE	PER CAPITA		RANK	STATE	PER CAPITA
14	Alabama	$357		1	New Jersey	$438
50	Alaska	216		2	West Virginia	428
37	Arizona	299		3	Pennsylvania	420
15	Arkansas	356		4	Florida	416
49	California	231		5	Connecticut	414
47	Colorado	244		6	Rhode Island	405
5	Connecticut	414		7	Delaware	403
7	Delaware	403		8	Kentucky	398
4	Florida	416		9	Michigan	396
30	Georgia	322		10	New York	392
46	Hawaii	261		10	Tennessee	392
43	Idaho	271		12	Nebraska	377
27	Illinois	328		13	Maine	366
18	Indiana	348		14	Alabama	357
25	Iowa	330		15	Arkansas	356
29	Kansas	324		16	Massachusetts	353
8	Kentucky	398		17	Mississippi	350
20	Louisiana	345		18	Indiana	348
13	Maine	366		19	Ohio	347
28	Maryland	327		20	Louisiana	345
16	Massachusetts	353		21	South Carolina	342
9	Michigan	396		22	North Carolina	340
32	Minnesota	315		23	Missouri	334
17	Mississippi	350		23	Wisconsin	334
23	Missouri	334		25	Iowa	330
45	Montana	266		25	New Hampshire	330
12	Nebraska	377		27	Illinois	328
42	Nevada	274		28	Maryland	327
25	New Hampshire	330		29	Kansas	324
1	New Jersey	438		30	Georgia	322
48	New Mexico	232		31	Oklahoma	316
10	New York	392		32	Minnesota	315
22	North Carolina	340		33	Virginia	314
36	North Dakota	301		34	Vermont	310
19	Ohio	347		35	Texas	306
31	Oklahoma	316		36	North Dakota	301
39	Oregon	280		37	Arizona	299
3	Pennsylvania	420		38	Washington	282
6	Rhode Island	405		39	Oregon	280
21	South Carolina	342		40	Wyoming	277
41	South Dakota	275		41	South Dakota	275
10	Tennessee	392		42	Nevada	274
35	Texas	306		43	Idaho	271
44	Utah	268		44	Utah	268
34	Vermont	310		45	Montana	266
33	Virginia	314		46	Hawaii	261
38	Washington	282		47	Colorado	244
2	West Virginia	428		48	New Mexico	232
23	Wisconsin	334		49	California	231
40	Wyoming	277		50	Alaska	216
					District of Columbia	345

Source: MQ Press using data from U.S. Dept of Health & Human Services, Centers for Medicare and Medicaid Services
    "State Health Care Expenditures" (http://www.cms.hhs.gov/statistics/nhe/)
*Purchases in retail outlets. By state of outlet. Revised figures.

Projected National Health Care Expenditures in 2005

Total Health Care Expenditures = $1,920,800,000,000*

The 1998 health care expenditures broken down to the state level and shown on pages 301 to 314 were released in August of 2000 and updated in 2002. The Centers for Medicare and Medicaid Services (CMS) plan to update these numbers but no updates were available as we went to press.

Given the high level of interest in health care finance data, we have assembled a table showing the most recent national level health care expenditure projections. We will continue to monitor CMS data releases and will include the state expenditure updates in forthcoming editions.

	PROJECTED EXPENDITURES IN 2005	PROJECTED PERCENT CHANGE: 2004 TO 2005
Total Health Care Expenditures	$1,920,800,000,000	7.1
Per Capita Total Health Care Expenditures	$6,541	
Personal Health Care Expenditures	$1,651,500,000,000	7.2
Per Capita Personal Health Care Expenditures	$5,624	
Hospital Care Expenditures	$585,800,000,000	6.2
Per Capita Hospital Care Expenditures	$1,995	
Physician Services Expenditures	$412,000,000,000	6.5
Per Capita Physician Services Expenditures	$1,403	
Dental Services Expenditures	$82,300,000,000	5.5
Per Capita Dental Services Expenditures	$280	
Other Professional Services	$54,200,000,000	6.3
Per Capita Other Professional Services	$185	
Home Health Care Expenditures	$43,200,000,000	6.4
Per Capita Home Health Care Expenditures	$147	
Prescription Drugs	$233,600,000,000	12.4
Per Capita Prescription Drugs	$795	
Nursing Home Care	$116,900,000,000	4.7
Per Capita Nursing Home Care	$398	
Other Personal Care Expenditures	$62,600,000,000	11.4
Per Capita Other Personal Care Expenditures	$213	

Source: U.S. Department of Health and Human Services, Centers for Medicare and Medicaid Services
    "National Health Expenditure Amounts and Average Annual Percent Change, by Type of Expenditure"
        http://www.cms.hhs.gov/statistics/nhe/projections-2003/t2.asp
*Per Capita figures calculated by Morgan Quitno Press using 2004 Census population estimates.
For definitions see the corresponding 1998 state tables in this chapter.

V. INCIDENCE OF DISEASE

V. INCIDENCE OF DISEASE (Continued)

Estimated New Cancer Cases in 2005

National Estimated Total = 1,372,910 New Cases*

ALPHA ORDER

RANK	STATE	CASES	% of USA
20	Alabama	24,320	1.8%
50	Alaska	1,930	0.1%
21	Arizona	23,880	1.7%
32	Arkansas	14,950	1.1%
1	California	135,030	9.8%
29	Colorado	16,080	1.2%
28	Connecticut	16,920	1.2%
46	Delaware	3,800	0.3%
2	Florida	96,200	7.0%
11	Georgia	35,650	2.6%
44	Hawaii	4,790	0.3%
42	Idaho	5,490	0.4%
6	Illinois	59,730	4.4%
14	Indiana	31,900	2.3%
30	Iowa	15,910	1.2%
33	Kansas	12,930	0.9%
23	Kentucky	23,020	1.7%
22	Louisiana	23,280	1.7%
38	Maine	7,750	0.6%
19	Maryland	25,450	1.9%
13	Massachusetts	33,030	2.4%
8	Michigan	50,220	3.7%
24	Minnesota	22,890	1.7%
31	Mississippi	14,970	1.1%
16	Missouri	30,210	2.2%
43	Montana	4,910	0.4%
36	Nebraska	8,330	0.6%
35	Nevada	11,120	0.8%
40	New Hampshire	6,310	0.5%
9	New Jersey	43,000	3.1%
37	New Mexico	7,780	0.6%
3	New York	87,050	6.3%
10	North Carolina	40,520	3.0%
47	North Dakota	3,080	0.2%
7	Ohio	59,680	4.3%
26	Oklahoma	18,460	1.3%
27	Oregon	17,720	1.3%
5	Pennsylvania	71,840	5.2%
41	Rhode Island	5,870	0.4%
25	South Carolina	21,860	1.6%
45	South Dakota	3,900	0.3%
15	Tennessee	31,080	2.3%
4	Texas	86,880	6.3%
39	Utah	6,380	0.5%
48	Vermont	3,030	0.2%
12	Virginia	33,680	2.5%
17	Washington	27,350	2.0%
34	West Virginia	11,190	0.8%
18	Wisconsin	26,340	1.9%
49	Wyoming	2,380	0.2%

RANK ORDER

RANK	STATE	CASES	% of USA
1	California	135,030	9.8%
2	Florida	96,200	7.0%
3	New York	87,050	6.3%
4	Texas	86,880	6.3%
5	Pennsylvania	71,840	5.2%
6	Illinois	59,730	4.4%
7	Ohio	59,680	4.3%
8	Michigan	50,220	3.7%
9	New Jersey	43,000	3.1%
10	North Carolina	40,520	3.0%
11	Georgia	35,650	2.6%
12	Virginia	33,680	2.5%
13	Massachusetts	33,030	2.4%
14	Indiana	31,900	2.3%
15	Tennessee	31,080	2.3%
16	Missouri	30,210	2.2%
17	Washington	27,350	2.0%
18	Wisconsin	26,340	1.9%
19	Maryland	25,450	1.9%
20	Alabama	24,320	1.8%
21	Arizona	23,880	1.7%
22	Louisiana	23,280	1.7%
23	Kentucky	23,020	1.7%
24	Minnesota	22,890	1.7%
25	South Carolina	21,860	1.6%
26	Oklahoma	18,460	1.3%
27	Oregon	17,720	1.3%
28	Connecticut	16,920	1.2%
29	Colorado	16,080	1.2%
30	Iowa	15,910	1.2%
31	Mississippi	14,970	1.1%
32	Arkansas	14,950	1.1%
33	Kansas	12,930	0.9%
34	West Virginia	11,190	0.8%
35	Nevada	11,120	0.8%
36	Nebraska	8,330	0.6%
37	New Mexico	7,780	0.6%
38	Maine	7,750	0.6%
39	Utah	6,380	0.5%
40	New Hampshire	6,310	0.5%
41	Rhode Island	5,870	0.4%
42	Idaho	5,490	0.4%
43	Montana	4,910	0.4%
44	Hawaii	4,790	0.3%
45	South Dakota	3,900	0.3%
46	Delaware	3,800	0.3%
47	North Dakota	3,080	0.2%
48	Vermont	3,030	0.2%
49	Wyoming	2,380	0.2%
50	Alaska	1,930	0.1%
	District of Columbia	2,820	0.2%

Source: American Cancer Society
   "Cancer Facts & Figures 2005" (Copyright 2005, American Cancer Society)
*These estimates are offered as a rough guide and should not be regarded as definitive. They are calculated according to the distribution of estimated 2005 cancer deaths by state. Totals do not include basal and squamous cell skin cancers or in situ carcinomas except urinary bladder.

Estimated Rate of New Cancer Cases in 2005

National Estimated Rate = 467.5 New Cases per 100,000 Population*

ALPHA ORDER

RANK	STATE	RATE
9	Alabama	536.8
49	Alaska	294.5
41	Arizona	415.8
7	Arkansas	543.1
47	California	376.2
48	Colorado	349.5
27	Connecticut	482.9
36	Delaware	457.6
5	Florida	553.0
43	Georgia	403.8
46	Hawaii	379.3
44	Idaho	394.0
34	Illinois	469.8
19	Indiana	511.4
8	Iowa	538.5
32	Kansas	472.7
4	Kentucky	555.2
17	Louisiana	515.5
2	Maine	588.3
35	Maryland	457.9
18	Massachusetts	514.8
21	Michigan	496.6
39	Minnesota	448.7
16	Mississippi	515.7
12	Missouri	525.0
10	Montana	529.7
29	Nebraska	476.8
30	Nevada	476.3
25	New Hampshire	485.6
22	New Jersey	494.3
42	New Mexico	408.8
37	New York	452.7
31	North Carolina	474.4
26	North Dakota	485.5
14	Ohio	520.8
13	Oklahoma	523.9
23	Oregon	493.0
3	Pennsylvania	579.1
6	Rhode Island	543.2
15	South Carolina	520.7
20	South Dakota	505.9
11	Tennessee	526.7
45	Texas	386.3
50	Utah	267.1
24	Vermont	487.6
38	Virginia	451.5
40	Washington	440.9
1	West Virginia	616.4
28	Wisconsin	478.1
33	Wyoming	469.9

RANK ORDER

RANK	STATE	RATE
1	West Virginia	616.4
2	Maine	588.3
3	Pennsylvania	579.1
4	Kentucky	555.2
5	Florida	553.0
6	Rhode Island	543.2
7	Arkansas	543.1
8	Iowa	538.5
9	Alabama	536.8
10	Montana	529.7
11	Tennessee	526.7
12	Missouri	525.0
13	Oklahoma	523.9
14	Ohio	520.8
15	South Carolina	520.7
16	Mississippi	515.7
17	Louisiana	515.5
18	Massachusetts	514.8
19	Indiana	511.4
20	South Dakota	505.9
21	Michigan	496.6
22	New Jersey	494.3
23	Oregon	493.0
24	Vermont	487.6
25	New Hampshire	485.6
26	North Dakota	485.5
27	Connecticut	482.9
28	Wisconsin	478.1
29	Nebraska	476.8
30	Nevada	476.3
31	North Carolina	474.4
32	Kansas	472.7
33	Wyoming	469.9
34	Illinois	469.8
35	Maryland	457.9
36	Delaware	457.6
37	New York	452.7
38	Virginia	451.5
39	Minnesota	448.7
40	Washington	440.9
41	Arizona	415.8
42	New Mexico	408.8
43	Georgia	403.8
44	Idaho	394.0
45	Texas	386.3
46	Hawaii	379.3
47	California	376.2
48	Colorado	349.5
49	Alaska	294.5
50	Utah	267.1

District of Columbia   509.5

Source: Morgan Quitno Press using data from American Cancer Society
        "Cancer Facts & Figures 2005" (Copyright 2005, American Cancer Society)
These estimates are offered as a rough guide and should not be regarded as definitive. They are calculated
according to the distribution of estimated 2005 cancer deaths by state. Totals do not include basal and squamous
cell skin cancers or in situ carcinomas except urinary bladder. Rates calculated using 2004 Census resident
population estimates.

Age-Adjusted Cancer Incidence Rates for Males in 2001

National Rate = 566.1 New Cases per 100,000 Male Population*

ALPHA ORDER

RANK	STATE	RATE
37	Alabama	505.5
18	Alaska	560.5
45	Arizona	466.3
30	Arkansas	533.7
33	California	525.4
36	Colorado	518.2
8	Connecticut	594.0
16	Delaware	566.2
14	Florida	569.1
26	Georgia	540.7
42	Hawaii	483.7
35	Idaho	520.0
12	Illinois	573.5
31	Indiana	532.0
19	Iowa	557.2
NA	Kansas**	NA
4	Kentucky	615.3
5	Louisiana	606.1
7	Maine	602.5
17	Maryland	565.0
6	Massachusetts	605.2
3	Michigan	615.4
21	Minnesota	554.3
NA	Mississippi**	NA
27	Missouri	539.3
23	Montana	552.7
25	Nebraska	545.9
40	Nevada	486.9
20	New Hampshire	555.0
2	New Jersey	628.7
44	New Mexico	470.7
15	New York	568.1
34	North Carolina	525.3
41	North Dakota	486.4
22	Ohio	553.6
29	Oklahoma	534.8
24	Oregon	546.3
NA	Pennsylvania**	NA
1	Rhode Island	634.9
11	South Carolina	576.7
39	South Dakota	492.5
NA	Tennessee**	NA
32	Texas	528.2
43	Utah	478.1
NA	Vermont**	NA
38	Virginia	498.7
10	Washington	579.1
9	West Virginia	583.9
13	Wisconsin	573.3
28	Wyoming	536.2

RANK ORDER

RANK	STATE	RATE
1	Rhode Island	634.9
2	New Jersey	628.7
3	Michigan	615.4
4	Kentucky	615.3
5	Louisiana	606.1
6	Massachusetts	605.2
7	Maine	602.5
8	Connecticut	594.0
9	West Virginia	583.9
10	Washington	579.1
11	South Carolina	576.7
12	Illinois	573.5
13	Wisconsin	573.3
14	Florida	569.1
15	New York	568.1
16	Delaware	566.2
17	Maryland	565.0
18	Alaska	560.5
19	Iowa	557.2
20	New Hampshire	555.0
21	Minnesota	554.3
22	Ohio	553.6
23	Montana	552.7
24	Oregon	546.3
25	Nebraska	545.9
26	Georgia	540.7
27	Missouri	539.3
28	Wyoming	536.2
29	Oklahoma	534.8
30	Arkansas	533.7
31	Indiana	532.0
32	Texas	528.2
33	California	525.4
34	North Carolina	525.3
35	Idaho	520.0
36	Colorado	518.2
37	Alabama	505.5
38	Virginia	498.7
39	South Dakota	492.5
40	Nevada	486.9
41	North Dakota	486.4
42	Hawaii	483.7
43	Utah	478.1
44	New Mexico	470.7
45	Arizona	466.3
NA	Kansas**	NA
NA	Mississippi**	NA
NA	Pennsylvania**	NA
NA	Tennessee**	NA
NA	Vermont**	NA
	District of Columbia	667.7

Source: American Cancer Society
    "Cancer Facts & Figures 2005" (Copyright 2005, American Cancer Society)
*For 1997 to 2001. Age-adjusted to the 2000 U.S. standard population.
**Not available.

Age-Adjusted Cancer Incidence Rates for Females in 2001

National Rate = 420.0 New Cases per 100,000 Female Population*

ALPHA ORDER

RANK	STATE	RATE
41	Alabama	353.6
7	Alaska	441.9
38	Arizona	370.3
35	Arkansas	380.4
30	California	394.8
26	Colorado	400.2
4	Connecticut	449.3
11	Delaware	433.0
19	Florida	419.8
37	Georgia	373.5
33	Hawaii	384.4
28	Idaho	396.9
15	Illinois	425.4
25	Indiana	408.3
17	Iowa	421.9
NA	Kansas**	NA
8	Kentucky	440.3
27	Louisiana	397.7
6	Maine	442.1
21	Maryland	411.9
5	Massachusetts	448.1
9	Michigan	435.3
22	Minnesota	410.3
NA	Mississippi**	NA
23	Missouri	409.7
20	Montana	416.1
24	Nebraska	408.6
29	Nevada	395.8
16	New Hampshire	422.1
2	New Jersey	452.3
42	New Mexico	352.9
12	New York	432.7
38	North Carolina	370.3
45	North Dakota	341.3
18	Ohio	420.5
31	Oklahoma	393.5
10	Oregon	435.2
NA	Pennsylvania**	NA
1	Rhode Island	453.3
34	South Carolina	381.0
43	South Dakota	350.0
NA	Tennessee**	NA
36	Texas	377.3
44	Utah	346.1
NA	Vermont**	NA
40	Virginia	362.5
3	Washington	449.8
13	West Virginia	430.3
14	Wisconsin	425.5
32	Wyoming	386.6

RANK ORDER

RANK	STATE	RATE
1	Rhode Island	453.3
2	New Jersey	452.3
3	Washington	449.8
4	Connecticut	449.3
5	Massachusetts	448.1
6	Maine	442.1
7	Alaska	441.9
8	Kentucky	440.3
9	Michigan	435.3
10	Oregon	435.2
11	Delaware	433.0
12	New York	432.7
13	West Virginia	430.3
14	Wisconsin	425.5
15	Illinois	425.4
16	New Hampshire	422.1
17	Iowa	421.9
18	Ohio	420.5
19	Florida	419.8
20	Montana	416.1
21	Maryland	411.9
22	Minnesota	410.3
23	Missouri	409.7
24	Nebraska	408.6
25	Indiana	408.3
26	Colorado	400.2
27	Louisiana	397.7
28	Idaho	396.9
29	Nevada	395.8
30	California	394.8
31	Oklahoma	393.5
32	Wyoming	386.6
33	Hawaii	384.4
34	South Carolina	381.0
35	Arkansas	380.4
36	Texas	377.3
37	Georgia	373.5
38	Arizona	370.3
38	North Carolina	370.3
40	Virginia	362.5
41	Alabama	353.6
42	New Mexico	352.9
43	South Dakota	350.0
44	Utah	346.1
45	North Dakota	341.3
NA	Kansas**	NA
NA	Mississippi**	NA
NA	Pennsylvania**	NA
NA	Tennessee**	NA
NA	Vermont**	NA
	District of Columbia	437.8

Source: American Cancer Society
    "Cancer Facts & Figures 2005" (Copyright 2005, American Cancer Society)
*For 1997 to 2001. Age-adjusted to the 2000 U.S. standard population.
**Not available.

Estimated New Cases of Bladder Cancer in 2005

National Estimated Total = 63,210 New Cases*

ALPHA ORDER

RANK ORDER

RANK	STATE	CASES	% of USA
24	Alabama	860	1.4%
49	Alaska	100	0.2%
17	Arizona	1,200	1.9%
32	Arkansas	620	1.0%
1	California	6,380	10.1%
29	Colorado	720	1.1%
24	Connecticut	860	1.4%
44	Delaware	190	0.3%
2	Florida	4,890	7.7%
12	Georgia	1,530	2.4%
44	Hawaii	190	0.3%
38	Idaho	340	0.5%
7	Illinois	2,640	4.2%
13	Indiana	1,390	2.2%
31	Iowa	670	1.1%
29	Kansas	720	1.1%
23	Kentucky	910	1.4%
28	Louisiana	770	1.2%
36	Maine	430	0.7%
18	Maryland	1,150	1.8%
10	Massachusetts	1,870	3.0%
8	Michigan	2,350	3.7%
18	Minnesota	1,150	1.8%
35	Mississippi	480	0.8%
18	Missouri	1,150	1.8%
43	Montana	240	0.4%
38	Nebraska	340	0.5%
34	Nevada	530	0.8%
37	New Hampshire	380	0.6%
9	New Jersey	2,060	3.3%
38	New Mexico	340	0.5%
3	New York	4,320	6.8%
11	North Carolina	1,580	2.5%
48	North Dakota	140	0.2%
6	Ohio	3,070	4.9%
27	Oklahoma	820	1.3%
22	Oregon	1,010	1.6%
4	Pennsylvania	3,600	5.7%
38	Rhode Island	340	0.5%
24	South Carolina	860	1.4%
44	South Dakota	190	0.3%
18	Tennessee	1,150	1.8%
5	Texas	3,410	5.4%
42	Utah	290	0.5%
44	Vermont	190	0.3%
13	Virginia	1,390	2.2%
16	Washington	1,250	2.0%
33	West Virginia	580	0.9%
15	Wisconsin	1,340	2.1%
49	Wyoming	100	0.2%

RANK	STATE	CASES	% of USA
1	California	6,380	10.1%
2	Florida	4,890	7.7%
3	New York	4,320	6.8%
4	Pennsylvania	3,600	5.7%
5	Texas	3,410	5.4%
6	Ohio	3,070	4.9%
7	Illinois	2,640	4.2%
8	Michigan	2,350	3.7%
9	New Jersey	2,060	3.3%
10	Massachusetts	1,870	3.0%
11	North Carolina	1,580	2.5%
12	Georgia	1,530	2.4%
13	Indiana	1,390	2.2%
13	Virginia	1,390	2.2%
15	Wisconsin	1,340	2.1%
16	Washington	1,250	2.0%
17	Arizona	1,200	1.9%
18	Maryland	1,150	1.8%
18	Minnesota	1,150	1.8%
18	Missouri	1,150	1.8%
18	Tennessee	1,150	1.8%
22	Oregon	1,010	1.6%
23	Kentucky	910	1.4%
24	Alabama	860	1.4%
24	Connecticut	860	1.4%
24	South Carolina	860	1.4%
27	Oklahoma	820	1.3%
28	Louisiana	770	1.2%
29	Colorado	720	1.1%
29	Kansas	720	1.1%
31	Iowa	670	1.1%
32	Arkansas	620	1.0%
33	West Virginia	580	0.9%
34	Nevada	530	0.8%
35	Mississippi	480	0.8%
36	Maine	430	0.7%
37	New Hampshire	380	0.6%
38	Idaho	340	0.5%
38	Nebraska	340	0.5%
38	New Mexico	340	0.5%
38	Rhode Island	340	0.5%
42	Utah	290	0.5%
43	Montana	240	0.4%
44	Delaware	190	0.3%
44	Hawaii	190	0.3%
44	South Dakota	190	0.3%
44	Vermont	190	0.3%
48	North Dakota	140	0.2%
49	Alaska	100	0.2%
49	Wyoming	100	0.2%
	District of Columbia	140	0.2%

Source: American Cancer Society
      "Cancer Facts & Figures 2005" (Copyright 2005, American Cancer Society)
*These estimates are offered as a rough guide and should be interpreted with caution. They are calculated according to the distribution of estimated 2005 cancer deaths by state.

Estimated Rate of New Bladder Cancer Cases in 2005

National Estimated Rate = 21.5 New Cases per 100,000 Population*

ALPHA ORDER

RANK	STATE	RATE
38	Alabama	19.0
47	Alaska	15.3
29	Arizona	20.9
23	Arkansas	22.5
42	California	17.8
46	Colorado	15.6
14	Connecticut	24.5
20	Delaware	22.9
8	Florida	28.1
43	Georgia	17.3
49	Hawaii	15.0
15	Idaho	24.4
30	Illinois	20.8
26	Indiana	22.3
21	Iowa	22.7
11	Kansas	26.3
28	Kentucky	21.9
44	Louisiana	17.1
1	Maine	32.6
31	Maryland	20.7
6	Massachusetts	29.1
19	Michigan	23.2
23	Minnesota	22.5
45	Mississippi	16.5
34	Missouri	20.0
12	Montana	25.9
36	Nebraska	19.5
21	Nevada	22.7
5	New Hampshire	29.2
17	New Jersey	23.7
41	New Mexico	17.9
23	New York	22.5
40	North Carolina	18.5
27	North Dakota	22.1
10	Ohio	26.8
18	Oklahoma	23.3
8	Oregon	28.1
7	Pennsylvania	29.0
3	Rhode Island	31.5
32	South Carolina	20.5
13	South Dakota	24.6
36	Tennessee	19.5
48	Texas	15.2
50	Utah	12.1
4	Vermont	30.6
39	Virginia	18.6
33	Washington	20.1
2	West Virginia	31.9
16	Wisconsin	24.3
35	Wyoming	19.7

RANK ORDER

RANK	STATE	RATE
1	Maine	32.6
2	West Virginia	31.9
3	Rhode Island	31.5
4	Vermont	30.6
5	New Hampshire	29.2
6	Massachusetts	29.1
7	Pennsylvania	29.0
8	Florida	28.1
8	Oregon	28.1
10	Ohio	26.8
11	Kansas	26.3
12	Montana	25.9
13	South Dakota	24.6
14	Connecticut	24.5
15	Idaho	24.4
16	Wisconsin	24.3
17	New Jersey	23.7
18	Oklahoma	23.3
19	Michigan	23.2
20	Delaware	22.9
21	Iowa	22.7
21	Nevada	22.7
23	Arkansas	22.5
23	Minnesota	22.5
23	New York	22.5
26	Indiana	22.3
27	North Dakota	22.1
28	Kentucky	21.9
29	Arizona	20.9
30	Illinois	20.8
31	Maryland	20.7
32	South Carolina	20.5
33	Washington	20.1
34	Missouri	20.0
35	Wyoming	19.7
36	Nebraska	19.5
36	Tennessee	19.5
38	Alabama	19.0
39	Virginia	18.6
40	North Carolina	18.5
41	New Mexico	17.9
42	California	17.8
43	Georgia	17.3
44	Louisiana	17.1
45	Mississippi	16.5
46	Colorado	15.6
47	Alaska	15.3
48	Texas	15.2
49	Hawaii	15.0
50	Utah	12.1
	District of Columbia	25.3

Source: Morgan Quitno Press using data from American Cancer Society
     "Cancer Facts & Figures 2005" (Copyright 2005, American Cancer Society)
*These estimates are offered as a rough guide and should be interpreted with caution. They are calculated according to the distribution of estimated 2005 cancer deaths by state. Rates calculated using 2004 Census resident population estimates.

Estimated New Female Breast Cancer Cases in 2005

National Estimated Total = 211,240 New Cases*

ALPHA ORDER

RANK	STATE	CASES	% of USA
21	Alabama	3,820	1.8%
49	Alaska	260	0.1%
22	Arizona	3,760	1.8%
32	Arkansas	2,090	1.0%
1	California	21,170	10.0%
29	Colorado	2,560	1.2%
27	Connecticut	2,720	1.3%
45	Delaware	630	0.3%
3	Florida	13,430	6.4%
12	Georgia	5,850	2.8%
43	Hawaii	680	0.3%
39	Idaho	940	0.4%
7	Illinois	9,300	4.4%
14	Indiana	4,600	2.2%
31	Iowa	2,300	1.1%
33	Kansas	1,990	0.9%
23	Kentucky	3,290	1.6%
20	Louisiana	3,870	1.8%
40	Maine	890	0.4%
16	Maryland	4,390	2.1%
13	Massachusetts	4,910	2.3%
9	Michigan	7,210	3.4%
25	Minnesota	3,240	1.5%
30	Mississippi	2,350	1.1%
15	Missouri	4,550	2.2%
43	Montana	680	0.3%
36	Nebraska	1,200	0.6%
34	Nevada	1,620	0.8%
40	New Hampshire	890	0.4%
8	New Jersey	7,740	3.7%
38	New Mexico	990	0.5%
2	New York	14,430	6.8%
10	North Carolina	6,330	3.0%
46	North Dakota	520	0.2%
6	Ohio	9,670	4.6%
26	Oklahoma	2,820	1.3%
28	Oregon	2,610	1.2%
5	Pennsylvania	11,340	5.4%
42	Rhode Island	780	0.4%
23	South Carolina	3,290	1.6%
46	South Dakota	520	0.2%
17	Tennessee	4,230	2.0%
4	Texas	12,860	6.1%
37	Utah	1,150	0.5%
48	Vermont	470	0.2%
11	Virginia	6,010	2.8%
19	Washington	3,920	1.9%
35	West Virginia	1,410	0.7%
18	Wisconsin	4,130	2.0%
49	Wyoming	260	0.1%

RANK ORDER

RANK	STATE	CASES	% of USA
1	California	21,170	10.0%
2	New York	14,430	6.8%
3	Florida	13,430	6.4%
4	Texas	12,860	6.1%
5	Pennsylvania	11,340	5.4%
6	Ohio	9,670	4.6%
7	Illinois	9,300	4.4%
8	New Jersey	7,740	3.7%
9	Michigan	7,210	3.4%
10	North Carolina	6,330	3.0%
11	Virginia	6,010	2.8%
12	Georgia	5,850	2.8%
13	Massachusetts	4,910	2.3%
14	Indiana	4,600	2.2%
15	Missouri	4,550	2.2%
16	Maryland	4,390	2.1%
17	Tennessee	4,230	2.0%
18	Wisconsin	4,130	2.0%
19	Washington	3,920	1.9%
20	Louisiana	3,870	1.8%
21	Alabama	3,820	1.8%
22	Arizona	3,760	1.8%
23	Kentucky	3,290	1.6%
23	South Carolina	3,290	1.6%
25	Minnesota	3,240	1.5%
26	Oklahoma	2,820	1.3%
27	Connecticut	2,720	1.3%
28	Oregon	2,610	1.2%
29	Colorado	2,560	1.2%
30	Mississippi	2,350	1.1%
31	Iowa	2,300	1.1%
32	Arkansas	2,090	1.0%
33	Kansas	1,990	0.9%
34	Nevada	1,620	0.8%
35	West Virginia	1,410	0.7%
36	Nebraska	1,200	0.6%
37	Utah	1,150	0.5%
38	New Mexico	990	0.5%
39	Idaho	940	0.4%
40	Maine	890	0.4%
40	New Hampshire	890	0.4%
42	Rhode Island	780	0.4%
43	Hawaii	680	0.3%
43	Montana	680	0.3%
45	Delaware	630	0.3%
46	North Dakota	520	0.2%
46	South Dakota	520	0.2%
48	Vermont	470	0.2%
49	Alaska	260	0.1%
49	Wyoming	260	0.1%
	District of Columbia	520	0.2%

Source: American Cancer Society
    "Cancer Facts & Figures 2005" (Copyright 2005, American Cancer Society)
*These estimates are offered as a rough guide and should be interpreted with caution. They are calculated
according to the distribution of estimated 2005 cancer deaths by state.

Age-Adjusted Incidence Rate of Female Breast Cancer Cases in 2001

National Rate = 132.2 New Cases per 100,000 Female Population*

ALPHA ORDER

RANK	STATE	RATE
44	Alabama	114.4
5	Alaska	139.0
36	Arizona	121.9
35	Arkansas	122.5
16	California	133.1
8	Colorado	135.8
3	Connecticut	143.8
12	Delaware	134.0
29	Florida	126.5
37	Georgia	121.7
11	Hawaii	134.2
24	Idaho	130.0
14	Illinois	133.4
26	Indiana	127.4
20	Iowa	131.5
NA	Kansas**	NA
27	Kentucky	127.2
34	Louisiana	122.9
22	Maine	131.4
17	Maryland	132.9
4	Massachusetts	143.4
13	Michigan	133.5
6	Minnesota	138.5
NA	Mississippi**	NA
28	Missouri	126.7
14	Montana	133.4
18	Nebraska	132.1
45	Nevada	113.8
10	New Hampshire	135.4
7	New Jersey	138.2
43	New Mexico	116.2
23	New York	130.9
32	North Carolina	123.2
42	North Dakota	117.4
20	Ohio	131.5
25	Oklahoma	128.5
2	Oregon	145.8
NA	Pennsylvania**	NA
19	Rhode Island	131.7
32	South Carolina	123.2
30	South Dakota	125.5
NA	Tennessee**	NA
41	Texas	118.9
39	Utah	119.4
NA	Vermont**	NA
31	Virginia	123.7
1	Washington	148.8
40	West Virginia	119.2
9	Wisconsin	135.6
38	Wyoming	121.5

RANK ORDER

RANK	STATE	RATE
1	Washington	148.8
2	Oregon	145.8
3	Connecticut	143.8
4	Massachusetts	143.4
5	Alaska	139.0
6	Minnesota	138.5
7	New Jersey	138.2
8	Colorado	135.8
9	Wisconsin	135.6
10	New Hampshire	135.4
11	Hawaii	134.2
12	Delaware	134.0
13	Michigan	133.5
14	Illinois	133.4
14	Montana	133.4
16	California	133.1
17	Maryland	132.9
18	Nebraska	132.1
19	Rhode Island	131.7
20	Iowa	131.5
20	Ohio	131.5
22	Maine	131.4
23	New York	130.9
24	Idaho	130.0
25	Oklahoma	128.5
26	Indiana	127.4
27	Kentucky	127.2
28	Missouri	126.7
29	Florida	126.5
30	South Dakota	125.5
31	Virginia	123.7
32	North Carolina	123.2
32	South Carolina	123.2
34	Louisiana	122.9
35	Arkansas	122.5
36	Arizona	121.9
37	Georgia	121.7
38	Wyoming	121.5
39	Utah	119.4
40	West Virginia	119.2
41	Texas	118.9
42	North Dakota	117.4
43	New Mexico	116.2
44	Alabama	114.4
45	Nevada	113.8
NA	Kansas**	NA
NA	Mississippi**	NA
NA	Pennsylvania**	NA
NA	Tennessee**	NA
NA	Vermont**	NA
	District of Columbia	143.3

Source: American Cancer Society
    "Cancer Facts & Figures 2005" (Copyright 2005, American Cancer Society)
*For 1997 to 2001. Age-adjusted to the 2000 U.S. standard population.
**Not available.

Percent of Women Who Have Ever Had a Mammogram: 2002

National Median = 63.4% of Women*

ALPHA ORDER

RANK	STATE	PERCENT
9	Alabama	66.6
48	Alaska	58.5
12	Arizona	66.1
41	Arkansas	62.0
47	California	59.1
42	Colorado	61.3
3	Connecticut	67.7
2	Delaware	69.1
1	Florida	69.5
32	Georgia	62.9
46	Hawaii	60.1
49	Idaho	57.8
32	Illinois	62.9
30	Indiana	63.3
15	Iowa	64.9
38	Kansas	62.2
18	Kentucky	64.8
21	Louisiana	64.1
4	Maine	67.4
13	Maryland	65.5
20	Massachusetts	64.4
11	Michigan	66.2
28	Minnesota	63.4
28	Mississippi	63.4
22	Missouri	64.0
24	Montana	63.8
38	Nebraska	62.2
31	Nevada	63.0
15	New Hampshire	64.9
23	New Jersey	63.9
44	New Mexico	60.4
26	New York	63.5
15	North Carolina	64.9
19	North Dakota	64.5
10	Ohio	66.4
38	Oklahoma	62.2
14	Oregon	65.1
7	Pennsylvania	66.9
8	Rhode Island	66.8
5	South Carolina	67.3
37	South Dakota	62.4
26	Tennessee	63.5
45	Texas	60.2
50	Utah	51.4
34	Vermont	62.7
25	Virginia	63.7
36	Washington	62.6
5	West Virginia	67.3
34	Wisconsin	62.7
43	Wyoming	60.5

RANK ORDER

RANK	STATE	PERCENT
1	Florida	69.5
2	Delaware	69.1
3	Connecticut	67.7
4	Maine	67.4
5	South Carolina	67.3
5	West Virginia	67.3
7	Pennsylvania	66.9
8	Rhode Island	66.8
9	Alabama	66.6
10	Ohio	66.4
11	Michigan	66.2
12	Arizona	66.1
13	Maryland	65.5
14	Oregon	65.1
15	Iowa	64.9
15	New Hampshire	64.9
15	North Carolina	64.9
18	Kentucky	64.8
19	North Dakota	64.5
20	Massachusetts	64.4
21	Louisiana	64.1
22	Missouri	64.0
23	New Jersey	63.9
24	Montana	63.8
25	Virginia	63.7
26	New York	63.5
26	Tennessee	63.5
28	Minnesota	63.4
28	Mississippi	63.4
30	Indiana	63.3
31	Nevada	63.0
32	Georgia	62.9
32	Illinois	62.9
34	Vermont	62.7
34	Wisconsin	62.7
36	Washington	62.6
37	South Dakota	62.4
38	Kansas	62.2
38	Nebraska	62.2
38	Oklahoma	62.2
41	Arkansas	62.0
42	Colorado	61.3
43	Wyoming	60.5
44	New Mexico	60.4
45	Texas	60.2
46	Hawaii	60.1
47	California	59.1
48	Alaska	58.5
49	Idaho	57.8
50	Utah	51.4
	District of Columbia	61.4

Source: U.S. Department of Health and Human Services, Centers for Disease Control and Prevention
*   "2002 Behavioral Risk Factor Surveillance Summary Prevalence Data" (http://apps.nccd.cdc.gov/brfss/)*
Percent of women 18 years and older.

Estimated New Colon and Rectum Cancer Cases in 2005

National Estimated Total = 145,290 New Cases*

ALPHA ORDER

RANK	STATE	CASES	% of USA
23	Alabama	2,300	1.6%
50	Alaska	210	0.1%
21	Arizona	2,500	1.7%
31	Arkansas	1,630	1.1%
1	California	14,070	9.7%
30	Colorado	1,650	1.1%
29	Connecticut	1,680	1.2%
46	Delaware	410	0.3%
2	Florida	9,860	6.8%
13	Georgia	3,480	2.4%
42	Hawaii	540	0.4%
42	Idaho	540	0.4%
6	Illinois	6,610	4.5%
14	Indiana	3,410	2.3%
28	Iowa	1,700	1.2%
33	Kansas	1,570	1.1%
22	Kentucky	2,350	1.6%
20	Louisiana	2,580	1.8%
38	Maine	800	0.6%
17	Maryland	2,760	1.9%
11	Massachusetts	3,560	2.5%
8	Michigan	4,830	3.3%
25	Minnesota	2,220	1.5%
31	Mississippi	1,630	1.1%
15	Missouri	3,230	2.2%
44	Montana	460	0.3%
36	Nebraska	1,030	0.7%
35	Nevada	1,240	0.9%
41	New Hampshire	620	0.4%
9	New Jersey	4,670	3.2%
37	New Mexico	880	0.6%
3	New York	9,700	6.7%
10	North Carolina	4,100	2.8%
47	North Dakota	360	0.2%
7	Ohio	6,500	4.5%
26	Oklahoma	2,010	1.4%
27	Oregon	1,760	1.2%
5	Pennsylvania	8,130	5.6%
40	Rhode Island	650	0.4%
23	South Carolina	2,300	1.6%
44	South Dakota	460	0.3%
16	Tennessee	3,150	2.2%
4	Texas	9,270	6.4%
39	Utah	670	0.5%
48	Vermont	340	0.2%
11	Virginia	3,560	2.5%
19	Washington	2,660	1.8%
34	West Virginia	1,260	0.9%
17	Wisconsin	2,760	1.9%
49	Wyoming	280	0.2%

RANK ORDER

RANK	STATE	CASES	% of USA
1	California	14,070	9.7%
2	Florida	9,860	6.8%
3	New York	9,700	6.7%
4	Texas	9,270	6.4%
5	Pennsylvania	8,130	5.6%
6	Illinois	6,610	4.5%
7	Ohio	6,500	4.5%
8	Michigan	4,830	3.3%
9	New Jersey	4,670	3.2%
10	North Carolina	4,100	2.8%
11	Massachusetts	3,560	2.5%
11	Virginia	3,560	2.5%
13	Georgia	3,480	2.4%
14	Indiana	3,410	2.3%
15	Missouri	3,230	2.2%
16	Tennessee	3,150	2.2%
17	Maryland	2,760	1.9%
17	Wisconsin	2,760	1.9%
19	Washington	2,660	1.8%
20	Louisiana	2,580	1.8%
21	Arizona	2,500	1.7%
22	Kentucky	2,350	1.6%
23	Alabama	2,300	1.6%
23	South Carolina	2,300	1.6%
25	Minnesota	2,220	1.5%
26	Oklahoma	2,010	1.4%
27	Oregon	1,760	1.2%
28	Iowa	1,700	1.2%
29	Connecticut	1,680	1.2%
30	Colorado	1,650	1.1%
31	Arkansas	1,630	1.1%
31	Mississippi	1,630	1.1%
33	Kansas	1,570	1.1%
34	West Virginia	1,260	0.9%
35	Nevada	1,240	0.9%
36	Nebraska	1,030	0.7%
37	New Mexico	880	0.6%
38	Maine	800	0.6%
39	Utah	670	0.5%
40	Rhode Island	650	0.4%
41	New Hampshire	620	0.4%
42	Hawaii	540	0.4%
42	Idaho	540	0.4%
44	Montana	460	0.3%
44	South Dakota	460	0.3%
46	Delaware	410	0.3%
47	North Dakota	360	0.2%
48	Vermont	340	0.2%
49	Wyoming	280	0.2%
50	Alaska	210	0.1%
	District of Columbia	340	0.2%

Source: American Cancer Society
      "Cancer Facts & Figures 2005" (Copyright 2005, American Cancer Society)
*These estimates are offered as a rough guide and should be interpreted with caution. They are calculated according to the distribution of estimated 2005 cancer deaths by state.

Estimated Rate of New Colon and Rectum Cancer Cases in 2005

National Estimated Rate = 49.5 New Cases per 100,000 Population*

ALPHA ORDER

RANK	STATE	RATE
27	Alabama	50.8
49	Alaska	32.0
40	Arizona	43.5
6	Arkansas	59.2
46	California	39.2
48	Colorado	35.9
34	Connecticut	48.0
32	Delaware	49.4
12	Florida	56.7
45	Georgia	39.4
43	Hawaii	42.8
47	Idaho	38.8
26	Illinois	52.0
21	Indiana	54.7
8	Iowa	57.5
9	Kansas	57.4
12	Kentucky	56.7
10	Louisiana	57.1
3	Maine	60.7
30	Maryland	49.7
18	Massachusetts	55.5
36	Michigan	47.8
40	Minnesota	43.5
16	Mississippi	56.1
16	Missouri	56.1
31	Montana	49.6
7	Nebraska	59.0
25	Nevada	53.1
37	New Hampshire	47.7
23	New Jersey	53.7
39	New Mexico	46.2
28	New York	50.4
34	North Carolina	48.0
12	North Dakota	56.7
12	Ohio	56.7
11	Oklahoma	57.0
33	Oregon	49.0
2	Pennsylvania	65.5
4	Rhode Island	60.1
20	South Carolina	54.8
5	South Dakota	59.7
24	Tennessee	53.4
44	Texas	41.2
50	Utah	28.0
21	Vermont	54.7
37	Virginia	47.7
42	Washington	42.9
1	West Virginia	69.4
29	Wisconsin	50.1
19	Wyoming	55.3

RANK ORDER

RANK	STATE	RATE
1	West Virginia	69.4
2	Pennsylvania	65.5
3	Maine	60.7
4	Rhode Island	60.1
5	South Dakota	59.7
6	Arkansas	59.2
7	Nebraska	59.0
8	Iowa	57.5
9	Kansas	57.4
10	Louisiana	57.1
11	Oklahoma	57.0
12	Florida	56.7
12	Kentucky	56.7
12	North Dakota	56.7
12	Ohio	56.7
16	Mississippi	56.1
16	Missouri	56.1
18	Massachusetts	55.5
19	Wyoming	55.3
20	South Carolina	54.8
21	Indiana	54.7
21	Vermont	54.7
23	New Jersey	53.7
24	Tennessee	53.4
25	Nevada	53.1
26	Illinois	52.0
27	Alabama	50.8
28	New York	50.4
29	Wisconsin	50.1
30	Maryland	49.7
31	Montana	49.6
32	Delaware	49.4
33	Oregon	49.0
34	Connecticut	48.0
34	North Carolina	48.0
36	Michigan	47.8
37	New Hampshire	47.7
37	Virginia	47.7
39	New Mexico	46.2
40	Arizona	43.5
40	Minnesota	43.5
42	Washington	42.9
43	Hawaii	42.8
44	Texas	41.2
45	Georgia	39.4
46	California	39.2
47	Idaho	38.8
48	Colorado	35.9
49	Alaska	32.0
50	Utah	28.0
	District of Columbia	61.4

Source: Morgan Quitno Press using data from American Cancer Society
"Cancer Facts & Figures 2005" (Copyright 2005, American Cancer Society)
*These estimates are offered as a rough guide and should be interpreted with caution. They are calculated according to the distribution of estimated 2005 cancer deaths by state. Rates calculated using 2004 Census resident population estimates.

Percent of Adults Receiving Recent Sigmoidoscopy or Colonoscopy Exam: 2002
National Median = 48.1% of Adults*

<table>
<tr><td colspan="3">ALPHA ORDER</td><td colspan="3">RANK ORDER</td></tr>
<tr><td>RANK</td><td>STATE</td><td>PERCENT</td><td>RANK</td><td>STATE</td><td>PERCENT</td></tr>
<tr><td>23</td><td>Alabama</td><td>48.7</td><td>1</td><td>Minnesota</td><td>64.8</td></tr>
<tr><td>15</td><td>Alaska</td><td>51.4</td><td>2</td><td>Delaware</td><td>57.4</td></tr>
<tr><td>12</td><td>Arizona</td><td>51.8</td><td>3</td><td>Connecticut</td><td>56.4</td></tr>
<tr><td>42</td><td>Arkansas</td><td>42.9</td><td>3</td><td>Wisconsin</td><td>56.4</td></tr>
<tr><td>16</td><td>California</td><td>50.7</td><td>5</td><td>Michigan</td><td>55.1</td></tr>
<tr><td>23</td><td>Colorado</td><td>48.7</td><td>6</td><td>Maryland</td><td>54.8</td></tr>
<tr><td>3</td><td>Connecticut</td><td>56.4</td><td>7</td><td>Washington</td><td>54.7</td></tr>
<tr><td>2</td><td>Delaware</td><td>57.4</td><td>8</td><td>Rhode Island</td><td>54.6</td></tr>
<tr><td>13</td><td>Florida</td><td>51.5</td><td>9</td><td>Massachusetts</td><td>53.4</td></tr>
<tr><td>21</td><td>Georgia</td><td>49.2</td><td>10</td><td>Vermont</td><td>52.9</td></tr>
<tr><td>50</td><td>Hawaii</td><td>39.2</td><td>11</td><td>Oregon</td><td>52.7</td></tr>
<tr><td>32</td><td>Idaho</td><td>46.3</td><td>12</td><td>Arizona</td><td>51.8</td></tr>
<tr><td>37</td><td>Illinois</td><td>45.1</td><td>13</td><td>Florida</td><td>51.5</td></tr>
<tr><td>40</td><td>Indiana</td><td>44.1</td><td>13</td><td>New York</td><td>51.5</td></tr>
<tr><td>25</td><td>Iowa</td><td>48.6</td><td>15</td><td>Alaska</td><td>51.4</td></tr>
<tr><td>29</td><td>Kansas</td><td>47.7</td><td>16</td><td>California</td><td>50.7</td></tr>
<tr><td>41</td><td>Kentucky</td><td>43.9</td><td>17</td><td>Utah</td><td>50.5</td></tr>
<tr><td>48</td><td>Louisiana</td><td>40.6</td><td>18</td><td>North Dakota</td><td>50.2</td></tr>
<tr><td>30</td><td>Maine</td><td>47.3</td><td>19</td><td>New Hampshire</td><td>50.1</td></tr>
<tr><td>6</td><td>Maryland</td><td>54.8</td><td>19</td><td>Virginia</td><td>50.1</td></tr>
<tr><td>9</td><td>Massachusetts</td><td>53.4</td><td>21</td><td>Georgia</td><td>49.2</td></tr>
<tr><td>5</td><td>Michigan</td><td>55.1</td><td>21</td><td>South Carolina</td><td>49.2</td></tr>
<tr><td>1</td><td>Minnesota</td><td>64.8</td><td>23</td><td>Alabama</td><td>48.7</td></tr>
<tr><td>42</td><td>Mississippi</td><td>42.9</td><td>23</td><td>Colorado</td><td>48.7</td></tr>
<tr><td>38</td><td>Missouri</td><td>44.2</td><td>25</td><td>Iowa</td><td>48.6</td></tr>
<tr><td>30</td><td>Montana</td><td>47.3</td><td>26</td><td>New Jersey</td><td>48.2</td></tr>
<tr><td>44</td><td>Nebraska</td><td>42.2</td><td>27</td><td>Pennsylvania</td><td>48.0</td></tr>
<tr><td>36</td><td>Nevada</td><td>45.4</td><td>28</td><td>North Carolina</td><td>47.8</td></tr>
<tr><td>19</td><td>New Hampshire</td><td>50.1</td><td>29</td><td>Kansas</td><td>47.7</td></tr>
<tr><td>26</td><td>New Jersey</td><td>48.2</td><td>30</td><td>Maine</td><td>47.3</td></tr>
<tr><td>38</td><td>New Mexico</td><td>44.2</td><td>30</td><td>Montana</td><td>47.3</td></tr>
<tr><td>13</td><td>New York</td><td>51.5</td><td>32</td><td>Idaho</td><td>46.3</td></tr>
<tr><td>28</td><td>North Carolina</td><td>47.8</td><td>33</td><td>Tennessee</td><td>46.1</td></tr>
<tr><td>18</td><td>North Dakota</td><td>50.2</td><td>34</td><td>Ohio</td><td>46.0</td></tr>
<tr><td>34</td><td>Ohio</td><td>46.0</td><td>35</td><td>Texas</td><td>45.5</td></tr>
<tr><td>47</td><td>Oklahoma</td><td>40.7</td><td>36</td><td>Nevada</td><td>45.4</td></tr>
<tr><td>11</td><td>Oregon</td><td>52.7</td><td>37</td><td>Illinois</td><td>45.1</td></tr>
<tr><td>27</td><td>Pennsylvania</td><td>48.0</td><td>38</td><td>Missouri</td><td>44.2</td></tr>
<tr><td>8</td><td>Rhode Island</td><td>54.6</td><td>38</td><td>New Mexico</td><td>44.2</td></tr>
<tr><td>21</td><td>South Carolina</td><td>49.2</td><td>40</td><td>Indiana</td><td>44.1</td></tr>
<tr><td>46</td><td>South Dakota</td><td>41.8</td><td>41</td><td>Kentucky</td><td>43.9</td></tr>
<tr><td>33</td><td>Tennessee</td><td>46.1</td><td>42</td><td>Arkansas</td><td>42.9</td></tr>
<tr><td>35</td><td>Texas</td><td>45.5</td><td>42</td><td>Mississippi</td><td>42.9</td></tr>
<tr><td>17</td><td>Utah</td><td>50.5</td><td>44</td><td>Nebraska</td><td>42.2</td></tr>
<tr><td>10</td><td>Vermont</td><td>52.9</td><td>45</td><td>Wyoming</td><td>42.1</td></tr>
<tr><td>19</td><td>Virginia</td><td>50.1</td><td>46</td><td>South Dakota</td><td>41.8</td></tr>
<tr><td>7</td><td>Washington</td><td>54.7</td><td>47</td><td>Oklahoma</td><td>40.7</td></tr>
<tr><td>49</td><td>West Virginia</td><td>40.4</td><td>48</td><td>Louisiana</td><td>40.6</td></tr>
<tr><td>3</td><td>Wisconsin</td><td>56.4</td><td>49</td><td>West Virginia</td><td>40.4</td></tr>
<tr><td>45</td><td>Wyoming</td><td>42.1</td><td>50</td><td>Hawaii</td><td>39.2</td></tr>
<tr><td></td><td></td><td></td><td></td><td>District of Columbia</td><td>61.4</td></tr>
</table>

Source: U.S. Department of Health and Human Services, Centers for Disease Control and Prevention
   "2002 Behavioral Risk Factor Surveillance Summary Prevalence Data" (http://apps.nccd.cdc.gov/brfss/)
*Persons 50 and older.

Estimated New Leukemia Cases in 2005

National Estimated Total = 34,810 New Cases*

ALPHA ORDER

RANK	STATE	CASES	% of USA
22	Alabama	560	1.6%
50	Alaska	50	0.1%
21	Arizona	620	1.8%
30	Arkansas	400	1.1%
1	California	3,380	9.7%
27	Colorado	460	1.3%
30	Connecticut	400	1.1%
43	Delaware	120	0.3%
2	Florida	2,620	7.5%
13	Georgia	820	2.4%
43	Hawaii	120	0.3%
40	Idaho	150	0.4%
6	Illinois	1,620	4.7%
13	Indiana	820	2.4%
26	Iowa	480	1.4%
33	Kansas	350	1.0%
25	Kentucky	490	1.4%
23	Louisiana	540	1.6%
40	Maine	150	0.4%
19	Maryland	680	2.0%
15	Massachusetts	770	2.2%
8	Michigan	1,250	3.6%
20	Minnesota	660	1.9%
32	Mississippi	370	1.1%
11	Missouri	830	2.4%
42	Montana	140	0.4%
35	Nebraska	250	0.7%
34	Nevada	260	0.7%
38	New Hampshire	170	0.5%
9	New Jersey	1,100	3.2%
38	New Mexico	170	0.5%
4	New York	2,170	6.2%
10	North Carolina	990	2.8%
46	North Dakota	110	0.3%
7	Ohio	1,510	4.3%
27	Oklahoma	460	1.3%
29	Oregon	420	1.2%
5	Pennsylvania	1,630	4.7%
43	Rhode Island	120	0.3%
24	South Carolina	510	1.5%
46	South Dakota	110	0.3%
17	Tennessee	760	2.2%
3	Texas	2,250	6.5%
36	Utah	220	0.6%
48	Vermont	90	0.3%
11	Virginia	830	2.4%
18	Washington	720	2.1%
36	West Virginia	220	0.6%
15	Wisconsin	770	2.2%
49	Wyoming	60	0.2%

RANK ORDER

RANK	STATE	CASES	% of USA
1	California	3,380	9.7%
2	Florida	2,620	7.5%
3	Texas	2,250	6.5%
4	New York	2,170	6.2%
5	Pennsylvania	1,630	4.7%
6	Illinois	1,620	4.7%
7	Ohio	1,510	4.3%
8	Michigan	1,250	3.6%
9	New Jersey	1,100	3.2%
10	North Carolina	990	2.8%
11	Missouri	830	2.4%
11	Virginia	830	2.4%
13	Georgia	820	2.4%
13	Indiana	820	2.4%
15	Massachusetts	770	2.2%
15	Wisconsin	770	2.2%
17	Tennessee	760	2.2%
18	Washington	720	2.1%
19	Maryland	680	2.0%
20	Minnesota	660	1.9%
21	Arizona	620	1.8%
22	Alabama	560	1.6%
23	Louisiana	540	1.6%
24	South Carolina	510	1.5%
25	Kentucky	490	1.4%
26	Iowa	480	1.4%
27	Colorado	460	1.3%
27	Oklahoma	460	1.3%
29	Oregon	420	1.2%
30	Arkansas	400	1.1%
30	Connecticut	400	1.1%
32	Mississippi	370	1.1%
33	Kansas	350	1.0%
34	Nevada	260	0.7%
35	Nebraska	250	0.7%
36	Utah	220	0.6%
36	West Virginia	220	0.6%
38	New Hampshire	170	0.5%
38	New Mexico	170	0.5%
40	Idaho	150	0.4%
40	Maine	150	0.4%
42	Montana	140	0.4%
43	Delaware	120	0.3%
43	Hawaii	120	0.3%
43	Rhode Island	120	0.3%
46	North Dakota	110	0.3%
46	South Dakota	110	0.3%
48	Vermont	90	0.3%
49	Wyoming	60	0.2%
50	Alaska	50	0.1%
	District of Columbia	50	0.1%

Source: American Cancer Society
    "Cancer Facts & Figures 2005" (Copyright 2005, American Cancer Society)
*These estimates are offered as a rough guide and should be interpreted with caution. They are calculated according to the distribution of estimated 2005 cancer deaths by state.
**Not available.

Estimated Rate of New Leukemia Cases in 2005

National Estimated Rate = 11.9 New Cases per 100,000 Population*

ALPHA ORDER

RANK	STATE	RATE
23	Alabama	12.4
50	Alaska	7.6
41	Arizona	10.8
5	Arkansas	14.5
46	California	9.4
43	Colorado	10.0
35	Connecticut	11.4
5	Delaware	14.5
3	Florida	15.1
47	Georgia	9.3
45	Hawaii	9.5
41	Idaho	10.8
20	Illinois	12.7
13	Indiana	13.1
2	Iowa	16.2
19	Kansas	12.8
30	Kentucky	11.8
28	Louisiana	12.0
35	Maine	11.4
25	Maryland	12.2
28	Massachusetts	12.0
23	Michigan	12.4
17	Minnesota	12.9
20	Mississippi	12.7
8	Missouri	14.4
3	Montana	15.1
9	Nebraska	14.3
38	Nevada	11.1
13	New Hampshire	13.1
22	New Jersey	12.6
49	New Mexico	8.9
37	New York	11.3
33	North Carolina	11.6
1	North Dakota	17.3
12	Ohio	13.2
13	Oklahoma	13.1
32	Oregon	11.7
13	Pennsylvania	13.1
38	Rhode Island	11.1
26	South Carolina	12.1
9	South Dakota	14.3
17	Tennessee	12.9
43	Texas	10.0
48	Utah	9.2
5	Vermont	14.5
38	Virginia	11.1
33	Washington	11.6
26	West Virginia	12.1
11	Wisconsin	14.0
30	Wyoming	11.8

RANK ORDER

RANK	STATE	RATE
1	North Dakota	17.3
2	Iowa	16.2
3	Florida	15.1
3	Montana	15.1
5	Arkansas	14.5
5	Delaware	14.5
5	Vermont	14.5
8	Missouri	14.4
9	Nebraska	14.3
9	South Dakota	14.3
11	Wisconsin	14.0
12	Ohio	13.2
13	Indiana	13.1
13	New Hampshire	13.1
13	Oklahoma	13.1
13	Pennsylvania	13.1
17	Minnesota	12.9
17	Tennessee	12.9
19	Kansas	12.8
20	Illinois	12.7
20	Mississippi	12.7
22	New Jersey	12.6
23	Alabama	12.4
23	Michigan	12.4
25	Maryland	12.2
26	South Carolina	12.1
26	West Virginia	12.1
28	Louisiana	12.0
28	Massachusetts	12.0
30	Kentucky	11.8
30	Wyoming	11.8
32	Oregon	11.7
33	North Carolina	11.6
33	Washington	11.6
35	Connecticut	11.4
35	Maine	11.4
37	New York	11.3
38	Nevada	11.1
38	Rhode Island	11.1
38	Virginia	11.1
41	Arizona	10.8
41	Idaho	10.8
43	Colorado	10.0
43	Texas	10.0
45	Hawaii	9.5
46	California	9.4
47	Georgia	9.3
48	Utah	9.2
49	New Mexico	8.9
50	Alaska	7.6

District of Columbia	9.0

Source: Morgan Quitno Press using data from American Cancer Society
   "Cancer Facts & Figures 2005" (Copyright 2005, American Cancer Society)
*These estimates are offered as a rough guide and should be interpreted with caution. They are calculated according to the distribution of estimated 2005 cancer deaths by state. Rates calculated using 2004 Census resident population estimates.

Estimated New Lung Cancer Cases in 2005

National Estimated Total = 172,570 New Cases*

ALPHA ORDER

RANK	STATE	CASES	% of USA
19	Alabama	3,340	1.9%
50	Alaska	220	0.1%
24	Arizona	2,870	1.7%
27	Arkansas	2,530	1.5%
1	California	15,150	8.8%
32	Colorado	1,750	1.0%
30	Connecticut	1,950	1.1%
44	Delaware	490	0.3%
2	Florida	13,130	7.6%
11	Georgia	4,800	2.8%
43	Hawaii	510	0.3%
41	Idaho	630	0.4%
7	Illinois	7,220	4.2%
13	Indiana	4,410	2.6%
31	Iowa	1,790	1.0%
34	Kansas	1,630	0.9%
17	Kentucky	3,680	2.1%
21	Louisiana	3,090	1.8%
37	Maine	990	0.6%
20	Maryland	3,210	1.9%
16	Massachusetts	4,010	2.3%
8	Michigan	6,110	3.5%
25	Minnesota	2,620	1.5%
28	Mississippi	2,180	1.3%
15	Missouri	4,070	2.4%
42	Montana	620	0.4%
36	Nebraska	1,000	0.6%
35	Nevada	1,530	0.9%
38	New Hampshire	790	0.5%
10	New Jersey	4,830	2.8%
39	New Mexico	760	0.4%
4	New York	9,870	5.7%
9	North Carolina	5,520	3.2%
48	North Dakota	330	0.2%
6	Ohio	7,790	4.5%
26	Oklahoma	2,580	1.5%
29	Oregon	2,160	1.3%
5	Pennsylvania	8,470	4.9%
40	Rhode Island	720	0.4%
23	South Carolina	2,880	1.7%
46	South Dakota	430	0.2%
12	Tennessee	4,630	2.7%
3	Texas	11,210	6.5%
45	Utah	460	0.3%
47	Vermont	390	0.2%
14	Virginia	4,400	2.5%
18	Washington	3,440	2.0%
33	West Virginia	1,700	1.0%
22	Wisconsin	3,060	1.8%
49	Wyoming	280	0.2%

RANK ORDER

RANK	STATE	CASES	% of USA
1	California	15,150	8.8%
2	Florida	13,130	7.6%
3	Texas	11,210	6.5%
4	New York	9,870	5.7%
5	Pennsylvania	8,470	4.9%
6	Ohio	7,790	4.5%
7	Illinois	7,220	4.2%
8	Michigan	6,110	3.5%
9	North Carolina	5,520	3.2%
10	New Jersey	4,830	2.8%
11	Georgia	4,800	2.8%
12	Tennessee	4,630	2.7%
13	Indiana	4,410	2.6%
14	Virginia	4,400	2.5%
15	Missouri	4,070	2.4%
16	Massachusetts	4,010	2.3%
17	Kentucky	3,680	2.1%
18	Washington	3,440	2.0%
19	Alabama	3,340	1.9%
20	Maryland	3,210	1.9%
21	Louisiana	3,090	1.8%
22	Wisconsin	3,060	1.8%
23	South Carolina	2,880	1.7%
24	Arizona	2,870	1.7%
25	Minnesota	2,620	1.5%
26	Oklahoma	2,580	1.5%
27	Arkansas	2,530	1.5%
28	Mississippi	2,180	1.3%
29	Oregon	2,160	1.3%
30	Connecticut	1,950	1.1%
31	Iowa	1,790	1.0%
32	Colorado	1,750	1.0%
33	West Virginia	1,700	1.0%
34	Kansas	1,630	0.9%
35	Nevada	1,530	0.9%
36	Nebraska	1,000	0.6%
37	Maine	990	0.6%
38	New Hampshire	790	0.5%
39	New Mexico	760	0.4%
40	Rhode Island	720	0.4%
41	Idaho	630	0.4%
42	Montana	620	0.4%
43	Hawaii	510	0.3%
44	Delaware	490	0.3%
45	Utah	460	0.3%
46	South Dakota	430	0.2%
47	Vermont	390	0.2%
48	North Dakota	330	0.2%
49	Wyoming	280	0.2%
50	Alaska	220	0.1%
	District of Columbia	310	0.2%

Source: American Cancer Society
    "Cancer Facts & Figures 2005" (Copyright 2005, American Cancer Society)
*These estimates are offered as a rough guide and should be interpreted with caution. They are calculated
according to the distribution of estimated 2005 cancer deaths by state.

Estimated Rate of New Lung Cancer Cases in 2005

National Estimated Rate = 58.8 New Cases per 100,000 Population*

ALPHA ORDER

RANK	STATE	RATE
8	Alabama	73.7
49	Alaska	33.6
42	Arizona	50.0
2	Arkansas	91.9
45	California	42.2
48	Colorado	38.0
33	Connecticut	55.7
27	Delaware	59.0
5	Florida	75.5
38	Georgia	54.4
46	Hawaii	40.4
44	Idaho	45.2
31	Illinois	56.8
10	Indiana	70.7
23	Iowa	60.6
26	Kansas	59.6
3	Kentucky	88.8
13	Louisiana	68.4
6	Maine	75.2
29	Maryland	57.8
21	Massachusetts	62.5
24	Michigan	60.4
40	Minnesota	51.4
7	Mississippi	75.1
10	Missouri	70.7
16	Montana	66.9
30	Nebraska	57.2
18	Nevada	65.5
22	New Hampshire	60.8
34	New Jersey	55.5
47	New Mexico	39.9
41	New York	51.3
19	North Carolina	64.6
39	North Dakota	52.0
15	Ohio	68.0
9	Oklahoma	73.2
25	Oregon	60.1
14	Pennsylvania	68.3
17	Rhode Island	66.6
12	South Carolina	68.6
32	South Dakota	55.8
4	Tennessee	78.5
43	Texas	49.8
50	Utah	19.3
20	Vermont	62.8
27	Virginia	59.0
36	Washington	55.4
1	West Virginia	93.6
34	Wisconsin	55.5
37	Wyoming	55.3

RANK ORDER

RANK	STATE	RATE
1	West Virginia	93.6
2	Arkansas	91.9
3	Kentucky	88.8
4	Tennessee	78.5
5	Florida	75.5
6	Maine	75.2
7	Mississippi	75.1
8	Alabama	73.7
9	Oklahoma	73.2
10	Indiana	70.7
10	Missouri	70.7
12	South Carolina	68.6
13	Louisiana	68.4
14	Pennsylvania	68.3
15	Ohio	68.0
16	Montana	66.9
17	Rhode Island	66.6
18	Nevada	65.5
19	North Carolina	64.6
20	Vermont	62.8
21	Massachusetts	62.5
22	New Hampshire	60.8
23	Iowa	60.6
24	Michigan	60.4
25	Oregon	60.1
26	Kansas	59.6
27	Delaware	59.0
27	Virginia	59.0
29	Maryland	57.8
30	Nebraska	57.2
31	Illinois	56.8
32	South Dakota	55.8
33	Connecticut	55.7
34	New Jersey	55.5
34	Wisconsin	55.5
36	Washington	55.4
37	Wyoming	55.3
38	Georgia	54.4
39	North Dakota	52.0
40	Minnesota	51.4
41	New York	51.3
42	Arizona	50.0
43	Texas	49.8
44	Idaho	45.2
45	California	42.2
46	Hawaii	40.4
47	New Mexico	39.9
48	Colorado	38.0
49	Alaska	33.6
50	Utah	19.3
	District of Columbia	56.0

*Source: Morgan Quitno Press using data from American Cancer Society
"Cancer Facts & Figures 2005" (Copyright 2005, American Cancer Society)*
*These estimates are offered as a rough guide and should be interpreted with caution. They are calculated according to the distribution of estimated 2005 cancer deaths by state. Rates calculated using 2004 Census resident population estimates.

Estimated New Non-Hodgkin's Lymphoma Cases in 2005

National Estimated Total = 56,390 New Cases*

ALPHA ORDER

RANK	STATE	CASES	% of USA
25	Alabama	940	1.7%
49	Alaska	90	0.2%
20	Arizona	1,060	1.9%
31	Arkansas	650	1.2%
1	California	5,700	10.1%
27	Colorado	880	1.6%
29	Connecticut	730	1.3%
44	Delaware	210	0.4%
2	Florida	3,470	6.2%
14	Georgia	1,380	2.4%
41	Hawaii	260	0.5%
44	Idaho	210	0.4%
6	Illinois	2,200	3.9%
12	Indiana	1,410	2.5%
28	Iowa	760	1.3%
31	Kansas	650	1.2%
24	Kentucky	970	1.7%
20	Louisiana	1,060	1.9%
41	Maine	260	0.5%
22	Maryland	1,030	1.8%
17	Massachusetts	1,260	2.2%
7	Michigan	2,140	3.8%
14	Minnesota	1,380	2.4%
33	Mississippi	530	0.9%
11	Missouri	1,530	2.7%
44	Montana	210	0.4%
36	Nebraska	380	0.7%
35	Nevada	440	0.8%
38	New Hampshire	320	0.6%
9	New Jersey	1,760	3.1%
38	New Mexico	320	0.6%
4	New York	2,940	5.2%
9	North Carolina	1,760	3.1%
47	North Dakota	180	0.3%
8	Ohio	1,970	3.5%
30	Oklahoma	680	1.2%
23	Oregon	1,000	1.8%
5	Pennsylvania	2,880	5.1%
40	Rhode Island	290	0.5%
25	South Carolina	940	1.7%
43	South Dakota	230	0.4%
16	Tennessee	1,350	2.4%
3	Texas	3,050	5.4%
36	Utah	380	0.7%
47	Vermont	180	0.3%
18	Virginia	1,170	2.1%
12	Washington	1,410	2.5%
34	West Virginia	500	0.9%
19	Wisconsin	1,120	2.0%
49	Wyoming	90	0.2%

RANK ORDER

RANK	STATE	CASES	% of USA
1	California	5,700	10.1%
2	Florida	3,470	6.2%
3	Texas	3,050	5.4%
4	New York	2,940	5.2%
5	Pennsylvania	2,880	5.1%
6	Illinois	2,200	3.9%
7	Michigan	2,140	3.8%
8	Ohio	1,970	3.5%
9	New Jersey	1,760	3.1%
9	North Carolina	1,760	3.1%
11	Missouri	1,530	2.7%
12	Indiana	1,410	2.5%
12	Washington	1,410	2.5%
14	Georgia	1,380	2.4%
14	Minnesota	1,380	2.4%
16	Tennessee	1,350	2.4%
17	Massachusetts	1,260	2.2%
18	Virginia	1,170	2.1%
19	Wisconsin	1,120	2.0%
20	Arizona	1,060	1.9%
20	Louisiana	1,060	1.9%
22	Maryland	1,030	1.8%
23	Oregon	1,000	1.8%
24	Kentucky	970	1.7%
25	Alabama	940	1.7%
25	South Carolina	940	1.7%
27	Colorado	880	1.6%
28	Iowa	760	1.3%
29	Connecticut	730	1.3%
30	Oklahoma	680	1.2%
31	Arkansas	650	1.2%
31	Kansas	650	1.2%
33	Mississippi	530	0.9%
34	West Virginia	500	0.9%
35	Nevada	440	0.8%
36	Nebraska	380	0.7%
36	Utah	380	0.7%
38	New Hampshire	320	0.6%
38	New Mexico	320	0.6%
40	Rhode Island	290	0.5%
41	Hawaii	260	0.5%
41	Maine	260	0.5%
43	South Dakota	230	0.4%
44	Delaware	210	0.4%
44	Idaho	210	0.4%
44	Montana	210	0.4%
47	North Dakota	180	0.3%
47	Vermont	180	0.3%
49	Alaska	90	0.2%
49	Wyoming	90	0.2%
	District of Columbia	90	0.2%

Source: American Cancer Society
    "Cancer Facts & Figures 2005" (Copyright 2005, American Cancer Society)
*These estimates are offered as a rough guide and should be interpreted with caution. They are calculated according to the distribution of estimated 2005 cancer deaths by state.

Estimated Rate of New Non-Hodgkin's Lymphoma Cases in 2005

National Estimated Rate = 19.2 New Cases per 100,000 Population*

ALPHA ORDER

RANK	STATE	RATE
25	Alabama	20.7
49	Alaska	13.7
36	Arizona	18.5
13	Arkansas	23.6
43	California	15.9
34	Colorado	19.1
24	Connecticut	20.8
10	Delaware	25.3
30	Florida	19.9
46	Georgia	15.6
26	Hawaii	20.6
48	Idaho	15.1
40	Illinois	17.3
20	Indiana	22.6
9	Iowa	25.7
12	Kansas	23.8
15	Kentucky	23.4
14	Louisiana	23.5
31	Maine	19.7
36	Maryland	18.5
32	Massachusetts	19.6
23	Michigan	21.2
6	Minnesota	27.1
38	Mississippi	18.3
8	Missouri	26.6
18	Montana	22.7
22	Nebraska	21.7
35	Nevada	18.8
11	New Hampshire	24.6
29	New Jersey	20.2
42	New Mexico	16.8
47	New York	15.3
26	North Carolina	20.6
3	North Dakota	28.4
41	Ohio	17.2
33	Oklahoma	19.3
4	Oregon	27.8
16	Pennsylvania	23.2
7	Rhode Island	26.8
21	South Carolina	22.4
1	South Dakota	29.8
17	Tennessee	22.9
50	Texas	13.6
43	Utah	15.9
2	Vermont	29.0
45	Virginia	15.7
18	Washington	22.7
5	West Virginia	27.5
28	Wisconsin	20.3
39	Wyoming	17.8

RANK ORDER

RANK	STATE	RATE
1	South Dakota	29.8
2	Vermont	29.0
3	North Dakota	28.4
4	Oregon	27.8
5	West Virginia	27.5
6	Minnesota	27.1
7	Rhode Island	26.8
8	Missouri	26.6
9	Iowa	25.7
10	Delaware	25.3
11	New Hampshire	24.6
12	Kansas	23.8
13	Arkansas	23.6
14	Louisiana	23.5
15	Kentucky	23.4
16	Pennsylvania	23.2
17	Tennessee	22.9
18	Montana	22.7
18	Washington	22.7
20	Indiana	22.6
21	South Carolina	22.4
22	Nebraska	21.7
23	Michigan	21.2
24	Connecticut	20.8
25	Alabama	20.7
26	Hawaii	20.6
26	North Carolina	20.6
28	Wisconsin	20.3
29	New Jersey	20.2
30	Florida	19.9
31	Maine	19.7
32	Massachusetts	19.6
33	Oklahoma	19.3
34	Colorado	19.1
35	Nevada	18.8
36	Arizona	18.5
36	Maryland	18.5
38	Mississippi	18.3
39	Wyoming	17.8
40	Illinois	17.3
41	Ohio	17.2
42	New Mexico	16.8
43	California	15.9
43	Utah	15.9
45	Virginia	15.7
46	Georgia	15.6
47	New York	15.3
48	Idaho	15.1
49	Alaska	13.7
50	Texas	13.6

District of Columbia 16.3

Source: Morgan Quitno Press using data from American Cancer Society
"Cancer Facts & Figures 2005" (Copyright 2005, American Cancer Society)
*These estimates are offered as a rough guide and should be interpreted with caution. They are calculated according to the distribution of estimated 2005 cancer deaths by state. Rates calculated using 2004 Census resident population estimates.

Estimated New Prostate Cancer Cases in 2005

National Estimated Total = 232,090 New Cases*

ALPHA ORDER

RANK	STATE	CASES	% of USA
16	Alabama	4,360	1.9%
50	Alaska	310	0.1%
22	Arizona	3,900	1.7%
32	Arkansas	2,060	0.9%
1	California	25,010	10.8%
29	Colorado	2,680	1.2%
24	Connecticut	3,360	1.4%
46	Delaware	610	0.3%
2	Florida	19,650	8.5%
12	Georgia	5,660	2.4%
43	Hawaii	920	0.4%
39	Idaho	1,150	0.5%
7	Illinois	9,410	4.1%
15	Indiana	4,890	2.1%
26	Iowa	3,060	1.3%
32	Kansas	2,060	0.9%
30	Kentucky	2,520	1.1%
23	Louisiana	3,440	1.5%
38	Maine	1,300	0.6%
19	Maryland	4,210	1.8%
14	Massachusetts	5,350	2.3%
8	Michigan	7,650	3.3%
16	Minnesota	4,360	1.9%
25	Mississippi	3,210	1.4%
26	Missouri	3,060	1.3%
42	Montana	990	0.4%
37	Nebraska	1,380	0.6%
34	Nevada	1,990	0.9%
39	New Hampshire	1,150	0.5%
10	New Jersey	6,420	2.8%
35	New Mexico	1,680	0.7%
3	New York	14,220	6.1%
9	North Carolina	6,810	2.9%
46	North Dakota	610	0.3%
6	Ohio	10,860	4.7%
31	Oklahoma	2,450	1.1%
28	Oregon	2,980	1.3%
5	Pennsylvania	13,150	5.7%
45	Rhode Island	840	0.4%
19	South Carolina	4,210	1.8%
43	South Dakota	920	0.4%
18	Tennessee	4,280	1.8%
4	Texas	13,380	5.8%
39	Utah	1,150	0.5%
49	Vermont	460	0.2%
11	Virginia	5,740	2.5%
13	Washington	5,510	2.4%
36	West Virginia	1,450	0.6%
21	Wisconsin	4,050	1.7%
46	Wyoming	610	0.3%

RANK ORDER

RANK	STATE	CASES	% of USA
1	California	25,010	10.8%
2	Florida	19,650	8.5%
3	New York	14,220	6.1%
4	Texas	13,380	5.8%
5	Pennsylvania	13,150	5.7%
6	Ohio	10,860	4.7%
7	Illinois	9,410	4.1%
8	Michigan	7,650	3.3%
9	North Carolina	6,810	2.9%
10	New Jersey	6,420	2.8%
11	Virginia	5,740	2.5%
12	Georgia	5,660	2.4%
13	Washington	5,510	2.4%
14	Massachusetts	5,350	2.3%
15	Indiana	4,890	2.1%
16	Alabama	4,360	1.9%
16	Minnesota	4,360	1.9%
18	Tennessee	4,280	1.8%
19	Maryland	4,210	1.8%
19	South Carolina	4,210	1.8%
21	Wisconsin	4,050	1.7%
22	Arizona	3,900	1.7%
23	Louisiana	3,440	1.5%
24	Connecticut	3,360	1.4%
25	Mississippi	3,210	1.4%
26	Iowa	3,060	1.3%
26	Missouri	3,060	1.3%
28	Oregon	2,980	1.3%
29	Colorado	2,680	1.2%
30	Kentucky	2,520	1.1%
31	Oklahoma	2,450	1.1%
32	Arkansas	2,060	0.9%
32	Kansas	2,060	0.9%
34	Nevada	1,990	0.9%
35	New Mexico	1,680	0.7%
36	West Virginia	1,450	0.6%
37	Nebraska	1,380	0.6%
38	Maine	1,300	0.6%
39	Idaho	1,150	0.5%
39	New Hampshire	1,150	0.5%
39	Utah	1,150	0.5%
42	Montana	990	0.4%
43	Hawaii	920	0.4%
43	South Dakota	920	0.4%
45	Rhode Island	840	0.4%
46	Delaware	610	0.3%
46	North Dakota	610	0.3%
46	Wyoming	610	0.3%
49	Vermont	460	0.2%
50	Alaska	310	0.1%
	District of Columbia	610	0.3%

Source: American Cancer Society
   "Cancer Facts & Figures 2005" (Copyright 2005, American Cancer Society)
These estimates are offered as a rough guide and should be interpreted with caution. They are calculated according to the distribution of estimated 2005 cancer deaths by state.

Age-Adjusted Incidence Rate of Prostate Cancer Cases in 2001

National Rate = 166.7 New Cases per 100,000 Male Population*

ALPHA ORDER

RANK	STATE	RATE
43	Alabama	128.7
20	Alaska	164.5
44	Arizona	128.0
38	Arkansas	144.0
27	California	157.6
22	Colorado	163.1
12	Connecticut	174.0
19	Delaware	165.1
30	Florida	154.8
26	Georgia	159.6
42	Hawaii	131.6
17	Idaho	167.9
25	Illinois	160.5
41	Indiana	132.9
32	Iowa	153.2
NA	Kansas**	NA
31	Kentucky	154.6
13	Louisiana	173.8
16	Maine	169.5
9	Maryland	177.6
4	Massachusetts	183.0
1	Michigan	198.2
3	Minnesota	184.5
NA	Mississippi**	NA
40	Missouri	137.0
14	Montana	172.7
24	Nebraska	162.4
45	Nevada	121.6
28	New Hampshire	155.1
2	New Jersey	198.0
37	New Mexico	146.5
23	New York	162.9
33	North Carolina	152.5
15	North Dakota	171.0
34	Ohio	150.0
39	Oklahoma	141.7
20	Oregon	164.5
NA	Pennsylvania**	NA
7	Rhode Island	177.9
11	South Carolina	174.2
5	South Dakota	180.2
NA	Tennessee**	NA
36	Texas	148.4
6	Utah	180.0
NA	Vermont**	NA
29	Virginia	155.0
10	Washington	175.6
35	West Virginia	149.3
18	Wisconsin	166.3
7	Wyoming	177.9

RANK ORDER

RANK	STATE	RATE
1	Michigan	198.2
2	New Jersey	198.0
3	Minnesota	184.5
4	Massachusetts	183.0
5	South Dakota	180.2
6	Utah	180.0
7	Rhode Island	177.9
7	Wyoming	177.9
9	Maryland	177.6
10	Washington	175.6
11	South Carolina	174.2
12	Connecticut	174.0
13	Louisiana	173.8
14	Montana	172.7
15	North Dakota	171.0
16	Maine	169.5
17	Idaho	167.9
18	Wisconsin	166.3
19	Delaware	165.1
20	Alaska	164.5
20	Oregon	164.5
22	Colorado	163.1
23	New York	162.9
24	Nebraska	162.4
25	Illinois	160.5
26	Georgia	159.6
27	California	157.6
28	New Hampshire	155.1
29	Virginia	155.0
30	Florida	154.8
31	Kentucky	154.6
32	Iowa	153.2
33	North Carolina	152.5
34	Ohio	150.0
35	West Virginia	149.3
36	Texas	148.4
37	New Mexico	146.5
38	Arkansas	144.0
39	Oklahoma	141.7
40	Missouri	137.0
41	Indiana	132.9
42	Hawaii	131.6
43	Alabama	128.7
44	Arizona	128.0
45	Nevada	121.6
NA	Kansas**	NA
NA	Mississippi**	NA
NA	Pennsylvania**	NA
NA	Tennessee**	NA
NA	Vermont**	NA
	District of Columbia	239.4

Source: American Cancer Society
    "Cancer Facts & Figures 2005" (Copyright 2005, American Cancer Society)
*For 1997 to 2001. Age-adjusted to the 2000 U.S. standard population.
**Not available.

Percent of Males Receiving Recent PSA Test for Prostate Cancer: 2001

National Median = 56.7% of Men 50 and Older*

ALPHA ORDER

ALPHA ORDER

RANK ORDER

RANK	STATE	PERCENT		RANK	STATE	PERCENT
26	Alabama	55.9		1	Florida	66.2
14	Alaska	60.5		2	Wyoming	65.4
11	Arizona	61.4		3	New Jersey	64.9
38	Arkansas	54.2		4	Delaware	64.1
42	California	53.8		4	Pennsylvania	64.1
24	Colorado	56.8		6	Massachusetts	63.8
17	Connecticut	58.7		7	Missouri	63.4
4	Delaware	64.1		8	Rhode Island	63.2
1	Florida	66.2		9	Ohio	62.8
12	Georgia	60.9		10	Michigan	61.9
48	Hawaii	49.5		11	Arizona	61.4
32	Idaho	54.9		12	Georgia	60.9
35	Illinois	54.6		13	South Carolina	60.6
33	Indiana	54.8		14	Alaska	60.5
35	Iowa	54.6		14	Maryland	60.5
19	Kansas	57.7		16	New York	60.0
40	Kentucky	54.0		17	Connecticut	58.7
28	Louisiana	55.8		18	West Virginia	58.5
48	Maine	49.5		19	Kansas	57.7
14	Maryland	60.5		20	New Hampshire	57.6
6	Massachusetts	63.8		21	Texas	57.1
10	Michigan	61.9		22	Montana	56.9
44	Minnesota	52.3		22	North Dakota	56.9
30	Mississippi	55.4		24	Colorado	56.8
7	Missouri	63.4		25	Virginia	56.7
22	Montana	56.9		26	Alabama	55.9
50	Nebraska	49.2		26	Nevada	55.9
26	Nevada	55.9		28	Louisiana	55.8
20	New Hampshire	57.6		29	South Dakota	55.6
3	New Jersey	64.9		30	Mississippi	55.4
45	New Mexico	51.9		31	Wisconsin	55.1
16	New York	60.0		32	Idaho	54.9
37	North Carolina	54.4		33	Indiana	54.8
22	North Dakota	56.9		33	Oregon	54.8
9	Ohio	62.8		35	Illinois	54.6
47	Oklahoma	50.7		35	Iowa	54.6
33	Oregon	54.8		37	North Carolina	54.4
4	Pennsylvania	64.1		38	Arkansas	54.2
8	Rhode Island	63.2		39	Vermont	54.1
13	South Carolina	60.6		40	Kentucky	54.0
29	South Dakota	55.6		40	Washington	54.0
46	Tennessee	51.8		42	California	53.8
21	Texas	57.1		42	Utah	53.8
42	Utah	53.8		44	Minnesota	52.3
39	Vermont	54.1		45	New Mexico	51.9
25	Virginia	56.7		46	Tennessee	51.8
40	Washington	54.0		47	Oklahoma	50.7
18	West Virginia	58.5		48	Hawaii	49.5
31	Wisconsin	55.1		48	Maine	49.5
2	Wyoming	65.4		50	Nebraska	49.2

District of Columbia   63.8

Source: U.S. Department of Health and Human Services, Centers for Disease Control and Prevention
"2001 Behavioral Risk Factor Surveillance System Public Use Data Tape"
*Men 50 and older receiving prostate-specific antigen (PSA) test within the past year.

Estimated New Skin Melanoma Cases in 2005

National Estimated Total = 59,580 New Cases*

ALPHA ORDER

RANK	STATE	CASES	% of USA
25	Alabama	920	1.5%
49	Alaska	80	0.1%
17	Arizona	1,300	2.2%
30	Arkansas	540	0.9%
1	California	5,440	9.1%
25	Colorado	920	1.5%
29	Connecticut	690	1.2%
43	Delaware	230	0.4%
2	Florida	4,600	7.7%
11	Georgia	1,610	2.7%
45	Hawaii	150	0.3%
37	Idaho	380	0.6%
7	Illinois	2,300	3.9%
14	Indiana	1,460	2.5%
30	Iowa	540	0.9%
30	Kansas	540	0.9%
20	Kentucky	1,150	1.9%
27	Louisiana	770	1.3%
37	Maine	380	0.6%
21	Maryland	1,070	1.8%
13	Massachusetts	1,530	2.6%
10	Michigan	1,840	3.1%
22	Minnesota	1,000	1.7%
34	Mississippi	460	0.8%
14	Missouri	1,460	2.5%
43	Montana	230	0.4%
37	Nebraska	380	0.6%
30	Nevada	540	0.9%
40	New Hampshire	310	0.5%
8	New Jersey	1,920	3.2%
40	New Mexico	310	0.5%
4	New York	3,220	5.4%
8	North Carolina	1,920	3.2%
49	North Dakota	80	0.1%
6	Ohio	2,450	4.1%
22	Oklahoma	1,000	1.7%
22	Oregon	1,000	1.7%
5	Pennsylvania	2,990	5.0%
40	Rhode Island	310	0.5%
27	South Carolina	770	1.3%
45	South Dakota	150	0.3%
17	Tennessee	1,300	2.2%
3	Texas	3,830	6.4%
34	Utah	460	0.8%
45	Vermont	150	0.3%
11	Virginia	1,610	2.7%
16	Washington	1,380	2.3%
34	West Virginia	460	0.8%
19	Wisconsin	1,230	2.1%
45	Wyoming	150	0.3%

RANK ORDER

RANK	STATE	CASES	% of USA
1	California	5,440	9.1%
2	Florida	4,600	7.7%
3	Texas	3,830	6.4%
4	New York	3,220	5.4%
5	Pennsylvania	2,990	5.0%
6	Ohio	2,450	4.1%
7	Illinois	2,300	3.9%
8	New Jersey	1,920	3.2%
8	North Carolina	1,920	3.2%
10	Michigan	1,840	3.1%
11	Georgia	1,610	2.7%
11	Virginia	1,610	2.7%
13	Massachusetts	1,530	2.6%
14	Indiana	1,460	2.5%
14	Missouri	1,460	2.5%
16	Washington	1,380	2.3%
17	Arizona	1,300	2.2%
17	Tennessee	1,300	2.2%
19	Wisconsin	1,230	2.1%
20	Kentucky	1,150	1.9%
21	Maryland	1,070	1.8%
22	Minnesota	1,000	1.7%
22	Oklahoma	1,000	1.7%
22	Oregon	1,000	1.7%
25	Alabama	920	1.5%
25	Colorado	920	1.5%
27	Louisiana	770	1.3%
27	South Carolina	770	1.3%
29	Connecticut	690	1.2%
30	Arkansas	540	0.9%
30	Iowa	540	0.9%
30	Kansas	540	0.9%
30	Nevada	540	0.9%
34	Mississippi	460	0.8%
34	Utah	460	0.8%
34	West Virginia	460	0.8%
37	Idaho	380	0.6%
37	Maine	380	0.6%
37	Nebraska	380	0.6%
40	New Hampshire	310	0.5%
40	New Mexico	310	0.5%
40	Rhode Island	310	0.5%
43	Delaware	230	0.4%
43	Montana	230	0.4%
45	Hawaii	150	0.3%
45	South Dakota	150	0.3%
45	Vermont	150	0.3%
45	Wyoming	150	0.3%
49	Alaska	80	0.1%
49	North Dakota	80	0.1%
	District of Columbia	80	0.1%

Source: American Cancer Society
    "Cancer Facts & Figures 2005" (Copyright 2005, American Cancer Society)
*These estimates are offered as a rough guide and should be interpreted with caution. They are calculated
according to the distribution of estimated 2005 cancer deaths by state.

Estimated Rate of New Skin Melanoma Cases in 2005

National Estimated Rate = 20.3 New Cases per 100,000 Population*

ALPHA ORDER

RANK ORDER

RANK	STATE	RATE		RANK	STATE	RATE
28	Alabama	20.3		1	Wyoming	29.6
49	Alaska	12.2		2	Maine	28.8
19	Arizona	22.6		3	Rhode Island	28.7
32	Arkansas	19.6		4	Oklahoma	28.4
47	California	15.2		5	Oregon	27.8
29	Colorado	20.0		6	Delaware	27.7
30	Connecticut	19.7		6	Kentucky	27.7
6	Delaware	27.7		8	Idaho	27.3
9	Florida	26.4		9	Florida	26.4
39	Georgia	18.2		10	Missouri	25.4
50	Hawaii	11.9		11	West Virginia	25.3
8	Idaho	27.3		12	Montana	24.8
41	Illinois	18.1		13	Pennsylvania	24.1
17	Indiana	23.4		13	Vermont	24.1
37	Iowa	18.3		15	New Hampshire	23.9
30	Kansas	19.7		16	Massachusetts	23.8
6	Kentucky	27.7		17	Indiana	23.4
42	Louisiana	17.1		18	Nevada	23.1
2	Maine	28.8		19	Arizona	22.6
35	Maryland	19.3		20	North Carolina	22.5
16	Massachusetts	23.8		21	Wisconsin	22.3
39	Michigan	18.2		22	Washington	22.2
32	Minnesota	19.6		23	New Jersey	22.1
46	Mississippi	15.8		24	Tennessee	22.0
10	Missouri	25.4		25	Nebraska	21.7
12	Montana	24.8		26	Virginia	21.6
25	Nebraska	21.7		27	Ohio	21.4
18	Nevada	23.1		28	Alabama	20.3
15	New Hampshire	23.9		29	Colorado	20.0
23	New Jersey	22.1		30	Connecticut	19.7
45	New Mexico	16.3		30	Kansas	19.7
44	New York	16.7		32	Arkansas	19.6
20	North Carolina	22.5		32	Minnesota	19.6
48	North Dakota	12.6		34	South Dakota	19.5
27	Ohio	21.4		35	Maryland	19.3
4	Oklahoma	28.4		35	Utah	19.3
5	Oregon	27.8		37	Iowa	18.3
13	Pennsylvania	24.1		37	South Carolina	18.3
3	Rhode Island	28.7		39	Georgia	18.2
37	South Carolina	18.3		39	Michigan	18.2
34	South Dakota	19.5		41	Illinois	18.1
24	Tennessee	22.0		42	Louisiana	17.1
43	Texas	17.0		43	Texas	17.0
35	Utah	19.3		44	New York	16.7
13	Vermont	24.1		45	New Mexico	16.3
26	Virginia	21.6		46	Mississippi	15.8
22	Washington	22.2		47	California	15.2
11	West Virginia	25.3		48	North Dakota	12.6
21	Wisconsin	22.3		49	Alaska	12.2
1	Wyoming	29.6		50	Hawaii	11.9

District of Columbia   14.5

Source: Morgan Quitno Press using data from American Cancer Society
"Cancer Facts & Figures 2005" (Copyright 2005, American Cancer Society)
These estimates are offered as a rough guide and should be interpreted with caution. They are calculated according to the distribution of estimated 2005 cancer deaths by state. Rates calculated using 2004 Census resident population estimates.

Estimated New Cervical Cancer Cases in 2005

National Estimated Total = 10,370 New Cases*

ALPHA ORDER

RANK ORDER

RANK	STATE	CASES	% of USA
17	Alabama	200	1.9%
NA	Alaska**	NA	NA
17	Arizona	200	1.9%
20	Arkansas	170	1.6%
1	California	1,090	10.5%
32	Colorado	80	0.8%
13	Connecticut	220	2.1%
NA	Delaware**	NA	NA
4	Florida	730	7.0%
8	Georgia	360	3.5%
36	Hawaii	60	0.6%
36	Idaho	60	0.6%
5	Illinois	500	4.8%
20	Indiana	170	1.6%
27	Iowa	110	1.1%
32	Kansas	80	0.8%
13	Kentucky	220	2.1%
13	Louisiana	220	2.1%
NA	Maine**	NA	NA
13	Maryland	220	2.1%
27	Massachusetts	110	1.1%
9	Michigan	340	3.3%
27	Minnesota	110	1.1%
24	Mississippi	140	1.4%
20	Missouri	170	1.6%
NA	Montana**	NA	NA
36	Nebraska	60	0.6%
32	Nevada	80	0.8%
NA	New Hampshire**	NA	NA
9	New Jersey	340	3.3%
36	New Mexico	60	0.6%
3	New York	840	8.1%
11	North Carolina	310	3.0%
NA	North Dakota**	NA	NA
6	Ohio	390	3.8%
24	Oklahoma	140	1.4%
24	Oregon	140	1.4%
6	Pennsylvania	390	3.8%
36	Rhode Island	60	0.6%
20	South Carolina	170	1.6%
NA	South Dakota**	NA	NA
12	Tennessee	280	2.7%
2	Texas	1,030	9.9%
NA	Utah**	NA	NA
NA	Vermont**	NA	NA
17	Virginia	200	1.9%
27	Washington	110	1.1%
27	West Virginia	110	1.1%
32	Wisconsin	80	0.8%
NA	Wyoming**	NA	NA

RANK	STATE	CASES	% of USA
1	California	1,090	10.5%
2	Texas	1,030	9.9%
3	New York	840	8.1%
4	Florida	730	7.0%
5	Illinois	500	4.8%
6	Ohio	390	3.8%
6	Pennsylvania	390	3.8%
8	Georgia	360	3.5%
9	Michigan	340	3.3%
9	New Jersey	340	3.3%
11	North Carolina	310	3.0%
12	Tennessee	280	2.7%
13	Connecticut	220	2.1%
13	Kentucky	220	2.1%
13	Louisiana	220	2.1%
13	Maryland	220	2.1%
17	Alabama	200	1.9%
17	Arizona	200	1.9%
17	Virginia	200	1.9%
20	Arkansas	170	1.6%
20	Indiana	170	1.6%
20	Missouri	170	1.6%
20	South Carolina	170	1.6%
24	Mississippi	140	1.4%
24	Oklahoma	140	1.4%
24	Oregon	140	1.4%
27	Iowa	110	1.1%
27	Massachusetts	110	1.1%
27	Minnesota	110	1.1%
27	Washington	110	1.1%
27	West Virginia	110	1.1%
32	Colorado	80	0.8%
32	Kansas	80	0.8%
32	Nevada	80	0.8%
32	Wisconsin	80	0.8%
36	Hawaii	60	0.6%
36	Idaho	60	0.6%
36	Nebraska	60	0.6%
36	New Mexico	60	0.6%
36	Rhode Island	60	0.6%
NA	Alaska**	NA	NA
NA	Delaware**	NA	NA
NA	Maine**	NA	NA
NA	Montana**	NA	NA
NA	New Hampshire**	NA	NA
NA	North Dakota**	NA	NA
NA	South Dakota**	NA	NA
NA	Utah**	NA	NA
NA	Vermont**	NA	NA
NA	Wyoming**	NA	NA
	District of Columbia**	NA	NA

Source: American Cancer Society
   "Cancer Facts & Figures 2005" (Copyright 2005, American Cancer Society)
*These estimates are offered as a rough guide and should be interpreted with caution. They are calculated according to the distribution of estimated 2004 cancer deaths by state.
**Not available.

Estimated Rate of New Cervical Cancer Cases in 2005

National Estimated Rate = 7.2 New Cases per 100,000 Female Population*

ALPHA ORDER

RANK	STATE	RATE
11	Alabama	9.2
NA	Alaska**	NA
24	Arizona	7.2
2	Arkansas	12.7
31	California	6.2
38	Colorado	3.5
1	Connecticut	13.0
NA	Delaware**	NA
13	Florida	8.8
15	Georgia	8.4
9	Hawaii	9.5
13	Idaho	8.8
18	Illinois	8.1
34	Indiana	5.6
22	Iowa	7.6
33	Kansas	5.9
5	Kentucky	10.9
6	Louisiana	10.1
NA	Maine**	NA
17	Maryland	8.3
38	Massachusetts	3.5
28	Michigan	6.9
36	Minnesota	4.4
7	Mississippi	10.0
32	Missouri	6.1
NA	Montana**	NA
25	Nebraska	7.0
25	Nevada	7.0
NA	New Hampshire**	NA
18	New Jersey	8.1
29	New Mexico	6.5
12	New York	9.1
23	North Carolina	7.5
NA	North Dakota**	NA
25	Ohio	7.0
18	Oklahoma	8.1
21	Oregon	7.9
29	Pennsylvania	6.5
4	Rhode Island	11.6
15	South Carolina	8.4
NA	South Dakota**	NA
8	Tennessee	9.8
10	Texas	9.4
NA	Utah**	NA
NA	Vermont**	NA
35	Virginia	5.5
37	Washington	3.6
3	West Virginia	12.5
40	Wisconsin	3.0
NA	Wyoming**	NA

RANK ORDER

RANK	STATE	RATE
1	Connecticut	13.0
2	Arkansas	12.7
3	West Virginia	12.5
4	Rhode Island	11.6
5	Kentucky	10.9
6	Louisiana	10.1
7	Mississippi	10.0
8	Tennessee	9.8
9	Hawaii	9.5
10	Texas	9.4
11	Alabama	9.2
12	New York	9.1
13	Florida	8.8
13	Idaho	8.8
15	Georgia	8.4
15	South Carolina	8.4
17	Maryland	8.3
18	Illinois	8.1
18	New Jersey	8.1
18	Oklahoma	8.1
21	Oregon	7.9
22	Iowa	7.6
23	North Carolina	7.5
24	Arizona	7.2
25	Nebraska	7.0
25	Nevada	7.0
25	Ohio	7.0
28	Michigan	6.9
29	New Mexico	6.5
29	Pennsylvania	6.5
31	California	6.2
32	Missouri	6.1
33	Kansas	5.9
34	Indiana	5.6
35	Virginia	5.5
36	Minnesota	4.4
37	Washington	3.6
38	Colorado	3.5
38	Massachusetts	3.5
40	Wisconsin	3.0
NA	Alaska**	NA
NA	Delaware**	NA
NA	Maine**	NA
NA	Montana**	NA
NA	New Hampshire**	NA
NA	North Dakota**	NA
NA	South Dakota**	NA
NA	Utah**	NA
NA	Vermont**	NA
NA	Wyoming**	NA
	District of Columbia**	NA

Source: Morgan Quitno Press using data from American Cancer Society
   "Cancer Facts & Figures 2005" (Copyright 2005, American Cancer Society)
*These estimates are offered as a rough guide and should be interpreted with caution. They are calculated according to the distribution of estimated 2005 cancer deaths by state. Rates calculated using 2003 Census female population estimates.
**Not available.

Percent of Women 18 Years Old and Older
Who Had a Pap Smear Within the Past Three Years: 2002
National Median = 87.5% of Women 18 Years and Older*

ALPHA ORDER

RANK ORDER

RANK	STATE	PERCENT
28	Alabama	88.0
11	Alaska	90.1
39	Arizona	85.7
50	Arkansas	80.5
31	California	87.2
19	Colorado	88.7
5	Connecticut	91.1
3	Delaware	91.6
19	Florida	88.7
7	Georgia	90.8
14	Hawaii	89.8
48	Idaho	82.8
33	Illinois	86.7
43	Indiana	84.7
25	Iowa	88.1
18	Kansas	89.2
14	Kentucky	89.8
11	Louisiana	90.1
19	Maine	88.7
1	Maryland	93.3
7	Massachusetts	90.8
19	Michigan	88.7
25	Minnesota	88.1
42	Mississippi	85.2
40	Missouri	85.5
46	Montana	84.3
29	Nebraska	87.8
36	Nevada	86.3
16	New Hampshire	89.7
7	New Jersey	90.8
38	New Mexico	86.2
6	New York	90.9
4	North Carolina	91.2
36	North Dakota	86.3
24	Ohio	88.2
49	Oklahoma	82.0
47	Oregon	82.9
32	Pennsylvania	87.1
7	Rhode Island	90.8
25	South Carolina	88.1
23	South Dakota	88.4
2	Tennessee	91.7
29	Texas	87.8
44	Utah	84.6
17	Vermont	89.3
13	Virginia	90.0
35	Washington	86.4
41	West Virginia	85.4
33	Wisconsin	86.7
45	Wyoming	84.4

RANK	STATE	PERCENT
1	Maryland	93.3
2	Tennessee	91.7
3	Delaware	91.6
4	North Carolina	91.2
5	Connecticut	91.1
6	New York	90.9
7	Georgia	90.8
7	Massachusetts	90.8
7	New Jersey	90.8
7	Rhode Island	90.8
11	Alaska	90.1
11	Louisiana	90.1
13	Virginia	90.0
14	Hawaii	89.8
14	Kentucky	89.8
16	New Hampshire	89.7
17	Vermont	89.3
18	Kansas	89.2
19	Colorado	88.7
19	Florida	88.7
19	Maine	88.7
19	Michigan	88.7
23	South Dakota	88.4
24	Ohio	88.2
25	Iowa	88.1
25	Minnesota	88.1
25	South Carolina	88.1
28	Alabama	88.0
29	Nebraska	87.8
29	Texas	87.8
31	California	87.2
32	Pennsylvania	87.1
33	Illinois	86.7
33	Wisconsin	86.7
35	Washington	86.4
36	Nevada	86.3
36	North Dakota	86.3
38	New Mexico	86.2
39	Arizona	85.7
40	Missouri	85.5
41	West Virginia	85.4
42	Mississippi	85.2
43	Indiana	84.7
44	Utah	84.6
45	Wyoming	84.4
46	Montana	84.3
47	Oregon	82.9
48	Idaho	82.8
49	Oklahoma	82.0
50	Arkansas	80.5

| | District of Columbia | 93.4 |

Source: Morgan Quitno Press using data from U.S. Dept of HHS, Centers for Disease Control and Prevention "2002 Behavioral Risk Factor Surveillance Summary Prevalence Data" (http://apps.nccd.cdc.gov/brfss/)
Of women with intact cervix. Pap smear is a test for cancer, especially of the female genital tract. Named after George Papanicolaou (1883-1962), American anatomist.

Estimated New Uterine Cancer Cases in 2005

National Estimated Total = 40,880 New Cases*

ALPHA ORDER

RANK	STATE	CASES	% of USA
20	Alabama	670	1.6%
49	Alaska	60	0.1%
22	Arizona	500	1.2%
32	Arkansas	340	0.8%
1	California	4,250	10.4%
28	Colorado	450	1.1%
22	Connecticut	500	1.2%
44	Delaware	110	0.3%
4	Florida	2,520	6.2%
14	Georgia	890	2.2%
40	Hawaii	170	0.4%
40	Idaho	170	0.4%
6	Illinois	2,010	4.9%
11	Indiana	1,010	2.5%
22	Iowa	500	1.2%
31	Kansas	390	1.0%
22	Kentucky	500	1.2%
22	Louisiana	500	1.2%
37	Maine	220	0.5%
18	Maryland	780	1.9%
11	Massachusetts	1,010	2.5%
9	Michigan	1,450	3.5%
20	Minnesota	670	1.6%
32	Mississippi	340	0.8%
16	Missouri	840	2.1%
40	Montana	170	0.4%
34	Nebraska	280	0.7%
37	Nevada	220	0.5%
40	New Hampshire	170	0.4%
8	New Jersey	1,790	4.4%
34	New Mexico	280	0.7%
2	New York	3,240	7.9%
10	North Carolina	1,170	2.9%
44	North Dakota	110	0.3%
7	Ohio	1,850	4.5%
28	Oklahoma	450	1.1%
28	Oregon	450	1.1%
3	Pennsylvania	2,570	6.3%
44	Rhode Island	110	0.3%
22	South Carolina	500	1.2%
44	South Dakota	110	0.3%
19	Tennessee	730	1.8%
5	Texas	2,400	5.9%
37	Utah	220	0.5%
44	Vermont	110	0.3%
11	Virginia	1,010	2.5%
14	Washington	890	2.2%
34	West Virginia	280	0.7%
16	Wisconsin	840	2.1%
49	Wyoming	60	0.1%

RANK ORDER

RANK	STATE	CASES	% of USA
1	California	4,250	10.4%
2	New York	3,240	7.9%
3	Pennsylvania	2,570	6.3%
4	Florida	2,520	6.2%
5	Texas	2,400	5.9%
6	Illinois	2,010	4.9%
7	Ohio	1,850	4.5%
8	New Jersey	1,790	4.4%
9	Michigan	1,450	3.5%
10	North Carolina	1,170	2.9%
11	Indiana	1,010	2.5%
11	Massachusetts	1,010	2.5%
11	Virginia	1,010	2.5%
14	Georgia	890	2.2%
14	Washington	890	2.2%
16	Missouri	840	2.1%
16	Wisconsin	840	2.1%
18	Maryland	780	1.9%
19	Tennessee	730	1.8%
20	Alabama	670	1.6%
20	Minnesota	670	1.6%
22	Arizona	500	1.2%
22	Connecticut	500	1.2%
22	Iowa	500	1.2%
22	Kentucky	500	1.2%
22	Louisiana	500	1.2%
22	South Carolina	500	1.2%
28	Colorado	450	1.1%
28	Oklahoma	450	1.1%
28	Oregon	450	1.1%
31	Kansas	390	1.0%
32	Arkansas	340	0.8%
32	Mississippi	340	0.8%
34	Nebraska	280	0.7%
34	New Mexico	280	0.7%
34	West Virginia	280	0.7%
37	Maine	220	0.5%
37	Nevada	220	0.5%
37	Utah	220	0.5%
40	Hawaii	170	0.4%
40	Idaho	170	0.4%
40	Montana	170	0.4%
40	New Hampshire	170	0.4%
44	Delaware	110	0.3%
44	North Dakota	110	0.3%
44	Rhode Island	110	0.3%
44	South Dakota	110	0.3%
44	Vermont	110	0.3%
49	Alaska	60	0.1%
49	Wyoming	60	0.1%
	District of Columbia	170	0.4%

Source: American Cancer Society
    "Cancer Facts & Figures 2005" (Copyright 2005, American Cancer Society)
*These estimates are offered as a rough guide and should be interpreted with caution. They are calculated according to the distribution of estimated 2005 cancer deaths by state.

Estimated Rate of New Uterine Cancer Cases in 2005

National Estimated Rate = 28.6 New Cases per 100,000 Female Population*

ALPHA ORDER

RANK	STATE	RATE
16	Alabama	30.7
49	Alaska	17.9
49	Arizona	17.9
34	Arkansas	25.5
40	California	24.0
46	Colorado	19.6
20	Connecticut	29.6
28	Delaware	27.6
18	Florida	30.2
45	Georgia	20.8
29	Hawaii	27.0
36	Idaho	24.8
13	Illinois	32.4
9	Indiana	33.2
8	Iowa	34.5
25	Kansas	28.9
36	Kentucky	24.8
42	Louisiana	22.9
7	Maine	34.6
21	Maryland	29.3
12	Massachusetts	32.5
21	Michigan	29.3
31	Minnesota	26.7
39	Mississippi	24.4
18	Missouri	30.2
3	Montana	37.2
11	Nebraska	32.6
47	Nevada	19.3
30	New Hampshire	26.8
2	New Jersey	42.6
17	New Mexico	30.4
5	New York	34.9
26	North Carolina	28.3
6	North Dakota	34.7
9	Ohio	33.2
32	Oklahoma	26.0
35	Oregon	25.4
1	Pennsylvania	42.9
44	Rhode Island	21.2
36	South Carolina	24.8
24	South Dakota	29.0
33	Tennessee	25.6
43	Texas	21.8
48	Utah	18.6
4	Vermont	36.2
27	Virginia	27.8
23	Washington	29.1
14	West Virginia	31.7
15	Wisconsin	31.0
41	Wyoming	23.8

RANK ORDER

RANK	STATE	RATE
1	Pennsylvania	42.9
2	New Jersey	42.6
3	Montana	37.2
4	Vermont	36.2
5	New York	34.9
6	North Dakota	34.7
7	Maine	34.6
8	Iowa	34.5
9	Indiana	33.2
9	Ohio	33.2
11	Nebraska	32.6
12	Massachusetts	32.5
13	Illinois	32.4
14	West Virginia	31.7
15	Wisconsin	31.0
16	Alabama	30.7
17	New Mexico	30.4
18	Florida	30.2
18	Missouri	30.2
20	Connecticut	29.6
21	Maryland	29.3
21	Michigan	29.3
23	Washington	29.1
24	South Dakota	29.0
25	Kansas	28.9
26	North Carolina	28.3
27	Virginia	27.8
28	Delaware	27.6
29	Hawaii	27.0
30	New Hampshire	26.8
31	Minnesota	26.7
32	Oklahoma	26.0
33	Tennessee	25.6
34	Arkansas	25.5
35	Oregon	25.4
36	Idaho	24.8
36	Kentucky	24.8
36	South Carolina	24.8
39	Mississippi	24.4
40	California	24.0
41	Wyoming	23.8
42	Louisiana	22.9
43	Texas	21.8
44	Rhode Island	21.2
45	Georgia	20.8
46	Colorado	19.6
47	Nevada	19.3
48	Utah	18.6
49	Alaska	17.9
49	Arizona	17.9

| | District of Columbia | 63.9 |

Source: Morgan Quitno Press using data from American Cancer Society "Cancer Facts & Figures 2005" (Copyright 2005, American Cancer Society)
*These estimates are offered as a rough guide and should be interpreted with caution. They are calculated according to the distribution of estimated 2005 cancer deaths by state. Rates calculated using 2003 Census female population estimates.

Percent of Women Who Have Had a Hysterectomy: 2002

National Median = 20.8% of Women*

ALPHA ORDER

RANK	STATE	PERCENT
4	Alabama	30.0
43	Alaska	16.6
11	Arizona	25.6
2	Arkansas	30.5
39	California	18.7
25	Colorado	21.1
46	Connecticut	15.6
1	Delaware	32.6
13	Florida	25.1
18	Georgia	23.8
50	Hawaii	14.6
16	Idaho	24.3
35	Illinois	19.4
21	Indiana	22.8
29	Iowa	20.7
14	Kansas	25.0
9	Kentucky	26.4
3	Louisiana	30.1
37	Maine	19.1
41	Maryland	17.3
46	Massachusetts	15.6
25	Michigan	21.1
42	Minnesota	17.0
6	Mississippi	29.1
27	Missouri	20.8
20	Montana	23.2
23	Nebraska	22.4
22	Nevada	22.7
44	New Hampshire	16.3
45	New Jersey	15.7
37	New Mexico	19.1
49	New York	14.7
19	North Carolina	23.5
27	North Dakota	20.8
29	Ohio	20.7
5	Oklahoma	29.6
12	Oregon	25.4
34	Pennsylvania	19.6
31	Rhode Island	20.3
7	South Carolina	26.5
33	South Dakota	19.8
7	Tennessee	26.5
17	Texas	23.9
24	Utah	21.5
48	Vermont	15.2
36	Virginia	19.3
32	Washington	20.2
14	West Virginia	25.0
40	Wisconsin	18.2
10	Wyoming	26.1

RANK ORDER

RANK	STATE	PERCENT
1	Delaware	32.6
2	Arkansas	30.5
3	Louisiana	30.1
4	Alabama	30.0
5	Oklahoma	29.6
6	Mississippi	29.1
7	South Carolina	26.5
7	Tennessee	26.5
9	Kentucky	26.4
10	Wyoming	26.1
11	Arizona	25.6
12	Oregon	25.4
13	Florida	25.1
14	Kansas	25.0
14	West Virginia	25.0
16	Idaho	24.3
17	Texas	23.9
18	Georgia	23.8
19	North Carolina	23.5
20	Montana	23.2
21	Indiana	22.8
22	Nevada	22.7
23	Nebraska	22.4
24	Utah	21.5
25	Colorado	21.1
25	Michigan	21.1
27	Missouri	20.8
27	North Dakota	20.8
29	Iowa	20.7
29	Ohio	20.7
31	Rhode Island	20.3
32	Washington	20.2
33	South Dakota	19.8
34	Pennsylvania	19.6
35	Illinois	19.4
36	Virginia	19.3
37	Maine	19.1
37	New Mexico	19.1
39	California	18.7
40	Wisconsin	18.2
41	Maryland	17.3
42	Minnesota	17.0
43	Alaska	16.6
44	New Hampshire	16.3
45	New Jersey	15.7
46	Connecticut	15.6
46	Massachusetts	15.6
48	Vermont	15.2
49	New York	14.7
50	Hawaii	14.6
	District of Columbia	16.5

Source: U.S. Department of Health and Human Services, Centers for Disease Control and Prevention
"2002 Behavioral Risk Factor Surveillance Summary Prevalence Data" (http://apps.nccd.cdc.gov/brfss/)
*Of women 18 years old and older.

AIDS Cases Reported in 2004

National Total = 39,097 New AIDS Cases*

ALPHA ORDER

RANK	STATE	CASES	% of USA
20	Alabama	442	1.1%
41	Alaska	56	0.1%
18	Arizona	550	1.4%
31	Arkansas	184	0.5%
3	California	4,383	11.2%
25	Colorado	313	0.8%
17	Connecticut	584	1.5%
34	Delaware	143	0.4%
2	Florida	5,380	13.8%
6	Georgia	1,558	4.0%
35	Hawaii	136	0.3%
45	Idaho	18	0.0%
5	Illinois	1,559	4.0%
23	Indiana	364	0.9%
40	Iowa	65	0.2%
37	Kansas	110	0.3%
28	Kentucky	232	0.6%
11	Louisiana	865	2.2%
43	Maine	48	0.1%
8	Maryland	1,363	3.5%
19	Massachusetts	495	1.3%
16	Michigan	614	1.6%
29	Minnesota	206	0.5%
21	Mississippi	437	1.1%
24	Missouri	338	0.9%
50	Montana	6	0.0%
42	Nebraska	54	0.1%
27	Nevada	260	0.7%
44	New Hampshire	44	0.1%
9	New Jersey	1,360	3.5%
32	New Mexico	178	0.5%
1	New York	6,210	15.9%
10	North Carolina	1,080	2.8%
45	North Dakota	18	0.0%
14	Ohio	617	1.6%
30	Oklahoma	202	0.5%
26	Oregon	282	0.7%
7	Pennsylvania	1,441	3.7%
36	Rhode Island	131	0.3%
13	South Carolina	709	1.8%
49	South Dakota	11	0.0%
12	Tennessee	722	1.8%
4	Texas	3,081	7.9%
39	Utah	72	0.2%
48	Vermont	16	0.0%
15	Virginia	615	1.6%
22	Washington	373	1.0%
38	West Virginia	86	0.2%
33	Wisconsin	157	0.4%
45	Wyoming	18	0.0%

RANK ORDER

RANK	STATE	CASES	% of USA
1	New York	6,210	15.9%
2	Florida	5,380	13.8%
3	California	4,383	11.2%
4	Texas	3,081	7.9%
5	Illinois	1,559	4.0%
6	Georgia	1,558	4.0%
7	Pennsylvania	1,441	3.7%
8	Maryland	1,363	3.5%
9	New Jersey	1,360	3.5%
10	North Carolina	1,080	2.8%
11	Louisiana	865	2.2%
12	Tennessee	722	1.8%
13	South Carolina	709	1.8%
14	Ohio	617	1.6%
15	Virginia	615	1.6%
16	Michigan	614	1.6%
17	Connecticut	584	1.5%
18	Arizona	550	1.4%
19	Massachusetts	495	1.3%
20	Alabama	442	1.1%
21	Mississippi	437	1.1%
22	Washington	373	1.0%
23	Indiana	364	0.9%
24	Missouri	338	0.9%
25	Colorado	313	0.8%
26	Oregon	282	0.7%
27	Nevada	260	0.7%
28	Kentucky	232	0.6%
29	Minnesota	206	0.5%
30	Oklahoma	202	0.5%
31	Arkansas	184	0.5%
32	New Mexico	178	0.5%
33	Wisconsin	157	0.4%
34	Delaware	143	0.4%
35	Hawaii	136	0.3%
36	Rhode Island	131	0.3%
37	Kansas	110	0.3%
38	West Virginia	86	0.2%
39	Utah	72	0.2%
40	Iowa	65	0.2%
41	Alaska	56	0.1%
42	Nebraska	54	0.1%
43	Maine	48	0.1%
44	New Hampshire	44	0.1%
45	Idaho	18	0.0%
45	North Dakota	18	0.0%
45	Wyoming	18	0.0%
48	Vermont	16	0.0%
49	South Dakota	11	0.0%
50	Montana	6	0.0%
	District of Columbia	911	2.3%

Source: U.S. Department of Health and Human Services, National Center for Health Statistics
    "Morbidity and Mortality Weekly Report" (January 7, 2005, Vol. 53, Nos. 51 & 52)
*Provisional data. AIDS is Acquired Immunodeficiency Syndrome. It is a specific group of diseases or conditions which are indicative of severe immunosuppression related to infection with the Human Immunodeficiency Virus (HIV). National total does not include 642 new cases in Puerto Rico.

AIDS Rate in 2004

National Rate = 13.3 New AIDS Cases Reported per 100,000 Population*

ALPHA ORDER

RANK	STATE	RATE
20	Alabama	9.8
23	Alaska	8.5
21	Arizona	9.6
28	Arkansas	6.7
14	California	12.2
27	Colorado	6.8
8	Connecticut	16.7
6	Delaware	17.2
2	Florida	30.9
5	Georgia	17.6
19	Hawaii	10.8
49	Idaho	1.3
13	Illinois	12.3
32	Indiana	5.8
47	Iowa	2.2
37	Kansas	4.0
34	Kentucky	5.6
4	Louisiana	19.2
39	Maine	3.6
3	Maryland	24.5
26	Massachusetts	7.7
29	Michigan	6.1
37	Minnesota	4.0
10	Mississippi	15.1
31	Missouri	5.9
50	Montana	0.6
42	Nebraska	3.1
18	Nevada	11.1
41	New Hampshire	3.4
9	New Jersey	15.6
22	New Mexico	9.4
1	New York	32.3
12	North Carolina	12.6
44	North Dakota	2.8
35	Ohio	5.4
33	Oklahoma	5.7
25	Oregon	7.8
17	Pennsylvania	11.6
16	Rhode Island	12.1
7	South Carolina	16.9
48	South Dakota	1.4
14	Tennessee	12.2
11	Texas	13.7
43	Utah	3.0
46	Vermont	2.6
24	Virginia	8.2
30	Washington	6.0
36	West Virginia	4.7
44	Wisconsin	2.8
39	Wyoming	3.6

RANK ORDER

RANK	STATE	RATE
1	New York	32.3
2	Florida	30.9
3	Maryland	24.5
4	Louisiana	19.2
5	Georgia	17.6
6	Delaware	17.2
7	South Carolina	16.9
8	Connecticut	16.7
9	New Jersey	15.6
10	Mississippi	15.1
11	Texas	13.7
12	North Carolina	12.6
13	Illinois	12.3
14	California	12.2
14	Tennessee	12.2
16	Rhode Island	12.1
17	Pennsylvania	11.6
18	Nevada	11.1
19	Hawaii	10.8
20	Alabama	9.8
21	Arizona	9.6
22	New Mexico	9.4
23	Alaska	8.5
24	Virginia	8.2
25	Oregon	7.8
26	Massachusetts	7.7
27	Colorado	6.8
28	Arkansas	6.7
29	Michigan	6.1
30	Washington	6.0
31	Missouri	5.9
32	Indiana	5.8
33	Oklahoma	5.7
34	Kentucky	5.6
35	Ohio	5.4
36	West Virginia	4.7
37	Kansas	4.0
37	Minnesota	4.0
39	Maine	3.6
39	Wyoming	3.6
41	New Hampshire	3.4
42	Nebraska	3.1
43	Utah	3.0
44	North Dakota	2.8
44	Wisconsin	2.8
46	Vermont	2.6
47	Iowa	2.2
48	South Dakota	1.4
49	Idaho	1.3
50	Montana	0.6

District of Columbia	164.6

Source: Morgan Quitno Press using data from U.S. Dept. of Health & Human Serv's, National Center for Health Statistics "Morbidity and Mortality Weekly Report" (January 7, 2005, Vol. 53, Nos. 51 & 52)
*Provisional data. AIDS is Acquired Immunodeficiency Syndrome. It is a specific group of diseases or conditions which are indicative of severe immunosuppression related to infection with the Human Immunodeficiency Virus (HIV). National rate does not include cases or population in U.S. territories.

AIDS Cases Reported Through December 2003

National Total = 872,629 Reported AIDS Cases*

ALPHA ORDER

RANK	STATE	CASES	% of USA
23	Alabama	7,607	0.9%
45	Alaska	565	0.1%
21	Arizona	9,208	1.1%
32	Arkansas	3,581	0.4%
2	California	133,292	15.3%
22	Colorado	8,073	0.9%
14	Connecticut	13,464	1.5%
33	Delaware	3,231	0.4%
3	Florida	94,725	10.9%
8	Georgia	27,915	3.2%
34	Hawaii	2,833	0.3%
44	Idaho	572	0.1%
6	Illinois	30,139	3.5%
24	Indiana	7,504	0.9%
39	Iowa	1,567	0.2%
35	Kansas	2,659	0.3%
30	Kentucky	4,192	0.5%
12	Louisiana	15,653	1.8%
42	Maine	1,084	0.1%
9	Maryland	26,918	3.1%
10	Massachusetts	18,525	2.1%
16	Michigan	13,326	1.5%
29	Minnesota	4,252	0.5%
25	Mississippi	5,799	0.7%
20	Missouri	10,406	1.2%
47	Montana	366	0.0%
41	Nebraska	1,296	0.1%
27	Nevada	5,237	0.6%
43	New Hampshire	995	0.1%
5	New Jersey	46,703	5.4%
36	New Mexico	2,389	0.3%
1	New York	162,446	18.6%
15	North Carolina	13,456	1.5%
50	North Dakota	115	0.0%
13	Ohio	13,502	1.5%
28	Oklahoma	4,441	0.5%
26	Oregon	5,599	0.6%
7	Pennsylvania	29,988	3.4%
37	Rhode Island	2,363	0.3%
17	South Carolina	11,818	1.4%
48	South Dakota	218	0.0%
19	Tennessee	10,740	1.2%
4	Texas	62,983	7.2%
38	Utah	2,176	0.2%
46	Vermont	457	0.1%
11	Virginia	15,723	1.8%
18	Washington	10,987	1.3%
40	West Virginia	1,352	0.2%
31	Wisconsin	4,136	0.5%
49	Wyoming	212	0.0%

RANK ORDER

RANK	STATE	CASES	% of USA
1	New York	162,446	18.6%
2	California	133,292	15.3%
3	Florida	94,725	10.9%
4	Texas	62,983	7.2%
5	New Jersey	46,703	5.4%
6	Illinois	30,139	3.5%
7	Pennsylvania	29,988	3.4%
8	Georgia	27,915	3.2%
9	Maryland	26,918	3.1%
10	Massachusetts	18,525	2.1%
11	Virginia	15,723	1.8%
12	Louisiana	15,653	1.8%
13	Ohio	13,502	1.5%
14	Connecticut	13,464	1.5%
15	North Carolina	13,456	1.5%
16	Michigan	13,326	1.5%
17	South Carolina	11,818	1.4%
18	Washington	10,987	1.3%
19	Tennessee	10,740	1.2%
20	Missouri	10,406	1.2%
21	Arizona	9,208	1.1%
22	Colorado	8,073	0.9%
23	Alabama	7,607	0.9%
24	Indiana	7,504	0.9%
25	Mississippi	5,799	0.7%
26	Oregon	5,599	0.6%
27	Nevada	5,237	0.6%
28	Oklahoma	4,441	0.5%
29	Minnesota	4,252	0.5%
30	Kentucky	4,192	0.5%
31	Wisconsin	4,136	0.5%
32	Arkansas	3,581	0.4%
33	Delaware	3,231	0.4%
34	Hawaii	2,833	0.3%
35	Kansas	2,659	0.3%
36	New Mexico	2,389	0.3%
37	Rhode Island	2,363	0.3%
38	Utah	2,176	0.2%
39	Iowa	1,567	0.2%
40	West Virginia	1,352	0.2%
41	Nebraska	1,296	0.1%
42	Maine	1,084	0.1%
43	New Hampshire	995	0.1%
44	Idaho	572	0.1%
45	Alaska	565	0.1%
46	Vermont	457	0.1%
47	Montana	366	0.0%
48	South Dakota	218	0.0%
49	Wyoming	212	0.0%
50	North Dakota	115	0.0%
	District of Columbia	15,841	1.8%

Source: U.S. Department of Health and Human Services, Centers for Disease Control and Prevention "HIV/AIDS Surveillance Report, 2003" (Vol. 15)

Cumulative through December 2003. AIDS is Acquired Immunodeficiency Syndrome. It is a specific group of diseases or conditions which are indicative of severe immunosuppression related to infection with the Human Immunodeficiency Virus (HIV). National total does not include 28,301 cases in Puerto Rico, 603 cases in the Virgin Islands and 67 cases in other U.S. territories.

AIDS Cases in Children 12 Years and Younger Through December 2003

National Total = 8,927 Juvenile AIDS Cases*

ALPHA ORDER

RANK	STATE	CASES	% of USA
18	Alabama	76	0.9%
44	Alaska	6	0.1%
23	Arizona	42	0.5%
24	Arkansas	38	0.4%
4	California	642	7.2%
27	Colorado	31	0.3%
11	Connecticut	180	2.0%
33	Delaware	25	0.3%
2	Florida	1,490	16.7%
9	Georgia	218	2.4%
36	Hawaii	17	0.2%
47	Idaho	3	0.0%
8	Illinois	282	3.2%
21	Indiana	54	0.6%
37	Iowa	13	0.1%
38	Kansas	12	0.1%
28	Kentucky	30	0.3%
13	Louisiana	134	1.5%
42	Maine	9	0.1%
7	Maryland	312	3.5%
10	Massachusetts	214	2.4%
16	Michigan	111	1.2%
30	Minnesota	27	0.3%
20	Mississippi	57	0.6%
19	Missouri	60	0.7%
47	Montana	3	0.0%
40	Nebraska	10	0.1%
29	Nevada	28	0.3%
40	New Hampshire	10	0.1%
3	New Jersey	767	8.6%
43	New Mexico	8	0.1%
1	New York	2,337	26.2%
15	North Carolina	121	1.4%
50	North Dakota	1	0.0%
14	Ohio	129	1.4%
30	Oklahoma	27	0.3%
35	Oregon	19	0.2%
6	Pennsylvania	349	3.9%
32	Rhode Island	26	0.3%
17	South Carolina	94	1.1%
46	South Dakota	4	0.0%
21	Tennessee	54	0.6%
5	Texas	391	4.4%
34	Utah	20	0.2%
44	Vermont	6	0.1%
12	Virginia	179	2.0%
25	Washington	34	0.4%
39	West Virginia	11	0.1%
26	Wisconsin	33	0.4%
49	Wyoming	2	0.0%

RANK ORDER

RANK	STATE	CASES	% of USA
1	New York	2,337	26.2%
2	Florida	1,490	16.7%
3	New Jersey	767	8.6%
4	California	642	7.2%
5	Texas	391	4.4%
6	Pennsylvania	349	3.9%
7	Maryland	312	3.5%
8	Illinois	282	3.2%
9	Georgia	218	2.4%
10	Massachusetts	214	2.4%
11	Connecticut	180	2.0%
12	Virginia	179	2.0%
13	Louisiana	134	1.5%
14	Ohio	129	1.4%
15	North Carolina	121	1.4%
16	Michigan	111	1.2%
17	South Carolina	94	1.1%
18	Alabama	76	0.9%
19	Missouri	60	0.7%
20	Mississippi	57	0.6%
21	Indiana	54	0.6%
21	Tennessee	54	0.6%
23	Arizona	42	0.5%
24	Arkansas	38	0.4%
25	Washington	34	0.4%
26	Wisconsin	33	0.4%
27	Colorado	31	0.3%
28	Kentucky	30	0.3%
29	Nevada	28	0.3%
30	Minnesota	27	0.3%
30	Oklahoma	27	0.3%
32	Rhode Island	26	0.3%
33	Delaware	25	0.3%
34	Utah	20	0.2%
35	Oregon	19	0.2%
36	Hawaii	17	0.2%
37	Iowa	13	0.1%
38	Kansas	12	0.1%
39	West Virginia	11	0.1%
40	Nebraska	10	0.1%
40	New Hampshire	10	0.1%
42	Maine	9	0.1%
43	New Mexico	8	0.1%
44	Alaska	6	0.1%
44	Vermont	6	0.1%
46	South Dakota	4	0.0%
47	Idaho	3	0.0%
47	Montana	3	0.0%
49	Wyoming	2	0.0%
50	North Dakota	1	0.0%
	District of Columbia	181	2.0%

Source: U.S. Department of Health and Human Services, Centers for Disease Control and Prevention
"HIV/AIDS Surveillance Report, 2003" (Vol. 15)

Cumulative through December 2003. AIDS is Acquired Immunodeficiency Syndrome. It is a specific group of diseases or conditions which are indicative of severe immunosuppression related to infection with the Human Immunodeficiency Virus (HIV). National total does not include 398 cases in Puerto Rico, 18 cases in the Virgin Islands and one case in Guam.

Chickenpox (Varicella) Cases Reported in 2004

National Total = 18,718 Cases*

ALPHA ORDER

RANK	STATE	CASES	% of USA
22	Alabama	0	0.0%
22	Alaska	0	0.0%
22	Arizona	0	0.0%
22	Arkansas	0	0.0%
22	California	0	0.0%
3	Colorado	1,958	10.5%
22	Connecticut	0	0.0%
19	Delaware	5	0.0%
22	Florida	0	0.0%
22	Georgia	0	0.0%
22	Hawaii	0	0.0%
22	Idaho	0	0.0%
21	Illinois	2	0.0%
12	Indiana	139	0.7%
NA	Iowa**	NA	NA
22	Kansas	0	0.0%
22	Kentucky	0	0.0%
17	Louisiana	51	0.3%
11	Maine	311	1.7%
22	Maryland	0	0.0%
22	Massachusetts	0	0.0%
2	Michigan	4,239	22.6%
22	Minnesota	0	0.0%
22	Mississippi	0	0.0%
19	Missouri	5	0.0%
22	Montana	0	0.0%
22	Nebraska	0	0.0%
22	Nevada	0	0.0%
22	New Hampshire	0	0.0%
22	New Jersey	0	0.0%
13	New Mexico	104	0.6%
22	New York	0	0.0%
NA	North Carolina**	NA	NA
15	North Dakota	82	0.4%
4	Ohio	1,572	8.4%
22	Oklahoma	0	0.0%
22	Oregon	0	0.0%
14	Pennsylvania	91	0.5%
22	Rhode Island	0	0.0%
10	South Carolina	318	1.7%
18	South Dakota	43	0.2%
22	Tennessee	0	0.0%
1	Texas	6,303	33.7%
8	Utah	472	2.5%
9	Vermont	411	2.2%
7	Virginia	626	3.3%
22	Washington	0	0.0%
5	West Virginia	1,276	6.8%
6	Wisconsin	628	3.4%
16	Wyoming	56	0.3%

RANK ORDER

RANK	STATE	CASES	% of USA
1	Texas	6,303	33.7%
2	Michigan	4,239	22.6%
3	Colorado	1,958	10.5%
4	Ohio	1,572	8.4%
5	West Virginia	1,276	6.8%
6	Wisconsin	628	3.4%
7	Virginia	626	3.3%
8	Utah	472	2.5%
9	Vermont	411	2.2%
10	South Carolina	318	1.7%
11	Maine	311	1.7%
12	Indiana	139	0.7%
13	New Mexico	104	0.6%
14	Pennsylvania	91	0.5%
15	North Dakota	82	0.4%
16	Wyoming	56	0.3%
17	Louisiana	51	0.3%
18	South Dakota	43	0.2%
19	Delaware	5	0.0%
19	Missouri	5	0.0%
21	Illinois	2	0.0%
22	Alabama	0	0.0%
22	Alaska	0	0.0%
22	Arizona	0	0.0%
22	Arkansas	0	0.0%
22	California	0	0.0%
22	Connecticut	0	0.0%
22	Florida	0	0.0%
22	Georgia	0	0.0%
22	Hawaii	0	0.0%
22	Idaho	0	0.0%
22	Kansas	0	0.0%
22	Kentucky	0	0.0%
22	Maryland	0	0.0%
22	Massachusetts	0	0.0%
22	Minnesota	0	0.0%
22	Mississippi	0	0.0%
22	Montana	0	0.0%
22	Nebraska	0	0.0%
22	Nevada	0	0.0%
22	New Hampshire	0	0.0%
22	New Jersey	0	0.0%
22	New York	0	0.0%
22	Oklahoma	0	0.0%
22	Oregon	0	0.0%
22	Rhode Island	0	0.0%
22	Tennessee	0	0.0%
22	Washington	0	0.0%
NA	Iowa**	NA	NA
NA	North Carolina**	NA	NA
	District of Columbia	26	0.1%

Source: U.S. Department of Health and Human Services, National Center for Health Statistics
    "Morbidity and Mortality Weekly Report" (January 7, 2005, Vol. 53, Nos. 51 & 52)
Provisional data. An illness with acute onset of generalized maculo-papulovesicular rash without other apparent cause.
**Not notifiable.*

350

Chickenpox (Varicella) Rate in 2004

National Rate = 6.4 Cases per 100,000 Population*

ALPHA ORDER

RANK	STATE	RATE
21	Alabama	0.0
21	Alaska	0.0
21	Arizona	0.0
21	Arkansas	0.0
21	California	0.0
3	Colorado	42.6
21	Connecticut	0.0
19	Delaware	0.6
21	Florida	0.0
21	Georgia	0.0
21	Hawaii	0.0
21	Idaho	0.0
21	Illinois	0.0
16	Indiana	2.2
NA	Iowa**	NA
21	Kansas	0.0
21	Kentucky	0.0
17	Louisiana	1.1
6	Maine	23.6
21	Maryland	0.0
21	Massachusetts	0.0
4	Michigan	41.9
21	Minnesota	0.0
21	Mississippi	0.0
20	Missouri	0.1
21	Montana	0.0
21	Nebraska	0.0
21	Nevada	0.0
21	New Hampshire	0.0
21	New Jersey	0.0
15	New Mexico	5.5
21	New York	0.0
NA	North Carolina**	NA
9	North Dakota	12.9
8	Ohio	13.7
21	Oklahoma	0.0
21	Oregon	0.0
18	Pennsylvania	0.7
21	Rhode Island	0.0
13	South Carolina	7.6
14	South Dakota	5.6
21	Tennessee	0.0
5	Texas	28.0
7	Utah	19.8
2	Vermont	66.1
12	Virginia	8.4
21	Washington	0.0
1	West Virginia	70.3
10	Wisconsin	11.4
11	Wyoming	11.1

RANK ORDER

RANK	STATE	RATE
1	West Virginia	70.3
2	Vermont	66.1
3	Colorado	42.6
4	Michigan	41.9
5	Texas	28.0
6	Maine	23.6
7	Utah	19.8
8	Ohio	13.7
9	North Dakota	12.9
10	Wisconsin	11.4
11	Wyoming	11.1
12	Virginia	8.4
13	South Carolina	7.6
14	South Dakota	5.6
15	New Mexico	5.5
16	Indiana	2.2
17	Louisiana	1.1
18	Pennsylvania	0.7
19	Delaware	0.6
20	Missouri	0.1
21	Alabama	0.0
21	Alaska	0.0
21	Arizona	0.0
21	Arkansas	0.0
21	California	0.0
21	Connecticut	0.0
21	Florida	0.0
21	Georgia	0.0
21	Hawaii	0.0
21	Idaho	0.0
21	Illinois	0.0
21	Kansas	0.0
21	Kentucky	0.0
21	Maryland	0.0
21	Massachusetts	0.0
21	Minnesota	0.0
21	Mississippi	0.0
21	Montana	0.0
21	Nebraska	0.0
21	Nevada	0.0
21	New Hampshire	0.0
21	New Jersey	0.0
21	New York	0.0
21	Oklahoma	0.0
21	Oregon	0.0
21	Rhode Island	0.0
21	Tennessee	0.0
21	Washington	0.0
NA	Iowa**	NA
NA	North Carolina**	NA

District of Columbia   4.7

Source: Morgan Quitno Press using data from U.S. Dept. of Health & Human Serv's, National Center for Health Statistics
    "Morbidity and Mortality Weekly Report" (January 7, 2005, Vol. 53, Nos. 51 & 52)
*Provisional data. An illness with acute onset of generalized maculo-papulovesicular rash without other apparent
cause.
**Not notifiable.

E-Coli Cases Reported in 2004

National Total = 2,993 Cases*

ALPHA ORDER

RANK	STATE	CASES	% of USA
30	Alabama	30	1.0%
50	Alaska	1	0.0%
32	Arizona	29	1.0%
37	Arkansas	17	0.6%
2	California	216	7.2%
24	Colorado	52	1.7%
20	Connecticut	61	2.0%
48	Delaware	3	0.1%
13	Florida	89	3.0%
29	Georgia	33	1.1%
44	Hawaii	10	0.3%
17	Idaho	66	2.2%
14	Illinois	78	2.6%
18	Indiana	62	2.1%
9	Iowa	123	4.1%
25	Kansas	44	1.5%
26	Kentucky	37	1.2%
47	Louisiana	6	0.2%
42	Maine	12	0.4%
30	Maryland	30	1.0%
10	Massachusetts	99	3.3%
10	Michigan	99	3.3%
6	Minnesota	134	4.5%
44	Mississippi	10	0.3%
8	Missouri	128	4.3%
38	Montana	16	0.5%
15	Nebraska	76	2.5%
33	Nevada	28	0.9%
33	New Hampshire	28	0.9%
18	New Jersey	62	2.1%
38	New Mexico	16	0.5%
1	New York	217	7.3%
3	North Carolina	152	5.1%
36	North Dakota	22	0.7%
7	Ohio	132	4.4%
35	Oklahoma	25	0.8%
16	Oregon	69	2.3%
12	Pennsylvania	98	3.3%
41	Rhode Island	14	0.5%
46	South Carolina	8	0.3%
28	South Dakota	35	1.2%
27	Tennessee	36	1.2%
23	Texas	54	1.8%
22	Utah	55	1.8%
42	Vermont	12	0.4%
21	Virginia	57	1.9%
4	Washington	149	5.0%
48	West Virginia	3	0.1%
5	Wisconsin	143	4.8%
38	Wyoming	16	0.5%

RANK ORDER

RANK	STATE	CASES	% of USA
1	New York	217	7.3%
2	California	216	7.2%
3	North Carolina	152	5.1%
4	Washington	149	5.0%
5	Wisconsin	143	4.8%
6	Minnesota	134	4.5%
7	Ohio	132	4.4%
8	Missouri	128	4.3%
9	Iowa	123	4.1%
10	Massachusetts	99	3.3%
10	Michigan	99	3.3%
12	Pennsylvania	98	3.3%
13	Florida	89	3.0%
14	Illinois	78	2.6%
15	Nebraska	76	2.5%
16	Oregon	69	2.3%
17	Idaho	66	2.2%
18	Indiana	62	2.1%
18	New Jersey	62	2.1%
20	Connecticut	61	2.0%
21	Virginia	57	1.9%
22	Utah	55	1.8%
23	Texas	54	1.8%
24	Colorado	52	1.7%
25	Kansas	44	1.5%
26	Kentucky	37	1.2%
27	Tennessee	36	1.2%
28	South Dakota	35	1.2%
29	Georgia	33	1.1%
30	Alabama	30	1.0%
30	Maryland	30	1.0%
32	Arizona	29	1.0%
33	Nevada	28	0.9%
33	New Hampshire	28	0.9%
35	Oklahoma	25	0.8%
36	North Dakota	22	0.7%
37	Arkansas	17	0.6%
38	Montana	16	0.5%
38	New Mexico	16	0.5%
38	Wyoming	16	0.5%
41	Rhode Island	14	0.5%
42	Maine	12	0.4%
42	Vermont	12	0.4%
44	Hawaii	10	0.3%
44	Mississippi	10	0.3%
46	South Carolina	8	0.3%
47	Louisiana	6	0.2%
48	Delaware	3	0.1%
48	West Virginia	3	0.1%
50	Alaska	1	0.0%
	District of Columbia	1	0.0%

Source: U.S. Department of Health and Human Services, National Center for Health Statistics
"Morbidity and Mortality Weekly Report" (January 7, 2005, Vol. 53, Nos. 51 & 52)
*Escherichia Coli is a common bacterium that normally inhabits the intestinal tracts of humans and animals but can cause infection in other parts of the body, especially the urinary tract. One strain, sometimes transmitted in hamburger meat, can cause serious infection resulting in sickness and death.

E-Coli Rate in 2004

National Rate = 1.0 Cases per 100,000 Population*

ALPHA ORDER

RANK	STATE	RATE
33	Alabama	0.7
46	Alaska	0.2
40	Arizona	0.5
36	Arkansas	0.6
36	California	0.6
23	Colorado	1.1
16	Connecticut	1.7
43	Delaware	0.4
40	Florida	0.5
43	Georgia	0.4
29	Hawaii	0.8
1	Idaho	4.7
36	Illinois	0.6
25	Indiana	1.0
4	Iowa	4.2
18	Kansas	1.6
27	Kentucky	0.9
50	Louisiana	0.1
27	Maine	0.9
40	Maryland	0.5
19	Massachusetts	1.5
25	Michigan	1.0
7	Minnesota	2.6
45	Mississippi	0.3
11	Missouri	2.2
16	Montana	1.7
3	Nebraska	4.3
21	Nevada	1.2
11	New Hampshire	2.2
33	New Jersey	0.7
29	New Mexico	0.8
23	New York	1.1
15	North Carolina	1.8
5	North Dakota	3.5
21	Ohio	1.2
33	Oklahoma	0.7
13	Oregon	1.9
29	Pennsylvania	0.8
20	Rhode Island	1.3
46	South Carolina	0.2
2	South Dakota	4.5
36	Tennessee	0.6
46	Texas	0.2
10	Utah	2.3
13	Vermont	1.9
29	Virginia	0.8
9	Washington	2.4
46	West Virginia	0.2
7	Wisconsin	2.6
6	Wyoming	3.2

RANK ORDER

RANK	STATE	RATE
1	Idaho	4.7
2	South Dakota	4.5
3	Nebraska	4.3
4	Iowa	4.2
5	North Dakota	3.5
6	Wyoming	3.2
7	Minnesota	2.6
7	Wisconsin	2.6
9	Washington	2.4
10	Utah	2.3
11	Missouri	2.2
11	New Hampshire	2.2
13	Oregon	1.9
13	Vermont	1.9
15	North Carolina	1.8
16	Connecticut	1.7
16	Montana	1.7
18	Kansas	1.6
19	Massachusetts	1.5
20	Rhode Island	1.3
21	Nevada	1.2
21	Ohio	1.2
23	Colorado	1.1
23	New York	1.1
25	Indiana	1.0
25	Michigan	1.0
27	Kentucky	0.9
27	Maine	0.9
29	Hawaii	0.8
29	New Mexico	0.8
29	Pennsylvania	0.8
29	Virginia	0.8
33	Alabama	0.7
33	New Jersey	0.7
33	Oklahoma	0.7
36	Arkansas	0.6
36	California	0.6
36	Illinois	0.6
36	Tennessee	0.6
40	Arizona	0.5
40	Florida	0.5
40	Maryland	0.5
43	Delaware	0.4
43	Georgia	0.4
45	Mississippi	0.3
46	Alaska	0.2
46	South Carolina	0.2
46	Texas	0.2
46	West Virginia	0.2
50	Louisiana	0.1

District of Columbia   0.2

Source: Morgan Quitno Press using data from U.S. Dept. of Health & Human Serv's, National Center for Health Statistics
"Morbidity and Mortality Weekly Report" (January 7, 2005, Vol. 53, Nos. 51 & 52)
*Escherichia Coli is a common bacterium that normally inhabits the intestinal tracts of humans and animals but can
cause infection in other parts of the body, especially the urinary tract. One strain, sometimes transmitted in
hamburger meat, can cause serious infection resulting in sickness and death.

Hepatitis A and B Cases Reported in 2004

National Total = 12,241 Cases*

ALPHA ORDER

RANK	STATE	CASES	% of USA
32	Alabama	76	0.6%
44	Alaska	20	0.2%
8	Arizona	595	4.9%
21	Arkansas	134	1.1%
1	California	1,313	10.7%
26	Colorado	112	0.9%
19	Connecticut	163	1.3%
37	Delaware	48	0.4%
6	Florida	822	6.7%
3	Georgia	902	7.4%
40	Hawaii	38	0.3%
42	Idaho	31	0.3%
14	Illinois	255	2.1%
20	Indiana	144	1.2%
33	Iowa	70	0.6%
38	Kansas	45	0.4%
28	Kentucky	103	0.8%
23	Louisiana	118	1.0%
45	Maine	15	0.1%
13	Maryland	276	2.3%
2	Massachusetts	1,101	9.0%
11	Michigan	388	3.2%
31	Minnesota	81	0.7%
22	Mississippi	130	1.1%
16	Missouri	233	1.9%
48	Montana	10	0.1%
36	Nebraska	53	0.4%
29	Nevada	85	0.7%
34	New Hampshire	67	0.5%
4	New Jersey	887	7.2%
40	New Mexico	38	0.3%
7	New York	612	5.0%
12	North Carolina	288	2.4%
49	North Dakota	5	0.0%
18	Ohio	171	1.4%
34	Oklahoma	67	0.5%
17	Oregon	179	1.5%
9	Pennsylvania	457	3.7%
43	Rhode Island	29	0.2%
24	South Carolina	116	0.9%
50	South Dakota	4	0.0%
15	Tennessee	254	2.1%
4	Texas	887	7.2%
27	Utah	107	0.9%
47	Vermont	13	0.1%
10	Virginia	417	3.4%
25	Washington	113	0.9%
38	West Virginia	45	0.4%
30	Wisconsin	84	0.7%
46	Wyoming	14	0.1%

RANK ORDER

RANK	STATE	CASES	% of USA
1	California	1,313	10.7%
2	Massachusetts	1,101	9.0%
3	Georgia	902	7.4%
4	New Jersey	887	7.2%
4	Texas	887	7.2%
6	Florida	822	6.7%
7	New York	612	5.0%
8	Arizona	595	4.9%
9	Pennsylvania	457	3.7%
10	Virginia	417	3.4%
11	Michigan	388	3.2%
12	North Carolina	288	2.4%
13	Maryland	276	2.3%
14	Illinois	255	2.1%
15	Tennessee	254	2.1%
16	Missouri	233	1.9%
17	Oregon	179	1.5%
18	Ohio	171	1.4%
19	Connecticut	163	1.3%
20	Indiana	144	1.2%
21	Arkansas	134	1.1%
22	Mississippi	130	1.1%
23	Louisiana	118	1.0%
24	South Carolina	116	0.9%
25	Washington	113	0.9%
26	Colorado	112	0.9%
27	Utah	107	0.9%
28	Kentucky	103	0.8%
29	Nevada	85	0.7%
30	Wisconsin	84	0.7%
31	Minnesota	81	0.7%
32	Alabama	76	0.6%
33	Iowa	70	0.6%
34	New Hampshire	67	0.5%
34	Oklahoma	67	0.5%
36	Nebraska	53	0.4%
37	Delaware	48	0.4%
38	Kansas	45	0.4%
38	West Virginia	45	0.4%
40	Hawaii	38	0.3%
40	New Mexico	38	0.3%
42	Idaho	31	0.3%
43	Rhode Island	29	0.2%
44	Alaska	20	0.2%
45	Maine	15	0.1%
46	Wyoming	14	0.1%
47	Vermont	13	0.1%
48	Montana	10	0.1%
49	North Dakota	5	0.0%
50	South Dakota	4	0.0%
	District of Columbia	26	0.2%

Source: U.S. Department of Health and Human Services, National Center for Health Statistics
"Morbidity and Mortality Weekly Report" (January 7, 2005, Vol. 53, Nos. 51 & 52)
*Provisional data. An inflammation of the liver.

Hepatitis A and B Rate in 2004

National Rate = 4.2 Cases per 100,000 Population*

ALPHA ORDER

RANK	STATE	RATE
42	Alabama	1.7
24	Alaska	3.1
2	Arizona	10.4
10	Arkansas	4.9
19	California	3.7
33	Colorado	2.4
11	Connecticut	4.7
5	Delaware	5.8
11	Florida	4.7
3	Georgia	10.2
25	Hawaii	3.0
36	Idaho	2.2
38	Illinois	2.0
35	Indiana	2.3
33	Iowa	2.4
43	Kansas	1.6
31	Kentucky	2.5
30	Louisiana	2.6
47	Maine	1.1
8	Maryland	5.0
1	Massachusetts	17.2
18	Michigan	3.8
43	Minnesota	1.6
13	Mississippi	4.5
16	Missouri	4.0
47	Montana	1.1
25	Nebraska	3.0
21	Nevada	3.6
7	New Hampshire	5.2
3	New Jersey	10.2
38	New Mexico	2.0
23	New York	3.2
22	North Carolina	3.4
49	North Dakota	0.8
45	Ohio	1.5
40	Oklahoma	1.9
8	Oregon	5.0
19	Pennsylvania	3.7
29	Rhode Island	2.7
27	South Carolina	2.8
50	South Dakota	0.5
15	Tennessee	4.3
17	Texas	3.9
13	Utah	4.5
37	Vermont	2.1
6	Virginia	5.6
41	Washington	1.8
31	West Virginia	2.5
45	Wisconsin	1.5
27	Wyoming	2.8

RANK ORDER

RANK	STATE	RATE
1	Massachusetts	17.2
2	Arizona	10.4
3	Georgia	10.2
3	New Jersey	10.2
5	Delaware	5.8
6	Virginia	5.6
7	New Hampshire	5.2
8	Maryland	5.0
8	Oregon	5.0
10	Arkansas	4.9
11	Connecticut	4.7
11	Florida	4.7
13	Mississippi	4.5
13	Utah	4.5
15	Tennessee	4.3
16	Missouri	4.0
17	Texas	3.9
18	Michigan	3.8
19	California	3.7
19	Pennsylvania	3.7
21	Nevada	3.6
22	North Carolina	3.4
23	New York	3.2
24	Alaska	3.1
25	Hawaii	3.0
25	Nebraska	3.0
27	South Carolina	2.8
27	Wyoming	2.8
29	Rhode Island	2.7
30	Louisiana	2.6
31	Kentucky	2.5
31	West Virginia	2.5
33	Colorado	2.4
33	Iowa	2.4
35	Indiana	2.3
36	Idaho	2.2
37	Vermont	2.1
38	Illinois	2.0
38	New Mexico	2.0
40	Oklahoma	1.9
41	Washington	1.8
42	Alabama	1.7
43	Kansas	1.6
43	Minnesota	1.6
45	Ohio	1.5
45	Wisconsin	1.5
47	Maine	1.1
47	Montana	1.1
49	North Dakota	0.8
50	South Dakota	0.5

District of Columbia 4.7

Source: Morgan Quitno Press using data from U.S. Dept. of Health & Human Serv's, National Center for Health Statistics "Morbidity and Mortality Weekly Report" (January 7, 2005, Vol. 53, Nos. 51 & 52)
*Provisional data. An inflammation of the liver.

Hepatitis C Cases Reported in 2004

National Total = 866 Cases*

ALPHA ORDER

RANK	STATE	CASES	% of USA
30	Alabama	5	0.6%
39	Alaska	0	0.0%
30	Arizona	5	0.6%
33	Arkansas	3	0.3%
8	California	33	3.8%
39	Colorado	0	0.0%
35	Connecticut	2	0.2%
9	Delaware	28	3.2%
4	Florida	63	7.3%
17	Georgia	17	2.0%
24	Hawaii	8	0.9%
39	Idaho	0	0.0%
21	Illinois	13	1.5%
23	Indiana	10	1.2%
39	Iowa	0	0.0%
39	Kansas	0	0.0%
13	Kentucky	23	2.7%
3	Louisiana	69	8.0%
39	Maine	0	0.0%
11	Maryland	26	3.0%
28	Massachusetts	6	0.7%
2	Michigan	78	9.0%
16	Minnesota	18	2.1%
9	Mississippi	28	3.2%
6	Missouri	36	4.2%
35	Montana	2	0.2%
38	Nebraska	1	0.1%
19	Nevada	15	1.7%
39	New Hampshire	0	0.0%
39	New Jersey	0	0.0%
27	New Mexico	7	0.8%
15	New York	19	2.2%
22	North Carolina	12	1.4%
39	North Dakota	0	0.0%
28	Ohio	6	0.7%
33	Oklahoma	3	0.3%
19	Oregon	15	1.7%
1	Pennsylvania	130	15.0%
39	Rhode Island	0	0.0%
24	South Carolina	8	0.9%
39	South Dakota	0	0.0%
7	Tennessee	35	4.0%
5	Texas	61	7.0%
30	Utah	5	0.6%
24	Vermont	8	0.9%
17	Virginia	17	2.0%
14	Washington	22	2.5%
12	West Virginia	24	2.8%
39	Wisconsin	0	0.0%
35	Wyoming	2	0.2%

RANK ORDER

RANK	STATE	CASES	% of USA
1	Pennsylvania	130	15.0%
2	Michigan	78	9.0%
3	Louisiana	69	8.0%
4	Florida	63	7.3%
5	Texas	61	7.0%
6	Missouri	36	4.2%
7	Tennessee	35	4.0%
8	California	33	3.8%
9	Delaware	28	3.2%
9	Mississippi	28	3.2%
11	Maryland	26	3.0%
12	West Virginia	24	2.8%
13	Kentucky	23	2.7%
14	Washington	22	2.5%
15	New York	19	2.2%
16	Minnesota	18	2.1%
17	Georgia	17	2.0%
17	Virginia	17	2.0%
19	Nevada	15	1.7%
19	Oregon	15	1.7%
21	Illinois	13	1.5%
22	North Carolina	12	1.4%
23	Indiana	10	1.2%
24	Hawaii	8	0.9%
24	South Carolina	8	0.9%
24	Vermont	8	0.9%
27	New Mexico	7	0.8%
28	Massachusetts	6	0.7%
28	Ohio	6	0.7%
30	Alabama	5	0.6%
30	Arizona	5	0.6%
30	Utah	5	0.6%
33	Arkansas	3	0.3%
33	Oklahoma	3	0.3%
35	Connecticut	2	0.2%
35	Montana	2	0.2%
35	Wyoming	2	0.2%
38	Nebraska	1	0.1%
39	Alaska	0	0.0%
39	Colorado	0	0.0%
39	Idaho	0	0.0%
39	Iowa	0	0.0%
39	Kansas	0	0.0%
39	Maine	0	0.0%
39	New Hampshire	0	0.0%
39	New Jersey	0	0.0%
39	North Dakota	0	0.0%
39	Rhode Island	0	0.0%
39	South Dakota	0	0.0%
39	Wisconsin	0	0.0%
	District of Columbia	3	0.3%

Source: U.S. Department of Health and Human Services, National Center for Health Statistics
    "Morbidity and Mortality Weekly Report" (January 7, 2005, Vol. 53, Nos. 51 & 52)
*Provisional data. An inflammation of the liver. It is the leading cause for liver transplantation and is transmitted by blood-to-blood contact. Most new cases of C are caused by high-risk drug behaviors.
**Not available.

Hepatitis C Rate in 2004

National Rate = 0.3 Cases per 100,000 Population*

ALPHA ORDER

RANK	STATE	RATE
27	Alabama	0.1
39	Alaska	0.0
27	Arizona	0.1
27	Arkansas	0.1
27	California	0.1
39	Colorado	0.0
27	Connecticut	0.1
1	Delaware	3.4
14	Florida	0.4
21	Georgia	0.2
8	Hawaii	0.6
39	Idaho	0.0
27	Illinois	0.1
21	Indiana	0.2
39	Iowa	0.0
39	Kansas	0.0
8	Kentucky	0.6
2	Louisiana	1.5
39	Maine	0.0
13	Maryland	0.5
27	Massachusetts	0.1
7	Michigan	0.8
14	Minnesota	0.4
5	Mississippi	1.0
8	Missouri	0.6
21	Montana	0.2
27	Nebraska	0.1
8	Nevada	0.6
39	New Hampshire	0.0
39	New Jersey	0.0
14	New Mexico	0.4
27	New York	0.1
27	North Carolina	0.1
39	North Dakota	0.0
27	Ohio	0.1
27	Oklahoma	0.1
14	Oregon	0.4
5	Pennsylvania	1.0
39	Rhode Island	0.0
21	South Carolina	0.2
39	South Dakota	0.0
8	Tennessee	0.6
20	Texas	0.3
21	Utah	0.2
3	Vermont	1.3
21	Virginia	0.2
14	Washington	0.4
3	West Virginia	1.3
39	Wisconsin	0.0
14	Wyoming	0.4

RANK ORDER

RANK	STATE	RATE
1	Delaware	3.4
2	Louisiana	1.5
3	Vermont	1.3
3	West Virginia	1.3
5	Mississippi	1.0
5	Pennsylvania	1.0
7	Michigan	0.8
8	Hawaii	0.6
8	Kentucky	0.6
8	Missouri	0.6
8	Nevada	0.6
8	Tennessee	0.6
13	Maryland	0.5
14	Florida	0.4
14	Minnesota	0.4
14	New Mexico	0.4
14	Oregon	0.4
14	Washington	0.4
14	Wyoming	0.4
20	Texas	0.3
21	Georgia	0.2
21	Indiana	0.2
21	Montana	0.2
21	South Carolina	0.2
21	Utah	0.2
21	Virginia	0.2
27	Alabama	0.1
27	Arizona	0.1
27	Arkansas	0.1
27	California	0.1
27	Connecticut	0.1
27	Illinois	0.1
27	Massachusetts	0.1
27	Nebraska	0.1
27	New York	0.1
27	North Carolina	0.1
27	Ohio	0.1
27	Oklahoma	0.1
39	Alaska	0.0
39	Colorado	0.0
39	Idaho	0.0
39	Iowa	0.0
39	Kansas	0.0
39	Maine	0.0
39	New Hampshire	0.0
39	New Jersey	0.0
39	North Dakota	0.0
39	Rhode Island	0.0
39	South Dakota	0.0
39	Wisconsin	0.0

District of Columbia	0.5

Source: Morgan Quitno Press using data from U.S. Dept. of Health & Human Serv's, National Center for Health Statistics
"Morbidity and Mortality Weekly Report" (January 7, 2005, Vol. 53, Nos. 51 & 52)
*Provisional data. An inflammation of the liver. It is the leading cause for liver transplantation and is transmitted by blood-to-blood contact. Most new cases of C are caused by high-risk drug behaviors.
**Not available.

Legionellosis Cases Reported in 2004

National Total = 1,917 Cases*

ALPHA ORDER

ALPHA ORDER

RANK	STATE	CASES	% of USA
27	Alabama	12	0.6%
46	Alaska	1	0.1%
21	Arizona	22	1.1%
47	Arkansas	0	0.0%
9	California	64	3.3%
22	Colorado	21	1.1%
20	Connecticut	23	1.2%
26	Delaware	13	0.7%
4	Florida	147	7.7%
14	Georgia	37	1.9%
47	Hawaii	0	0.0%
29	Idaho	9	0.5%
15	Illinois	35	1.8%
8	Indiana	78	4.1%
35	Iowa	6	0.3%
39	Kansas	4	0.2%
12	Kentucky	40	2.1%
35	Louisiana	6	0.3%
47	Maine	0	0.0%
7	Maryland	82	4.3%
17	Massachusetts	34	1.8%
5	Michigan	134	7.0%
33	Minnesota	7	0.4%
43	Mississippi	3	0.2%
15	Missouri	35	1.8%
43	Montana	3	0.2%
39	Nebraska	4	0.2%
39	Nevada	4	0.2%
28	New Hampshire	11	0.6%
6	New Jersey	100	5.2%
39	New Mexico	4	0.2%
3	New York	174	9.1%
12	North Carolina	40	2.1%
45	North Dakota	2	0.1%
2	Ohio	220	11.5%
31	Oklahoma	8	0.4%
NA	Oregon**	NA	NA
1	Pennsylvania	265	13.8%
23	Rhode Island	18	0.9%
31	South Carolina	8	0.4%
38	South Dakota	5	0.3%
18	Tennessee	33	1.7%
9	Texas	64	3.3%
19	Utah	24	1.3%
35	Vermont	6	0.3%
11	Virginia	53	2.8%
25	Washington	14	0.7%
29	West Virginia	9	0.5%
24	Wisconsin	17	0.9%
33	Wyoming	7	0.4%

RANK ORDER

RANK	STATE	CASES	% of USA
1	Pennsylvania	265	13.8%
2	Ohio	220	11.5%
3	New York	174	9.1%
4	Florida	147	7.7%
5	Michigan	134	7.0%
6	New Jersey	100	5.2%
7	Maryland	82	4.3%
8	Indiana	78	4.1%
9	California	64	3.3%
9	Texas	64	3.3%
11	Virginia	53	2.8%
12	Kentucky	40	2.1%
12	North Carolina	40	2.1%
14	Georgia	37	1.9%
15	Illinois	35	1.8%
15	Missouri	35	1.8%
17	Massachusetts	34	1.8%
18	Tennessee	33	1.7%
19	Utah	24	1.3%
20	Connecticut	23	1.2%
21	Arizona	22	1.1%
22	Colorado	21	1.1%
23	Rhode Island	18	0.9%
24	Wisconsin	17	0.9%
25	Washington	14	0.7%
26	Delaware	13	0.7%
27	Alabama	12	0.6%
28	New Hampshire	11	0.6%
29	Idaho	9	0.5%
29	West Virginia	9	0.5%
31	Oklahoma	8	0.4%
31	South Carolina	8	0.4%
33	Minnesota	7	0.4%
33	Wyoming	7	0.4%
35	Iowa	6	0.3%
35	Louisiana	6	0.3%
35	Vermont	6	0.3%
38	South Dakota	5	0.3%
39	Kansas	4	0.2%
39	Nebraska	4	0.2%
39	Nevada	4	0.2%
39	New Mexico	4	0.2%
43	Mississippi	3	0.2%
43	Montana	3	0.2%
45	North Dakota	2	0.1%
46	Alaska	1	0.1%
47	Arkansas	0	0.0%
47	Hawaii	0	0.0%
47	Maine	0	0.0%
NA	Oregon**	NA	NA
	District of Columbia	11	0.6%

Source: U.S. Department of Health and Human Services, National Center for Health Statistics "Morbidity and Mortality Weekly Report" (January 7, 2005, Vol. 53, Nos. 51 & 52)
Provisional data. A pneumonia-like disease (Legionnaire's Disease).
**Not notifiable.*

Legionellosis Rate in 2004

National Rate = 0.7 Cases per 100,000 Population*

ALPHA ORDER

RANK	STATE	RATE
28	Alabama	0.3
34	Alaska	0.2
26	Arizona	0.4
47	Arkansas	0.0
34	California	0.2
22	Colorado	0.5
16	Connecticut	0.7
4	Delaware	1.6
14	Florida	0.8
26	Georgia	0.4
47	Hawaii	0.0
18	Idaho	0.6
28	Illinois	0.3
7	Indiana	1.3
34	Iowa	0.2
43	Kansas	0.1
10	Kentucky	1.0
43	Louisiana	0.1
47	Maine	0.0
5	Maryland	1.5
22	Massachusetts	0.5
7	Michigan	1.3
43	Minnesota	0.1
43	Mississippi	0.1
18	Missouri	0.6
28	Montana	0.3
34	Nebraska	0.2
34	Nevada	0.2
14	New Hampshire	0.8
9	New Jersey	1.1
34	New Mexico	0.2
13	New York	0.9
22	North Carolina	0.5
28	North Dakota	0.3
2	Ohio	1.9
34	Oklahoma	0.2
NA	Oregon**	NA
1	Pennsylvania	2.1
3	Rhode Island	1.7
34	South Carolina	0.2
18	South Dakota	0.6
18	Tennessee	0.6
28	Texas	0.3
10	Utah	1.0
10	Vermont	1.0
16	Virginia	0.7
34	Washington	0.2
22	West Virginia	0.5
28	Wisconsin	0.3
6	Wyoming	1.4

RANK ORDER

RANK	STATE	RATE
1	Pennsylvania	2.1
2	Ohio	1.9
3	Rhode Island	1.7
4	Delaware	1.6
5	Maryland	1.5
6	Wyoming	1.4
7	Indiana	1.3
7	Michigan	1.3
9	New Jersey	1.1
10	Kentucky	1.0
10	Utah	1.0
10	Vermont	1.0
13	New York	0.9
14	Florida	0.8
14	New Hampshire	0.8
16	Connecticut	0.7
16	Virginia	0.7
18	Idaho	0.6
18	Missouri	0.6
18	South Dakota	0.6
18	Tennessee	0.6
22	Colorado	0.5
22	Massachusetts	0.5
22	North Carolina	0.5
22	West Virginia	0.5
26	Arizona	0.4
26	Georgia	0.4
28	Alabama	0.3
28	Illinois	0.3
28	Montana	0.3
28	North Dakota	0.3
28	Texas	0.3
28	Wisconsin	0.3
34	Alaska	0.2
34	California	0.2
34	Iowa	0.2
34	Nebraska	0.2
34	Nevada	0.2
34	New Mexico	0.2
34	Oklahoma	0.2
34	South Carolina	0.2
34	Washington	0.2
43	Kansas	0.1
43	Louisiana	0.1
43	Minnesota	0.1
43	Mississippi	0.1
47	Arkansas	0.0
47	Hawaii	0.0
47	Maine	0.0
NA	Oregon**	NA
	District of Columbia	2.0

Source: Morgan Quitno Press using data from U.S. Dept. of Health & Human Serv's, National Center for Health Statistics
        "Morbidity and Mortality Weekly Report" (January 7, 2005, Vol. 53, Nos. 51 & 52)
*Provisional data. A pneumonia-like disease (Legionnaire's Disease).
**Not notifiable.

Lyme Disease Cases in 2004

National Total = 18,523 Cases*

ALPHA ORDER

RANK	STATE	CASES	% of USA
37	Alabama	5	0.0%
41	Alaska	2	0.0%
35	Arizona	7	0.0%
33	Arkansas	8	0.0%
19	California	52	0.3%
46	Colorado	0	0.0%
4	Connecticut	1,171	6.3%
9	Delaware	301	1.6%
15	Florida	61	0.3%
31	Georgia	13	0.1%
NA	Hawaii**	NA	NA
36	Idaho	6	0.0%
42	Illinois	1	0.0%
25	Indiana	22	0.1%
21	Iowa	45	0.2%
40	Kansas	3	0.0%
28	Kentucky	15	0.1%
37	Louisiana	5	0.0%
18	Maine	53	0.3%
7	Maryland	809	4.4%
5	Massachusetts	1,134	6.1%
24	Michigan	27	0.1%
8	Minnesota	735	4.0%
32	Mississippi	11	0.1%
17	Missouri	56	0.3%
46	Montana	0	0.0%
33	Nebraska	8	0.0%
42	Nevada	1	0.0%
11	New Hampshire	216	1.2%
3	New Jersey	3,271	17.7%
42	New Mexico	1	0.0%
2	New York	4,156	22.4%
13	North Carolina	123	0.7%
46	North Dakota	0	0.0%
15	Ohio	61	0.3%
46	Oklahoma	0	0.0%
22	Oregon	33	0.2%
1	Pennsylvania	4,541	24.5%
10	Rhode Island	234	1.3%
27	South Carolina	16	0.1%
42	South Dakota	1	0.0%
26	Tennessee	17	0.1%
14	Texas	79	0.4%
29	Utah	14	0.1%
20	Vermont	51	0.3%
12	Virginia	179	1.0%
29	Washington	14	0.1%
23	West Virginia	28	0.2%
6	Wisconsin	922	5.0%
39	Wyoming	4	0.0%

RANK ORDER

RANK	STATE	CASES	% of USA
1	Pennsylvania	4,541	24.5%
2	New York	4,156	22.4%
3	New Jersey	3,271	17.7%
4	Connecticut	1,171	6.3%
5	Massachusetts	1,134	6.1%
6	Wisconsin	922	5.0%
7	Maryland	809	4.4%
8	Minnesota	735	4.0%
9	Delaware	301	1.6%
10	Rhode Island	234	1.3%
11	New Hampshire	216	1.2%
12	Virginia	179	1.0%
13	North Carolina	123	0.7%
14	Texas	79	0.4%
15	Florida	61	0.3%
15	Ohio	61	0.3%
17	Missouri	56	0.3%
18	Maine	53	0.3%
19	California	52	0.3%
20	Vermont	51	0.3%
21	Iowa	45	0.2%
22	Oregon	33	0.2%
23	West Virginia	28	0.2%
24	Michigan	27	0.1%
25	Indiana	22	0.1%
26	Tennessee	17	0.1%
27	South Carolina	16	0.1%
28	Kentucky	15	0.1%
29	Utah	14	0.1%
29	Washington	14	0.1%
31	Georgia	13	0.1%
32	Mississippi	11	0.1%
33	Arkansas	8	0.0%
33	Nebraska	8	0.0%
35	Arizona	7	0.0%
36	Idaho	6	0.0%
37	Alabama	5	0.0%
37	Louisiana	5	0.0%
39	Wyoming	4	0.0%
40	Kansas	3	0.0%
41	Alaska	2	0.0%
42	Illinois	1	0.0%
42	Nevada	1	0.0%
42	New Mexico	1	0.0%
42	South Dakota	1	0.0%
46	Colorado	0	0.0%
46	Montana	0	0.0%
46	North Dakota	0	0.0%
46	Oklahoma	0	0.0%
NA	Hawaii**	NA	NA
	District of Columbia	11	0.1%

Source: U.S. Department of Health and Human Services, National Center for Health Statistics
    "Morbidity and Mortality Weekly Report" (January 7, 2005, Vol. 53, Nos. 51 & 52)
*Provisional data. Caused by ticks-lesions, followed by arthritis of large joints, myalgia, malaise and neurologic
and cardiac manifestations. Named after Old Lyme, CT, where the disease was first reported.
**Not notifiable.

Lyme Disease Rate in 2004

National Rate = 6.3 Cases per 100,000 Population*

ALPHA ORDER

RANK	STATE	RATE
36	Alabama	0.1
31	Alaska	0.3
36	Arizona	0.1
31	Arkansas	0.3
36	California	0.1
44	Colorado	0.0
4	Connecticut	33.4
3	Delaware	36.2
24	Florida	0.4
36	Georgia	0.1
NA	Hawaii**	NA
24	Idaho	0.4
44	Illinois	0.0
24	Indiana	0.4
15	Iowa	1.5
36	Kansas	0.1
24	Kentucky	0.4
36	Louisiana	0.1
13	Maine	4.0
10	Maryland	14.6
7	Massachusetts	17.7
31	Michigan	0.3
11	Minnesota	14.4
24	Mississippi	0.4
18	Missouri	1.0
44	Montana	0.0
22	Nebraska	0.5
44	Nevada	0.0
9	New Hampshire	16.6
1	New Jersey	37.6
36	New Mexico	0.1
6	New York	21.6
17	North Carolina	1.4
44	North Dakota	0.0
22	Ohio	0.5
44	Oklahoma	0.0
19	Oregon	0.9
2	Pennsylvania	36.6
5	Rhode Island	21.7
24	South Carolina	0.4
36	South Dakota	0.1
31	Tennessee	0.3
24	Texas	0.4
21	Utah	0.6
12	Vermont	8.2
14	Virginia	2.4
35	Washington	0.2
15	West Virginia	1.5
8	Wisconsin	16.7
20	Wyoming	0.8

RANK ORDER

RANK	STATE	RATE
1	New Jersey	37.6
2	Pennsylvania	36.6
3	Delaware	36.2
4	Connecticut	33.4
5	Rhode Island	21.7
6	New York	21.6
7	Massachusetts	17.7
8	Wisconsin	16.7
9	New Hampshire	16.6
10	Maryland	14.6
11	Minnesota	14.4
12	Vermont	8.2
13	Maine	4.0
14	Virginia	2.4
15	Iowa	1.5
15	West Virginia	1.5
17	North Carolina	1.4
18	Missouri	1.0
19	Oregon	0.9
20	Wyoming	0.8
21	Utah	0.6
22	Nebraska	0.5
22	Ohio	0.5
24	Florida	0.4
24	Idaho	0.4
24	Indiana	0.4
24	Kentucky	0.4
24	Mississippi	0.4
24	South Carolina	0.4
24	Texas	0.4
31	Alaska	0.3
31	Arkansas	0.3
31	Michigan	0.3
31	Tennessee	0.3
35	Washington	0.2
36	Alabama	0.1
36	Arizona	0.1
36	California	0.1
36	Georgia	0.1
36	Kansas	0.1
36	Louisiana	0.1
36	New Mexico	0.1
36	South Dakota	0.1
44	Colorado	0.0
44	Illinois	0.0
44	Montana	0.0
44	Nevada	0.0
44	North Dakota	0.0
44	Oklahoma	0.0
NA	Hawaii**	NA

District of Columbia   2.0

Source: Morgan Quitno Press using data from U.S. Dept. of Health & Human Serv's, National Center for Health Statistics
"Morbidity and Mortality Weekly Report" (January 7, 2005, Vol. 53, Nos. 51 & 52)
*Provisional data. Caused by ticks-lesions, followed by arthritis of large joints, myalgia, malaise and neurologic
and cardiac manifestations. Named after Old Lyme, CT, where the disease was first reported.
**Not notifiable.

Malaria Cases Reported in 2004

National Total = 1,300 Cases*

ALPHA ORDER

RANK	STATE	CASES	% of USA
24	Alabama	12	0.9%
45	Alaska	2	0.2%
23	Arizona	13	1.0%
28	Arkansas	8	0.6%
2	California	132	10.2%
20	Colorado	16	1.2%
21	Connecticut	15	1.2%
32	Delaware	6	0.5%
3	Florida	95	7.3%
7	Georgia	54	4.2%
43	Hawaii	3	0.2%
47	Idaho	1	0.1%
13	Illinois	24	1.8%
18	Indiana	18	1.4%
39	Iowa	4	0.3%
26	Kansas	9	0.7%
35	Kentucky	5	0.4%
35	Louisiana	5	0.4%
32	Maine	6	0.5%
5	Maryland	78	6.0%
9	Massachusetts	48	3.7%
15	Michigan	21	1.6%
12	Minnesota	25	1.9%
35	Mississippi	5	0.4%
16	Missouri	20	1.5%
47	Montana	1	0.1%
39	Nebraska	4	0.3%
32	Nevada	6	0.5%
35	New Hampshire	5	0.4%
6	New Jersey	59	4.5%
39	New Mexico	4	0.3%
1	New York	236	18.2%
14	North Carolina	23	1.8%
43	North Dakota	3	0.2%
11	Ohio	30	2.3%
29	Oklahoma	7	0.5%
18	Oregon	18	1.4%
10	Pennsylvania	46	3.5%
29	Rhode Island	7	0.5%
25	South Carolina	10	0.8%
47	South Dakota	1	0.1%
29	Tennessee	7	0.5%
4	Texas	92	7.1%
26	Utah	9	0.7%
39	Vermont	4	0.3%
8	Virginia	53	4.1%
16	Washington	20	1.5%
45	West Virginia	2	0.2%
22	Wisconsin	14	1.1%
47	Wyoming	1	0.1%

RANK ORDER

RANK	STATE	CASES	% of USA
1	New York	236	18.2%
2	California	132	10.2%
3	Florida	95	7.3%
4	Texas	92	7.1%
5	Maryland	78	6.0%
6	New Jersey	59	4.5%
7	Georgia	54	4.2%
8	Virginia	53	4.1%
9	Massachusetts	48	3.7%
10	Pennsylvania	46	3.5%
11	Ohio	30	2.3%
12	Minnesota	25	1.9%
13	Illinois	24	1.8%
14	North Carolina	23	1.8%
15	Michigan	21	1.6%
16	Missouri	20	1.5%
16	Washington	20	1.5%
18	Indiana	18	1.4%
18	Oregon	18	1.4%
20	Colorado	16	1.2%
21	Connecticut	15	1.2%
22	Wisconsin	14	1.1%
23	Arizona	13	1.0%
24	Alabama	12	0.9%
25	South Carolina	10	0.8%
26	Kansas	9	0.7%
26	Utah	9	0.7%
28	Arkansas	8	0.6%
29	Oklahoma	7	0.5%
29	Rhode Island	7	0.5%
29	Tennessee	7	0.5%
32	Delaware	6	0.5%
32	Maine	6	0.5%
32	Nevada	6	0.5%
35	Kentucky	5	0.4%
35	Louisiana	5	0.4%
35	Mississippi	5	0.4%
35	New Hampshire	5	0.4%
39	Iowa	4	0.3%
39	Nebraska	4	0.3%
39	New Mexico	4	0.3%
39	Vermont	4	0.3%
43	Hawaii	3	0.2%
43	North Dakota	3	0.2%
45	Alaska	2	0.2%
45	West Virginia	2	0.2%
47	Idaho	1	0.1%
47	Montana	1	0.1%
47	South Dakota	1	0.1%
47	Wyoming	1	0.1%
	District of Columbia	13	1.0%

Source: U.S. Department of Health and Human Services, National Center for Health Statistics
"Morbidity and Mortality Weekly Report" (January 7, 2005, Vol. 53, Nos. 51 & 52)
*Provisional data. Infectious disease usually transmitted by bites of infected mosquitoes. Symptoms include high fever, shaking chills, sweating and anemia.

Malaria Rate in 2004

National Rate = 0.4 Cases per 100,000 Population*

ALPHA ORDER

RANK	STATE	RATE
21	Alabama	0.3
21	Alaska	0.3
33	Arizona	0.2
21	Arkansas	0.3
15	California	0.4
21	Colorado	0.3
15	Connecticut	0.4
3	Delaware	0.7
10	Florida	0.5
7	Georgia	0.6
33	Hawaii	0.2
43	Idaho	0.1
33	Illinois	0.2
21	Indiana	0.3
43	Iowa	0.1
21	Kansas	0.3
43	Kentucky	0.1
43	Louisiana	0.1
10	Maine	0.5
1	Maryland	1.4
3	Massachusetts	0.7
33	Michigan	0.2
10	Minnesota	0.5
33	Mississippi	0.2
21	Missouri	0.3
43	Montana	0.1
33	Nebraska	0.2
21	Nevada	0.3
15	New Hampshire	0.4
3	New Jersey	0.7
33	New Mexico	0.2
2	New York	1.2
21	North Carolina	0.3
10	North Dakota	0.5
21	Ohio	0.3
33	Oklahoma	0.2
10	Oregon	0.5
15	Pennsylvania	0.4
7	Rhode Island	0.6
33	South Carolina	0.2
43	South Dakota	0.1
43	Tennessee	0.1
15	Texas	0.4
15	Utah	0.4
7	Vermont	0.6
3	Virginia	0.7
21	Washington	0.3
43	West Virginia	0.1
21	Wisconsin	0.3
33	Wyoming	0.2

RANK ORDER

RANK	STATE	RATE
1	Maryland	1.4
2	New York	1.2
3	Delaware	0.7
3	Massachusetts	0.7
3	New Jersey	0.7
3	Virginia	0.7
7	Georgia	0.6
7	Rhode Island	0.6
7	Vermont	0.6
10	Florida	0.5
10	Maine	0.5
10	Minnesota	0.5
10	North Dakota	0.5
10	Oregon	0.5
15	California	0.4
15	Connecticut	0.4
15	New Hampshire	0.4
15	Pennsylvania	0.4
15	Texas	0.4
15	Utah	0.4
21	Alabama	0.3
21	Alaska	0.3
21	Arkansas	0.3
21	Colorado	0.3
21	Indiana	0.3
21	Kansas	0.3
21	Missouri	0.3
21	Nevada	0.3
21	North Carolina	0.3
21	Ohio	0.3
21	Washington	0.3
21	Wisconsin	0.3
33	Arizona	0.2
33	Hawaii	0.2
33	Illinois	0.2
33	Michigan	0.2
33	Mississippi	0.2
33	Nebraska	0.2
33	New Mexico	0.2
33	Oklahoma	0.2
33	South Carolina	0.2
33	Wyoming	0.2
43	Idaho	0.1
43	Iowa	0.1
43	Kentucky	0.1
43	Louisiana	0.1
43	Montana	0.1
43	South Dakota	0.1
43	Tennessee	0.1
43	West Virginia	0.1

| District of Columbia | 2.3 |

*Source: Morgan Quitno Press using data from U.S. Dept. of Health & Human Serv's, National Center for Health Statistics
"Morbidity and Mortality Weekly Report" (January 7, 2005, Vol. 53, Nos. 51 & 52)*
*Provisional data. Infectious disease usually transmitted by bites of infected mosquitoes. Symptoms include high fever, shaking chills, sweating and anemia.

Meningococcal Infections Reported in 2004

National Total = 1,254 Cases*

RANK	STATE	CASES	% of USA
21	Alabama	17	1.4%
44	Alaska	3	0.2%
28	Arizona	12	1.0%
17	Arkansas	20	1.6%
1	California	189	15.1%
24	Colorado	15	1.2%
33	Connecticut	10	0.8%
44	Delaware	3	0.2%
2	Florida	107	8.5%
23	Georgia	16	1.3%
35	Hawaii	9	0.7%
37	Idaho	7	0.6%
16	Illinois	22	1.8%
14	Indiana	31	2.5%
20	Iowa	18	1.4%
27	Kansas	14	1.1%
28	Kentucky	12	1.0%
10	Louisiana	36	2.9%
31	Maine	11	0.9%
31	Maryland	11	0.9%
10	Massachusetts	36	2.9%
8	Michigan	49	3.9%
15	Minnesota	23	1.8%
21	Mississippi	17	1.4%
17	Missouri	20	1.6%
44	Montana	3	0.2%
42	Nebraska	4	0.3%
37	Nevada	7	0.6%
37	New Hampshire	7	0.6%
9	New Jersey	37	3.0%
35	New Mexico	9	0.7%
4	New York	64	5.1%
10	North Carolina	36	2.9%
48	North Dakota	2	0.2%
3	Ohio	73	5.8%
33	Oklahoma	10	0.8%
5	Oregon	58	4.6%
7	Pennsylvania	56	4.5%
48	Rhode Island	2	0.2%
28	South Carolina	12	1.0%
48	South Dakota	2	0.2%
24	Tennessee	15	1.2%
5	Texas	58	4.6%
37	Utah	7	0.6%
42	Vermont	4	0.3%
17	Virginia	20	1.6%
13	Washington	32	2.6%
41	West Virginia	6	0.5%
24	Wisconsin	15	1.2%
44	Wyoming	3	0.2%

RANK	STATE	CASES	% of USA
1	California	189	15.1%
2	Florida	107	8.5%
3	Ohio	73	5.8%
4	New York	64	5.1%
5	Oregon	58	4.6%
5	Texas	58	4.6%
7	Pennsylvania	56	4.5%
8	Michigan	49	3.9%
9	New Jersey	37	3.0%
10	Louisiana	36	2.9%
10	Massachusetts	36	2.9%
10	North Carolina	36	2.9%
13	Washington	32	2.6%
14	Indiana	31	2.5%
15	Minnesota	23	1.8%
16	Illinois	22	1.8%
17	Arkansas	20	1.6%
17	Missouri	20	1.6%
17	Virginia	20	1.6%
20	Iowa	18	1.4%
21	Alabama	17	1.4%
21	Mississippi	17	1.4%
23	Georgia	16	1.3%
24	Colorado	15	1.2%
24	Tennessee	15	1.2%
24	Wisconsin	15	1.2%
27	Kansas	14	1.1%
28	Arizona	12	1.0%
28	Kentucky	12	1.0%
28	South Carolina	12	1.0%
31	Maine	11	0.9%
31	Maryland	11	0.9%
33	Connecticut	10	0.8%
33	Oklahoma	10	0.8%
35	Hawaii	9	0.7%
35	New Mexico	9	0.7%
37	Idaho	7	0.6%
37	Nevada	7	0.6%
37	New Hampshire	7	0.6%
37	Utah	7	0.6%
41	West Virginia	6	0.5%
42	Nebraska	4	0.3%
42	Vermont	4	0.3%
44	Alaska	3	0.2%
44	Delaware	3	0.2%
44	Montana	3	0.2%
44	Wyoming	3	0.2%
48	North Dakota	2	0.2%
48	Rhode Island	2	0.2%
48	South Dakota	2	0.2%
	District of Columbia	4	0.3%

Source: U.S. Department of Health and Human Services, National Center for Health Statistics
"Morbidity and Mortality Weekly Report" (January 7, 2005, Vol. 53, Nos. 51 & 52)
*Provisional data. A bacterium (Neisseria meningitidis) that causes cerebrospinal meningitis.

Meningococcal Infection Rate in 2004

National Rate = 0.4 Cases per 100,000 Population*

ALPHA ORDER

RANK	STATE	RATE
24	Alabama	0.4
13	Alaska	0.5
45	Arizona	0.2
4	Arkansas	0.7
13	California	0.5
28	Colorado	0.3
28	Connecticut	0.3
24	Delaware	0.4
6	Florida	0.6
45	Georgia	0.2
4	Hawaii	0.7
13	Idaho	0.5
45	Illinois	0.2
13	Indiana	0.5
6	Iowa	0.6
13	Kansas	0.5
28	Kentucky	0.3
2	Louisiana	0.8
2	Maine	0.8
45	Maryland	0.2
6	Massachusetts	0.6
13	Michigan	0.5
13	Minnesota	0.5
6	Mississippi	0.6
28	Missouri	0.3
28	Montana	0.3
45	Nebraska	0.2
28	Nevada	0.3
13	New Hampshire	0.5
24	New Jersey	0.4
13	New Mexico	0.5
28	New York	0.3
24	North Carolina	0.4
28	North Dakota	0.3
6	Ohio	0.6
28	Oklahoma	0.3
1	Oregon	1.6
13	Pennsylvania	0.5
45	Rhode Island	0.2
28	South Carolina	0.3
28	South Dakota	0.3
28	Tennessee	0.3
28	Texas	0.3
28	Utah	0.3
6	Vermont	0.6
28	Virginia	0.3
13	Washington	0.5
28	West Virginia	0.3
28	Wisconsin	0.3
6	Wyoming	0.6

RANK ORDER

RANK	STATE	RATE
1	Oregon	1.6
2	Louisiana	0.8
2	Maine	0.8
4	Arkansas	0.7
4	Hawaii	0.7
6	Florida	0.6
6	Iowa	0.6
6	Massachusetts	0.6
6	Mississippi	0.6
6	Ohio	0.6
6	Vermont	0.6
6	Wyoming	0.6
13	Alaska	0.5
13	California	0.5
13	Idaho	0.5
13	Indiana	0.5
13	Kansas	0.5
13	Michigan	0.5
13	Minnesota	0.5
13	New Hampshire	0.5
13	New Mexico	0.5
13	Pennsylvania	0.5
13	Washington	0.5
24	Alabama	0.4
24	Delaware	0.4
24	New Jersey	0.4
24	North Carolina	0.4
28	Colorado	0.3
28	Connecticut	0.3
28	Kentucky	0.3
28	Missouri	0.3
28	Montana	0.3
28	Nevada	0.3
28	New York	0.3
28	North Dakota	0.3
28	Oklahoma	0.3
28	South Carolina	0.3
28	South Dakota	0.3
28	Tennessee	0.3
28	Texas	0.3
28	Utah	0.3
28	Virginia	0.3
28	West Virginia	0.3
28	Wisconsin	0.3
45	Arizona	0.2
45	Georgia	0.2
45	Illinois	0.2
45	Maryland	0.2
45	Nebraska	0.2
45	Rhode Island	0.2
	District of Columbia	0.7

Source: Morgan Quitno Press using data from U.S. Dept. of Health & Human Serv's, National Center for Health Statistics
"Morbidity and Mortality Weekly Report" (January 7, 2005, Vol. 53, Nos. 51 & 52)
*Provisional data. A bacterium (Neisseria meningitidis) that causes cerebrospinal meningitis.

Rabies (Animal) Cases Reported in 2004

National Total = 5,851 Cases*

ALPHA ORDER

RANK	STATE	CASES	% of USA
21	Alabama	66	1.1%
40	Alaska	8	0.1%
12	Arizona	115	2.0%
26	Arkansas	49	0.8%
10	California	166	2.8%
27	Colorado	43	0.7%
9	Connecticut	218	3.7%
38	Delaware	9	0.2%
46	Florida	2	0.0%
8	Georgia	298	5.1%
47	Hawaii	0	0.0%
40	Idaho	8	0.1%
25	Illinois	51	0.9%
35	Indiana	11	0.2%
13	Iowa	104	1.8%
15	Kansas	96	1.6%
33	Kentucky	23	0.4%
47	Louisiana	0	0.0%
23	Maine	55	0.9%
6	Maryland	323	5.5%
7	Massachusetts	320	5.5%
34	Michigan	15	0.3%
16	Minnesota	90	1.5%
35	Mississippi	11	0.2%
22	Missouri	59	1.0%
32	Montana	26	0.4%
24	Nebraska	53	0.9%
45	Nevada	3	0.1%
31	New Hampshire	31	0.5%
47	New Jersey	0	0.0%
44	New Mexico	5	0.1%
3	New York	531	9.1%
2	North Carolina	581	9.9%
19	North Dakota	69	1.2%
18	Ohio	77	1.3%
13	Oklahoma	104	1.8%
43	Oregon	6	0.1%
5	Pennsylvania	405	6.9%
29	Rhode Island	38	0.6%
11	South Carolina	151	2.6%
16	South Dakota	90	1.5%
30	Tennessee	36	0.6%
1	Texas	906	15.5%
37	Utah	10	0.2%
28	Vermont	40	0.7%
4	Virginia	464	7.9%
47	Washington	0	0.0%
19	West Virginia	69	1.2%
38	Wisconsin	9	0.2%
42	Wyoming	7	0.1%

RANK ORDER

RANK	STATE	CASES	% of USA
1	Texas	906	15.5%
2	North Carolina	581	9.9%
3	New York	531	9.1%
4	Virginia	464	7.9%
5	Pennsylvania	405	6.9%
6	Maryland	323	5.5%
7	Massachusetts	320	5.5%
8	Georgia	298	5.1%
9	Connecticut	218	3.7%
10	California	166	2.8%
11	South Carolina	151	2.6%
12	Arizona	115	2.0%
13	Iowa	104	1.8%
13	Oklahoma	104	1.8%
15	Kansas	96	1.6%
16	Minnesota	90	1.5%
16	South Dakota	90	1.5%
18	Ohio	77	1.3%
19	North Dakota	69	1.2%
19	West Virginia	69	1.2%
21	Alabama	66	1.1%
22	Missouri	59	1.0%
23	Maine	55	0.9%
24	Nebraska	53	0.9%
25	Illinois	51	0.9%
26	Arkansas	49	0.8%
27	Colorado	43	0.7%
28	Vermont	40	0.7%
29	Rhode Island	38	0.6%
30	Tennessee	36	0.6%
31	New Hampshire	31	0.5%
32	Montana	26	0.4%
33	Kentucky	23	0.4%
34	Michigan	15	0.3%
35	Indiana	11	0.2%
35	Mississippi	11	0.2%
37	Utah	10	0.2%
38	Delaware	9	0.2%
38	Wisconsin	9	0.2%
40	Alaska	8	0.1%
40	Idaho	8	0.1%
42	Wyoming	7	0.1%
43	Oregon	6	0.1%
44	New Mexico	5	0.1%
45	Nevada	3	0.1%
46	Florida	2	0.0%
47	Hawaii	0	0.0%
47	Louisiana	0	0.0%
47	New Jersey	0	0.0%
47	Washington	0	0.0%
	District of Columbia	0	0.0%

Source: U.S. Department of Health and Human Services, National Center for Health Statistics
"Morbidity and Mortality Weekly Report" (January 7, 2005, Vol. 53, Nos. 51 & 52)
*Provisional data. An acute, infectious, often fatal viral disease of most warm-blooded animals, especially wolves, cats, and dogs, that attacks the central nervous system and is transmitted by the bite of infected animals.

Rabies (Animal) Rate in 2004

National Rate = 2.0 Cases per 100,000 Human Population*

ALPHA ORDER

RANK	STATE	RATE
26	Alabama	1.5
28	Alaska	1.2
23	Arizona	2.0
24	Arkansas	1.8
36	California	0.5
31	Colorado	0.9
5	Connecticut	6.2
29	Delaware	1.1
46	Florida	0.0
16	Georgia	3.4
46	Hawaii	0.0
33	Idaho	0.6
37	Illinois	0.4
41	Indiana	0.2
13	Iowa	3.5
13	Kansas	3.5
33	Kentucky	0.6
46	Louisiana	0.0
9	Maine	4.2
7	Maryland	5.8
8	Massachusetts	5.0
44	Michigan	0.1
24	Minnesota	1.8
37	Mississippi	0.4
30	Missouri	1.0
20	Montana	2.8
18	Nebraska	3.0
44	Nevada	0.1
22	New Hampshire	2.4
46	New Jersey	0.0
40	New Mexico	0.3
20	New York	2.8
3	North Carolina	6.8
2	North Dakota	10.9
32	Ohio	0.7
18	Oklahoma	3.0
41	Oregon	0.2
17	Pennsylvania	3.3
13	Rhode Island	3.5
12	South Carolina	3.6
1	South Dakota	11.7
33	Tennessee	0.6
10	Texas	4.0
37	Utah	0.4
4	Vermont	6.4
5	Virginia	6.2
46	Washington	0.0
11	West Virginia	3.8
41	Wisconsin	0.2
27	Wyoming	1.4

RANK ORDER

RANK	STATE	RATE
1	South Dakota	11.7
2	North Dakota	10.9
3	North Carolina	6.8
4	Vermont	6.4
5	Connecticut	6.2
5	Virginia	6.2
7	Maryland	5.8
8	Massachusetts	5.0
9	Maine	4.2
10	Texas	4.0
11	West Virginia	3.8
12	South Carolina	3.6
13	Iowa	3.5
13	Kansas	3.5
13	Rhode Island	3.5
16	Georgia	3.4
17	Pennsylvania	3.3
18	Nebraska	3.0
18	Oklahoma	3.0
20	Montana	2.8
20	New York	2.8
22	New Hampshire	2.4
23	Arizona	2.0
24	Arkansas	1.8
24	Minnesota	1.8
26	Alabama	1.5
27	Wyoming	1.4
28	Alaska	1.2
29	Delaware	1.1
30	Missouri	1.0
31	Colorado	0.9
32	Ohio	0.7
33	Idaho	0.6
33	Kentucky	0.6
33	Tennessee	0.6
36	California	0.5
37	Illinois	0.4
37	Mississippi	0.4
37	Utah	0.4
40	New Mexico	0.3
41	Indiana	0.2
41	Oregon	0.2
41	Wisconsin	0.2
44	Michigan	0.1
44	Nevada	0.1
46	Florida	0.0
46	Hawaii	0.0
46	Louisiana	0.0
46	New Jersey	0.0
46	Washington	0.0

District of Columbia   0.0

Source: Morgan Quitno Press using data from U.S. Dept. of Health & Human Serv's, National Center for Health Statistics
"Morbidity and Mortality Weekly Report" (January 7, 2005, Vol. 53, Nos. 51 & 52)
*Provisional data. An acute, infectious, often fatal viral disease of most warm-blooded animals, especially wolves,
cats, and dogs, that attacks the central nervous system and is transmitted by the bite of infected animals.

Rocky Mountain Spotted Fever Cases Reported in 2004

National Total = 1,514 Cases*

ALPHA ORDER

RANK	STATE	CASES	% of USA
8	Alabama	48	3.2%
42	Alaska	0	0.0%
26	Arizona	4	0.3%
2	Arkansas	154	10.2%
34	California	2	0.1%
39	Colorado	1	0.1%
34	Connecticut	2	0.1%
21	Delaware	6	0.4%
14	Florida	26	1.7%
7	Georgia	67	4.4%
42	Hawaii	0	0.0%
26	Idaho	4	0.3%
34	Illinois	2	0.1%
21	Indiana	6	0.4%
39	Iowa	1	0.1%
42	Kansas	0	0.0%
34	Kentucky	2	0.1%
23	Louisiana	5	0.3%
42	Maine	0	0.0%
5	Maryland	79	5.2%
16	Massachusetts	21	1.4%
26	Michigan	4	0.3%
26	Minnesota	4	0.3%
11	Mississippi	36	2.4%
3	Missouri	106	7.0%
31	Montana	3	0.2%
17	Nebraska	19	1.3%
42	Nevada	0	0.0%
42	New Hampshire	0	0.0%
12	New Jersey	33	2.2%
34	New Mexico	2	0.1%
13	New York	29	1.9%
1	North Carolina	535	35.3%
42	North Dakota	0	0.0%
18	Ohio	12	0.8%
6	Oklahoma	71	4.7%
31	Oregon	3	0.2%
9	Pennsylvania	40	2.6%
31	Rhode Island	3	0.2%
15	South Carolina	24	1.6%
26	South Dakota	4	0.3%
4	Tennessee	88	5.8%
19	Texas	10	0.7%
20	Utah	9	0.6%
39	Vermont	1	0.1%
10	Virginia	38	2.5%
42	Washington	0	0.0%
23	West Virginia	5	0.3%
42	Wisconsin	0	0.0%
23	Wyoming	5	0.3%

RANK ORDER

RANK	STATE	CASES	% of USA
1	North Carolina	535	35.3%
2	Arkansas	154	10.2%
3	Missouri	106	7.0%
4	Tennessee	88	5.8%
5	Maryland	79	5.2%
6	Oklahoma	71	4.7%
7	Georgia	67	4.4%
8	Alabama	48	3.2%
9	Pennsylvania	40	2.6%
10	Virginia	38	2.5%
11	Mississippi	36	2.4%
12	New Jersey	33	2.2%
13	New York	29	1.9%
14	Florida	26	1.7%
15	South Carolina	24	1.6%
16	Massachusetts	21	1.4%
17	Nebraska	19	1.3%
18	Ohio	12	0.8%
19	Texas	10	0.7%
20	Utah	9	0.6%
21	Delaware	6	0.4%
21	Indiana	6	0.4%
23	Louisiana	5	0.3%
23	West Virginia	5	0.3%
23	Wyoming	5	0.3%
26	Arizona	4	0.3%
26	Idaho	4	0.3%
26	Michigan	4	0.3%
26	Minnesota	4	0.3%
26	South Dakota	4	0.3%
31	Montana	3	0.2%
31	Oregon	3	0.2%
31	Rhode Island	3	0.2%
34	California	2	0.1%
34	Connecticut	2	0.1%
34	Illinois	2	0.1%
34	Kentucky	2	0.1%
34	New Mexico	2	0.1%
39	Colorado	1	0.1%
39	Iowa	1	0.1%
39	Vermont	1	0.1%
42	Alaska	0	0.0%
42	Hawaii	0	0.0%
42	Kansas	0	0.0%
42	Maine	0	0.0%
42	Nevada	0	0.0%
42	New Hampshire	0	0.0%
42	North Dakota	0	0.0%
42	Washington	0	0.0%
42	Wisconsin	0	0.0%
	District of Columbia	0	0.0%

Source: U.S. Department of Health and Human Services, National Center for Health Statistics
   "Morbidity and Mortality Weekly Report" (January 7, 2005, Vol. 53, Nos. 51 & 52)
Provisional data. An illness caused by Rickettsia rickettsii, a bacterial pathogen transmitted to humans through contact with ticks. Characterized by acute onset of fever, and may be accompanied by headache, malaise, myalgia, nausea/vomiting, or neurologic signs. A rash is often present on the palms and soles.

Rocky Mountain Spotted Fever Rate in 2004

National Rate = 0.5 Cases per 100,000 Population*

ALPHA ORDER

RANK	STATE	RATE
8	Alabama	1.1
35	Alaska	0.0
26	Arizona	0.1
2	Arkansas	5.6
35	California	0.0
35	Colorado	0.0
26	Connecticut	0.1
12	Delaware	0.7
26	Florida	0.1
11	Georgia	0.8
35	Hawaii	0.0
18	Idaho	0.3
35	Illinois	0.0
26	Indiana	0.1
35	Iowa	0.0
35	Kansas	0.0
35	Kentucky	0.0
26	Louisiana	0.1
35	Maine	0.0
6	Maryland	1.4
18	Massachusetts	0.3
35	Michigan	0.0
26	Minnesota	0.1
7	Mississippi	1.2
4	Missouri	1.8
18	Montana	0.3
8	Nebraska	1.1
35	Nevada	0.0
35	New Hampshire	0.0
16	New Jersey	0.4
26	New Mexico	0.1
24	New York	0.2
1	North Carolina	6.3
35	North Dakota	0.0
26	Ohio	0.1
3	Oklahoma	2.0
26	Oregon	0.1
18	Pennsylvania	0.3
18	Rhode Island	0.3
13	South Carolina	0.6
14	South Dakota	0.5
5	Tennessee	1.5
35	Texas	0.0
16	Utah	0.4
24	Vermont	0.2
14	Virginia	0.5
35	Washington	0.0
18	West Virginia	0.3
35	Wisconsin	0.0
10	Wyoming	1.0

RANK ORDER

RANK	STATE	RATE
1	North Carolina	6.3
2	Arkansas	5.6
3	Oklahoma	2.0
4	Missouri	1.8
5	Tennessee	1.5
6	Maryland	1.4
7	Mississippi	1.2
8	Alabama	1.1
8	Nebraska	1.1
10	Wyoming	1.0
11	Georgia	0.8
12	Delaware	0.7
13	South Carolina	0.6
14	South Dakota	0.5
14	Virginia	0.5
16	New Jersey	0.4
16	Utah	0.4
18	Idaho	0.3
18	Massachusetts	0.3
18	Montana	0.3
18	Pennsylvania	0.3
18	Rhode Island	0.3
18	West Virginia	0.3
24	New York	0.2
24	Vermont	0.2
26	Arizona	0.1
26	Connecticut	0.1
26	Florida	0.1
26	Indiana	0.1
26	Louisiana	0.1
26	Minnesota	0.1
26	New Mexico	0.1
26	Ohio	0.1
26	Oregon	0.1
35	Alaska	0.0
35	California	0.0
35	Colorado	0.0
35	Hawaii	0.0
35	Illinois	0.0
35	Iowa	0.0
35	Kansas	0.0
35	Kentucky	0.0
35	Maine	0.0
35	Michigan	0.0
35	Nevada	0.0
35	New Hampshire	0.0
35	North Dakota	0.0
35	Texas	0.0
35	Washington	0.0
35	Wisconsin	0.0
	District of Columbia	0.0

Source: Morgan Quitno Press using data from U.S. Dept. of Health & Human Serv's, National Center for Health Statistics
    "Morbidity and Mortality Weekly Report" (January 7, 2005, Vol. 53, Nos. 51 & 52)
*Provisional data. An illness caused by Rickettsia rickettsii, a bacterial pathogen transmitted to humans through contact with ticks. Characterized by acute onset of fever, and may be accompanied by headache, malaise, myalgia, nausea/vomiting, or neurologic signs. A rash is often present on the palms and soles.

Salmonellosis Cases Reported in 2004

National Total = 40,252 Cases*

ALPHA ORDER

RANK	STATE	CASES	% of USA
19	Alabama	760	1.9%
48	Alaska	64	0.2%
20	Arizona	757	1.9%
25	Arkansas	575	1.4%
2	California	4,057	10.1%
26	Colorado	536	1.3%
28	Connecticut	453	1.1%
45	Delaware	101	0.3%
1	Florida	4,280	10.6%
6	Georgia	1,869	4.6%
33	Hawaii	371	0.9%
41	Idaho	145	0.4%
8	Illinois	1,357	3.4%
22	Indiana	637	1.6%
29	Iowa	429	1.1%
32	Kansas	392	1.0%
34	Kentucky	353	0.9%
16	Louisiana	815	2.0%
46	Maine	90	0.2%
18	Maryland	809	2.0%
11	Massachusetts	1,142	2.8%
17	Michigan	812	2.0%
23	Minnesota	633	1.6%
14	Mississippi	844	2.1%
21	Missouri	641	1.6%
39	Montana	184	0.5%
38	Nebraska	185	0.5%
40	Nevada	180	0.4%
42	New Hampshire	138	0.3%
12	New Jersey	968	2.4%
35	New Mexico	271	0.7%
3	New York	2,436	6.1%
7	North Carolina	1,648	4.1%
50	North Dakota	42	0.1%
9	Ohio	1,208	3.0%
30	Oklahoma	404	1.0%
30	Oregon	404	1.0%
5	Pennsylvania	2,008	5.0%
44	Rhode Island	136	0.3%
13	South Carolina	956	2.4%
43	South Dakota	137	0.3%
27	Tennessee	523	1.3%
4	Texas	2,285	5.7%
36	Utah	239	0.6%
47	Vermont	65	0.2%
10	Virginia	1,159	2.9%
24	Washington	581	1.4%
37	West Virginia	225	0.6%
15	Wisconsin	832	2.1%
49	Wyoming	54	0.1%

RANK ORDER

RANK	STATE	CASES	% of USA
1	Florida	4,280	10.6%
2	California	4,057	10.1%
3	New York	2,436	6.1%
4	Texas	2,285	5.7%
5	Pennsylvania	2,008	5.0%
6	Georgia	1,869	4.6%
7	North Carolina	1,648	4.1%
8	Illinois	1,357	3.4%
9	Ohio	1,208	3.0%
10	Virginia	1,159	2.9%
11	Massachusetts	1,142	2.8%
12	New Jersey	968	2.4%
13	South Carolina	956	2.4%
14	Mississippi	844	2.1%
15	Wisconsin	832	2.1%
16	Louisiana	815	2.0%
17	Michigan	812	2.0%
18	Maryland	809	2.0%
19	Alabama	760	1.9%
20	Arizona	757	1.9%
21	Missouri	641	1.6%
22	Indiana	637	1.6%
23	Minnesota	633	1.6%
24	Washington	581	1.4%
25	Arkansas	575	1.4%
26	Colorado	536	1.3%
27	Tennessee	523	1.3%
28	Connecticut	453	1.1%
29	Iowa	429	1.1%
30	Oklahoma	404	1.0%
30	Oregon	404	1.0%
32	Kansas	392	1.0%
33	Hawaii	371	0.9%
34	Kentucky	353	0.9%
35	New Mexico	271	0.7%
36	Utah	239	0.6%
37	West Virginia	225	0.6%
38	Nebraska	185	0.5%
39	Montana	184	0.5%
40	Nevada	180	0.4%
41	Idaho	145	0.4%
42	New Hampshire	138	0.3%
43	South Dakota	137	0.3%
44	Rhode Island	136	0.3%
45	Delaware	101	0.3%
46	Maine	90	0.2%
47	Vermont	65	0.2%
48	Alaska	64	0.2%
49	Wyoming	54	0.1%
50	North Dakota	42	0.1%
	District of Columbia	62	0.2%

Source: U.S. Department of Health and Human Services, National Center for Health Statistics
"Morbidity and Mortality Weekly Report" (January 7, 2005, Vol. 53, Nos. 51 & 52)
*Provisional data. Any disease caused by a salmonella infection, which may be manifested as food poisoning with acute gastroenteritis, vomiting and diarrhea.

Salmonellosis Rate in 2004

National Rate = 13.7 Cases per 100,000 Population*

ALPHA ORDER

RANK	STATE	RATE
12	Alabama	16.8
43	Alaska	9.8
20	Arizona	13.2
6	Arkansas	20.9
29	California	11.3
27	Colorado	11.6
21	Connecticut	12.9
26	Delaware	12.2
3	Florida	24.6
5	Georgia	21.2
1	Hawaii	29.4
39	Idaho	10.4
33	Illinois	10.7
40	Indiana	10.2
17	Iowa	14.5
18	Kansas	14.3
46	Kentucky	8.5
9	Louisiana	18.0
49	Maine	6.8
16	Maryland	14.6
10	Massachusetts	17.8
47	Michigan	8.0
24	Minnesota	12.4
2	Mississippi	29.1
31	Missouri	11.1
7	Montana	19.9
35	Nebraska	10.6
48	Nevada	7.7
35	New Hampshire	10.6
31	New Jersey	11.1
19	New Mexico	14.2
22	New York	12.7
8	North Carolina	19.3
50	North Dakota	6.6
37	Ohio	10.5
28	Oklahoma	11.5
30	Oregon	11.2
13	Pennsylvania	16.2
23	Rhode Island	12.6
4	South Carolina	22.8
10	South Dakota	17.8
45	Tennessee	8.9
40	Texas	10.2
42	Utah	10.0
37	Vermont	10.5
14	Virginia	15.5
44	Washington	9.4
24	West Virginia	12.4
15	Wisconsin	15.1
33	Wyoming	10.7

RANK ORDER

RANK	STATE	RATE
1	Hawaii	29.4
2	Mississippi	29.1
3	Florida	24.6
4	South Carolina	22.8
5	Georgia	21.2
6	Arkansas	20.9
7	Montana	19.9
8	North Carolina	19.3
9	Louisiana	18.0
10	Massachusetts	17.8
10	South Dakota	17.8
12	Alabama	16.8
13	Pennsylvania	16.2
14	Virginia	15.5
15	Wisconsin	15.1
16	Maryland	14.6
17	Iowa	14.5
18	Kansas	14.3
19	New Mexico	14.2
20	Arizona	13.2
21	Connecticut	12.9
22	New York	12.7
23	Rhode Island	12.6
24	Minnesota	12.4
24	West Virginia	12.4
26	Delaware	12.2
27	Colorado	11.6
28	Oklahoma	11.5
29	California	11.3
30	Oregon	11.2
31	Missouri	11.1
31	New Jersey	11.1
33	Illinois	10.7
33	Wyoming	10.7
35	Nebraska	10.6
35	New Hampshire	10.6
37	Ohio	10.5
37	Vermont	10.5
39	Idaho	10.4
40	Indiana	10.2
40	Texas	10.2
42	Utah	10.0
43	Alaska	9.8
44	Washington	9.4
45	Tennessee	8.9
46	Kentucky	8.5
47	Michigan	8.0
48	Nevada	7.7
49	Maine	6.8
50	North Dakota	6.6

District of Columbia   11.2

Source: Morgan Quitno Press using data from U.S. Dept. of Health & Human Serv's, National Center for Health Statistics
"Morbidity and Mortality Weekly Report" (January 7, 2005, Vol. 53, Nos. 51 & 52)
*Provisional data. Any disease caused by a salmonella infection, which may be manifested as food poisoning with acute gastroenteritis, vomiting and diarrhea.

Shigellosis Cases Reported in 2004

National Total = 12,735 Cases*

ALPHA ORDER

RANK	STATE	CASES	% of USA
12	Alabama	323	2.5%
46	Alaska	6	0.0%
8	Arizona	425	3.3%
28	Arkansas	81	0.6%
2	California	1,679	13.2%
22	Colorado	158	1.2%
31	Connecticut	68	0.5%
43	Delaware	9	0.1%
3	Florida	965	7.6%
5	Georgia	620	4.9%
37	Hawaii	47	0.4%
40	Idaho	13	0.1%
9	Illinois	330	2.6%
16	Indiana	225	1.8%
32	Iowa	66	0.5%
27	Kansas	82	0.6%
30	Kentucky	75	0.6%
13	Louisiana	278	2.2%
43	Maine	9	0.1%
23	Maryland	151	1.2%
18	Massachusetts	175	1.4%
14	Michigan	234	1.8%
32	Minnesota	66	0.5%
36	Mississippi	48	0.4%
17	Missouri	186	1.5%
48	Montana	4	0.0%
37	Nebraska	47	0.4%
34	Nevada	65	0.5%
42	New Hampshire	10	0.1%
15	New Jersey	231	1.8%
24	New Mexico	122	1.0%
4	New York	799	6.3%
7	North Carolina	476	3.7%
50	North Dakota	3	0.0%
20	Ohio	171	1.3%
6	Oklahoma	526	4.1%
28	Oregon	81	0.6%
26	Pennsylvania	103	0.8%
39	Rhode Island	20	0.2%
11	South Carolina	326	2.6%
40	South Dakota	13	0.1%
10	Tennessee	327	2.6%
1	Texas	2,528	19.9%
35	Utah	50	0.4%
48	Vermont	4	0.0%
21	Virginia	166	1.3%
25	Washington	115	0.9%
43	West Virginia	9	0.1%
19	Wisconsin	174	1.4%
46	Wyoming	6	0.0%

RANK ORDER

RANK	STATE	CASES	% of USA
1	Texas	2,528	19.9%
2	California	1,679	13.2%
3	Florida	965	7.6%
4	New York	799	6.3%
5	Georgia	620	4.9%
6	Oklahoma	526	4.1%
7	North Carolina	476	3.7%
8	Arizona	425	3.3%
9	Illinois	330	2.6%
10	Tennessee	327	2.6%
11	South Carolina	326	2.6%
12	Alabama	323	2.5%
13	Louisiana	278	2.2%
14	Michigan	234	1.8%
15	New Jersey	231	1.8%
16	Indiana	225	1.8%
17	Missouri	186	1.5%
18	Massachusetts	175	1.4%
19	Wisconsin	174	1.4%
20	Ohio	171	1.3%
21	Virginia	166	1.3%
22	Colorado	158	1.2%
23	Maryland	151	1.2%
24	New Mexico	122	1.0%
25	Washington	115	0.9%
26	Pennsylvania	103	0.8%
27	Kansas	82	0.6%
28	Arkansas	81	0.6%
28	Oregon	81	0.6%
30	Kentucky	75	0.6%
31	Connecticut	68	0.5%
32	Iowa	66	0.5%
32	Minnesota	66	0.5%
34	Nevada	65	0.5%
35	Utah	50	0.4%
36	Mississippi	48	0.4%
37	Hawaii	47	0.4%
37	Nebraska	47	0.4%
39	Rhode Island	20	0.2%
40	Idaho	13	0.1%
40	South Dakota	13	0.1%
42	New Hampshire	10	0.1%
43	Delaware	9	0.1%
43	Maine	9	0.1%
43	West Virginia	9	0.1%
46	Alaska	6	0.0%
46	Wyoming	6	0.0%
48	Montana	4	0.0%
48	Vermont	4	0.0%
50	North Dakota	3	0.0%
	District of Columbia	40	0.3%

Source: U.S. Department of Health and Human Services, National Center for Health Statistics
"Morbidity and Mortality Weekly Report" (January 7, 2005, Vol. 53, Nos. 51 & 52)
*Provisional data. Dysentery caused by any of various species of shigellae, occurring most frequently in areas where poor sanitation and malnutrition are prevalent and commonly affecting children and infants.

Shigellosis Rate in 2004

National Rate = 4.3 Cases per 100,000 Population*

ALPHA ORDER

RANK	STATE	RATE
5	Alabama	7.1
42	Alaska	0.9
4	Arizona	7.4
20	Arkansas	2.9
12	California	4.7
16	Colorado	3.4
32	Connecticut	1.9
41	Delaware	1.1
10	Florida	5.5
6	Georgia	7.0
14	Hawaii	3.7
42	Idaho	0.9
26	Illinois	2.6
15	Indiana	3.6
29	Iowa	2.2
19	Kansas	3.0
35	Kentucky	1.8
8	Louisiana	6.2
46	Maine	0.7
22	Maryland	2.7
22	Massachusetts	2.7
27	Michigan	2.3
39	Minnesota	1.3
36	Mississippi	1.7
17	Missouri	3.2
50	Montana	0.4
22	Nebraska	2.7
21	Nevada	2.8
44	New Hampshire	0.8
22	New Jersey	2.7
7	New Mexico	6.4
13	New York	4.2
9	North Carolina	5.6
48	North Dakota	0.5
38	Ohio	1.5
1	Oklahoma	14.9
27	Oregon	2.3
44	Pennsylvania	0.8
32	Rhode Island	1.9
3	South Carolina	7.8
36	South Dakota	1.7
10	Tennessee	5.5
2	Texas	11.2
31	Utah	2.1
47	Vermont	0.6
29	Virginia	2.2
32	Washington	1.9
48	West Virginia	0.5
17	Wisconsin	3.2
40	Wyoming	1.2

RANK ORDER

RANK	STATE	RATE
1	Oklahoma	14.9
2	Texas	11.2
3	South Carolina	7.8
4	Arizona	7.4
5	Alabama	7.1
6	Georgia	7.0
7	New Mexico	6.4
8	Louisiana	6.2
9	North Carolina	5.6
10	Florida	5.5
10	Tennessee	5.5
12	California	4.7
13	New York	4.2
14	Hawaii	3.7
15	Indiana	3.6
16	Colorado	3.4
17	Missouri	3.2
17	Wisconsin	3.2
19	Kansas	3.0
20	Arkansas	2.9
21	Nevada	2.8
22	Maryland	2.7
22	Massachusetts	2.7
22	Nebraska	2.7
22	New Jersey	2.7
26	Illinois	2.6
27	Michigan	2.3
27	Oregon	2.3
29	Iowa	2.2
29	Virginia	2.2
31	Utah	2.1
32	Connecticut	1.9
32	Rhode Island	1.9
32	Washington	1.9
35	Kentucky	1.8
36	Mississippi	1.7
36	South Dakota	1.7
38	Ohio	1.5
39	Minnesota	1.3
40	Wyoming	1.2
41	Delaware	1.1
42	Alaska	0.9
42	Idaho	0.9
44	New Hampshire	0.8
44	Pennsylvania	0.8
46	Maine	0.7
47	Vermont	0.6
48	North Dakota	0.5
48	West Virginia	0.5
50	Montana	0.4
	District of Columbia	7.2

Source: Morgan Quitno Press using data from U.S. Dept. of Health & Human Serv's, National Center for Health Statistics
"Morbidity and Mortality Weekly Report" (January 7, 2005, Vol. 53, Nos. 51 & 52)
*Provisional data. Dysentery caused by any of various species of shigellae, occurring most frequently in areas
where poor sanitation and malnutrition are prevalent and commonly affecting children and infants.

Tuberculosis Cases Reported in 2004

National Total = 11,178 Cases*

ALPHA ORDER

RANK	STATE	CASES	% of USA
20	Alabama	153	1.4%
37	Alaska	35	0.3%
16	Arizona	229	2.0%
24	Arkansas	118	1.1%
1	California	1,979	17.7%
26	Colorado	111	1.0%
30	Connecticut	75	0.7%
42	Delaware	17	0.2%
3	Florida	956	8.6%
7	Georgia	416	3.7%
26	Hawaii	111	1.0%
46	Idaho	4	0.0%
5	Illinois	541	4.8%
22	Indiana	127	1.1%
33	Iowa	42	0.4%
32	Kansas	59	0.5%
23	Kentucky	123	1.1%
49	Louisiana	0	0.0%
49	Maine	0	0.0%
12	Maryland	250	2.2%
11	Massachusetts	273	2.4%
13	Michigan	240	2.1%
18	Minnesota	181	1.6%
39	Mississippi	33	0.3%
25	Missouri	116	1.0%
43	Montana	14	0.1%
36	Nebraska	36	0.3%
29	Nevada	80	0.7%
41	New Hampshire	18	0.2%
6	New Jersey	440	3.9%
37	New Mexico	35	0.3%
2	New York	1,282	11.5%
9	North Carolina	334	3.0%
46	North Dakota	4	0.0%
17	Ohio	208	1.9%
21	Oklahoma	152	1.4%
31	Oregon	74	0.7%
8	Pennsylvania	345	3.1%
34	Rhode Island	38	0.3%
19	South Carolina	167	1.5%
44	South Dakota	8	0.1%
15	Tennessee	230	2.1%
4	Texas	785	7.0%
35	Utah	37	0.3%
46	Vermont	4	0.0%
10	Virginia	277	2.5%
14	Washington	234	2.1%
40	West Virginia	24	0.2%
28	Wisconsin	87	0.8%
45	Wyoming	5	0.0%

RANK ORDER

RANK	STATE	CASES	% of USA
1	California	1,979	17.7%
2	New York	1,282	11.5%
3	Florida	956	8.6%
4	Texas	785	7.0%
5	Illinois	541	4.8%
6	New Jersey	440	3.9%
7	Georgia	416	3.7%
8	Pennsylvania	345	3.1%
9	North Carolina	334	3.0%
10	Virginia	277	2.5%
11	Massachusetts	273	2.4%
12	Maryland	250	2.2%
13	Michigan	240	2.1%
14	Washington	234	2.1%
15	Tennessee	230	2.1%
16	Arizona	229	2.0%
17	Ohio	208	1.9%
18	Minnesota	181	1.6%
19	South Carolina	167	1.5%
20	Alabama	153	1.4%
21	Oklahoma	152	1.4%
22	Indiana	127	1.1%
23	Kentucky	123	1.1%
24	Arkansas	118	1.1%
25	Missouri	116	1.0%
26	Colorado	111	1.0%
26	Hawaii	111	1.0%
28	Wisconsin	87	0.8%
29	Nevada	80	0.7%
30	Connecticut	75	0.7%
31	Oregon	74	0.7%
32	Kansas	59	0.5%
33	Iowa	42	0.4%
34	Rhode Island	38	0.3%
35	Utah	37	0.3%
36	Nebraska	36	0.3%
37	Alaska	35	0.3%
37	New Mexico	35	0.3%
39	Mississippi	33	0.3%
40	West Virginia	24	0.2%
41	New Hampshire	18	0.2%
42	Delaware	17	0.2%
43	Montana	14	0.1%
44	South Dakota	8	0.1%
45	Wyoming	5	0.0%
46	Idaho	4	0.0%
46	North Dakota	4	0.0%
46	Vermont	4	0.0%
49	Louisiana	0	0.0%
49	Maine	0	0.0%
	District of Columbia	71	0.6%

Source: U.S. Department of Health and Human Services, National Center for Health Statistics
"Morbidity and Mortality Weekly Report" (January 7, 2005, Vol. 53, Nos. 51 & 52)
*Provisional data. An infectious disease caused by the tubercle bacillus and causing the formation of tubercles on the lungs and other tissues of the body, often developing long after the initial infection. Characterized by the coughing up of mucus and sputum, fever, weight loss, and chest pain.

Tuberculosis Rate in 2004

National Rate = 38 Cases per 100,000 Population*

ALPHA ORDER			RANK ORDER		
RANK	**STATE**	**RATE**	**RANK**	**STATE**	**RATE**
22	Alabama	3.4	1	Hawaii	8.8
5	Alaska	5.3	2	New York	6.7
13	Arizona	4.0	3	California	5.5
9	Arkansas	4.3	3	Florida	5.5
3	California	5.5	5	Alaska	5.3
26	Colorado	2.4	6	New Jersey	5.1
29	Connecticut	2.1	7	Georgia	4.7
32	Delaware	2.0	8	Maryland	4.5
3	Florida	5.5	9	Arkansas	4.3
7	Georgia	4.7	9	Illinois	4.3
1	Hawaii	8.8	9	Massachusetts	4.3
48	Idaho	0.3	9	Oklahoma	4.3
9	Illinois	4.3	13	Arizona	4.0
32	Indiana	2.0	13	South Carolina	4.0
40	Iowa	1.4	15	North Carolina	3.9
28	Kansas	2.2	15	Tennessee	3.9
24	Kentucky	3.0	17	Washington	3.8
49	Louisiana	0.0	18	Virginia	3.7
49	Maine	0.0	19	Minnesota	3.5
8	Maryland	4.5	19	Rhode Island	3.5
9	Massachusetts	4.3	19	Texas	3.5
26	Michigan	2.4	22	Alabama	3.4
19	Minnesota	3.5	22	Nevada	3.4
43	Mississippi	1.1	24	Kentucky	3.0
32	Missouri	2.0	25	Pennsylvania	2.8
38	Montana	1.5	26	Colorado	2.4
29	Nebraska	2.1	26	Michigan	2.4
22	Nevada	3.4	28	Kansas	2.2
40	New Hampshire	1.4	29	Connecticut	2.1
6	New Jersey	5.1	29	Nebraska	2.1
35	New Mexico	1.8	29	Oregon	2.1
2	New York	6.7	32	Delaware	2.0
15	North Carolina	3.9	32	Indiana	2.0
46	North Dakota	0.6	32	Missouri	2.0
35	Ohio	1.8	35	New Mexico	1.8
9	Oklahoma	4.3	35	Ohio	1.8
29	Oregon	2.1	37	Wisconsin	1.6
25	Pennsylvania	2.8	38	Montana	1.5
19	Rhode Island	3.5	38	Utah	1.5
13	South Carolina	4.0	40	Iowa	1.4
44	South Dakota	1.0	40	New Hampshire	1.4
15	Tennessee	3.9	42	West Virginia	1.3
19	Texas	3.5	43	Mississippi	1.1
38	Utah	1.5	44	South Dakota	1.0
46	Vermont	0.6	44	Wyoming	1.0
18	Virginia	3.7	46	North Dakota	0.6
17	Washington	3.8	46	Vermont	0.6
42	West Virginia	1.3	48	Idaho	0.3
37	Wisconsin	1.6	49	Louisiana	0.0
44	Wyoming	1.0	49	Maine	0.0

District of Columbia   12.8

Source: Morgan Quitno Press using data from U.S. Dept. of Health & Human Serv's, National Center for Health Statistics
       "Morbidity and Mortality Weekly Report" (January 7, 2005, Vol. 53, Nos. 51 & 52)
*Provisional data. An infectious disease caused by the tubercle bacillus and causing the formation of tubercles on
the lungs and other tissues of the body, often developing long after the initial infection. Characterized by the
coughing up of mucus and sputum, fever, weight loss, and chest pain.

West Nile Encephalitis and Meningitis Cases Reported in 2004

National Total = 888 Cases*

<table>
<thead>
<tr><th colspan="4">ALPHA ORDER</th><th colspan="4">RANK ORDER</th></tr>
<tr><th>RANK</th><th>STATE</th><th>CASES</th><th>% of USA</th><th>RANK</th><th>STATE</th><th>CASES</th><th>% of USA</th></tr>
</thead>
<tbody>
<tr><td>13</td><td>Alabama</td><td>15</td><td>1.7%</td><td>1</td><td>California</td><td>154</td><td>17.3%</td></tr>
<tr><td>37</td><td>Alaska</td><td>0</td><td>0.0%</td><td>2</td><td>Arizona</td><td>129</td><td>14.5%</td></tr>
<tr><td>2</td><td>Arizona</td><td>129</td><td>14.5%</td><td>3</td><td>Texas</td><td>108</td><td>12.2%</td></tr>
<tr><td>18</td><td>Arkansas</td><td>12</td><td>1.4%</td><td>4</td><td>Louisiana</td><td>81</td><td>9.1%</td></tr>
<tr><td>1</td><td>California</td><td>154</td><td>17.3%</td><td>5</td><td>Colorado</td><td>39</td><td>4.4%</td></tr>
<tr><td>5</td><td>Colorado</td><td>39</td><td>4.4%</td><td>6</td><td>Florida</td><td>31</td><td>3.5%</td></tr>
<tr><td>37</td><td>Connecticut</td><td>0</td><td>0.0%</td><td>6</td><td>Mississippi</td><td>31</td><td>3.5%</td></tr>
<tr><td>37</td><td>Delaware</td><td>0</td><td>0.0%</td><td>6</td><td>New Mexico</td><td>31</td><td>3.5%</td></tr>
<tr><td>6</td><td>Florida</td><td>31</td><td>3.5%</td><td>9</td><td>Illinois</td><td>28</td><td>3.2%</td></tr>
<tr><td>18</td><td>Georgia</td><td>12</td><td>1.4%</td><td>10</td><td>Missouri</td><td>26</td><td>2.9%</td></tr>
<tr><td>37</td><td>Hawaii</td><td>0</td><td>0.0%</td><td>11</td><td>Nevada</td><td>25</td><td>2.8%</td></tr>
<tr><td>37</td><td>Idaho</td><td>0</td><td>0.0%</td><td>12</td><td>Kansas</td><td>18</td><td>2.0%</td></tr>
<tr><td>9</td><td>Illinois</td><td>28</td><td>3.2%</td><td>13</td><td>Alabama</td><td>15</td><td>1.7%</td></tr>
<tr><td>23</td><td>Indiana</td><td>8</td><td>0.9%</td><td>14</td><td>Oklahoma</td><td>14</td><td>1.6%</td></tr>
<tr><td>15</td><td>Iowa</td><td>13</td><td>1.5%</td><td>15</td><td>Iowa</td><td>13</td><td>1.5%</td></tr>
<tr><td>12</td><td>Kansas</td><td>18</td><td>2.0%</td><td>15</td><td>Minnesota</td><td>13</td><td>1.5%</td></tr>
<tr><td>35</td><td>Kentucky</td><td>1</td><td>0.1%</td><td>15</td><td>Tennessee</td><td>13</td><td>1.5%</td></tr>
<tr><td>4</td><td>Louisiana</td><td>81</td><td>9.1%</td><td>18</td><td>Arkansas</td><td>12</td><td>1.4%</td></tr>
<tr><td>37</td><td>Maine</td><td>0</td><td>0.0%</td><td>18</td><td>Georgia</td><td>12</td><td>1.4%</td></tr>
<tr><td>23</td><td>Maryland</td><td>8</td><td>0.9%</td><td>18</td><td>Michigan</td><td>12</td><td>1.4%</td></tr>
<tr><td>37</td><td>Massachusetts</td><td>0</td><td>0.0%</td><td>21</td><td>Ohio</td><td>11</td><td>1.2%</td></tr>
<tr><td>18</td><td>Michigan</td><td>12</td><td>1.4%</td><td>22</td><td>Pennsylvania</td><td>9</td><td>1.0%</td></tr>
<tr><td>15</td><td>Minnesota</td><td>13</td><td>1.5%</td><td>23</td><td>Indiana</td><td>8</td><td>0.9%</td></tr>
<tr><td>6</td><td>Mississippi</td><td>31</td><td>3.5%</td><td>23</td><td>Maryland</td><td>8</td><td>0.9%</td></tr>
<tr><td>10</td><td>Missouri</td><td>26</td><td>2.9%</td><td>25</td><td>Nebraska</td><td>7</td><td>0.8%</td></tr>
<tr><td>32</td><td>Montana</td><td>2</td><td>0.2%</td><td>25</td><td>New York</td><td>7</td><td>0.8%</td></tr>
<tr><td>25</td><td>Nebraska</td><td>7</td><td>0.8%</td><td>27</td><td>South Dakota</td><td>6</td><td>0.7%</td></tr>
<tr><td>11</td><td>Nevada</td><td>25</td><td>2.8%</td><td>27</td><td>Utah</td><td>6</td><td>0.7%</td></tr>
<tr><td>37</td><td>New Hampshire</td><td>0</td><td>0.0%</td><td>29</td><td>Wisconsin</td><td>5</td><td>0.6%</td></tr>
<tr><td>35</td><td>New Jersey</td><td>1</td><td>0.1%</td><td>30</td><td>Virginia</td><td>4</td><td>0.5%</td></tr>
<tr><td>6</td><td>New Mexico</td><td>31</td><td>3.5%</td><td>31</td><td>North Carolina</td><td>3</td><td>0.3%</td></tr>
<tr><td>25</td><td>New York</td><td>7</td><td>0.8%</td><td>32</td><td>Montana</td><td>2</td><td>0.2%</td></tr>
<tr><td>31</td><td>North Carolina</td><td>3</td><td>0.3%</td><td>32</td><td>North Dakota</td><td>2</td><td>0.2%</td></tr>
<tr><td>32</td><td>North Dakota</td><td>2</td><td>0.2%</td><td>32</td><td>Wyoming</td><td>2</td><td>0.2%</td></tr>
<tr><td>21</td><td>Ohio</td><td>11</td><td>1.2%</td><td>35</td><td>Kentucky</td><td>1</td><td>0.1%</td></tr>
<tr><td>14</td><td>Oklahoma</td><td>14</td><td>1.6%</td><td>35</td><td>New Jersey</td><td>1</td><td>0.1%</td></tr>
<tr><td>37</td><td>Oregon</td><td>0</td><td>0.0%</td><td>37</td><td>Alaska</td><td>0</td><td>0.0%</td></tr>
<tr><td>22</td><td>Pennsylvania</td><td>9</td><td>1.0%</td><td>37</td><td>Connecticut</td><td>0</td><td>0.0%</td></tr>
<tr><td>37</td><td>Rhode Island</td><td>0</td><td>0.0%</td><td>37</td><td>Delaware</td><td>0</td><td>0.0%</td></tr>
<tr><td>37</td><td>South Carolina</td><td>0</td><td>0.0%</td><td>37</td><td>Hawaii</td><td>0</td><td>0.0%</td></tr>
<tr><td>27</td><td>South Dakota</td><td>6</td><td>0.7%</td><td>37</td><td>Idaho</td><td>0</td><td>0.0%</td></tr>
<tr><td>15</td><td>Tennessee</td><td>13</td><td>1.5%</td><td>37</td><td>Maine</td><td>0</td><td>0.0%</td></tr>
<tr><td>3</td><td>Texas</td><td>108</td><td>12.2%</td><td>37</td><td>Massachusetts</td><td>0</td><td>0.0%</td></tr>
<tr><td>27</td><td>Utah</td><td>6</td><td>0.7%</td><td>37</td><td>New Hampshire</td><td>0</td><td>0.0%</td></tr>
<tr><td>37</td><td>Vermont</td><td>0</td><td>0.0%</td><td>37</td><td>Oregon</td><td>0</td><td>0.0%</td></tr>
<tr><td>30</td><td>Virginia</td><td>4</td><td>0.5%</td><td>37</td><td>Rhode Island</td><td>0</td><td>0.0%</td></tr>
<tr><td>37</td><td>Washington</td><td>0</td><td>0.0%</td><td>37</td><td>South Carolina</td><td>0</td><td>0.0%</td></tr>
<tr><td>37</td><td>West Virginia</td><td>0</td><td>0.0%</td><td>37</td><td>Vermont</td><td>0</td><td>0.0%</td></tr>
<tr><td>29</td><td>Wisconsin</td><td>5</td><td>0.6%</td><td>37</td><td>Washington</td><td>0</td><td>0.0%</td></tr>
<tr><td>32</td><td>Wyoming</td><td>2</td><td>0.2%</td><td>37</td><td>West Virginia</td><td>0</td><td>0.0%</td></tr>
<tr><td></td><td></td><td></td><td></td><td></td><td>District of Columbia</td><td>1</td><td>0.1%</td></tr>
</tbody>
</table>

Source: U.S. Department of Health and Human Services, Centers for Disease Control and Prevention
    "West Nile Virus 2004 Human Cases" (January 9, 2005, http://www.cdc.gov/ncidod/dvbid/westnile/index.htm)
*Provisional data as of 12/28/04. A flavivirus typically carried by mosquitoes. Figures do not include 1,101 West Nile Fever cases caused by the West Nile virus that result in mild, flu-like symptoms. Encephalitis refers to an inflammation of the brain, meningitis is an inflammation of the membrane around the brain and the spinal cord, and meningoencephalitis refers to inflammation of the brain and the membrane surrounding it.

West Nile Encephalitis and Meningitis Rate in 2004

National Rate = 0.3 Cases per 100,000 Population

ALPHA ORDER

RANK	STATE	RATE
17	Alabama	0.3
33	Alaska	0.0
1	Arizona	2.2
11	Arkansas	0.4
11	California	0.4
6	Colorado	0.8
33	Connecticut	0.0
33	Delaware	0.0
21	Florida	0.2
25	Georgia	0.1
33	Hawaii	0.0
33	Idaho	0.0
21	Illinois	0.2
25	Indiana	0.1
11	Iowa	0.4
8	Kansas	0.7
33	Kentucky	0.0
2	Louisiana	1.8
33	Maine	0.0
25	Maryland	0.1
33	Massachusetts	0.0
25	Michigan	0.1
17	Minnesota	0.3
4	Mississippi	1.1
9	Missouri	0.5
21	Montana	0.2
11	Nebraska	0.4
4	Nevada	1.1
33	New Hampshire	0.0
33	New Jersey	0.0
3	New Mexico	1.6
33	New York	0.0
33	North Carolina	0.0
17	North Dakota	0.3
25	Ohio	0.1
11	Oklahoma	0.4
33	Oregon	0.0
25	Pennsylvania	0.1
33	Rhode Island	0.0
33	South Carolina	0.0
6	South Dakota	0.8
21	Tennessee	0.2
9	Texas	0.5
17	Utah	0.3
33	Vermont	0.0
25	Virginia	0.1
33	Washington	0.0
33	West Virginia	0.0
25	Wisconsin	0.1
11	Wyoming	0.4

RANK ORDER

RANK	STATE	RATE
1	Arizona	2.2
2	Louisiana	1.8
3	New Mexico	1.6
4	Mississippi	1.1
4	Nevada	1.1
6	Colorado	0.8
6	South Dakota	0.8
8	Kansas	0.7
9	Missouri	0.5
9	Texas	0.5
11	Arkansas	0.4
11	California	0.4
11	Iowa	0.4
11	Nebraska	0.4
11	Oklahoma	0.4
11	Wyoming	0.4
17	Alabama	0.3
17	Minnesota	0.3
17	North Dakota	0.3
17	Utah	0.3
21	Florida	0.2
21	Illinois	0.2
21	Montana	0.2
21	Tennessee	0.2
25	Georgia	0.1
25	Indiana	0.1
25	Maryland	0.1
25	Michigan	0.1
25	Ohio	0.1
25	Pennsylvania	0.1
25	Virginia	0.1
25	Wisconsin	0.1
33	Alaska	0.0
33	Connecticut	0.0
33	Delaware	0.0
33	Hawaii	0.0
33	Idaho	0.0
33	Kentucky	0.0
33	Maine	0.0
33	Massachusetts	0.0
33	New Hampshire	0.0
33	New Jersey	0.0
33	New York	0.0
33	North Carolina	0.0
33	Oregon	0.0
33	Rhode Island	0.0
33	South Carolina	0.0
33	Vermont	0.0
33	Washington	0.0
33	West Virginia	0.0

District of Columbia   0.2

Source: Morgan Quitno Press using data from U.S. Dept. of Health & Human Serv's, CDC
"West Nile Virus 2004 Human Cases" (January 9, 2005, http://www.cdc.gov/ncidod/dvbid/westnile/index.htm)
*Provisional data as of 12/28/04. A flavivirus typically carried by mosquitoes. Figures do not include 1,101 West Nile Fever cases caused by the West Nile virus that result in mild, flu-like symptoms. Encephalitis refers to an inflammation of the brain, meningitis is an inflammation of the membrane around the brain and the spinal cord, and meningoencephalitis refers to inflammation of the brain and the membrane surrounding it.

Whooping Cough (Pertussis) Cases Reported in 2004

National Total = 18,957 Cases*

RANK	STATE	CASES	% of USA
38	Alabama	45	0.2%
48	Alaska	12	0.1%
21	Arizona	240	1.3%
31	Arkansas	78	0.4%
12	California	521	2.7%
4	Colorado	1,072	5.7%
48	Connecticut	12	0.1%
50	Delaware	5	0.0%
26	Florida	133	0.7%
45	Georgia	23	0.1%
43	Hawaii	27	0.1%
39	Idaho	37	0.2%
13	Illinois	503	2.7%
16	Indiana	293	1.5%
15	Iowa	308	1.6%
22	Kansas	230	1.2%
30	Kentucky	87	0.5%
47	Louisiana	16	0.1%
41	Maine	34	0.2%
24	Maryland	139	0.7%
3	Massachusetts	1,589	8.4%
17	Michigan	288	1.5%
14	Minnesota	497	2.6%
46	Mississippi	17	0.1%
10	Missouri	553	2.9%
33	Montana	74	0.4%
32	Nebraska	75	0.4%
36	Nevada	48	0.3%
29	New Hampshire	98	0.5%
20	New Jersey	247	1.3%
23	New Mexico	146	0.8%
2	New York	2,059	10.9%
28	North Carolina	101	0.5%
8	North Dakota	754	4.0%
7	Ohio	764	4.0%
42	Oklahoma	33	0.2%
11	Oregon	535	2.8%
9	Pennsylvania	590	3.1%
37	Rhode Island	47	0.2%
35	South Carolina	57	0.3%
34	South Dakota	73	0.4%
25	Tennessee	135	0.7%
5	Texas	845	4.5%
19	Utah	250	1.3%
27	Vermont	125	0.7%
18	Virginia	261	1.4%
6	Washington	765	4.0%
44	West Virginia	24	0.1%
1	Wisconsin	4,048	21.4%
40	Wyoming	35	0.2%

RANK	STATE	CASES	% of USA
1	Wisconsin	4,048	21.4%
2	New York	2,059	10.9%
3	Massachusetts	1,589	8.4%
4	Colorado	1,072	5.7%
5	Texas	845	4.5%
6	Washington	765	4.0%
7	Ohio	764	4.0%
8	North Dakota	754	4.0%
9	Pennsylvania	590	3.1%
10	Missouri	553	2.9%
11	Oregon	535	2.8%
12	California	521	2.7%
13	Illinois	503	2.7%
14	Minnesota	497	2.6%
15	Iowa	308	1.6%
16	Indiana	293	1.5%
17	Michigan	288	1.5%
18	Virginia	261	1.4%
19	Utah	250	1.3%
20	New Jersey	247	1.3%
21	Arizona	240	1.3%
22	Kansas	230	1.2%
23	New Mexico	146	0.8%
24	Maryland	139	0.7%
25	Tennessee	135	0.7%
26	Florida	133	0.7%
27	Vermont	125	0.7%
28	North Carolina	101	0.5%
29	New Hampshire	98	0.5%
30	Kentucky	87	0.5%
31	Arkansas	78	0.4%
32	Nebraska	75	0.4%
33	Montana	74	0.4%
34	South Dakota	73	0.4%
35	South Carolina	57	0.3%
36	Nevada	48	0.3%
37	Rhode Island	47	0.2%
38	Alabama	45	0.2%
39	Idaho	37	0.2%
40	Wyoming	35	0.2%
41	Maine	34	0.2%
42	Oklahoma	33	0.2%
43	Hawaii	27	0.1%
44	West Virginia	24	0.1%
45	Georgia	23	0.1%
46	Mississippi	17	0.1%
47	Louisiana	16	0.1%
48	Alaska	12	0.1%
48	Connecticut	12	0.1%
50	Delaware	5	0.0%
	District of Columbia	9	0.0%

Source: U.S. Department of Health and Human Services, National Center for Health Statistics
"Morbidity and Mortality Weekly Report" (January 7, 2005, Vol. 53, Nos. 51 & 52)
*Provisional data. Acute, highly contagious infection of respiratory tract.

Whooping Cough (Pertussis) Rate in 2004

National Rate = 6.5 Cases per 100,000 Population*

ALPHA ORDER

RANK	STATE	RATE
43	Alabama	1.0
38	Alaska	1.8
24	Arizona	4.2
28	Arkansas	2.8
39	California	1.5
4	Colorado	23.3
49	Connecticut	0.3
46	Delaware	0.6
45	Florida	0.8
49	Georgia	0.3
35	Hawaii	2.1
31	Idaho	2.7
25	Illinois	4.0
21	Indiana	4.7
10	Iowa	10.4
14	Kansas	8.4
35	Kentucky	2.1
48	Louisiana	0.4
32	Maine	2.6
33	Maryland	2.5
3	Massachusetts	24.8
28	Michigan	2.8
11	Minnesota	9.7
46	Mississippi	0.6
12	Missouri	9.6
15	Montana	8.0
22	Nebraska	4.3
35	Nevada	2.1
17	New Hampshire	7.5
28	New Jersey	2.8
16	New Mexico	7.7
8	New York	10.7
42	North Carolina	1.2
1	North Dakota	118.9
19	Ohio	6.7
44	Oklahoma	0.9
6	Oregon	14.9
20	Pennsylvania	4.8
22	Rhode Island	4.3
40	South Carolina	1.4
13	South Dakota	9.5
34	Tennessee	2.3
26	Texas	3.8
9	Utah	10.5
5	Vermont	20.1
27	Virginia	3.5
7	Washington	12.3
41	West Virginia	1.3
2	Wisconsin	73.5
18	Wyoming	6.9

RANK ORDER

RANK	STATE	RATE
1	North Dakota	118.9
2	Wisconsin	73.5
3	Massachusetts	24.8
4	Colorado	23.3
5	Vermont	20.1
6	Oregon	14.9
7	Washington	12.3
8	New York	10.7
9	Utah	10.5
10	Iowa	10.4
11	Minnesota	9.7
12	Missouri	9.6
13	South Dakota	9.5
14	Kansas	8.4
15	Montana	8.0
16	New Mexico	7.7
17	New Hampshire	7.5
18	Wyoming	6.9
19	Ohio	6.7
20	Pennsylvania	4.8
21	Indiana	4.7
22	Nebraska	4.3
22	Rhode Island	4.3
24	Arizona	4.2
25	Illinois	4.0
26	Texas	3.8
27	Virginia	3.5
28	Arkansas	2.8
28	Michigan	2.8
28	New Jersey	2.8
31	Idaho	2.7
32	Maine	2.6
33	Maryland	2.5
34	Tennessee	2.3
35	Hawaii	2.1
35	Kentucky	2.1
35	Nevada	2.1
38	Alaska	1.8
39	California	1.5
40	South Carolina	1.4
41	West Virginia	1.3
42	North Carolina	1.2
43	Alabama	1.0
44	Oklahoma	0.9
45	Florida	0.8
46	Delaware	0.6
46	Mississippi	0.6
48	Louisiana	0.4
49	Connecticut	0.3
49	Georgia	0.3

District of Columbia	1.6

Source: Morgan Quitno Press using data from U.S. Dept. of Health & Human Serv's, National Center for Health Statistics "Morbidity and Mortality Weekly Report" (January 7, 2005, Vol. 53, Nos. 51 & 52)
Provisional data. Acute, highly contagious infection of respiratory tract.

Percent of Children Aged 19 to 35 Months Immunized in 2003

National Percent = 81.3%*

ALPHA ORDER

RANK	STATE	PERCENT	RANK	STATE	PERCENT
24	Alabama	82.2	1	Connecticut	94.6
30	Alaska	81.4	2	Massachusetts	91.7
39	Arizona	78.8	3	Vermont	89.5
37	Arkansas	79.5	4	North Carolina	88.6
35	California	79.6	5	New Hampshire	88.4
50	Colorado	68.6	6	Rhode Island	87.3
1	Connecticut	94.6	7	Pennsylvania	86.9
35	Delaware	79.6	8	Virginia	84.8
20	Florida	82.7	9	Illinois	84.6
46	Georgia	76.6	9	Montana	84.6
19	Hawaii	82.8	9	South Carolina	84.6
29	Idaho	81.6	12	Minnesota	84.4
9	Illinois	84.6	13	Maryland	84.3
28	Indiana	81.7	14	Missouri	84.2
22	Iowa	82.6	14	Ohio	84.2
41	Kansas	77.7	16	Mississippi	84.0
31	Kentucky	81.2	17	South Dakota	83.4
48	Louisiana	72.4	18	Michigan	82.9
27	Maine	81.8	19	Hawaii	82.8
13	Maryland	84.3	20	Florida	82.7
2	Massachusetts	91.7	20	Wisconsin	82.7
18	Michigan	82.9	22	Iowa	82.6
12	Minnesota	84.4	23	North Dakota	82.5
16	Mississippi	84.0	24	Alabama	82.2
14	Missouri	84.2	25	Nebraska	82.0
9	Montana	84.6	26	New York	81.9
25	Nebraska	82.0	27	Maine	81.8
40	Nevada	78.1	28	Indiana	81.7
5	New Hampshire	88.4	29	Idaho	81.6
47	New Jersey	75.8	30	Alaska	81.4
45	New Mexico	77.0	31	Kentucky	81.2
26	New York	81.9	32	Tennessee	80.5
4	North Carolina	88.6	33	Utah	80.2
23	North Dakota	82.5	34	Washington	79.7
14	Ohio	84.2	35	California	79.6
49	Oklahoma	72.3	35	Delaware	79.6
38	Oregon	79.3	37	Arkansas	79.5
7	Pennsylvania	86.9	38	Oregon	79.3
6	Rhode Island	87.3	39	Arizona	78.8
9	South Carolina	84.6	40	Nevada	78.1
17	South Dakota	83.4	41	Kansas	77.7
32	Tennessee	80.5	42	West Virginia	77.4
43	Texas	77.2	43	Texas	77.2
33	Utah	80.2	43	Wyoming	77.2
3	Vermont	89.5	45	New Mexico	77.0
8	Virginia	84.8	46	Georgia	76.6
34	Washington	79.7	47	New Jersey	75.8
42	West Virginia	77.4	48	Louisiana	72.4
20	Wisconsin	82.7	49	Oklahoma	72.3
43	Wyoming	77.2	50	Colorado	68.6

District of Columbia 77.2

Source: U.S. Department of Health and Human Services, Centers for Disease Control and Prevention
"State Vaccination Coverage Levels" (Morbidity and Mortality Weekly Report, Vol. 53, No. 29, July 30, 2004)
This table is consistent with previous tables showing "fully" immunized children. Figures here are for the 4:3:1:3
series. Children received four doses of DTP/DT/DTaP (Diphtheria, Tetanus, Pertussis (Whooping Cough), Acellular
Pertussis), three doses of OPV (Oral Poliovirus Vaccine), one dose of MCV (Measles-Containing Vaccine) and three
doses of Hib (Haemophilus influenzae type b). Hepatitis B and Varicella vaccines are not included in this series.

Percent of Children Aged 19 to 35 Months Fully Immunized in 2003

National Percent = 72.5%*

ALPHA ORDER

RANK	STATE	PERCENT
6	Alabama	79.1
23	Alaska	72.9
32	Arizona	68.4
17	Arkansas	74.5
15	California	75.6
44	Colorado	63.0
1	Connecticut	89.1
35	Delaware	66.1
19	Florida	73.7
16	Georgia	74.6
8	Hawaii	78.7
47	Idaho	61.4
30	Illinois	69.1
46	Indiana	62.3
41	Iowa	63.4
45	Kansas	62.8
10	Kentucky	78.5
38	Louisiana	64.7
31	Maine	68.6
12	Maryland	77.4
2	Massachusetts	82.5
9	Michigan	78.6
26	Minnesota	70.7
11	Mississippi	78.2
18	Missouri	74.4
38	Montana	64.7
33	Nebraska	67.8
36	Nevada	65.5
14	New Hampshire	76.1
40	New Jersey	63.6
25	New Mexico	70.8
22	New York	73.1
13	North Carolina	77.3
43	North Dakota	63.1
24	Ohio	71.0
34	Oklahoma	67.0
27	Oregon	70.3
6	Pennsylvania	79.1
4	Rhode Island	79.8
3	South Carolina	80.3
48	South Dakota	60.0
20	Tennessee	73.5
29	Texas	69.8
28	Utah	70.1
37	Vermont	65.3
4	Virginia	79.8
50	Washington	56.2
42	West Virginia	63.2
21	Wisconsin	73.4
49	Wyoming	56.8

RANK ORDER

RANK	STATE	PERCENT
1	Connecticut	89.1
2	Massachusetts	82.5
3	South Carolina	80.3
4	Rhode Island	79.8
4	Virginia	79.8
6	Alabama	79.1
6	Pennsylvania	79.1
8	Hawaii	78.7
9	Michigan	78.6
10	Kentucky	78.5
11	Mississippi	78.2
12	Maryland	77.4
13	North Carolina	77.3
14	New Hampshire	76.1
15	California	75.6
16	Georgia	74.6
17	Arkansas	74.5
18	Missouri	74.4
19	Florida	73.7
20	Tennessee	73.5
21	Wisconsin	73.4
22	New York	73.1
23	Alaska	72.9
24	Ohio	71.0
25	New Mexico	70.8
26	Minnesota	70.7
27	Oregon	70.3
28	Utah	70.1
29	Texas	69.8
30	Illinois	69.1
31	Maine	68.6
32	Arizona	68.4
33	Nebraska	67.8
34	Oklahoma	67.0
35	Delaware	66.1
36	Nevada	65.5
37	Vermont	65.3
38	Louisiana	64.7
38	Montana	64.7
40	New Jersey	63.6
41	Iowa	63.4
42	West Virginia	63.2
43	North Dakota	63.1
44	Colorado	63.0
45	Kansas	62.8
46	Indiana	62.3
47	Idaho	61.4
48	South Dakota	60.0
49	Wyoming	56.8
50	Washington	56.2

District of Columbia   71.9

Source: U.S. Department of Health and Human Services, Centers for Disease Control and Prevention
"State Vaccination Coverage Levels" (Morbidity and Mortality Weekly Report, Vol. 53, No. 29, July 30, 2004)
*Fully immunized (4:3:1:3:3:1 series) children received four doses of DTP/DT/DTaP (Diphtheria, Tetanus, Pertussis (Whooping Cough), Acellular Pertussis), three doses of OPV (Oral Poliovirus Vaccine), one dose of MCV (Measles-Containing Vaccine), three doses of Hib (Haemophilus influenzae type b), three doses of Hepatitis B vaccine and one dose of Varicella (chickenpox) vaccine. This differs from previous "fully" immunized tables.

Percent of Adults Aged 65 Years and Older Who Received Flu Shots in 2003

National Median = 69.9%*

ALPHA ORDER

RANK	STATE	PERCENT
26	Alabama	70.2
46	Alaska	66.5
36	Arizona	68.9
22	Arkansas	71.0
19	California	72.5
11	Colorado	74.2
10	Connecticut	74.3
27	Delaware	70.0
48	Florida	65.9
45	Georgia	67.0
4	Hawaii	76.4
25	Idaho	70.3
49	Illinois	62.2
47	Indiana	66.1
3	Iowa	77.5
23	Kansas	70.8
31	Kentucky	69.1
39	Louisiana	68.3
8	Maine	74.8
38	Maryland	68.4
7	Massachusetts	74.9
43	Michigan	67.5
1	Minnesota	80.3
35	Mississippi	69.0
28	Missouri	69.9
17	Montana	72.8
14	Nebraska	73.6
50	Nevada	60.0
13	New Hampshire	73.9
44	New Jersey	67.2
20	New Mexico	72.4
40	New York	68.0
37	North Carolina	68.8
16	North Dakota	73.0
40	Ohio	68.0
6	Oklahoma	75.8
24	Oregon	70.5
31	Pennsylvania	69.1
5	Rhode Island	76.2
30	South Carolina	69.3
2	South Dakota	77.9
31	Tennessee	69.1
42	Texas	67.7
8	Utah	74.8
12	Vermont	74.1
29	Virginia	69.6
15	Washington	73.4
31	West Virginia	69.1
21	Wisconsin	72.1
18	Wyoming	72.6

RANK ORDER

RANK	STATE	PERCENT
1	Minnesota	80.3
2	South Dakota	77.9
3	Iowa	77.5
4	Hawaii	76.4
5	Rhode Island	76.2
6	Oklahoma	75.8
7	Massachusetts	74.9
8	Maine	74.8
8	Utah	74.8
10	Connecticut	74.3
11	Colorado	74.2
12	Vermont	74.1
13	New Hampshire	73.9
14	Nebraska	73.6
15	Washington	73.4
16	North Dakota	73.0
17	Montana	72.8
18	Wyoming	72.6
19	California	72.5
20	New Mexico	72.4
21	Wisconsin	72.1
22	Arkansas	71.0
23	Kansas	70.8
24	Oregon	70.5
25	Idaho	70.3
26	Alabama	70.2
27	Delaware	70.0
28	Missouri	69.9
29	Virginia	69.6
30	South Carolina	69.3
31	Kentucky	69.1
31	Pennsylvania	69.1
31	Tennessee	69.1
31	West Virginia	69.1
35	Mississippi	69.0
36	Arizona	68.9
37	North Carolina	68.8
38	Maryland	68.4
39	Louisiana	68.3
40	New York	68.0
40	Ohio	68.0
42	Texas	67.7
43	Michigan	67.5
44	New Jersey	67.2
45	Georgia	67.0
46	Alaska	66.5
47	Indiana	66.1
48	Florida	65.9
49	Illinois	62.2
50	Nevada	60.0
	District of Columbia	63.0

Source: U.S. Department of Health and Human Services, Centers for Disease Control and Prevention
"2003 Behavioral Risk Factor Surveillance Summary Prevalence Data" (http://apps.nccd.cdc.gov/brfss/)
*Percent of adults 65 years old and older who reported receiving influenza vaccine during the preceding 12 months.

Sexually Transmitted Diseases in 2003

National Total = 1,219,813 Cases*

ALPHA ORDER

RANK	STATE	CASES	% of USA
18	Alabama	23,626	1.9%
38	Alaska	4,474	0.4%
23	Arizona	16,587	1.4%
29	Arkansas	12,158	1.0%
1	California	144,690	11.9%
24	Colorado	15,932	1.3%
28	Connecticut	12,537	1.0%
40	Delaware	4,170	0.3%
6	Florida	62,016	5.1%
7	Georgia	53,957	4.4%
36	Hawaii	6,757	0.6%
45	Idaho	2,449	0.2%
4	Illinois	70,485	5.8%
17	Indiana	23,806	2.0%
35	Iowa	8,057	0.7%
31	Kansas	9,921	0.8%
30	Kentucky	11,593	1.0%
11	Louisiana	33,003	2.7%
46	Maine	2,271	0.2%
15	Maryland	25,176	2.1%
26	Massachusetts	14,338	1.2%
9	Michigan	46,786	3.8%
27	Minnesota	13,963	1.1%
22	Mississippi	18,561	1.5%
14	Missouri	27,423	2.2%
44	Montana	2,669	0.2%
37	Nebraska	6,372	0.5%
34	Nevada	8,063	0.7%
47	New Hampshire	1,760	0.1%
16	New Jersey	24,283	2.0%
33	New Mexico	8,720	0.7%
3	New York	79,982	6.6%
10	North Carolina	41,457	3.4%
47	North Dakota	1,760	0.1%
5	Ohio	65,256	5.3%
25	Oklahoma	15,629	1.3%
32	Oregon	8,738	0.7%
8	Pennsylvania	49,317	4.0%
41	Rhode Island	4,006	0.3%
20	South Carolina	23,259	1.9%
43	South Dakota	2,836	0.2%
12	Tennessee	29,034	2.4%
2	Texas	94,452	7.7%
39	Utah	4,321	0.4%
49	Vermont	1,158	0.1%
13	Virginia	28,587	2.3%
21	Washington	19,632	1.6%
42	West Virginia	3,434	0.3%
19	Wisconsin	23,621	1.9%
50	Wyoming	1,007	0.1%

RANK ORDER

RANK	STATE	CASES	% of USA
1	California	144,690	11.9%
2	Texas	94,452	7.7%
3	New York	79,982	6.6%
4	Illinois	70,485	5.8%
5	Ohio	65,256	5.3%
6	Florida	62,016	5.1%
7	Georgia	53,957	4.4%
8	Pennsylvania	49,317	4.0%
9	Michigan	46,786	3.8%
10	North Carolina	41,457	3.4%
11	Louisiana	33,003	2.7%
12	Tennessee	29,034	2.4%
13	Virginia	28,587	2.3%
14	Missouri	27,423	2.2%
15	Maryland	25,176	2.1%
16	New Jersey	24,283	2.0%
17	Indiana	23,806	2.0%
18	Alabama	23,626	1.9%
19	Wisconsin	23,621	1.9%
20	South Carolina	23,259	1.9%
21	Washington	19,632	1.6%
22	Mississippi	18,561	1.5%
23	Arizona	16,587	1.4%
24	Colorado	15,932	1.3%
25	Oklahoma	15,629	1.3%
26	Massachusetts	14,338	1.2%
27	Minnesota	13,963	1.1%
28	Connecticut	12,537	1.0%
29	Arkansas	12,158	1.0%
30	Kentucky	11,593	1.0%
31	Kansas	9,921	0.8%
32	Oregon	8,738	0.7%
33	New Mexico	8,720	0.7%
34	Nevada	8,063	0.7%
35	Iowa	8,057	0.7%
36	Hawaii	6,757	0.6%
37	Nebraska	6,372	0.5%
38	Alaska	4,474	0.4%
39	Utah	4,321	0.4%
40	Delaware	4,170	0.3%
41	Rhode Island	4,006	0.3%
42	West Virginia	3,434	0.3%
43	South Dakota	2,836	0.2%
44	Montana	2,669	0.2%
45	Idaho	2,449	0.2%
46	Maine	2,271	0.2%
47	New Hampshire	1,760	0.1%
47	North Dakota	1,760	0.1%
49	Vermont	1,158	0.1%
50	Wyoming	1,007	0.1%

District of Columbia 5,724 0.5%

Source: Morgan Quitno Press using data from U.S. Dept. of Health and Human Services, Nat'l Center for Health Statistics
"Sexually Transmitted Disease Surveillance 2003" (http://www.cdc.gov/std/stats/TOC2003.htm)
*Includes chancroid, chlamydia, gonorrhea and primary and secondary syphilis.

Sexually Transmitted Disease Rate in 2003

National Rate = 423.0 Cases per 100,000 Population*

ALPHA ORDER

RANK	STATE	RATE
9	Alabama	526.6
2	Alaska	695.0
35	Arizona	303.9
17	Arkansas	448.7
22	California	412.0
33	Colorado	353.5
32	Connecticut	362.3
10	Delaware	516.5
29	Florida	371.0
4	Georgia	630.3
8	Hawaii	542.8
48	Idaho	182.6
7	Illinois	559.4
25	Indiana	386.5
41	Iowa	274.3
31	Kansas	365.3
37	Kentucky	283.2
1	Louisiana	736.3
49	Maine	175.4
16	Maryland	461.3
43	Massachusetts	223.0
15	Michigan	465.5
39	Minnesota	278.1
3	Mississippi	646.4
13	Missouri	483.5
36	Montana	293.5
30	Nebraska	368.6
28	Nevada	371.0
50	New Hampshire	138.0
38	New Jersey	282.7
14	New Mexico	470.0
21	New York	417.5
12	North Carolina	498.2
40	North Dakota	277.5
5	Ohio	571.3
18	Oklahoma	447.3
42	Oregon	248.2
23	Pennsylvania	399.8
26	Rhode Island	374.5
6	South Carolina	566.3
27	South Dakota	372.7
11	Tennessee	500.7
20	Texas	433.6
47	Utah	186.6
46	Vermont	187.8
24	Virginia	391.9
34	Washington	323.6
45	West Virginia	190.6
19	Wisconsin	434.1
44	Wyoming	201.9

RANK ORDER

RANK	STATE	RATE
1	Louisiana	736.3
2	Alaska	695.0
3	Mississippi	646.4
4	Georgia	630.3
5	Ohio	571.3
6	South Carolina	566.3
7	Illinois	559.4
8	Hawaii	542.8
9	Alabama	526.6
10	Delaware	516.5
11	Tennessee	500.7
12	North Carolina	498.2
13	Missouri	483.5
14	New Mexico	470.0
15	Michigan	465.5
16	Maryland	461.3
17	Arkansas	448.7
18	Oklahoma	447.3
19	Wisconsin	434.1
20	Texas	433.6
21	New York	417.5
22	California	412.0
23	Pennsylvania	399.8
24	Virginia	391.9
25	Indiana	386.5
26	Rhode Island	374.5
27	South Dakota	372.7
28	Nevada	371.0
29	Florida	371.0
30	Nebraska	368.6
31	Kansas	365.3
32	Connecticut	362.3
33	Colorado	353.5
34	Washington	323.6
35	Arizona	303.9
36	Montana	293.5
37	Kentucky	283.2
38	New Jersey	282.7
39	Minnesota	278.1
40	North Dakota	277.5
41	Iowa	274.3
42	Oregon	248.2
43	Massachusetts	223.0
44	Wyoming	201.9
45	West Virginia	190.6
46	Vermont	187.8
47	Utah	186.6
48	Idaho	182.6
49	Maine	175.4
50	New Hampshire	138.0

District of Columbia 1,026.5

Source: Morgan Quitno Press using data from U.S. Dept. of Health and Human Services, Nat'l Center for Health Statistics "Sexually Transmitted Disease Surveillance 2003" (http://www.cdc.gov/std/stats/TOC2003.htm)
*Includes chancroid, chlamydia, gonorrhea and primary and secondary syphilis.

Chlamydia Cases Reported in 2003

National Total = 877,478 Cases*

ALPHA ORDER

RANK	STATE	CASES	% of USA
21	Alabama	14,209	1.6%
38	Alaska	3,900	0.4%
23	Arizona	12,819	1.5%
30	Arkansas	7,856	0.9%
1	California	117,428	13.4%
22	Colorado	13,039	1.5%
28	Connecticut	9,393	1.1%
40	Delaware	3,035	0.3%
6	Florida	42,382	4.8%
8	Georgia	35,686	4.1%
36	Hawaii	5,480	0.6%
45	Idaho	2,366	0.3%
4	Illinois	48,294	5.5%
16	Indiana	17,075	1.9%
34	Iowa	6,491	0.7%
33	Kansas	7,249	0.8%
29	Kentucky	7,981	0.9%
11	Louisiana	20,970	2.4%
46	Maine	2,030	0.2%
17	Maryland	16,831	1.9%
25	Massachusetts	11,301	1.3%
9	Michigan	32,572	3.7%
27	Minnesota	10,714	1.2%
24	Mississippi	12,193	1.4%
14	Missouri	18,570	2.1%
44	Montana	2,547	0.3%
37	Nebraska	4,739	0.5%
35	Nevada	5,830	0.7%
48	New Hampshire	1,616	0.2%
19	New Jersey	16,169	1.8%
32	New Mexico	7,480	0.9%
3	New York	57,222	6.5%
10	North Carolina	26,187	3.0%
47	North Dakota	1,655	0.2%
5	Ohio	42,522	4.8%
26	Oklahoma	11,013	1.3%
31	Oregon	7,688	0.9%
7	Pennsylvania	37,291	4.2%
41	Rhode Island	3,000	0.3%
20	South Carolina	14,623	1.7%
42	South Dakota	2,608	0.3%
12	Tennessee	20,380	2.3%
2	Texas	69,200	7.9%
39	Utah	3,893	0.4%
49	Vermont	1,060	0.1%
13	Virginia	19,439	2.2%
18	Washington	16,797	1.9%
43	West Virginia	2,585	0.3%
15	Wisconsin	17,942	2.0%
50	Wyoming	960	0.1%

RANK ORDER

RANK	STATE	CASES	% of USA
1	California	117,428	13.4%
2	Texas	69,200	7.9%
3	New York	57,222	6.5%
4	Illinois	48,294	5.5%
5	Ohio	42,522	4.8%
6	Florida	42,382	4.8%
7	Pennsylvania	37,291	4.2%
8	Georgia	35,686	4.1%
9	Michigan	32,572	3.7%
10	North Carolina	26,187	3.0%
11	Louisiana	20,970	2.4%
12	Tennessee	20,380	2.3%
13	Virginia	19,439	2.2%
14	Missouri	18,570	2.1%
15	Wisconsin	17,942	2.0%
16	Indiana	17,075	1.9%
17	Maryland	16,831	1.9%
18	Washington	16,797	1.9%
19	New Jersey	16,169	1.8%
20	South Carolina	14,623	1.7%
21	Alabama	14,209	1.6%
22	Colorado	13,039	1.5%
23	Arizona	12,819	1.5%
24	Mississippi	12,193	1.4%
25	Massachusetts	11,301	1.3%
26	Oklahoma	11,013	1.3%
27	Minnesota	10,714	1.2%
28	Connecticut	9,393	1.1%
29	Kentucky	7,981	0.9%
30	Arkansas	7,856	0.9%
31	Oregon	7,688	0.9%
32	New Mexico	7,480	0.9%
33	Kansas	7,249	0.8%
34	Iowa	6,491	0.7%
35	Nevada	5,830	0.7%
36	Hawaii	5,480	0.6%
37	Nebraska	4,739	0.5%
38	Alaska	3,900	0.4%
39	Utah	3,893	0.4%
40	Delaware	3,035	0.3%
41	Rhode Island	3,000	0.3%
42	South Dakota	2,608	0.3%
43	West Virginia	2,585	0.3%
44	Montana	2,547	0.3%
45	Idaho	2,366	0.3%
46	Maine	2,030	0.2%
47	North Dakota	1,655	0.2%
48	New Hampshire	1,616	0.2%
49	Vermont	1,060	0.1%
50	Wyoming	960	0.1%
	District of Columbia	3,168	0.4%

Source: U.S. Department of Health and Human Services, National Center for Health Statistics "Sexually Transmitted Disease Surveillance 2003" (http://www.cdc.gov/std/stats/TOC2003.htm)
*Any of several common, often asymptomatic, sexually transmitted diseases caused by the microorganism Chlamydia trachomatis, including nonspecific urethritis in men.

Chlamydia Rate in 2003

National Rate = 304.3 Cases per 100,000 Population*

ALPHA ORDER

RANK	STATE	RATE
18	Alabama	316.7
1	Alaska	605.8
37	Arizona	234.9
24	Arkansas	289.9
13	California	334.4
25	Colorado	289.3
31	Connecticut	271.4
8	Delaware	375.9
36	Florida	253.6
5	Georgia	416.9
3	Hawaii	440.2
44	Idaho	176.4
7	Illinois	383.3
28	Indiana	277.2
38	Iowa	221.0
33	Kansas	266.9
41	Kentucky	195.0
2	Louisiana	467.8
48	Maine	156.8
21	Maryland	308.4
45	Massachusetts	175.8
16	Michigan	324.1
40	Minnesota	213.4
4	Mississippi	424.6
15	Missouri	327.4
27	Montana	280.1
30	Nebraska	274.1
32	Nevada	268.2
50	New Hampshire	126.7
43	New Jersey	188.2
6	New Mexico	403.2
23	New York	298.7
20	North Carolina	314.7
35	North Dakota	261.0
9	Ohio	372.3
19	Oklahoma	315.2
39	Oregon	218.3
22	Pennsylvania	302.3
26	Rhode Island	280.4
10	South Carolina	356.0
12	South Dakota	342.7
11	Tennessee	351.5
17	Texas	317.7
47	Utah	168.1
46	Vermont	171.9
34	Virginia	266.5
29	Washington	276.8
49	West Virginia	143.5
14	Wisconsin	329.7
42	Wyoming	192.5

RANK ORDER

RANK	STATE	RATE
1	Alaska	605.8
2	Louisiana	467.8
3	Hawaii	440.2
4	Mississippi	424.6
5	Georgia	416.9
6	New Mexico	403.2
7	Illinois	383.3
8	Delaware	375.9
9	Ohio	372.3
10	South Carolina	356.0
11	Tennessee	351.5
12	South Dakota	342.7
13	California	334.4
14	Wisconsin	329.7
15	Missouri	327.4
16	Michigan	324.1
17	Texas	317.7
18	Alabama	316.7
19	Oklahoma	315.2
20	North Carolina	314.7
21	Maryland	308.4
22	Pennsylvania	302.3
23	New York	298.7
24	Arkansas	289.9
25	Colorado	289.3
26	Rhode Island	280.4
27	Montana	280.1
28	Indiana	277.2
29	Washington	276.8
30	Nebraska	274.1
31	Connecticut	271.4
32	Nevada	268.2
33	Kansas	266.9
34	Virginia	266.5
35	North Dakota	261.0
36	Florida	253.6
37	Arizona	234.9
38	Iowa	221.0
39	Oregon	218.3
40	Minnesota	213.4
41	Kentucky	195.0
42	Wyoming	192.5
43	New Jersey	188.2
44	Idaho	176.4
45	Massachusetts	175.8
46	Vermont	171.9
47	Utah	168.1
48	Maine	156.8
49	West Virginia	143.5
50	New Hampshire	126.7
	District of Columbia	568.1

Source: U.S. Department of Health and Human Services, National Center for Health Statistics
  "Sexually Transmitted Disease Surveillance 2003" (http://www.cdc.gov/std/stats/TOC2003.htm)
*Any of several common, often asymptomatic, sexually transmitted diseases caused by the microorganism Chlamydia trachomatis, including nonspecific urethritis in men.

Gonorrhea Cases Reported in 2003

National Total = 335,104 Cases*

ALPHA ORDER

RANK	STATE	CASES	% of USA
12	Alabama	9,303	2.8%
41	Alaska	573	0.2%
24	Arizona	3,580	1.1%
23	Arkansas	4,251	1.3%
1	California	25,963	7.7%
29	Colorado	2,854	0.9%
27	Connecticut	3,114	0.9%
37	Delaware	1,128	0.3%
6	Florida	18,974	5.7%
7	Georgia	17,686	5.3%
35	Hawaii	1,263	0.4%
49	Idaho	68	0.0%
5	Illinois	21,817	6.5%
19	Indiana	6,681	2.0%
34	Iowa	1,554	0.5%
31	Kansas	2,647	0.8%
25	Kentucky	3,578	1.1%
11	Louisiana	11,850	3.5%
43	Maine	233	0.1%
17	Maryland	8,032	2.4%
28	Massachusetts	2,901	0.9%
9	Michigan	13,965	4.2%
26	Minnesota	3,202	1.0%
20	Mississippi	6,328	1.9%
14	Missouri	8,792	2.6%
46	Montana	122	0.0%
33	Nebraska	1,623	0.5%
32	Nevada	2,221	0.7%
45	New Hampshire	125	0.0%
18	New Jersey	7,944	2.4%
36	New Mexico	1,169	0.3%
4	New York	22,166	6.6%
8	North Carolina	15,116	4.5%
47	North Dakota	103	0.0%
3	Ohio	22,537	6.7%
22	Oklahoma	4,552	1.4%
38	Oregon	1,000	0.3%
10	Pennsylvania	11,866	3.5%
39	Rhode Island	973	0.3%
16	South Carolina	8,518	2.5%
44	South Dakota	226	0.1%
15	Tennessee	8,519	2.5%
2	Texas	24,595	7.3%
42	Utah	412	0.1%
48	Vermont	97	0.0%
13	Virginia	9,066	2.7%
30	Washington	2,753	0.8%
40	West Virginia	847	0.3%
21	Wisconsin	5,663	1.7%
50	Wyoming	46	0.0%

RANK ORDER

RANK	STATE	CASES	% of USA
1	California	25,963	7.7%
2	Texas	24,595	7.3%
3	Ohio	22,537	6.7%
4	New York	22,166	6.6%
5	Illinois	21,817	6.5%
6	Florida	18,974	5.7%
7	Georgia	17,686	5.3%
8	North Carolina	15,116	4.5%
9	Michigan	13,965	4.2%
10	Pennsylvania	11,866	3.5%
11	Louisiana	11,850	3.5%
12	Alabama	9,303	2.8%
13	Virginia	9,066	2.7%
14	Missouri	8,792	2.6%
15	Tennessee	8,519	2.5%
16	South Carolina	8,518	2.5%
17	Maryland	8,032	2.4%
18	New Jersey	7,944	2.4%
19	Indiana	6,681	2.0%
20	Mississippi	6,328	1.9%
21	Wisconsin	5,663	1.7%
22	Oklahoma	4,552	1.4%
23	Arkansas	4,251	1.3%
24	Arizona	3,580	1.1%
25	Kentucky	3,578	1.1%
26	Minnesota	3,202	1.0%
27	Connecticut	3,114	0.9%
28	Massachusetts	2,901	0.9%
29	Colorado	2,854	0.9%
30	Washington	2,753	0.8%
31	Kansas	2,647	0.8%
32	Nevada	2,221	0.7%
33	Nebraska	1,623	0.5%
34	Iowa	1,554	0.5%
35	Hawaii	1,263	0.4%
36	New Mexico	1,169	0.3%
37	Delaware	1,128	0.3%
38	Oregon	1,000	0.3%
39	Rhode Island	973	0.3%
40	West Virginia	847	0.3%
41	Alaska	573	0.2%
42	Utah	412	0.1%
43	Maine	233	0.1%
44	South Dakota	226	0.1%
45	New Hampshire	125	0.0%
46	Montana	122	0.0%
47	North Dakota	103	0.0%
48	Vermont	97	0.0%
49	Idaho	68	0.0%
50	Wyoming	46	0.0%
	District of Columbia	2,508	0.7%

Source: U.S. Department of Health and Human Services, National Center for Health Statistics
"Sexually Transmitted Disease Surveillance 2003" (http://www.cdc.gov/std/stats/TOC2003.htm)
*Gonorrhea is a sexually transmitted disease caused by gonococcal bacteria that affects the mucous membrane chiefly of the genital and urinary tracts and is characterized by an acute purulent discharge and painful or difficult urination, though women often have no symptoms.

Gonorrhea Rate in 2003

National Rate = 116.2 Cases per 100,000 Population*

ALPHA ORDER

RANK	STATE	RATE
3	Alabama	207.4
30	Alaska	89.0
33	Arizona	65.6
9	Arkansas	156.9
32	California	73.9
35	Colorado	63.3
29	Connecticut	90.0
13	Delaware	139.7
18	Florida	113.5
5	Georgia	206.6
23	Hawaii	101.5
50	Idaho	5.1
8	Illinois	173.1
20	Indiana	108.5
37	Iowa	52.9
24	Kansas	97.5
31	Kentucky	87.4
1	Louisiana	264.4
43	Maine	18.0
11	Maryland	147.2
40	Massachusetts	45.1
14	Michigan	138.9
34	Minnesota	63.8
2	Mississippi	220.4
10	Missouri	155.0
47	Montana	13.4
26	Nebraska	93.9
22	Nevada	102.2
48	New Hampshire	9.8
27	New Jersey	92.5
36	New Mexico	63.0
17	New York	115.7
7	North Carolina	181.7
45	North Dakota	16.2
6	Ohio	197.3
15	Oklahoma	130.3
42	Oregon	28.4
25	Pennsylvania	96.2
28	Rhode Island	91.0
3	South Carolina	207.4
41	South Dakota	29.7
12	Tennessee	146.9
19	Texas	112.9
44	Utah	17.8
46	Vermont	15.7
16	Virginia	124.3
39	Washington	45.4
38	West Virginia	47.0
21	Wisconsin	104.1
49	Wyoming	9.2

RANK ORDER

RANK	STATE	RATE
1	Louisiana	264.4
2	Mississippi	220.4
3	Alabama	207.4
3	South Carolina	207.4
5	Georgia	206.6
6	Ohio	197.3
7	North Carolina	181.7
8	Illinois	173.1
9	Arkansas	156.9
10	Missouri	155.0
11	Maryland	147.2
12	Tennessee	146.9
13	Delaware	139.7
14	Michigan	138.9
15	Oklahoma	130.3
16	Virginia	124.3
17	New York	115.7
18	Florida	113.5
19	Texas	112.9
20	Indiana	108.5
21	Wisconsin	104.1
22	Nevada	102.2
23	Hawaii	101.5
24	Kansas	97.5
25	Pennsylvania	96.2
26	Nebraska	93.9
27	New Jersey	92.5
28	Rhode Island	91.0
29	Connecticut	90.0
30	Alaska	89.0
31	Kentucky	87.4
32	California	73.9
33	Arizona	65.6
34	Minnesota	63.8
35	Colorado	63.3
36	New Mexico	63.0
37	Iowa	52.9
38	West Virginia	47.0
39	Washington	45.4
40	Massachusetts	45.1
41	South Dakota	29.7
42	Oregon	28.4
43	Maine	18.0
44	Utah	17.8
45	North Dakota	16.2
46	Vermont	15.7
47	Montana	13.4
48	New Hampshire	9.8
49	Wyoming	9.2
50	Idaho	5.1

| | District of Columbia | 449.8 |

Source: U.S. Department of Health and Human Services, National Center for Health Statistics
"Sexually Transmitted Disease Surveillance 2003" (http://www.cdc.gov/std/stats/TOC2003.htm)
*Gonorrhea is a sexually transmitted disease caused by gonococcal bacteria that affects the mucous membrane chiefly of the genital and urinary tracts and is characterized by an acute purulent discharge and painful or difficult urination, though women often have no symptoms.

Syphilis Cases Reported in 2003

National Total = 7,177 Cases*

ALPHA ORDER

RANK	STATE	CASES	% of USA
17	Alabama	114	1.6%
47	Alaska	1	0.0%
10	Arizona	186	2.6%
24	Arkansas	51	0.7%
1	California	1,299	18.1%
29	Colorado	39	0.5%
32	Connecticut	30	0.4%
43	Delaware	7	0.1%
2	Florida	658	9.2%
4	Georgia	585	8.2%
37	Hawaii	14	0.2%
36	Idaho	15	0.2%
6	Illinois	374	5.2%
25	Indiana	50	0.7%
39	Iowa	12	0.2%
33	Kansas	25	0.3%
30	Kentucky	33	0.5%
11	Louisiana	183	2.5%
42	Maine	8	0.1%
7	Maryland	312	4.3%
16	Massachusetts	133	1.9%
8	Michigan	249	3.5%
27	Minnesota	47	0.7%
28	Mississippi	40	0.6%
23	Missouri	61	0.8%
49	Montana	0	0.0%
41	Nebraska	10	0.1%
39	Nevada	12	0.2%
34	New Hampshire	19	0.3%
12	New Jersey	170	2.4%
21	New Mexico	71	1.0%
5	New York	584	8.1%
14	North Carolina	152	2.1%
44	North Dakota	2	0.0%
9	Ohio	197	2.7%
22	Oklahoma	64	0.9%
26	Oregon	48	0.7%
13	Pennsylvania	159	2.2%
30	Rhode Island	33	0.5%
18	South Carolina	94	1.3%
44	South Dakota	2	0.0%
15	Tennessee	135	1.9%
3	Texas	654	9.1%
37	Utah	14	0.2%
47	Vermont	1	0.0%
19	Virginia	82	1.1%
19	Washington	82	1.1%
44	West Virginia	2	0.0%
35	Wisconsin	16	0.2%
49	Wyoming	0	0.0%

RANK ORDER

RANK	STATE	CASES	% of USA
1	California	1,299	18.1%
2	Florida	658	9.2%
3	Texas	654	9.1%
4	Georgia	585	8.2%
5	New York	584	8.1%
6	Illinois	374	5.2%
7	Maryland	312	4.3%
8	Michigan	249	3.5%
9	Ohio	197	2.7%
10	Arizona	186	2.6%
11	Louisiana	183	2.5%
12	New Jersey	170	2.4%
13	Pennsylvania	159	2.2%
14	North Carolina	152	2.1%
15	Tennessee	135	1.9%
16	Massachusetts	133	1.9%
17	Alabama	114	1.6%
18	South Carolina	94	1.3%
19	Virginia	82	1.1%
19	Washington	82	1.1%
21	New Mexico	71	1.0%
22	Oklahoma	64	0.9%
23	Missouri	61	0.8%
24	Arkansas	51	0.7%
25	Indiana	50	0.7%
26	Oregon	48	0.7%
27	Minnesota	47	0.7%
28	Mississippi	40	0.6%
29	Colorado	39	0.5%
30	Kentucky	33	0.5%
30	Rhode Island	33	0.5%
32	Connecticut	30	0.4%
33	Kansas	25	0.3%
34	New Hampshire	19	0.3%
35	Wisconsin	16	0.2%
36	Idaho	15	0.2%
37	Hawaii	14	0.2%
37	Utah	14	0.2%
39	Iowa	12	0.2%
39	Nevada	12	0.2%
41	Nebraska	10	0.1%
42	Maine	8	0.1%
43	Delaware	7	0.1%
44	North Dakota	2	0.0%
44	South Dakota	2	0.0%
44	West Virginia	2	0.0%
47	Alaska	1	0.0%
47	Vermont	1	0.0%
49	Montana	0	0.0%
49	Wyoming	0	0.0%
	District of Columbia	48	0.7%

Source: U.S. Department of Health and Human Services, National Center for Health Statistics
"Sexually Transmitted Disease Surveillance 2003" (http://www.cdc.gov/std/stats/TOC2003.htm)
*Includes only primary and secondary cases. Does not include 27,093 cases in other stages. A chronic infectious disease caused by a spirochete (Treponema pallidum), either transmitted by direct contact, usually in sexual intercourse, or passed from mother to child in utero, and progressing through three stages characterized respectively by local formation of chancres, ulcerous skin eruptions, and systemic infection leading to general paresis.

Syphilis Rate in 2003

National Rate = 2.5 Cases per 100,000 Population*

ALPHA ORDER

RANK ORDER

RANK	STATE	RATE	RANK	STATE	RATE
12	Alabama	2.5	1	Georgia	6.8
46	Alaska	0.2	2	Maryland	5.7
7	Arizona	3.4	3	Louisiana	4.1
18	Arkansas	1.9	4	Florida	3.9
6	California	3.7	5	New Mexico	3.8
31	Colorado	0.9	6	California	3.7
31	Connecticut	0.9	7	Arizona	3.4
31	Delaware	0.9	8	Rhode Island	3.1
4	Florida	3.9	9	Illinois	3.0
1	Georgia	6.8	9	New York	3.0
27	Hawaii	1.1	9	Texas	3.0
27	Idaho	1.1	12	Alabama	2.5
9	Illinois	3.0	12	Michigan	2.5
36	Indiana	0.8	14	South Carolina	2.3
42	Iowa	0.4	14	Tennessee	2.3
31	Kansas	0.9	16	Massachusetts	2.1
36	Kentucky	0.8	17	New Jersey	2.0
3	Louisiana	4.1	18	Arkansas	1.9
38	Maine	0.6	19	North Carolina	1.8
2	Maryland	5.7	19	Oklahoma	1.8
16	Massachusetts	2.1	21	Ohio	1.7
12	Michigan	2.5	22	New Hampshire	1.5
31	Minnesota	0.9	23	Mississippi	1.4
23	Mississippi	1.4	23	Oregon	1.4
27	Missouri	1.1	23	Washington	1.4
49	Montana	0.0	26	Pennsylvania	1.3
38	Nebraska	0.6	27	Hawaii	1.1
38	Nevada	0.6	27	Idaho	1.1
22	New Hampshire	1.5	27	Missouri	1.1
17	New Jersey	2.0	27	Virginia	1.1
5	New Mexico	3.8	31	Colorado	0.9
9	New York	3.0	31	Connecticut	0.9
19	North Carolina	1.8	31	Delaware	0.9
43	North Dakota	0.3	31	Kansas	0.9
21	Ohio	1.7	31	Minnesota	0.9
19	Oklahoma	1.8	36	Indiana	0.8
23	Oregon	1.4	36	Kentucky	0.8
26	Pennsylvania	1.3	38	Maine	0.6
8	Rhode Island	3.1	38	Nebraska	0.6
14	South Carolina	2.3	38	Nevada	0.6
43	South Dakota	0.3	38	Utah	0.6
14	Tennessee	2.3	42	Iowa	0.4
9	Texas	3.0	43	North Dakota	0.3
38	Utah	0.6	43	South Dakota	0.3
46	Vermont	0.2	43	Wisconsin	0.3
27	Virginia	1.1	46	Alaska	0.2
23	Washington	1.4	46	Vermont	0.2
48	West Virginia	0.1	48	West Virginia	0.1
43	Wisconsin	0.3	49	Montana	0.0
49	Wyoming	0.0	49	Wyoming	0.0

District of Columbia   8.6

Source: U.S. Department of Health and Human Services, National Center for Health Statistics
"Sexually Transmitted Disease Surveillance 2003" (http://www.cdc.gov/std/stats/TOC2003.htm)
*Includes only primary and secondary cases. Does not include 27,093 cases in other stages. A chronic infectious disease caused by a spirochete (Treponema pallidum), either transmitted by direct contact, usually in sexual intercourse, or passed from mother to child in utero, and progressing through three stages characterized respectively by local formation of chancres, ulcerous skin eruptions, and systemic infection leading to general paresis.

Percent of Adults Who Have Asthma: 2003

National Median = 7.6% of Adults*

ALPHA ORDER

RANK	STATE	PERCENT
26	Alabama	7.5
7	Alaska	9.1
12	Arizona	8.3
33	Arkansas	7.3
10	California	8.4
12	Colorado	8.3
12	Connecticut	8.3
26	Delaware	7.5
48	Florida	6.1
39	Georgia	7.0
50	Hawaii	5.6
19	Idaho	7.9
31	Illinois	7.4
16	Indiana	8.1
46	Iowa	6.2
26	Kansas	7.5
3	Kentucky	9.8
46	Louisiana	6.2
1	Maine	9.9
22	Maryland	7.8
1	Massachusetts	9.9
5	Michigan	9.3
43	Minnesota	6.8
41	Mississippi	6.9
18	Missouri	8.0
19	Montana	7.9
35	Nebraska	7.1
45	Nevada	6.6
9	New Hampshire	8.5
35	New Jersey	7.1
44	New Mexico	6.7
23	New York	7.6
35	North Carolina	7.1
39	North Dakota	7.0
35	Ohio	7.1
23	Oklahoma	7.6
5	Oregon	9.3
12	Pennsylvania	8.3
4	Rhode Island	9.6
48	South Carolina	6.1
33	South Dakota	7.3
19	Tennessee	7.9
41	Texas	6.9
31	Utah	7.4
10	Vermont	8.4
23	Virginia	7.6
7	Washington	9.1
16	West Virginia	8.1
26	Wisconsin	7.5
26	Wyoming	7.5

RANK ORDER

RANK	STATE	PERCENT
1	Maine	9.9
1	Massachusetts	9.9
3	Kentucky	9.8
4	Rhode Island	9.6
5	Michigan	9.3
5	Oregon	9.3
7	Alaska	9.1
7	Washington	9.1
9	New Hampshire	8.5
10	California	8.4
10	Vermont	8.4
12	Arizona	8.3
12	Colorado	8.3
12	Connecticut	8.3
12	Pennsylvania	8.3
16	Indiana	8.1
16	West Virginia	8.1
18	Missouri	8.0
19	Idaho	7.9
19	Montana	7.9
19	Tennessee	7.9
22	Maryland	7.8
23	New York	7.6
23	Oklahoma	7.6
23	Virginia	7.6
26	Alabama	7.5
26	Delaware	7.5
26	Kansas	7.5
26	Wisconsin	7.5
26	Wyoming	7.5
31	Illinois	7.4
31	Utah	7.4
33	Arkansas	7.3
33	South Dakota	7.3
35	Nebraska	7.1
35	New Jersey	7.1
35	North Carolina	7.1
35	Ohio	7.1
39	Georgia	7.0
39	North Dakota	7.0
41	Mississippi	6.9
41	Texas	6.9
43	Minnesota	6.8
44	New Mexico	6.7
45	Nevada	6.6
46	Iowa	6.2
46	Louisiana	6.2
48	Florida	6.1
48	South Carolina	6.1
50	Hawaii	5.6

	District of Columbia	7.8

Source: U.S. Department of Health and Human Services, Centers for Disease Control and Prevention
   "2003 Behavioral Risk Factor Surveillance Summary Prevalence Data" (http://apps.nccd.cdc.gov/brfss/)
*Percent of adults who answered yes to the questions "Have you ever been told by a doctor, nurse or other health professional that you had asthma?" and "Do you still have asthma?"

Percent of Adults Who Have Been Told They Have Diabetes: 2003

National Median = 7.2% of Adults*

ALPHA ORDER

RANK	STATE	PERCENT
6	Alabama	8.7
49	Alaska	5.0
33	Arizona	6.3
18	Arkansas	7.4
22	California	7.2
50	Colorado	4.7
41	Connecticut	5.9
16	Delaware	7.7
7	Florida	8.5
14	Georgia	7.8
17	Hawaii	7.6
33	Idaho	6.3
21	Illinois	7.3
14	Indiana	7.8
30	Iowa	6.7
39	Kansas	6.0
7	Kentucky	8.5
7	Louisiana	8.5
18	Maine	7.4
27	Maryland	7.0
37	Massachusetts	6.2
13	Michigan	7.9
46	Minnesota	5.5
1	Mississippi	11.0
28	Missouri	6.9
46	Montana	5.5
32	Nebraska	6.4
33	Nevada	6.3
45	New Hampshire	5.6
25	New Jersey	7.1
44	New Mexico	5.7
18	New York	7.4
10	North Carolina	8.1
37	North Dakota	6.2
5	Ohio	8.9
22	Oklahoma	7.2
33	Oregon	6.3
12	Pennsylvania	8.0
29	Rhode Island	6.8
4	South Carolina	9.3
25	South Dakota	7.1
3	Tennessee	9.4
10	Texas	8.1
46	Utah	5.5
42	Vermont	5.8
22	Virginia	7.2
31	Washington	6.6
2	West Virginia	9.8
39	Wisconsin	6.0
42	Wyoming	5.8

RANK ORDER

RANK	STATE	PERCENT
1	Mississippi	11.0
2	West Virginia	9.8
3	Tennessee	9.4
4	South Carolina	9.3
5	Ohio	8.9
6	Alabama	8.7
7	Florida	8.5
7	Kentucky	8.5
7	Louisiana	8.5
10	North Carolina	8.1
10	Texas	8.1
12	Pennsylvania	8.0
13	Michigan	7.9
14	Georgia	7.8
14	Indiana	7.8
16	Delaware	7.7
17	Hawaii	7.6
18	Arkansas	7.4
18	Maine	7.4
18	New York	7.4
21	Illinois	7.3
22	California	7.2
22	Oklahoma	7.2
22	Virginia	7.2
25	New Jersey	7.1
25	South Dakota	7.1
27	Maryland	7.0
28	Missouri	6.9
29	Rhode Island	6.8
30	Iowa	6.7
31	Washington	6.6
32	Nebraska	6.4
33	Arizona	6.3
33	Idaho	6.3
33	Nevada	6.3
33	Oregon	6.3
37	Massachusetts	6.2
37	North Dakota	6.2
39	Kansas	6.0
39	Wisconsin	6.0
41	Connecticut	5.9
42	Vermont	5.8
42	Wyoming	5.8
44	New Mexico	5.7
45	New Hampshire	5.6
46	Minnesota	5.5
46	Montana	5.5
46	Utah	5.5
49	Alaska	5.0
50	Colorado	4.7

	District of Columbia	8.2

Source: U.S. Department of Health and Human Services, Centers for Disease Control and Prevention
"2003 Behavioral Risk Factor Surveillance Summary Prevalence Data" (http://apps.nccd.cdc.gov/brfss/)
*Of population 18 years old and older. Does not include pregnancy-related diabetes.

Percent of Population Reporting Serious Mental Illness: 2002

National Percent = 8.3% of Population*

ALPHA ORDER

RANK	STATE	PERCENT
6	Alabama	10.4
11	Alaska	9.8
35	Arizona	8.1
2	Arkansas	11.0
49	California	7.0
46	Colorado	7.4
45	Connecticut	7.5
27	Delaware	8.7
44	Florida	7.6
20	Georgia	9.1
40	Hawaii	7.9
10	Idaho	10.0
47	Illinois	7.3
25	Indiana	8.8
42	Iowa	7.7
27	Kansas	8.7
4	Kentucky	10.5
30	Louisiana	8.5
16	Maine	9.4
40	Maryland	7.9
35	Massachusetts	8.1
35	Michigan	8.1
30	Minnesota	8.5
22	Mississippi	8.9
13	Missouri	9.6
3	Montana	10.6
38	Nebraska	8.0
27	Nevada	8.7
33	New Hampshire	8.2
50	New Jersey	6.5
38	New Mexico	8.0
25	New York	8.8
16	North Carolina	9.4
18	North Dakota	9.3
14	Ohio	9.5
1	Oklahoma	11.4
11	Oregon	9.8
42	Pennsylvania	7.7
6	Rhode Island	10.4
21	South Carolina	9.0
14	South Dakota	9.5
22	Tennessee	8.9
48	Texas	7.2
4	Utah	10.5
22	Vermont	8.9
33	Virginia	8.2
6	Washington	10.4
6	West Virginia	10.4
30	Wisconsin	8.5
18	Wyoming	9.3

RANK ORDER

RANK	STATE	PERCENT
1	Oklahoma	11.4
2	Arkansas	11.0
3	Montana	10.6
4	Kentucky	10.5
4	Utah	10.5
6	Alabama	10.4
6	Rhode Island	10.4
6	Washington	10.4
6	West Virginia	10.4
10	Idaho	10.0
11	Alaska	9.8
11	Oregon	9.8
13	Missouri	9.6
14	Ohio	9.5
14	South Dakota	9.5
16	Maine	9.4
16	North Carolina	9.4
18	North Dakota	9.3
18	Wyoming	9.3
20	Georgia	9.1
21	South Carolina	9.0
22	Mississippi	8.9
22	Tennessee	8.9
22	Vermont	8.9
25	Indiana	8.8
25	New York	8.8
27	Delaware	8.7
27	Kansas	8.7
27	Nevada	8.7
30	Louisiana	8.5
30	Minnesota	8.5
30	Wisconsin	8.5
33	New Hampshire	8.2
33	Virginia	8.2
35	Arizona	8.1
35	Massachusetts	8.1
35	Michigan	8.1
38	Nebraska	8.0
38	New Mexico	8.0
40	Hawaii	7.9
40	Maryland	7.9
42	Iowa	7.7
42	Pennsylvania	7.7
44	Florida	7.6
45	Connecticut	7.5
46	Colorado	7.4
47	Illinois	7.3
48	Texas	7.2
49	California	7.0
50	New Jersey	6.5
	District of Columbia	9.5

Source: U.S. Department of Health and Human Services, Substance Abuse and Mental Health Services Administration "2002 National Survey on Drug Use and Health" (July 2004)
Population 12 years and older. Serious mental illness is defined as having a diagnosable mental, behavioral or emotional disorder that resulted in functional impairment that substantially interfered with or limited one or more major life activities.

VI. PROVIDERS

VI. PROVIDERS (continued)

Health Care Practitioners and Technicians in 2003

National Total = 6,213,490 Practitioners and Technicians*

ALPHA ORDER

RANK ORDER

RANK	STATE	PRACTITIONERS	% of USA
22	Alabama	101,200	1.6%
49	Alaska	12,010	0.2%
24	Arizona	95,260	1.5%
33	Arkansas	61,380	1.0%
1	California	566,760	9.1%
27	Colorado	85,960	1.4%
26	Connecticut	86,260	1.4%
46	Delaware	18,920	0.3%
4	Florida	370,510	6.0%
12	Georgia	163,150	2.6%
43	Hawaii	22,200	0.4%
42	Idaho	26,740	0.4%
7	Illinois	278,770	4.5%
16	Indiana	144,380	2.3%
30	Iowa	67,730	1.1%
31	Kansas	64,590	1.0%
23	Kentucky	96,410	1.6%
21	Louisiana	107,460	1.7%
39	Maine	32,050	0.5%
19	Maryland	120,380	1.9%
10	Massachusetts	182,360	2.9%
8	Michigan	215,960	3.5%
17	Minnesota	135,000	2.2%
32	Mississippi	62,730	1.0%
14	Missouri	145,490	2.3%
45	Montana	19,800	0.3%
34	Nebraska	46,240	0.7%
37	Nevada	37,790	0.6%
40	New Hampshire	29,370	0.5%
11	New Jersey	180,150	2.9%
38	New Mexico	34,990	0.6%
2	New York	425,410	6.8%
9	North Carolina	182,810	2.9%
47	North Dakota	17,690	0.3%
6	Ohio	284,170	4.6%
28	Oklahoma	74,930	1.2%
29	Oregon	67,990	1.1%
5	Pennsylvania	319,930	5.1%
41	Rhode Island	28,110	0.5%
25	South Carolina	87,510	1.4%
44	South Dakota	21,080	0.3%
15	Tennessee	144,430	2.3%
3	Texas	412,030	6.6%
36	Utah	42,990	0.7%
48	Vermont	15,240	0.2%
13	Virginia	146,890	2.4%
20	Washington	118,990	1.9%
35	West Virginia	45,170	0.7%
18	Wisconsin	129,280	2.1%
50	Wyoming	10,440	0.2%

RANK	STATE	PRACTITIONERS	% of USA
1	California	566,760	9.1%
2	New York	425,410	6.8%
3	Texas	412,030	6.6%
4	Florida	370,510	6.0%
5	Pennsylvania	319,930	5.1%
6	Ohio	284,170	4.6%
7	Illinois	278,770	4.5%
8	Michigan	215,960	3.5%
9	North Carolina	182,810	2.9%
10	Massachusetts	182,360	2.9%
11	New Jersey	180,150	2.9%
12	Georgia	163,150	2.6%
13	Virginia	146,890	2.4%
14	Missouri	145,490	2.3%
15	Tennessee	144,430	2.3%
16	Indiana	144,380	2.3%
17	Minnesota	135,000	2.2%
18	Wisconsin	129,280	2.1%
19	Maryland	120,380	1.9%
20	Washington	118,990	1.9%
21	Louisiana	107,460	1.7%
22	Alabama	101,200	1.6%
23	Kentucky	96,410	1.6%
24	Arizona	95,260	1.5%
25	South Carolina	87,510	1.4%
26	Connecticut	86,260	1.4%
27	Colorado	85,960	1.4%
28	Oklahoma	74,930	1.2%
29	Oregon	67,990	1.1%
30	Iowa	67,730	1.1%
31	Kansas	64,590	1.0%
32	Mississippi	62,730	1.0%
33	Arkansas	61,380	1.0%
34	Nebraska	46,240	0.7%
35	West Virginia	45,170	0.7%
36	Utah	42,990	0.7%
37	Nevada	37,790	0.6%
38	New Mexico	34,990	0.6%
39	Maine	32,050	0.5%
40	New Hampshire	29,370	0.5%
41	Rhode Island	28,110	0.5%
42	Idaho	26,740	0.4%
43	Hawaii	22,200	0.4%
44	South Dakota	21,080	0.3%
45	Montana	19,800	0.3%
46	Delaware	18,920	0.3%
47	North Dakota	17,690	0.3%
48	Vermont	15,240	0.2%
49	Alaska	12,010	0.2%
50	Wyoming	10,440	0.2%
	District of Columbia	26,380	0.4%

Source: U.S. Department of Labor, Bureau of Labor Statistics
"Occupational Employment and Wages, 2003" (http://www.bls.gov/oes/)
*Does not include self-employed. Includes various doctors, dentists, nurses, therapists, optometrists, paramedics and technicians. Does not include assistants and aides listed under health care support occupations. Veterinarians have been subtracted from the totals.

Rate of Health Care Practitioners and Technicians in 2003

National Rate = 2,137 Practitioners and Technicians per 100,000 Population*

ALPHA ORDER

RANK	STATE	RATE
24	Alabama	2,247
45	Alaska	1,853
48	Arizona	1,707
23	Arkansas	2,250
50	California	1,598
41	Colorado	1,890
11	Connecticut	2,474
20	Delaware	2,312
28	Florida	2,180
42	Georgia	1,880
47	Hawaii	1,778
38	Idaho	1,956
26	Illinois	2,204
19	Indiana	2,329
21	Iowa	2,302
16	Kansas	2,370
18	Kentucky	2,341
15	Louisiana	2,391
14	Maine	2,448
27	Maryland	2,184
1	Massachusetts	2,840
32	Michigan	2,142
4	Minnesota	2,666
29	Mississippi	2,176
8	Missouri	2,544
31	Montana	2,156
5	Nebraska	2,661
49	Nevada	1,685
22	New Hampshire	2,279
35	New Jersey	2,084
44	New Mexico	1,863
25	New York	2,214
30	North Carolina	2,171
2	North Dakota	2,793
10	Ohio	2,485
33	Oklahoma	2,137
40	Oregon	1,908
7	Pennsylvania	2,586
6	Rhode Island	2,612
34	South Carolina	2,109
3	South Dakota	2,756
12	Tennessee	2,471
43	Texas	1,864
46	Utah	1,828
13	Vermont	2,461
37	Virginia	1,994
39	Washington	1,941
9	West Virginia	2,494
17	Wisconsin	2,362
36	Wyoming	2,079

RANK ORDER

RANK	STATE	RATE
1	Massachusetts	2,840
2	North Dakota	2,793
3	South Dakota	2,756
4	Minnesota	2,666
5	Nebraska	2,661
6	Rhode Island	2,612
7	Pennsylvania	2,586
8	Missouri	2,544
9	West Virginia	2,494
10	Ohio	2,485
11	Connecticut	2,474
12	Tennessee	2,471
13	Vermont	2,461
14	Maine	2,448
15	Louisiana	2,391
16	Kansas	2,370
17	Wisconsin	2,362
18	Kentucky	2,341
19	Indiana	2,329
20	Delaware	2,312
21	Iowa	2,302
22	New Hampshire	2,279
23	Arkansas	2,250
24	Alabama	2,247
25	New York	2,214
26	Illinois	2,204
27	Maryland	2,184
28	Florida	2,180
29	Mississippi	2,176
30	North Carolina	2,171
31	Montana	2,156
32	Michigan	2,142
33	Oklahoma	2,137
34	South Carolina	2,109
35	New Jersey	2,084
36	Wyoming	2,079
37	Virginia	1,994
38	Idaho	1,956
39	Washington	1,941
40	Oregon	1,908
41	Colorado	1,890
42	Georgia	1,880
43	Texas	1,864
44	New Mexico	1,863
45	Alaska	1,853
46	Utah	1,828
47	Hawaii	1,778
48	Arizona	1,707
49	Nevada	1,685
50	California	1,598

	District of Columbia	4,731

Source: Morgan Quitno Press using data from U.S. Department of Labor, Bureau of Labor Statistics
    "Occupational Employment and Wages, 2003" (http://www.bls.gov/oes/)
*Does not include self-employed. Includes various doctors, dentists, nurses, therapists, optometrists, paramedics
and technicians. Does not include assistants and aides listed under health care support occupations.
Veterinarians have been subtracted from the totals.

Average Annual Wages of Health Care Practitioners and Technicians in 2003

National Average = $56,240*

RANK	STATE	WAGES
47	Alabama	$47,240
7	Alaska	62,370
18	Arizona	57,640
48	Arkansas	45,440
2	California	65,650
17	Colorado	59,090
6	Connecticut	62,680
8	Delaware	61,900
26	Florida	54,480
32	Georgia	52,390
16	Hawaii	59,250
38	Idaho	49,440
34	Illinois	50,830
33	Indiana	51,210
41	Iowa	48,740
45	Kansas	47,640
39	Kentucky	49,100
40	Louisiana	49,030
25	Maine	54,610
4	Maryland	64,480
9	Massachusetts	61,160
15	Michigan	59,260
21	Minnesota	56,910
50	Mississippi	44,390
37	Missouri	49,730
49	Montana	45,020
35	Nebraska	50,230
1	Nevada	66,820
12	New Hampshire	59,790
3	New Jersey	64,550
22	New Mexico	55,990
5	New York	63,050
30	North Carolina	52,730
44	North Dakota	47,980
20	Ohio	57,220
36	Oklahoma	49,960
13	Oregon	59,670
31	Pennsylvania	52,670
10	Rhode Island	60,540
29	South Carolina	52,980
45	South Dakota	47,640
43	Tennessee	48,380
24	Texas	54,840
14	Utah	59,330
19	Vermont	57,360
27	Virginia	54,190
11	Washington	60,400
42	West Virginia	48,580
23	Wisconsin	54,970
28	Wyoming	53,590

RANK	STATE	WAGES
1	Nevada	$66,820
2	California	65,650
3	New Jersey	64,550
4	Maryland	64,480
5	New York	63,050
6	Connecticut	62,680
7	Alaska	62,370
8	Delaware	61,900
9	Massachusetts	61,160
10	Rhode Island	60,540
11	Washington	60,400
12	New Hampshire	59,790
13	Oregon	59,670
14	Utah	59,330
15	Michigan	59,260
16	Hawaii	59,250
17	Colorado	59,090
18	Arizona	57,640
19	Vermont	57,360
20	Ohio	57,220
21	Minnesota	56,910
22	New Mexico	55,990
23	Wisconsin	54,970
24	Texas	54,840
25	Maine	54,610
26	Florida	54,480
27	Virginia	54,190
28	Wyoming	53,590
29	South Carolina	52,980
30	North Carolina	52,730
31	Pennsylvania	52,670
32	Georgia	52,390
33	Indiana	51,210
34	Illinois	50,830
35	Nebraska	50,230
36	Oklahoma	49,960
37	Missouri	49,730
38	Idaho	49,440
39	Kentucky	49,100
40	Louisiana	49,030
41	Iowa	48,740
42	West Virginia	48,580
43	Tennessee	48,380
44	North Dakota	47,980
45	Kansas	47,640
45	South Dakota	47,640
47	Alabama	47,240
48	Arkansas	45,440
49	Montana	45,020
50	Mississippi	44,390
	District of Columbia	62,340

Source: U.S. Department of Labor, Bureau of Labor Statistics
   "Occupational Employment and Wages, 2003" (http://www.bls.gov/oes/)
*Does not include self-employed. Includes various doctors, dentists, nurses, therapists, optometrists, paramedics and technicians. Does not include assistants and aides listed under health care support occupations.

Physicians in 2003

National Total = 858,510 Physicians*

ALPHA ORDER

RANK	STATE	PHYSICIANS	% of USA
27	Alabama	10,434	1.2%
49	Alaska	1,545	0.2%
22	Arizona	13,641	1.6%
32	Arkansas	6,121	0.7%
1	California	104,261	12.1%
23	Colorado	13,051	1.5%
21	Connecticut	13,834	1.6%
46	Delaware	2,284	0.3%
4	Florida	50,000	5.8%
14	Georgia	21,075	2.5%
39	Hawaii	4,358	0.5%
43	Idaho	2,642	0.3%
6	Illinois	37,608	4.4%
20	Indiana	14,716	1.7%
31	Iowa	6,318	0.7%
30	Kansas	6,743	0.8%
28	Kentucky	10,215	1.2%
24	Louisiana	12,878	1.5%
41	Maine	3,995	0.5%
11	Maryland	24,806	2.9%
8	Massachusetts	30,603	3.6%
10	Michigan	26,459	3.1%
17	Minnesota	15,591	1.8%
33	Mississippi	5,820	0.7%
19	Missouri	14,779	1.7%
45	Montana	2,425	0.3%
37	Nebraska	4,643	0.5%
36	Nevada	4,691	0.5%
42	New Hampshire	3,846	0.4%
9	New Jersey	29,053	3.4%
35	New Mexico	5,031	0.6%
2	New York	81,199	9.5%
12	North Carolina	23,530	2.7%
48	North Dakota	1,691	0.2%
7	Ohio	32,150	3.7%
29	Oklahoma	6,792	0.8%
25	Oregon	10,741	1.3%
5	Pennsylvania	40,542	4.7%
40	Rhode Island	4,091	0.5%
26	South Carolina	10,510	1.2%
47	South Dakota	1,831	0.2%
16	Tennessee	16,547	1.9%
3	Texas	50,840	5.9%
34	Utah	5,514	0.6%
44	Vermont	2,578	0.3%
13	Virginia	22,373	2.6%
15	Washington	18,580	2.2%
38	West Virginia	4,587	0.5%
18	Wisconsin	15,246	1.8%
50	Wyoming	1,095	0.1%

RANK ORDER

RANK	STATE	PHYSICIANS	% of USA
1	California	104,261	12.1%
2	New York	81,199	9.5%
3	Texas	50,840	5.9%
4	Florida	50,000	5.8%
5	Pennsylvania	40,542	4.7%
6	Illinois	37,608	4.4%
7	Ohio	32,150	3.7%
8	Massachusetts	30,603	3.6%
9	New Jersey	29,053	3.4%
10	Michigan	26,459	3.1%
11	Maryland	24,806	2.9%
12	North Carolina	23,530	2.7%
13	Virginia	22,373	2.6%
14	Georgia	21,075	2.5%
15	Washington	18,580	2.2%
16	Tennessee	16,547	1.9%
17	Minnesota	15,591	1.8%
18	Wisconsin	15,246	1.8%
19	Missouri	14,779	1.7%
20	Indiana	14,716	1.7%
21	Connecticut	13,834	1.6%
22	Arizona	13,641	1.6%
23	Colorado	13,051	1.5%
24	Louisiana	12,878	1.5%
25	Oregon	10,741	1.3%
26	South Carolina	10,510	1.2%
27	Alabama	10,434	1.2%
28	Kentucky	10,215	1.2%
29	Oklahoma	6,792	0.8%
30	Kansas	6,743	0.8%
31	Iowa	6,318	0.7%
32	Arkansas	6,121	0.7%
33	Mississippi	5,820	0.7%
34	Utah	5,514	0.6%
35	New Mexico	5,031	0.6%
36	Nevada	4,691	0.5%
37	Nebraska	4,643	0.5%
38	West Virginia	4,587	0.5%
39	Hawaii	4,358	0.5%
40	Rhode Island	4,091	0.5%
41	Maine	3,995	0.5%
42	New Hampshire	3,846	0.4%
43	Idaho	2,642	0.3%
44	Vermont	2,578	0.3%
45	Montana	2,425	0.3%
46	Delaware	2,284	0.3%
47	South Dakota	1,831	0.2%
48	North Dakota	1,691	0.2%
49	Alaska	1,545	0.2%
50	Wyoming	1,095	0.1%
	District of Columbia	4,607	0.5%

Source: American Medical Association (Chicago, Illinois)
   "Physician Characteristics and Distribution in the U.S." (2005 Edition)
*As of December 31, 2003. Total does not include 13,025 physicians in the U.S. territories and possessions, at APO's and FPO's and whose addresses are unknown.

Rate of Physicians in 2003

National Rate = 295 Physicians per 100,000 Population*

ALPHA ORDER

RANK	STATE	RATE
42	Alabama	232
39	Alaska	238
36	Arizona	244
44	Arkansas	224
17	California	294
19	Colorado	287
5	Connecticut	397
23	Delaware	279
17	Florida	294
37	Georgia	243
7	Hawaii	349
50	Idaho	193
16	Illinois	297
40	Indiana	237
46	Iowa	215
35	Kansas	247
34	Kentucky	248
19	Louisiana	287
11	Maine	305
2	Maryland	450
1	Massachusetts	477
30	Michigan	262
10	Minnesota	308
48	Mississippi	202
31	Missouri	258
29	Montana	264
27	Nebraska	267
47	Nevada	209
15	New Hampshire	298
8	New Jersey	336
26	New Mexico	268
3	New York	423
23	North Carolina	279
27	North Dakota	267
22	Ohio	281
49	Oklahoma	194
14	Oregon	301
9	Pennsylvania	328
6	Rhode Island	380
32	South Carolina	253
38	South Dakota	239
21	Tennessee	283
43	Texas	230
41	Utah	234
4	Vermont	416
12	Virginia	304
13	Washington	303
32	West Virginia	253
23	Wisconsin	279
45	Wyoming	218

RANK ORDER

RANK	STATE	RATE
1	Massachusetts	477
2	Maryland	450
3	New York	423
4	Vermont	416
5	Connecticut	397
6	Rhode Island	380
7	Hawaii	349
8	New Jersey	336
9	Pennsylvania	328
10	Minnesota	308
11	Maine	305
12	Virginia	304
13	Washington	303
14	Oregon	301
15	New Hampshire	298
16	Illinois	297
17	California	294
17	Florida	294
19	Colorado	287
19	Louisiana	287
21	Tennessee	283
22	Ohio	281
23	Delaware	279
23	North Carolina	279
23	Wisconsin	279
26	New Mexico	268
27	Nebraska	267
27	North Dakota	267
29	Montana	264
30	Michigan	262
31	Missouri	258
32	South Carolina	253
32	West Virginia	253
34	Kentucky	248
35	Kansas	247
36	Arizona	244
37	Georgia	243
38	South Dakota	239
39	Alaska	238
40	Indiana	237
41	Utah	234
42	Alabama	232
43	Texas	230
44	Arkansas	224
45	Wyoming	218
46	Iowa	215
47	Nevada	209
48	Mississippi	202
49	Oklahoma	194
50	Idaho	193
	District of Columbia	826

Source: Morgan Quitno Press using data from American Medical Association (Chicago, Illinois)
"Physician Characteristics and Distribution in the U.S." (2005 Edition)
As of December 31, 2003. National rate does not include physicians in the U.S. territories and possessions, at APO's and FPO's and whose addresses are unknown.

Female Physicians in 2003

National Total = 221,314 Physicians*

ALPHA ORDER

RANK	STATE	PHYSICIANS	% of USA
28	Alabama	2,122	1.0%
47	Alaska	430	0.2%
23	Arizona	3,158	1.4%
34	Arkansas	1,201	0.5%
1	California	27,069	12.2%
20	Colorado	3,508	1.6%
18	Connecticut	3,751	1.7%
44	Delaware	633	0.3%
6	Florida	9,861	4.5%
14	Georgia	5,136	2.3%
36	Hawaii	1,080	0.5%
46	Idaho	431	0.2%
4	Illinois	11,179	5.1%
22	Indiana	3,361	1.5%
32	Iowa	1,336	0.6%
29	Kansas	1,577	0.7%
26	Kentucky	2,339	1.1%
24	Louisiana	2,962	1.3%
39	Maine	996	0.5%
10	Maryland	7,480	3.4%
7	Massachusetts	9,675	4.4%
11	Michigan	7,156	3.2%
16	Minnesota	4,121	1.9%
35	Mississippi	1,103	0.5%
19	Missouri	3,709	1.7%
45	Montana	457	0.2%
37	Nebraska	1,053	0.5%
41	Nevada	954	0.4%
42	New Hampshire	945	0.4%
8	New Jersey	8,571	3.9%
30	New Mexico	1,460	0.7%
2	New York	24,375	11.0%
13	North Carolina	5,817	2.6%
49	North Dakota	333	0.2%
9	Ohio	8,345	3.8%
31	Oklahoma	1,385	0.6%
25	Oregon	2,757	1.2%
5	Pennsylvania	10,731	4.8%
33	Rhode Island	1,215	0.5%
27	South Carolina	2,196	1.0%
48	South Dakota	347	0.2%
21	Tennessee	3,468	1.6%
3	Texas	12,461	5.6%
38	Utah	1,032	0.5%
43	Vermont	727	0.3%
12	Virginia	6,014	2.7%
15	Washington	4,868	2.2%
40	West Virginia	970	0.4%
17	Wisconsin	3,754	1.7%
50	Wyoming	202	0.1%

RANK ORDER

RANK	STATE	PHYSICIANS	% of USA
1	California	27,069	12.2%
2	New York	24,375	11.0%
3	Texas	12,461	5.6%
4	Illinois	11,179	5.1%
5	Pennsylvania	10,731	4.8%
6	Florida	9,861	4.5%
7	Massachusetts	9,675	4.4%
8	New Jersey	8,571	3.9%
9	Ohio	8,345	3.8%
10	Maryland	7,480	3.4%
11	Michigan	7,156	3.2%
12	Virginia	6,014	2.7%
13	North Carolina	5,817	2.6%
14	Georgia	5,136	2.3%
15	Washington	4,868	2.2%
16	Minnesota	4,121	1.9%
17	Wisconsin	3,754	1.7%
18	Connecticut	3,751	1.7%
19	Missouri	3,709	1.7%
20	Colorado	3,508	1.6%
21	Tennessee	3,468	1.6%
22	Indiana	3,361	1.5%
23	Arizona	3,158	1.4%
24	Louisiana	2,962	1.3%
25	Oregon	2,757	1.2%
26	Kentucky	2,339	1.1%
27	South Carolina	2,196	1.0%
28	Alabama	2,122	1.0%
29	Kansas	1,577	0.7%
30	New Mexico	1,460	0.7%
31	Oklahoma	1,385	0.6%
32	Iowa	1,336	0.6%
33	Rhode Island	1,215	0.5%
34	Arkansas	1,201	0.5%
35	Mississippi	1,103	0.5%
36	Hawaii	1,080	0.5%
37	Nebraska	1,053	0.5%
38	Utah	1,032	0.5%
39	Maine	996	0.5%
40	West Virginia	970	0.4%
41	Nevada	954	0.4%
42	New Hampshire	945	0.4%
43	Vermont	727	0.3%
44	Delaware	633	0.3%
45	Montana	457	0.2%
46	Idaho	431	0.2%
47	Alaska	430	0.2%
48	South Dakota	347	0.2%
49	North Dakota	333	0.2%
50	Wyoming	202	0.1%
	District of Columbia	1,503	0.7%

Source: American Medical Association (Chicago, Illinois)
    "Physician Characteristics and Distribution in the U.S." (2005 Edition)
*As of December 31, 2003. Total does not include 3,728 female physicians in the U.S. territories and possessions, at APO's and FPO's and whose addresses are unknown.

Percent of Physicians Who Are Female: 2003

National Percent = 25.8% of Physicians*

ALPHA ORDER

RANK ORDER

RANK	STATE	PERCENT	RANK	STATE	PERCENT
40	Alabama	20.3	1	Massachusetts	31.6
9	Alaska	27.8	2	Maryland	30.2
30	Arizona	23.2	3	New York	30.0
44	Arkansas	19.6	4	Illinois	29.7
18	California	26.0	4	Rhode Island	29.7
13	Colorado	26.9	6	New Jersey	29.5
11	Connecticut	27.1	7	New Mexico	29.0
10	Delaware	27.7	8	Vermont	28.2
42	Florida	19.7	9	Alaska	27.8
28	Georgia	24.4	10	Delaware	27.7
23	Hawaii	24.8	11	Connecticut	27.1
50	Idaho	16.3	12	Michigan	27.0
4	Illinois	29.7	13	Colorado	26.9
33	Indiana	22.8	13	Virginia	26.9
35	Iowa	21.1	15	Pennsylvania	26.5
29	Kansas	23.4	16	Minnesota	26.4
32	Kentucky	22.9	17	Washington	26.2
31	Louisiana	23.0	18	California	26.0
22	Maine	24.9	18	Ohio	26.0
2	Maryland	30.2	20	Oregon	25.7
1	Massachusetts	31.6	21	Missouri	25.1
12	Michigan	27.0	22	Maine	24.9
16	Minnesota	26.4	23	Hawaii	24.8
45	Mississippi	19.0	24	North Carolina	24.7
21	Missouri	25.1	25	New Hampshire	24.6
47	Montana	18.8	25	Wisconsin	24.6
34	Nebraska	22.7	27	Texas	24.5
40	Nevada	20.3	28	Georgia	24.4
25	New Hampshire	24.6	29	Kansas	23.4
6	New Jersey	29.5	30	Arizona	23.2
7	New Mexico	29.0	31	Louisiana	23.0
3	New York	30.0	32	Kentucky	22.9
24	North Carolina	24.7	33	Indiana	22.8
42	North Dakota	19.7	34	Nebraska	22.7
18	Ohio	26.0	35	Iowa	21.1
39	Oklahoma	20.4	35	West Virginia	21.1
20	Oregon	25.7	37	Tennessee	21.0
15	Pennsylvania	26.5	38	South Carolina	20.9
4	Rhode Island	29.7	39	Oklahoma	20.4
38	South Carolina	20.9	40	Alabama	20.3
45	South Dakota	19.0	40	Nevada	20.3
37	Tennessee	21.0	42	Florida	19.7
27	Texas	24.5	42	North Dakota	19.7
48	Utah	18.7	44	Arkansas	19.6
8	Vermont	28.2	45	Mississippi	19.0
13	Virginia	26.9	45	South Dakota	19.0
17	Washington	26.2	47	Montana	18.8
35	West Virginia	21.1	48	Utah	18.7
25	Wisconsin	24.6	49	Wyoming	18.4
49	Wyoming	18.4	50	Idaho	16.3

District of Columbia   32.6

Source: Morgan Quitno Press using data from American Medical Association (Chicago, Illinois)
"Physician Characteristics and Distribution in the U.S." (2005 Edition)
As of December 31, 2003. National percent does not include physicians in the U.S. territories and possessions, at APO's and FPO's and whose addresses are unknown.

Physicians Under 35 Years Old in 2003

National Total = 137,979 Physicians*

ALPHA ORDER

RANK	STATE	PHYSICIANS	% of USA
26	Alabama	1,620	1.2%
48	Alaska	142	0.1%
25	Arizona	1,649	1.2%
31	Arkansas	979	0.7%
2	California	14,284	10.4%
23	Colorado	1,811	1.3%
22	Connecticut	2,226	1.6%
44	Delaware	353	0.3%
9	Florida	4,888	3.5%
14	Georgia	3,122	2.3%
39	Hawaii	569	0.4%
47	Idaho	175	0.1%
4	Illinois	7,940	5.8%
21	Indiana	2,239	1.6%
29	Iowa	1,082	0.8%
30	Kansas	1,045	0.8%
27	Kentucky	1,608	1.2%
18	Louisiana	2,503	1.8%
42	Maine	387	0.3%
12	Maryland	4,030	2.9%
7	Massachusetts	6,011	4.4%
8	Michigan	5,154	3.7%
16	Minnesota	2,694	2.0%
35	Mississippi	819	0.6%
15	Missouri	2,841	2.1%
48	Montana	142	0.1%
33	Nebraska	880	0.6%
40	Nevada	470	0.3%
41	New Hampshire	455	0.3%
10	New Jersey	4,099	3.0%
38	New Mexico	699	0.5%
1	New York	15,967	11.6%
11	North Carolina	4,086	3.0%
45	North Dakota	215	0.2%
6	Ohio	6,145	4.5%
32	Oklahoma	933	0.7%
28	Oregon	1,266	0.9%
5	Pennsylvania	6,996	5.1%
36	Rhode Island	814	0.6%
24	South Carolina	1,719	1.2%
46	South Dakota	184	0.1%
17	Tennessee	2,599	1.9%
3	Texas	8,732	6.3%
34	Utah	857	0.6%
43	Vermont	373	0.3%
13	Virginia	3,750	2.7%
20	Washington	2,259	1.6%
37	West Virginia	760	0.6%
19	Wisconsin	2,307	1.7%
50	Wyoming	84	0.1%

RANK ORDER

RANK	STATE	PHYSICIANS	% of USA
1	New York	15,967	11.6%
2	California	14,284	10.4%
3	Texas	8,732	6.3%
4	Illinois	7,940	5.8%
5	Pennsylvania	6,996	5.1%
6	Ohio	6,145	4.5%
7	Massachusetts	6,011	4.4%
8	Michigan	5,154	3.7%
9	Florida	4,888	3.5%
10	New Jersey	4,099	3.0%
11	North Carolina	4,086	3.0%
12	Maryland	4,030	2.9%
13	Virginia	3,750	2.7%
14	Georgia	3,122	2.3%
15	Missouri	2,841	2.1%
16	Minnesota	2,694	2.0%
17	Tennessee	2,599	1.9%
18	Louisiana	2,503	1.8%
19	Wisconsin	2,307	1.7%
20	Washington	2,259	1.6%
21	Indiana	2,239	1.6%
22	Connecticut	2,226	1.6%
23	Colorado	1,811	1.3%
24	South Carolina	1,719	1.2%
25	Arizona	1,649	1.2%
26	Alabama	1,620	1.2%
27	Kentucky	1,608	1.2%
28	Oregon	1,266	0.9%
29	Iowa	1,082	0.8%
30	Kansas	1,045	0.8%
31	Arkansas	979	0.7%
32	Oklahoma	933	0.7%
33	Nebraska	880	0.6%
34	Utah	857	0.6%
35	Mississippi	819	0.6%
36	Rhode Island	814	0.6%
37	West Virginia	760	0.6%
38	New Mexico	699	0.5%
39	Hawaii	569	0.4%
40	Nevada	470	0.3%
41	New Hampshire	455	0.3%
42	Maine	387	0.3%
43	Vermont	373	0.3%
44	Delaware	353	0.3%
45	North Dakota	215	0.2%
46	South Dakota	184	0.1%
47	Idaho	175	0.1%
48	Alaska	142	0.1%
48	Montana	142	0.1%
50	Wyoming	84	0.1%
	District of Columbia	1,017	0.7%

Source: American Medical Association (Chicago, Illinois)
   "Physician Characteristics and Distribution in the U.S." (2005 Edition)
*As of December 31, 2003. Total does not include 1,888 physicians in the U.S. territories and possessions, at APO's and FPO's and whose addresses are unknown.

Percent of Physicians Under 35 Years Old in 2003

National Percent = 16.1% of Physicians*

ALPHA ORDER				RANK ORDER		
RANK	STATE	PERCENT		RANK	STATE	PERCENT
23	Alabama	15.5		1	Illinois	21.1
47	Alaska	9.2		2	Rhode Island	19.9
40	Arizona	12.1		3	New York	19.7
20	Arkansas	16.0		4	Massachusetts	19.6
35	California	13.7		5	Michigan	19.5
33	Colorado	13.9		6	Louisiana	19.4
19	Connecticut	16.1		7	Missouri	19.2
23	Delaware	15.5		8	Ohio	19.1
45	Florida	9.8		9	Nebraska	19.0
29	Georgia	14.8		10	North Carolina	17.4
37	Hawaii	13.1		11	Minnesota	17.3
49	Idaho	6.6		11	Pennsylvania	17.3
1	Illinois	21.1		13	Texas	17.2
27	Indiana	15.2		14	Iowa	17.1
14	Iowa	17.1		15	Virginia	16.8
23	Kansas	15.5		16	West Virginia	16.6
21	Kentucky	15.7		17	South Carolina	16.4
6	Louisiana	19.4		18	Maryland	16.2
46	Maine	9.7		19	Connecticut	16.1
18	Maryland	16.2		20	Arkansas	16.0
4	Massachusetts	19.6		21	Kentucky	15.7
5	Michigan	19.5		21	Tennessee	15.7
11	Minnesota	17.3		23	Alabama	15.5
31	Mississippi	14.1		23	Delaware	15.5
7	Missouri	19.2		23	Kansas	15.5
50	Montana	5.9		23	Utah	15.5
9	Nebraska	19.0		27	Indiana	15.2
43	Nevada	10.0		28	Wisconsin	15.1
41	New Hampshire	11.8		29	Georgia	14.8
31	New Jersey	14.1		30	Vermont	14.5
33	New Mexico	13.9		31	Mississippi	14.1
3	New York	19.7		31	New Jersey	14.1
10	North Carolina	17.4		33	Colorado	13.9
38	North Dakota	12.7		33	New Mexico	13.9
8	Ohio	19.1		35	California	13.7
35	Oklahoma	13.7		35	Oklahoma	13.7
41	Oregon	11.8		37	Hawaii	13.1
11	Pennsylvania	17.3		38	North Dakota	12.7
2	Rhode Island	19.9		39	Washington	12.2
17	South Carolina	16.4		40	Arizona	12.1
43	South Dakota	10.0		41	New Hampshire	11.8
21	Tennessee	15.7		41	Oregon	11.8
13	Texas	17.2		43	Nevada	10.0
23	Utah	15.5		43	South Dakota	10.0
30	Vermont	14.5		45	Florida	9.8
15	Virginia	16.8		46	Maine	9.7
39	Washington	12.2		47	Alaska	9.2
16	West Virginia	16.6		48	Wyoming	7.7
28	Wisconsin	15.1		49	Idaho	6.6
48	Wyoming	7.7		50	Montana	5.9

	District of Columbia	22.1

Source: Morgan Quitno Press using data from American Medical Association (Chicago, Illinois)
    "Physician Characteristics and Distribution in the U.S." (2005 Edition)
As of December 31, 2003. National percent does not include physicians in the U.S. territories and possessions, at APO's and FPO's and whose addresses are unknown.

Physicians 65 Years Old and Older in 2003

National Total = 159,320 Physicians*

RANK	STATE	PHYSICIANS	% of USA	RANK	STATE	PHYSICIANS	% of USA
27	Alabama	1,653	1.0%	1	California	23,215	14.6%
50	Alaska	200	0.1%	2	New York	15,221	9.6%
16	Arizona	3,061	1.9%	3	Florida	13,067	8.2%
33	Arkansas	1,050	0.7%	4	Texas	8,196	5.1%
1	California	23,215	14.6%	5	Pennsylvania	7,546	4.7%
22	Colorado	2,296	1.4%	6	Illinois	5,793	3.6%
17	Connecticut	2,644	1.7%	7	Ohio	5,482	3.4%
46	Delaware	432	0.3%	8	New Jersey	5,246	3.3%
3	Florida	13,067	8.2%	9	Massachusetts	5,001	3.1%
15	Georgia	3,342	2.1%	10	Michigan	4,511	2.8%
37	Hawaii	856	0.5%	11	Maryland	4,419	2.8%
43	Idaho	550	0.3%	12	Virginia	4,085	2.6%
6	Illinois	5,793	3.6%	13	North Carolina	3,813	2.4%
20	Indiana	2,512	1.6%	14	Washington	3,514	2.2%
31	Iowa	1,101	0.7%	15	Georgia	3,342	2.1%
30	Kansas	1,290	0.8%	16	Arizona	3,061	1.9%
28	Kentucky	1,603	1.0%	17	Connecticut	2,644	1.7%
24	Louisiana	2,136	1.3%	18	Tennessee	2,617	1.6%
38	Maine	849	0.5%	19	Wisconsin	2,523	1.6%
11	Maryland	4,419	2.8%	20	Indiana	2,512	1.6%
9	Massachusetts	5,001	3.1%	21	Minnesota	2,466	1.5%
10	Michigan	4,511	2.8%	22	Colorado	2,296	1.4%
21	Minnesota	2,466	1.5%	23	Missouri	2,232	1.4%
32	Mississippi	1,096	0.7%	24	Louisiana	2,136	1.3%
23	Missouri	2,232	1.4%	25	Oregon	2,079	1.3%
44	Montana	526	0.3%	26	South Carolina	1,783	1.1%
42	Nebraska	744	0.5%	27	Alabama	1,653	1.0%
34	Nevada	982	0.6%	28	Kentucky	1,603	1.0%
40	New Hampshire	780	0.5%	29	Oklahoma	1,324	0.8%
8	New Jersey	5,246	3.3%	30	Kansas	1,290	0.8%
35	New Mexico	872	0.5%	31	Iowa	1,101	0.7%
2	New York	15,221	9.6%	32	Mississippi	1,096	0.7%
13	North Carolina	3,813	2.4%	33	Arkansas	1,050	0.7%
48	North Dakota	274	0.2%	34	Nevada	982	0.6%
7	Ohio	5,482	3.4%	35	New Mexico	872	0.5%
29	Oklahoma	1,324	0.8%	35	Utah	872	0.5%
25	Oregon	2,079	1.3%	37	Hawaii	856	0.5%
5	Pennsylvania	7,546	4.7%	38	Maine	849	0.5%
41	Rhode Island	751	0.5%	39	West Virginia	807	0.5%
26	South Carolina	1,783	1.1%	40	New Hampshire	780	0.5%
47	South Dakota	299	0.2%	41	Rhode Island	751	0.5%
18	Tennessee	2,617	1.6%	42	Nebraska	744	0.5%
4	Texas	8,196	5.1%	43	Idaho	550	0.3%
35	Utah	872	0.5%	44	Montana	526	0.3%
45	Vermont	517	0.3%	45	Vermont	517	0.3%
12	Virginia	4,085	2.6%	46	Delaware	432	0.3%
14	Washington	3,514	2.2%	47	South Dakota	299	0.2%
39	West Virginia	807	0.5%	48	North Dakota	274	0.2%
19	Wisconsin	2,523	1.6%	49	Wyoming	218	0.1%
49	Wyoming	218	0.1%	50	Alaska	200	0.1%
					District of Columbia	874	0.5%

Source: American Medical Association (Chicago, Illinois)
"Physician Characteristics and Distribution in the U.S." (2005 Edition)
*As of December 31, 2003. Total does not include 2,853 physicians in the U.S. territories and possessions, at APO's and FPO's and whose addresses are unknown.

Percent of Physicians 65 Years Old and Older in 2003

National Percent = 18.6% of Physicians*

RANK	STATE	PERCENT
43	Alabama	15.8
50	Alaska	12.9
2	Arizona	22.4
29	Arkansas	17.2
3	California	22.3
25	Colorado	17.6
14	Connecticut	19.1
16	Delaware	18.9
1	Florida	26.1
42	Georgia	15.9
11	Hawaii	19.6
7	Idaho	20.8
48	Illinois	15.4
30	Indiana	17.1
27	Iowa	17.4
14	Kansas	19.1
47	Kentucky	15.7
34	Louisiana	16.6
5	Maine	21.3
24	Maryland	17.8
36	Massachusetts	16.3
32	Michigan	17.0
43	Minnesota	15.8
18	Mississippi	18.8
49	Missouri	15.1
4	Montana	21.7
41	Nebraska	16.0
6	Nevada	20.9
8	New Hampshire	20.3
23	New Jersey	18.1
28	New Mexico	17.3
19	New York	18.7
38	North Carolina	16.2
38	North Dakota	16.2
30	Ohio	17.1
12	Oklahoma	19.5
13	Oregon	19.4
20	Pennsylvania	18.6
21	Rhode Island	18.4
32	South Carolina	17.0
36	South Dakota	16.3
43	Tennessee	15.8
40	Texas	16.1
43	Utah	15.8
9	Vermont	20.1
22	Virginia	18.3
16	Washington	18.9
25	West Virginia	17.6
35	Wisconsin	16.5
10	Wyoming	19.9

RANK	STATE	PERCENT
1	Florida	26.1
2	Arizona	22.4
3	California	22.3
4	Montana	21.7
5	Maine	21.3
6	Nevada	20.9
7	Idaho	20.8
8	New Hampshire	20.3
9	Vermont	20.1
10	Wyoming	19.9
11	Hawaii	19.6
12	Oklahoma	19.5
13	Oregon	19.4
14	Connecticut	19.1
14	Kansas	19.1
16	Delaware	18.9
16	Washington	18.9
18	Mississippi	18.8
19	New York	18.7
20	Pennsylvania	18.6
21	Rhode Island	18.4
22	Virginia	18.3
23	New Jersey	18.1
24	Maryland	17.8
25	Colorado	17.6
25	West Virginia	17.6
27	Iowa	17.4
28	New Mexico	17.3
29	Arkansas	17.2
30	Indiana	17.1
30	Ohio	17.1
32	Michigan	17.0
32	South Carolina	17.0
34	Louisiana	16.6
35	Wisconsin	16.5
36	Massachusetts	16.3
36	South Dakota	16.3
38	North Carolina	16.2
38	North Dakota	16.2
40	Texas	16.1
41	Nebraska	16.0
42	Georgia	15.9
43	Alabama	15.8
43	Minnesota	15.8
43	Tennessee	15.8
43	Utah	15.8
47	Kentucky	15.7
48	Illinois	15.4
49	Missouri	15.1
50	Alaska	12.9

	District of Columbia	19.0

Source: Morgan Quitno Press using data from American Medical Association (Chicago, Illinois)
 "Physician Characteristics and Distribution in the U.S." (2005 Edition)
*As of December 31, 2003. National percent does not include physicians in the U.S. territories and possessions, at APO's and FPO's and whose addresses are unknown.

Physicians in Patient Care in 2003

National Total = 682,581 Physicians*

ALPHA ORDER

RANK	STATE	PHYSICIANS	% of USA
26	Alabama	8,677	1.3%
49	Alaska	1,327	0.2%
23	Arizona	10,567	1.5%
31	Arkansas	5,077	0.7%
1	California	81,013	11.9%
24	Colorado	10,401	1.5%
21	Connecticut	10,875	1.6%
46	Delaware	1,847	0.3%
4	Florida	38,121	5.6%
14	Georgia	17,187	2.5%
39	Hawaii	3,538	0.5%
43	Idaho	2,198	0.3%
6	Illinois	30,264	4.4%
19	Indiana	12,195	1.8%
32	Iowa	4,887	0.7%
30	Kansas	5,407	0.8%
27	Kentucky	8,471	1.2%
22	Louisiana	10,643	1.6%
41	Maine	3,148	0.5%
12	Maryland	18,545	2.7%
9	Massachusetts	23,459	3.4%
10	Michigan	21,089	3.1%
17	Minnesota	12,568	1.8%
33	Mississippi	4,819	0.7%
20	Missouri	12,151	1.8%
45	Montana	1,964	0.3%
37	Nebraska	3,809	0.6%
36	Nevada	3,852	0.6%
42	New Hampshire	3,090	0.5%
8	New Jersey	23,587	3.5%
35	New Mexico	3,962	0.6%
2	New York	63,604	9.3%
11	North Carolina	18,999	2.8%
48	North Dakota	1,381	0.2%
7	Ohio	25,857	3.8%
29	Oklahoma	5,455	0.8%
28	Oregon	8,379	1.2%
5	Pennsylvania	31,788	4.7%
40	Rhode Island	3,301	0.5%
25	South Carolina	8,693	1.3%
47	South Dakota	1,522	0.2%
16	Tennessee	13,610	2.0%
3	Texas	41,750	6.1%
34	Utah	4,480	0.7%
44	Vermont	1,984	0.3%
13	Virginia	18,002	2.6%
15	Washington	14,537	2.1%
38	West Virginia	3,704	0.5%
18	Wisconsin	12,496	1.8%
50	Wyoming	906	0.1%

RANK ORDER

RANK	STATE	PHYSICIANS	% of USA
1	California	81,013	11.9%
2	New York	63,604	9.3%
3	Texas	41,750	6.1%
4	Florida	38,121	5.6%
5	Pennsylvania	31,788	4.7%
6	Illinois	30,264	4.4%
7	Ohio	25,857	3.8%
8	New Jersey	23,587	3.5%
9	Massachusetts	23,459	3.4%
10	Michigan	21,089	3.1%
11	North Carolina	18,999	2.8%
12	Maryland	18,545	2.7%
13	Virginia	18,002	2.6%
14	Georgia	17,187	2.5%
15	Washington	14,537	2.1%
16	Tennessee	13,610	2.0%
17	Minnesota	12,568	1.8%
18	Wisconsin	12,496	1.8%
19	Indiana	12,195	1.8%
20	Missouri	12,151	1.8%
21	Connecticut	10,875	1.6%
22	Louisiana	10,643	1.6%
23	Arizona	10,567	1.5%
24	Colorado	10,401	1.5%
25	South Carolina	8,693	1.3%
26	Alabama	8,677	1.3%
27	Kentucky	8,471	1.2%
28	Oregon	8,379	1.2%
29	Oklahoma	5,455	0.8%
30	Kansas	5,407	0.8%
31	Arkansas	5,077	0.7%
32	Iowa	4,887	0.7%
33	Mississippi	4,819	0.7%
34	Utah	4,480	0.7%
35	New Mexico	3,962	0.6%
36	Nevada	3,852	0.6%
37	Nebraska	3,809	0.6%
38	West Virginia	3,704	0.5%
39	Hawaii	3,538	0.5%
40	Rhode Island	3,301	0.5%
41	Maine	3,148	0.5%
42	New Hampshire	3,090	0.5%
43	Idaho	2,198	0.3%
44	Vermont	1,984	0.3%
45	Montana	1,964	0.3%
46	Delaware	1,847	0.3%
47	South Dakota	1,522	0.2%
48	North Dakota	1,381	0.2%
49	Alaska	1,327	0.2%
50	Wyoming	906	0.1%
	District of Columbia	3,395	0.5%

Source: American Medical Association (Chicago, Illinois)
    "Physician Characteristics and Distribution in the U.S." (2005 Edition)
*As of December 31, 2003. Total does not include 9,292 physicians in U.S. territories and possessions.

Rate of Physicians in Patient Care in 2003

National Rate = 235 Physicians per 100,000 Population*

RANK	STATE	RATE
40	Alabama	193
34	Alaska	205
42	Arizona	189
44	Arkansas	186
20	California	228
19	Colorado	229
5	Connecticut	312
22	Delaware	226
25	Florida	224
37	Georgia	198
7	Hawaii	283
49	Idaho	161
14	Illinois	239
39	Indiana	197
48	Iowa	166
37	Kansas	198
33	Kentucky	206
15	Louisiana	237
12	Maine	240
2	Maryland	336
1	Massachusetts	365
32	Michigan	209
10	Minnesota	248
47	Mississippi	167
29	Missouri	212
28	Montana	214
26	Nebraska	219
46	Nevada	172
12	New Hampshire	240
8	New Jersey	273
30	New Mexico	211
3	New York	331
22	North Carolina	226
27	North Dakota	218
22	Ohio	226
50	Oklahoma	156
17	Oregon	235
9	Pennsylvania	257
6	Rhode Island	307
31	South Carolina	210
36	South Dakota	199
18	Tennessee	233
42	Texas	189
41	Utah	190
4	Vermont	320
11	Virginia	244
15	Washington	237
35	West Virginia	204
20	Wisconsin	228
45	Wyoming	180

RANK	STATE	RATE
1	Massachusetts	365
2	Maryland	336
3	New York	331
4	Vermont	320
5	Connecticut	312
6	Rhode Island	307
7	Hawaii	283
8	New Jersey	273
9	Pennsylvania	257
10	Minnesota	248
11	Virginia	244
12	Maine	240
12	New Hampshire	240
14	Illinois	239
15	Louisiana	237
15	Washington	237
17	Oregon	235
18	Tennessee	233
19	Colorado	229
20	California	228
20	Wisconsin	228
22	Delaware	226
22	North Carolina	226
22	Ohio	226
25	Florida	224
26	Nebraska	219
27	North Dakota	218
28	Montana	214
29	Missouri	212
30	New Mexico	211
31	South Carolina	210
32	Michigan	209
33	Kentucky	206
34	Alaska	205
35	West Virginia	204
36	South Dakota	199
37	Georgia	198
37	Kansas	198
39	Indiana	197
40	Alabama	193
41	Utah	190
42	Arizona	189
42	Texas	189
44	Arkansas	186
45	Wyoming	180
46	Nevada	172
47	Mississippi	167
48	Iowa	166
49	Idaho	161
50	Oklahoma	156
	District of Columbia	609

Source: Morgan Quitno Press using data from American Medical Association (Chicago, Illinois)
"Physician Characteristics and Distribution in the U.S." (2005 Edition)
As of December 31, 2003. National rate does not include physicians in U.S. territories and possessions.

Physicians in Primary Care in 2003

National Total = 288,653 Physicians*

ALPHA ORDER

RANK	STATE	PHYSICIANS	% of USA
26	Alabama	3,776	1.3%
49	Alaska	660	0.2%
23	Arizona	4,320	1.5%
31	Arkansas	2,230	0.8%
1	California	34,956	12.1%
21	Colorado	4,422	1.5%
22	Connecticut	4,402	1.5%
46	Delaware	749	0.3%
4	Florida	14,989	5.2%
13	Georgia	7,609	2.6%
39	Hawaii	1,573	0.5%
43	Idaho	968	0.3%
5	Illinois	13,535	4.7%
19	Indiana	5,189	1.8%
32	Iowa	2,118	0.7%
29	Kansas	2,375	0.8%
28	Kentucky	3,580	1.2%
24	Louisiana	4,276	1.5%
40	Maine	1,393	0.5%
14	Maryland	7,593	2.6%
9	Massachusetts	9,176	3.2%
10	Michigan	9,101	3.2%
16	Minnesota	5,699	2.0%
33	Mississippi	2,052	0.7%
20	Missouri	4,930	1.7%
45	Montana	847	0.3%
36	Nebraska	1,751	0.6%
37	Nevada	1,627	0.6%
42	New Hampshire	1,338	0.5%
8	New Jersey	10,038	3.5%
35	New Mexico	1,800	0.6%
2	New York	26,700	9.2%
11	North Carolina	8,011	2.8%
48	North Dakota	664	0.2%
7	Ohio	10,954	3.8%
30	Oklahoma	2,371	0.8%
27	Oregon	3,704	1.3%
6	Pennsylvania	12,527	4.3%
41	Rhode Island	1,380	0.5%
25	South Carolina	3,816	1.3%
47	South Dakota	698	0.2%
17	Tennessee	5,659	2.0%
3	Texas	17,229	6.0%
34	Utah	1,824	0.6%
44	Vermont	907	0.3%
12	Virginia	7,848	2.7%
15	Washington	6,422	2.2%
38	West Virginia	1,609	0.6%
18	Wisconsin	5,461	1.9%
50	Wyoming	442	0.2%

RANK ORDER

RANK	STATE	PHYSICIANS	% of USA
1	California	34,956	12.1%
2	New York	26,700	9.2%
3	Texas	17,229	6.0%
4	Florida	14,989	5.2%
5	Illinois	13,535	4.7%
6	Pennsylvania	12,527	4.3%
7	Ohio	10,954	3.8%
8	New Jersey	10,038	3.5%
9	Massachusetts	9,176	3.2%
10	Michigan	9,101	3.2%
11	North Carolina	8,011	2.8%
12	Virginia	7,848	2.7%
13	Georgia	7,609	2.6%
14	Maryland	7,593	2.6%
15	Washington	6,422	2.2%
16	Minnesota	5,699	2.0%
17	Tennessee	5,659	2.0%
18	Wisconsin	5,461	1.9%
19	Indiana	5,189	1.8%
20	Missouri	4,930	1.7%
21	Colorado	4,422	1.5%
22	Connecticut	4,402	1.5%
23	Arizona	4,320	1.5%
24	Louisiana	4,276	1.5%
25	South Carolina	3,816	1.3%
26	Alabama	3,776	1.3%
27	Oregon	3,704	1.3%
28	Kentucky	3,580	1.2%
29	Kansas	2,375	0.8%
30	Oklahoma	2,371	0.8%
31	Arkansas	2,230	0.8%
32	Iowa	2,118	0.7%
33	Mississippi	2,052	0.7%
34	Utah	1,824	0.6%
35	New Mexico	1,800	0.6%
36	Nebraska	1,751	0.6%
37	Nevada	1,627	0.6%
38	West Virginia	1,609	0.6%
39	Hawaii	1,573	0.5%
40	Maine	1,393	0.5%
41	Rhode Island	1,380	0.5%
42	New Hampshire	1,338	0.5%
43	Idaho	968	0.3%
44	Vermont	907	0.3%
45	Montana	847	0.3%
46	Delaware	749	0.3%
47	South Dakota	698	0.2%
48	North Dakota	664	0.2%
49	Alaska	660	0.2%
50	Wyoming	442	0.2%
	District of Columbia	1,355	0.5%

Source: American Medical Association (Chicago, Illinois)
    "Physician Characteristics and Distribution in the U.S." (2005 Edition)
*As of December 31, 2003. National total does not include 5,048 physicians in U.S. territories and possessions.
Primary Care Specialties include Family Practice, General Practice, Internal Medicine, Obstetrics/Gynecology and Pediatrics excluding subspecialties within each category.

Rate of Physicians in Primary Care in 2003

National Rate = 99 Physicians per 100,000 Population*

ALPHA ORDER

RANK	STATE	RATE
40	Alabama	84
17	Alaska	102
45	Arizona	77
42	Arkansas	82
21	California	99
22	Colorado	97
6	Connecticut	126
28	Delaware	92
34	Florida	88
34	Georgia	88
6	Hawaii	126
48	Idaho	71
10	Illinois	107
40	Indiana	84
47	Iowa	72
37	Kansas	87
37	Kentucky	87
26	Louisiana	95
12	Maine	106
4	Maryland	138
2	Massachusetts	143
32	Michigan	90
9	Minnesota	113
48	Mississippi	71
39	Missouri	86
28	Montana	92
18	Nebraska	101
46	Nevada	73
15	New Hampshire	104
8	New Jersey	116
24	New Mexico	96
3	New York	139
26	North Carolina	95
13	North Dakota	105
24	Ohio	96
50	Oklahoma	68
15	Oregon	104
18	Pennsylvania	101
5	Rhode Island	128
28	South Carolina	92
31	South Dakota	91
22	Tennessee	97
43	Texas	78
43	Utah	78
1	Vermont	146
10	Virginia	107
13	Washington	105
33	West Virginia	89
20	Wisconsin	100
34	Wyoming	88

RANK ORDER

RANK	STATE	RATE
1	Vermont	146
2	Massachusetts	143
3	New York	139
4	Maryland	138
5	Rhode Island	128
6	Connecticut	126
6	Hawaii	126
8	New Jersey	116
9	Minnesota	113
10	Illinois	107
10	Virginia	107
12	Maine	106
13	North Dakota	105
13	Washington	105
15	New Hampshire	104
15	Oregon	104
17	Alaska	102
18	Nebraska	101
18	Pennsylvania	101
20	Wisconsin	100
21	California	99
22	Colorado	97
22	Tennessee	97
24	New Mexico	96
24	Ohio	96
26	Louisiana	95
26	North Carolina	95
28	Delaware	92
28	Montana	92
28	South Carolina	92
31	South Dakota	91
32	Michigan	90
33	West Virginia	89
34	Florida	88
34	Georgia	88
34	Wyoming	88
37	Kansas	87
37	Kentucky	87
39	Missouri	86
40	Alabama	84
40	Indiana	84
42	Arkansas	82
43	Texas	78
43	Utah	78
45	Arizona	77
46	Nevada	73
47	Iowa	72
48	Idaho	71
48	Mississippi	71
50	Oklahoma	68

District of Columbia	243

Source: Morgan Quitno Press using data from American Medical Association (Chicago, Illinois)
"Physician Characteristics and Distribution in the U.S." (2005 Edition)
As of December 31, 2003. National rate does not include physicians in U.S. territories and possessions. Primary Care Specialties include Family Practice, General Practice, Internal Medicine, Obstetrics/Gynecology and Pediatrics excluding subspecialties within each category.

Percent of Physicians in Primary Care in 2003

National Percent = 33.6% of Physicians*

<table>
<tr><td colspan="3">ALPHA ORDER</td><td colspan="3">RANK ORDER</td></tr>
<tr><td>RANK</td><td>STATE</td><td>PERCENT</td><td>RANK</td><td>STATE</td><td>PERCENT</td></tr>
<tr><td>10</td><td>Alabama</td><td>36.2</td><td>1</td><td>Alaska</td><td>42.7</td></tr>
<tr><td>1</td><td>Alaska</td><td>42.7</td><td>2</td><td>Wyoming</td><td>40.4</td></tr>
<tr><td>46</td><td>Arizona</td><td>31.7</td><td>3</td><td>North Dakota</td><td>39.3</td></tr>
<tr><td>8</td><td>Arkansas</td><td>36.4</td><td>4</td><td>South Dakota</td><td>38.1</td></tr>
<tr><td>38</td><td>California</td><td>33.5</td><td>5</td><td>Nebraska</td><td>37.7</td></tr>
<tr><td>35</td><td>Colorado</td><td>33.9</td><td>6</td><td>Idaho</td><td>36.6</td></tr>
<tr><td>45</td><td>Connecticut</td><td>31.8</td><td>6</td><td>Minnesota</td><td>36.6</td></tr>
<tr><td>44</td><td>Delaware</td><td>32.8</td><td>8</td><td>Arkansas</td><td>36.4</td></tr>
<tr><td>49</td><td>Florida</td><td>30.0</td><td>9</td><td>South Carolina</td><td>36.3</td></tr>
<tr><td>11</td><td>Georgia</td><td>36.1</td><td>10</td><td>Alabama</td><td>36.2</td></tr>
<tr><td>11</td><td>Hawaii</td><td>36.1</td><td>11</td><td>Georgia</td><td>36.1</td></tr>
<tr><td>6</td><td>Idaho</td><td>36.6</td><td>11</td><td>Hawaii</td><td>36.1</td></tr>
<tr><td>13</td><td>Illinois</td><td>36.0</td><td>13</td><td>Illinois</td><td>36.0</td></tr>
<tr><td>16</td><td>Indiana</td><td>35.3</td><td>14</td><td>New Mexico</td><td>35.8</td></tr>
<tr><td>38</td><td>Iowa</td><td>33.5</td><td>14</td><td>Wisconsin</td><td>35.8</td></tr>
<tr><td>18</td><td>Kansas</td><td>35.2</td><td>16</td><td>Indiana</td><td>35.3</td></tr>
<tr><td>22</td><td>Kentucky</td><td>35.0</td><td>16</td><td>Mississippi</td><td>35.3</td></tr>
<tr><td>41</td><td>Louisiana</td><td>33.2</td><td>18</td><td>Kansas</td><td>35.2</td></tr>
<tr><td>23</td><td>Maine</td><td>34.9</td><td>18</td><td>Vermont</td><td>35.2</td></tr>
<tr><td>48</td><td>Maryland</td><td>30.6</td><td>20</td><td>Virginia</td><td>35.1</td></tr>
<tr><td>49</td><td>Massachusetts</td><td>30.0</td><td>20</td><td>West Virginia</td><td>35.1</td></tr>
<tr><td>31</td><td>Michigan</td><td>34.4</td><td>22</td><td>Kentucky</td><td>35.0</td></tr>
<tr><td>6</td><td>Minnesota</td><td>36.6</td><td>23</td><td>Maine</td><td>34.9</td></tr>
<tr><td>16</td><td>Mississippi</td><td>35.3</td><td>23</td><td>Montana</td><td>34.9</td></tr>
<tr><td>40</td><td>Missouri</td><td>33.4</td><td>23</td><td>Oklahoma</td><td>34.9</td></tr>
<tr><td>23</td><td>Montana</td><td>34.9</td><td>26</td><td>New Hampshire</td><td>34.8</td></tr>
<tr><td>5</td><td>Nebraska</td><td>37.7</td><td>27</td><td>Nevada</td><td>34.7</td></tr>
<tr><td>27</td><td>Nevada</td><td>34.7</td><td>28</td><td>New Jersey</td><td>34.6</td></tr>
<tr><td>26</td><td>New Hampshire</td><td>34.8</td><td>28</td><td>Washington</td><td>34.6</td></tr>
<tr><td>28</td><td>New Jersey</td><td>34.6</td><td>30</td><td>Oregon</td><td>34.5</td></tr>
<tr><td>14</td><td>New Mexico</td><td>35.8</td><td>31</td><td>Michigan</td><td>34.4</td></tr>
<tr><td>43</td><td>New York</td><td>32.9</td><td>32</td><td>Tennessee</td><td>34.2</td></tr>
<tr><td>34</td><td>North Carolina</td><td>34.0</td><td>33</td><td>Ohio</td><td>34.1</td></tr>
<tr><td>3</td><td>North Dakota</td><td>39.3</td><td>34</td><td>North Carolina</td><td>34.0</td></tr>
<tr><td>33</td><td>Ohio</td><td>34.1</td><td>35</td><td>Colorado</td><td>33.9</td></tr>
<tr><td>23</td><td>Oklahoma</td><td>34.9</td><td>35</td><td>Texas</td><td>33.9</td></tr>
<tr><td>30</td><td>Oregon</td><td>34.5</td><td>37</td><td>Rhode Island</td><td>33.7</td></tr>
<tr><td>47</td><td>Pennsylvania</td><td>30.9</td><td>38</td><td>California</td><td>33.5</td></tr>
<tr><td>37</td><td>Rhode Island</td><td>33.7</td><td>38</td><td>Iowa</td><td>33.5</td></tr>
<tr><td>9</td><td>South Carolina</td><td>36.3</td><td>40</td><td>Missouri</td><td>33.4</td></tr>
<tr><td>4</td><td>South Dakota</td><td>38.1</td><td>41</td><td>Louisiana</td><td>33.2</td></tr>
<tr><td>32</td><td>Tennessee</td><td>34.2</td><td>42</td><td>Utah</td><td>33.1</td></tr>
<tr><td>35</td><td>Texas</td><td>33.9</td><td>43</td><td>New York</td><td>32.9</td></tr>
<tr><td>42</td><td>Utah</td><td>33.1</td><td>44</td><td>Delaware</td><td>32.8</td></tr>
<tr><td>18</td><td>Vermont</td><td>35.2</td><td>45</td><td>Connecticut</td><td>31.8</td></tr>
<tr><td>20</td><td>Virginia</td><td>35.1</td><td>46</td><td>Arizona</td><td>31.7</td></tr>
<tr><td>28</td><td>Washington</td><td>34.6</td><td>47</td><td>Pennsylvania</td><td>30.9</td></tr>
<tr><td>20</td><td>West Virginia</td><td>35.1</td><td>48</td><td>Maryland</td><td>30.6</td></tr>
<tr><td>14</td><td>Wisconsin</td><td>35.8</td><td>49</td><td>Florida</td><td>30.0</td></tr>
<tr><td>2</td><td>Wyoming</td><td>40.4</td><td>49</td><td>Massachusetts</td><td>30.0</td></tr>
<tr><td></td><td></td><td></td><td></td><td>District of Columbia</td><td>29.4</td></tr>
</table>

Source: Morgan Quitno Press using data from American Medical Association (Chicago, Illinois)
"Physician Characteristics and Distribution in the U.S." (2005 Edition)
As of December 31, 2003. National percent does not include physicians in U.S. territories and possessions.
Primary Care Specialties include Family Practice, General Practice, Internal Medicine, Obstetrics/Gynecology and Pediatrics excluding subspecialties within each category.

Percent of Population Lacking Access to Primary Care in 2004

National Percent = 11.6% of Population*

ALPHA ORDER

RANK	STATE	PERCENT
3	Alabama	25.9
21	Alaska	13.2
17	Arizona	13.9
31	Arkansas	9.8
29	California	9.9
31	Colorado	9.8
43	Connecticut	6.6
36	Delaware	8.1
13	Florida	15.5
11	Georgia	16.2
48	Hawaii	4.4
10	Idaho	18.4
23	Illinois	13.0
35	Indiana	8.5
33	Iowa	9.2
14	Kansas	15.4
16	Kentucky	14.3
7	Louisiana	19.8
36	Maine	8.1
41	Maryland	7.2
47	Massachusetts	5.1
27	Michigan	10.9
25	Minnesota	11.7
1	Mississippi	27.7
5	Missouri	23.9
8	Montana	19.6
46	Nebraska	5.7
20	Nevada	13.5
45	New Hampshire	5.9
50	New Jersey	2.9
2	New Mexico	26.5
29	New York	9.9
39	North Carolina	7.9
6	North Dakota	20.4
41	Ohio	7.2
12	Oklahoma	15.6
36	Oregon	8.1
44	Pennsylvania	6.3
34	Rhode Island	8.7
14	South Carolina	15.4
4	South Dakota	24.7
24	Tennessee	11.8
17	Texas	13.9
19	Utah	13.7
49	Vermont	3.6
40	Virginia	7.6
26	Washington	11.5
21	West Virginia	13.2
28	Wisconsin	10.3
9	Wyoming	18.8

RANK ORDER

RANK	STATE	PERCENT
1	Mississippi	27.7
2	New Mexico	26.5
3	Alabama	25.9
4	South Dakota	24.7
5	Missouri	23.9
6	North Dakota	20.4
7	Louisiana	19.8
8	Montana	19.6
9	Wyoming	18.8
10	Idaho	18.4
11	Georgia	16.2
12	Oklahoma	15.6
13	Florida	15.5
14	Kansas	15.4
14	South Carolina	15.4
16	Kentucky	14.3
17	Arizona	13.9
17	Texas	13.9
19	Utah	13.7
20	Nevada	13.5
21	Alaska	13.2
21	West Virginia	13.2
23	Illinois	13.0
24	Tennessee	11.8
25	Minnesota	11.7
26	Washington	11.5
27	Michigan	10.9
28	Wisconsin	10.3
29	California	9.9
29	New York	9.9
31	Arkansas	9.8
31	Colorado	9.8
33	Iowa	9.2
34	Rhode Island	8.7
35	Indiana	8.5
36	Delaware	8.1
36	Maine	8.1
36	Oregon	8.1
39	North Carolina	7.9
40	Virginia	7.6
41	Maryland	7.2
41	Ohio	7.2
43	Connecticut	6.6
44	Pennsylvania	6.3
45	New Hampshire	5.9
46	Nebraska	5.7
47	Massachusetts	5.1
48	Hawaii	4.4
49	Vermont	3.6
50	New Jersey	2.9

District of Columbia   26.6

Source: Morgan Quitno Press using data from U.S. Dept. of Health and Human Services, Div. of Shortage Designation "Selected Statistics on Health Professional Shortage Areas" (as of September 30, 2004)
*Percent of population considered under-served by primary medical practitioners (Family & General Practice doctors, Internists, Ob/Gyns and Pediatricians). An under-served population does not have primary medical care within reasonable economic and geographic bounds.

Physicians in General/Family Practice in 2003

National Total = 89,918 Physicians*

ALPHA ORDER

RANK ORDER

RANK	STATE	PHYSICIANS	% of USA	RANK	STATE	PHYSICIANS	% of USA
26	Alabama	1,288	1.4%	1	California	10,804	12.0%
44	Alaska	378	0.4%	2	Texas	6,237	6.9%
20	Arizona	1,485	1.7%	3	Florida	4,916	5.5%
28	Arkansas	1,196	1.3%	4	New York	3,929	4.4%
1	California	10,804	12.0%	5	Pennsylvania	3,851	4.3%
17	Colorado	1,743	1.9%	6	Illinois	3,822	4.3%
37	Connecticut	614	0.7%	7	Ohio	3,462	3.9%
50	Delaware	231	0.3%	8	Washington	2,904	3.2%
3	Florida	4,916	5.5%	9	North Carolina	2,853	3.2%
15	Georgia	2,230	2.5%	10	Minnesota	2,736	3.0%
42	Hawaii	426	0.5%	11	Michigan	2,733	3.0%
39	Idaho	541	0.6%	12	Virginia	2,653	3.0%
6	Illinois	3,822	4.3%	13	Indiana	2,448	2.7%
13	Indiana	2,448	2.7%	14	Wisconsin	2,357	2.6%
29	Iowa	1,161	1.3%	15	Georgia	2,230	2.5%
30	Kansas	1,104	1.2%	16	Tennessee	1,901	2.1%
23	Kentucky	1,368	1.5%	17	Colorado	1,743	1.9%
24	Louisiana	1,328	1.5%	18	New Jersey	1,653	1.8%
38	Maine	597	0.7%	19	South Carolina	1,567	1.7%
21	Maryland	1,383	1.5%	20	Arizona	1,485	1.7%
27	Massachusetts	1,279	1.4%	21	Maryland	1,383	1.5%
11	Michigan	2,733	3.0%	22	Missouri	1,369	1.5%
10	Minnesota	2,736	3.0%	23	Kentucky	1,368	1.5%
33	Mississippi	817	0.9%	24	Louisiana	1,328	1.5%
22	Missouri	1,369	1.5%	25	Oregon	1,302	1.4%
43	Montana	421	0.5%	26	Alabama	1,288	1.4%
32	Nebraska	903	1.0%	27	Massachusetts	1,279	1.4%
40	Nevada	524	0.6%	28	Arkansas	1,196	1.3%
41	New Hampshire	472	0.5%	29	Iowa	1,161	1.3%
18	New Jersey	1,653	1.8%	30	Kansas	1,104	1.2%
34	New Mexico	760	0.8%	31	Oklahoma	1,058	1.2%
4	New York	3,929	4.4%	32	Nebraska	903	1.0%
9	North Carolina	2,853	3.2%	33	Mississippi	817	0.9%
45	North Dakota	376	0.4%	34	New Mexico	760	0.8%
7	Ohio	3,462	3.9%	35	Utah	694	0.8%
31	Oklahoma	1,058	1.2%	36	West Virginia	662	0.7%
25	Oregon	1,302	1.4%	37	Connecticut	614	0.7%
5	Pennsylvania	3,851	4.3%	38	Maine	597	0.7%
49	Rhode Island	241	0.3%	39	Idaho	541	0.6%
19	South Carolina	1,567	1.7%	40	Nevada	524	0.6%
46	South Dakota	372	0.4%	41	New Hampshire	472	0.5%
16	Tennessee	1,901	2.1%	42	Hawaii	426	0.5%
2	Texas	6,237	6.9%	43	Montana	421	0.5%
35	Utah	694	0.8%	44	Alaska	378	0.4%
47	Vermont	324	0.4%	45	North Dakota	376	0.4%
12	Virginia	2,653	3.0%	46	South Dakota	372	0.4%
8	Washington	2,904	3.2%	47	Vermont	324	0.4%
36	West Virginia	662	0.7%	48	Wyoming	246	0.3%
14	Wisconsin	2,357	2.6%	49	Rhode Island	241	0.3%
48	Wyoming	246	0.3%	50	Delaware	231	0.3%
					District of Columbia	199	0.2%

Source: American Medical Association (Chicago, Illinois)
   "Physician Characteristics and Distribution in the U.S." (2005 Edition)
*As of December 31, 2003. Total does not include 2,388 physicians in U.S. territories and possessions.

Rate of Physicians in General/Family Practice in 2003

National Rate = 31 Physicians per 100,000 Population*

ALPHA ORDER

RANK ORDER

RANK	STATE	RATE		RANK	STATE	RATE
35	Alabama	29		1	North Dakota	59
2	Alaska	58		2	Alaska	58
40	Arizona	27		3	Minnesota	54
11	Arkansas	44		4	Nebraska	52
29	California	30		4	Vermont	52
18	Colorado	38		6	South Dakota	49
50	Connecticut	18		6	Wyoming	49
37	Delaware	28		8	Washington	47
35	Florida	29		9	Maine	46
42	Georgia	26		9	Montana	46
24	Hawaii	34		11	Arkansas	44
14	Idaho	40		12	Wisconsin	43
29	Illinois	30		13	Kansas	41
16	Indiana	39		14	Idaho	40
16	Iowa	39		14	New Mexico	40
13	Kansas	41		16	Indiana	39
26	Kentucky	33		16	Iowa	39
29	Louisiana	30		18	Colorado	38
9	Maine	46		18	South Carolina	38
43	Maryland	25		20	New Hampshire	37
47	Massachusetts	20		20	Oregon	37
40	Michigan	27		20	West Virginia	37
3	Minnesota	54		23	Virginia	36
37	Mississippi	28		24	Hawaii	34
44	Missouri	24		24	North Carolina	34
9	Montana	46		26	Kentucky	33
4	Nebraska	52		26	Tennessee	33
45	Nevada	23		28	Pennsylvania	31
20	New Hampshire	37		29	California	30
49	New Jersey	19		29	Illinois	30
14	New Mexico	40		29	Louisiana	30
47	New York	20		29	Ohio	30
24	North Carolina	34		29	Oklahoma	30
1	North Dakota	59		29	Utah	30
29	Ohio	30		35	Alabama	29
29	Oklahoma	30		35	Florida	29
20	Oregon	37		37	Delaware	28
28	Pennsylvania	31		37	Mississippi	28
46	Rhode Island	22		37	Texas	28
18	South Carolina	38		40	Arizona	27
6	South Dakota	49		40	Michigan	27
26	Tennessee	33		42	Georgia	26
37	Texas	28		43	Maryland	25
29	Utah	30		44	Missouri	24
4	Vermont	52		45	Nevada	23
23	Virginia	36		46	Rhode Island	22
8	Washington	47		47	Massachusetts	20
20	West Virginia	37		47	New York	20
12	Wisconsin	43		49	New Jersey	19
6	Wyoming	49		50	Connecticut	18
					District of Columbia	36

Source: Morgan Quitno Press using data from American Medical Association (Chicago, Illinois)
    "Physician Characteristics and Distribution in the U.S." (2005 Edition)
*As of December 31, 2003. National rate does not include physicians in U.S. territories and possessions.

Average Annual Wages of Family and General Practitioners in 2003

National Average = $139,860*

ALPHA ORDER

RANK	STATE	WAGES
23	Alabama	$145,650
43	Alaska	122,030
11	Arizona	157,540
19	Arkansas	149,240
47	California	115,070
35	Colorado	133,260
20	Connecticut	147,640
48	Delaware	111,680
12	Florida	156,640
17	Georgia	152,060
21	Hawaii	147,420
28	Idaho	138,520
40	Illinois	127,630
18	Indiana	150,050
9	Iowa	159,390
10	Kansas	158,450
27	Kentucky	140,670
3	Louisiana	169,100
46	Maine	118,260
4	Maryland	167,410
5	Massachusetts	167,070
45	Michigan	120,060
13	Minnesota	156,170
25	Mississippi	144,280
29	Missouri	137,450
32	Montana	135,420
31	Nebraska	135,860
1	Nevada	193,290
7	New Hampshire	162,080
37	New Jersey	129,870
39	New Mexico	128,320
26	New York	140,880
36	North Carolina	130,350
8	North Dakota	159,690
16	Ohio	152,650
14	Oklahoma	154,760
NA	Oregon**	NA
30	Pennsylvania	136,380
2	Rhode Island	182,700
33	South Carolina	134,680
41	South Dakota	124,720
49	Tennessee	89,860
34	Texas	134,650
15	Utah	154,250
44	Vermont	120,740
42	Virginia	123,240
24	Washington	145,050
22	West Virginia	146,150
6	Wisconsin	164,150
38	Wyoming	129,270

RANK ORDER

RANK	STATE	WAGES
1	Nevada	$193,290
2	Rhode Island	182,700
3	Louisiana	169,100
4	Maryland	167,410
5	Massachusetts	167,070
6	Wisconsin	164,150
7	New Hampshire	162,080
8	North Dakota	159,690
9	Iowa	159,390
10	Kansas	158,450
11	Arizona	157,540
12	Florida	156,640
13	Minnesota	156,170
14	Oklahoma	154,760
15	Utah	154,250
16	Ohio	152,650
17	Georgia	152,060
18	Indiana	150,050
19	Arkansas	149,240
20	Connecticut	147,640
21	Hawaii	147,420
22	West Virginia	146,150
23	Alabama	145,650
24	Washington	145,050
25	Mississippi	144,280
26	New York	140,880
27	Kentucky	140,670
28	Idaho	138,520
29	Missouri	137,450
30	Pennsylvania	136,380
31	Nebraska	135,860
32	Montana	135,420
33	South Carolina	134,680
34	Texas	134,650
35	Colorado	133,260
36	North Carolina	130,350
37	New Jersey	129,870
38	Wyoming	129,270
39	New Mexico	128,320
40	Illinois	127,630
41	South Dakota	124,720
42	Virginia	123,240
43	Alaska	122,030
44	Vermont	120,740
45	Michigan	120,060
46	Maine	118,260
47	California	115,070
48	Delaware	111,680
49	Tennessee	89,860
NA	Oregon**	NA
	District of Columbia	71,400

Source: U.S. Department of Labor, Bureau of Labor Statistics
"Occupational Employment and Wages, 2003" (http://www.bls.gov/oes/)
*Does not include self-employed.
**Not available.

Percent of Physicians Who Are Specialists in 2003

National Percent = 74.1% of Physicians*

ALPHA ORDER

RANK	STATE	PERCENT
14	Alabama	74.9
45	Alaska	65.8
29	Arizona	70.9
43	Arkansas	67.0
24	California	72.5
28	Colorado	71.6
1	Connecticut	81.0
11	Delaware	75.4
35	Florida	70.0
9	Georgia	76.1
10	Hawaii	76.0
47	Idaho	65.1
13	Illinois	75.0
31	Indiana	70.5
48	Iowa	64.1
41	Kansas	67.8
22	Kentucky	73.3
8	Louisiana	76.4
37	Maine	68.8
6	Maryland	79.1
4	Massachusetts	80.0
16	Michigan	74.2
39	Minnesota	68.1
25	Mississippi	72.2
7	Missouri	78.0
44	Montana	66.1
42	Nebraska	67.1
19	Nevada	73.9
26	New Hampshire	72.1
2	New Jersey	80.7
36	New Mexico	69.2
5	New York	79.3
21	North Carolina	73.7
50	North Dakota	63.0
18	Ohio	74.0
38	Oklahoma	68.7
31	Oregon	70.5
14	Pennsylvania	74.9
3	Rhode Island	80.4
27	South Carolina	71.8
46	South Dakota	65.4
12	Tennessee	75.1
16	Texas	74.2
20	Utah	73.8
34	Vermont	70.1
22	Virginia	73.3
39	Washington	68.1
33	West Virginia	70.4
29	Wisconsin	70.9
49	Wyoming	63.7

RANK ORDER

RANK	STATE	PERCENT
1	Connecticut	81.0
2	New Jersey	80.7
3	Rhode Island	80.4
4	Massachusetts	80.0
5	New York	79.3
6	Maryland	79.1
7	Missouri	78.0
8	Louisiana	76.4
9	Georgia	76.1
10	Hawaii	76.0
11	Delaware	75.4
12	Tennessee	75.1
13	Illinois	75.0
14	Alabama	74.9
14	Pennsylvania	74.9
16	Michigan	74.2
16	Texas	74.2
18	Ohio	74.0
19	Nevada	73.9
20	Utah	73.8
21	North Carolina	73.7
22	Kentucky	73.3
22	Virginia	73.3
24	California	72.5
25	Mississippi	72.2
26	New Hampshire	72.1
27	South Carolina	71.8
28	Colorado	71.6
29	Arizona	70.9
29	Wisconsin	70.9
31	Indiana	70.5
31	Oregon	70.5
33	West Virginia	70.4
34	Vermont	70.1
35	Florida	70.0
36	New Mexico	69.2
37	Maine	68.8
38	Oklahoma	68.7
39	Minnesota	68.1
39	Washington	68.1
41	Kansas	67.8
42	Nebraska	67.1
43	Arkansas	67.0
44	Montana	66.1
45	Alaska	65.8
46	South Dakota	65.4
47	Idaho	65.1
48	Iowa	64.1
49	Wyoming	63.7
50	North Dakota	63.0

District of Columbia 80.9

Source: Morgan Quitno Press using data from American Medical Association (Chicago, Illinois)
"Physician Characteristics and Distribution in the U.S." (2005 Edition)
*As of December 31, 2003. National percent does not include physicians in U.S. territories and possessions.
Includes physicians in medical, surgical and other specialties.

Physicians in Medical Specialties in 2003

National Total = 273,105 Physicians*

<u>ALPHA ORDER</u>

RANK	STATE	PHYSICIANS	% of USA
25	Alabama	3,276	1.2%
49	Alaska	318	0.1%
23	Arizona	3,884	1.4%
33	Arkansas	1,583	0.6%
1	California	32,001	11.7%
24	Colorado	3,678	1.3%
16	Connecticut	5,168	1.9%
43	Delaware	759	0.3%
4	Florida	14,993	5.5%
14	Georgia	6,662	2.4%
38	Hawaii	1,377	0.5%
45	Idaho	556	0.2%
6	Illinois	12,747	4.7%
22	Indiana	4,016	1.5%
35	Iowa	1,509	0.6%
30	Kansas	1,754	0.6%
26	Kentucky	3,040	1.1%
21	Louisiana	4,056	1.5%
42	Maine	1,051	0.4%
10	Maryland	8,919	3.3%
7	Massachusetts	11,538	4.2%
11	Michigan	8,497	3.1%
19	Minnesota	4,580	1.7%
31	Mississippi	1,637	0.6%
17	Missouri	5,081	1.9%
46	Montana	549	0.2%
40	Nebraska	1,182	0.4%
37	Nevada	1,402	0.5%
41	New Hampshire	1,113	0.4%
8	New Jersey	11,310	4.1%
36	New Mexico	1,423	0.5%
2	New York	30,607	11.2%
12	North Carolina	7,232	2.6%
48	North Dakota	402	0.1%
9	Ohio	10,319	3.8%
29	Oklahoma	1,835	0.7%
27	Oregon	3,020	1.1%
5	Pennsylvania	12,999	4.8%
32	Rhode Island	1,601	0.6%
28	South Carolina	2,913	1.1%
47	South Dakota	457	0.2%
15	Tennessee	5,323	1.9%
3	Texas	15,233	5.6%
34	Utah	1,566	0.6%
44	Vermont	729	0.3%
13	Virginia	6,748	2.5%
18	Washington	4,974	1.8%
39	West Virginia	1,284	0.5%
20	Wisconsin	4,343	1.6%
50	Wyoming	214	0.1%

<u>RANK ORDER</u>

RANK	STATE	PHYSICIANS	% of USA
1	California	32,001	11.7%
2	New York	30,607	11.2%
3	Texas	15,233	5.6%
4	Florida	14,993	5.5%
5	Pennsylvania	12,999	4.8%
6	Illinois	12,747	4.7%
7	Massachusetts	11,538	4.2%
8	New Jersey	11,310	4.1%
9	Ohio	10,319	3.8%
10	Maryland	8,919	3.3%
11	Michigan	8,497	3.1%
12	North Carolina	7,232	2.6%
13	Virginia	6,748	2.5%
14	Georgia	6,662	2.4%
15	Tennessee	5,323	1.9%
16	Connecticut	5,168	1.9%
17	Missouri	5,081	1.9%
18	Washington	4,974	1.8%
19	Minnesota	4,580	1.7%
20	Wisconsin	4,343	1.6%
21	Louisiana	4,056	1.5%
22	Indiana	4,016	1.5%
23	Arizona	3,884	1.4%
24	Colorado	3,678	1.3%
25	Alabama	3,276	1.2%
26	Kentucky	3,040	1.1%
27	Oregon	3,020	1.1%
28	South Carolina	2,913	1.1%
29	Oklahoma	1,835	0.7%
30	Kansas	1,754	0.6%
31	Mississippi	1,637	0.6%
32	Rhode Island	1,601	0.6%
33	Arkansas	1,583	0.6%
34	Utah	1,566	0.6%
35	Iowa	1,509	0.6%
36	New Mexico	1,423	0.5%
37	Nevada	1,402	0.5%
38	Hawaii	1,377	0.5%
39	West Virginia	1,284	0.5%
40	Nebraska	1,182	0.4%
41	New Hampshire	1,113	0.4%
42	Maine	1,051	0.4%
43	Delaware	759	0.3%
44	Vermont	729	0.3%
45	Idaho	556	0.2%
46	Montana	549	0.2%
47	South Dakota	457	0.2%
48	North Dakota	402	0.1%
49	Alaska	318	0.1%
50	Wyoming	214	0.1%
	District of Columbia	1,647	0.6%

Source: American Medical Association (Chicago, Illinois)
   "Physician Characteristics and Distribution in the U.S." (2005 Edition)
*As of December 31, 2003. Total does not include 3,161 physicians in U.S. territories and possessions. Medical Specialties are Allergy/Immunology, Cardiovascular Diseases, Dermatology, Gastroenterology, Internal Medicine, Pediatrics, Pediatric Cardiology and Pulmonary Diseases.

Rate of Nonfederal Physicians in Medical Specialties in 2003

National Rate = 94 Physicians per 100,000 Population*

ALPHA ORDER

RANK	STATE	RATE
31	Alabama	73
48	Alaska	49
33	Arizona	70
44	Arkansas	58
14	California	90
24	Colorado	81
5	Connecticut	148
11	Delaware	93
19	Florida	88
28	Georgia	77
8	Hawaii	110
50	Idaho	41
10	Illinois	101
38	Indiana	65
47	Iowa	51
39	Kansas	64
30	Kentucky	74
14	Louisiana	90
26	Maine	80
2	Maryland	162
1	Massachusetts	180
23	Michigan	84
14	Minnesota	90
45	Mississippi	57
18	Missouri	89
42	Montana	60
36	Nebraska	68
40	Nevada	63
20	New Hampshire	86
6	New Jersey	131
29	New Mexico	76
3	New York	159
20	North Carolina	86
40	North Dakota	63
14	Ohio	90
46	Oklahoma	52
22	Oregon	85
9	Pennsylvania	105
4	Rhode Island	149
33	South Carolina	70
42	South Dakota	60
13	Tennessee	91
35	Texas	69
37	Utah	67
7	Vermont	118
12	Virginia	92
24	Washington	81
32	West Virginia	71
27	Wisconsin	79
49	Wyoming	43

RANK ORDER

RANK	STATE	RATE
1	Massachusetts	180
2	Maryland	162
3	New York	159
4	Rhode Island	149
5	Connecticut	148
6	New Jersey	131
7	Vermont	118
8	Hawaii	110
9	Pennsylvania	105
10	Illinois	101
11	Delaware	93
12	Virginia	92
13	Tennessee	91
14	California	90
14	Louisiana	90
14	Minnesota	90
14	Ohio	90
18	Missouri	89
19	Florida	88
20	New Hampshire	86
20	North Carolina	86
22	Oregon	85
23	Michigan	84
24	Colorado	81
24	Washington	81
26	Maine	80
27	Wisconsin	79
28	Georgia	77
29	New Mexico	76
30	Kentucky	74
31	Alabama	73
32	West Virginia	71
33	Arizona	70
33	South Carolina	70
35	Texas	69
36	Nebraska	68
37	Utah	67
38	Indiana	65
39	Kansas	64
40	Nevada	63
40	North Dakota	63
42	Montana	60
42	South Dakota	60
44	Arkansas	58
45	Mississippi	57
46	Oklahoma	52
47	Iowa	51
48	Alaska	49
49	Wyoming	43
50	Idaho	41

District of Columbia — 295

Source: Morgan Quitno Press using data from American Medical Association (Chicago, Illinois)
    "Physician Characteristics and Distribution in the U.S." (2005 Edition)
*As of December 31, 2003. National rate does not include physicians in U.S. territories and possessions. Medical Specialties are Allergy/Immunology, Cardiovascular Diseases, Dermatology, Gastroenterology, Internal Medicine, Pediatrics, Pediatric Cardiology and Pulmonary Diseases.

Physicians in Internal Medicine in 2003

National Total = 146,146 Physicians*

ALPHA ORDER

RANK ORDER

RANK	STATE	PHYSICIANS	% of USA
26	Alabama	1,762	1.2%
49	Alaska	147	0.1%
23	Arizona	1,931	1.3%
36	Arkansas	728	0.5%
2	California	16,933	11.6%
24	Colorado	1,905	1.3%
15	Connecticut	3,012	2.1%
44	Delaware	357	0.2%
3	Florida	7,465	5.1%
14	Georgia	3,511	2.4%
35	Hawaii	771	0.5%
46	Idaho	284	0.2%
5	Illinois	7,247	5.0%
21	Indiana	2,022	1.4%
37	Iowa	712	0.5%
30	Kansas	900	0.6%
27	Kentucky	1,517	1.0%
22	Louisiana	2,016	1.4%
42	Maine	576	0.4%
10	Maryland	4,961	3.4%
7	Massachusetts	6,749	4.6%
11	Michigan	4,761	3.3%
19	Minnesota	2,483	1.7%
32	Mississippi	825	0.6%
17	Missouri	2,710	1.9%
45	Montana	300	0.2%
40	Nebraska	592	0.4%
33	Nevada	792	0.5%
41	New Hampshire	583	0.4%
8	New Jersey	6,066	4.2%
34	New Mexico	787	0.5%
1	New York	17,576	12.0%
12	North Carolina	3,662	2.5%
48	North Dakota	247	0.2%
9	Ohio	5,303	3.6%
29	Oklahoma	935	0.6%
25	Oregon	1,789	1.2%
6	Pennsylvania	7,065	4.8%
31	Rhode Island	873	0.6%
28	South Carolina	1,459	1.0%
47	South Dakota	262	0.2%
16	Tennessee	2,739	1.9%
4	Texas	7,417	5.1%
39	Utah	682	0.5%
43	Vermont	419	0.3%
13	Virginia	3,543	2.4%
18	Washington	2,673	1.8%
38	West Virginia	694	0.5%
20	Wisconsin	2,360	1.6%
50	Wyoming	119	0.1%

RANK	STATE	PHYSICIANS	% of USA
1	New York	17,576	12.0%
2	California	16,933	11.6%
3	Florida	7,465	5.1%
4	Texas	7,417	5.1%
5	Illinois	7,247	5.0%
6	Pennsylvania	7,065	4.8%
7	Massachusetts	6,749	4.6%
8	New Jersey	6,066	4.2%
9	Ohio	5,303	3.6%
10	Maryland	4,961	3.4%
11	Michigan	4,761	3.3%
12	North Carolina	3,662	2.5%
13	Virginia	3,543	2.4%
14	Georgia	3,511	2.4%
15	Connecticut	3,012	2.1%
16	Tennessee	2,739	1.9%
17	Missouri	2,710	1.9%
18	Washington	2,673	1.8%
19	Minnesota	2,483	1.7%
20	Wisconsin	2,360	1.6%
21	Indiana	2,022	1.4%
22	Louisiana	2,016	1.4%
23	Arizona	1,931	1.3%
24	Colorado	1,905	1.3%
25	Oregon	1,789	1.2%
26	Alabama	1,762	1.2%
27	Kentucky	1,517	1.0%
28	South Carolina	1,459	1.0%
29	Oklahoma	935	0.6%
30	Kansas	900	0.6%
31	Rhode Island	873	0.6%
32	Mississippi	825	0.6%
33	Nevada	792	0.5%
34	New Mexico	787	0.5%
35	Hawaii	771	0.5%
36	Arkansas	728	0.5%
37	Iowa	712	0.5%
38	West Virginia	694	0.5%
39	Utah	682	0.5%
40	Nebraska	592	0.4%
41	New Hampshire	583	0.4%
42	Maine	576	0.4%
43	Vermont	419	0.3%
44	Delaware	357	0.2%
45	Montana	300	0.2%
46	Idaho	284	0.2%
47	South Dakota	262	0.2%
48	North Dakota	247	0.2%
49	Alaska	147	0.1%
50	Wyoming	119	0.1%
	District of Columbia	924	0.6%

Source: American Medical Association (Chicago, Illinois)
   "Physician Characteristics and Distribution in the U.S." (2005 Edition)
As of December 31, 2003. Total does not include 1,500 physicians in U.S. territories and possessions. Internal Medicine includes Diabetes, Endocrinology, Geriatrics, Hematology, Infectious Diseases, Nephrology, Nutrition, Medical Oncology and Rheumatology.

Rate of Physicians in Internal Medicine in 2003

National Rate = 50 Physicians per 100,000 Population*

ALPHA ORDER

RANK	STATE	RATE
30	Alabama	39
49	Alaska	23
34	Arizona	35
45	Arkansas	27
13	California	48
27	Colorado	42
4	Connecticut	86
21	Delaware	44
21	Florida	44
29	Georgia	40
8	Hawaii	62
50	Idaho	21
9	Illinois	57
40	Indiana	33
47	Iowa	24
40	Kansas	33
33	Kentucky	37
19	Louisiana	45
21	Maine	44
3	Maryland	90
1	Massachusetts	105
15	Michigan	47
12	Minnesota	49
43	Mississippi	29
15	Missouri	47
40	Montana	33
37	Nebraska	34
34	Nevada	35
19	New Hampshire	45
6	New Jersey	70
27	New Mexico	42
2	New York	91
25	North Carolina	43
30	North Dakota	39
18	Ohio	46
45	Oklahoma	27
11	Oregon	50
9	Pennsylvania	57
5	Rhode Island	81
34	South Carolina	35
37	South Dakota	34
15	Tennessee	47
37	Texas	34
43	Utah	29
7	Vermont	68
13	Virginia	48
21	Washington	44
32	West Virginia	38
25	Wisconsin	43
47	Wyoming	24

RANK ORDER

RANK	STATE	RATE
1	Massachusetts	105
2	New York	91
3	Maryland	90
4	Connecticut	86
5	Rhode Island	81
6	New Jersey	70
7	Vermont	68
8	Hawaii	62
9	Illinois	57
9	Pennsylvania	57
11	Oregon	50
12	Minnesota	49
13	California	48
13	Virginia	48
15	Michigan	47
15	Missouri	47
15	Tennessee	47
18	Ohio	46
19	Louisiana	45
19	New Hampshire	45
21	Delaware	44
21	Florida	44
21	Maine	44
21	Washington	44
25	North Carolina	43
25	Wisconsin	43
27	Colorado	42
27	New Mexico	42
29	Georgia	40
30	Alabama	39
30	North Dakota	39
32	West Virginia	38
33	Kentucky	37
34	Arizona	35
34	Nevada	35
34	South Carolina	35
37	Nebraska	34
37	South Dakota	34
37	Texas	34
40	Indiana	33
40	Kansas	33
40	Montana	33
43	Mississippi	29
43	Utah	29
45	Arkansas	27
45	Oklahoma	27
47	Iowa	24
47	Wyoming	24
49	Alaska	23
50	Idaho	21

| | District of Columbia | 166 |

Source: Morgan Quitno Press using data from American Medical Association (Chicago, Illinois)
    "Physician Characteristics and Distribution in the U.S." (2005 Edition)

*As of December 31, 2003. National rate does not include physicians in U.S. territories and possessions. Internal Medicine includes Diabetes, Endocrinology, Geriatrics, Hematology, Infectious Diseases, Nephrology, Nutrition, Medical Oncology and Rheumatology.

Physicians in Pediatrics in 2003

National Total = 67,634 Physicians*

RANK	STATE	PHYSICIANS	% of USA	RANK	STATE	PHYSICIANS	% of USA
26	Alabama	778	1.2%	1	California	8,214	12.1%
45	Alaska	113	0.2%	2	New York	7,215	10.7%
23	Arizona	1,009	1.5%	3	Texas	4,229	6.3%
30	Arkansas	447	0.7%	4	Florida	3,497	5.2%
1	California	8,214	12.1%	5	Illinois	3,002	4.4%
24	Colorado	946	1.4%	6	Ohio	2,880	4.3%
19	Connecticut	1,086	1.6%	7	New Jersey	2,865	4.2%
43	Delaware	249	0.4%	8	Pennsylvania	2,810	4.2%
4	Florida	3,497	5.2%	9	Massachusetts	2,523	3.7%
14	Georgia	1,755	2.6%	10	Maryland	2,184	3.2%
35	Hawaii	380	0.6%	11	Michigan	2,054	3.0%
45	Idaho	113	0.2%	12	North Carolina	1,891	2.8%
5	Illinois	3,002	4.4%	13	Virginia	1,786	2.6%
22	Indiana	1,023	1.5%	14	Georgia	1,755	2.6%
37	Iowa	355	0.5%	15	Tennessee	1,389	2.1%
31	Kansas	442	0.7%	16	Missouri	1,253	1.9%
25	Kentucky	821	1.2%	17	Washington	1,214	1.8%
18	Louisiana	1,096	1.6%	18	Louisiana	1,096	1.6%
42	Maine	258	0.4%	19	Connecticut	1,086	1.6%
10	Maryland	2,184	3.2%	20	Wisconsin	1,061	1.6%
9	Massachusetts	2,523	3.7%	21	Minnesota	1,034	1.5%
11	Michigan	2,054	3.0%	22	Indiana	1,023	1.5%
21	Minnesota	1,034	1.5%	23	Arizona	1,009	1.5%
33	Mississippi	421	0.6%	24	Colorado	946	1.4%
16	Missouri	1,253	1.9%	25	Kentucky	821	1.2%
47	Montana	112	0.2%	26	Alabama	778	1.2%
38	Nebraska	314	0.5%	27	South Carolina	773	1.1%
40	Nevada	300	0.4%	28	Oregon	639	0.9%
41	New Hampshire	282	0.4%	29	Utah	496	0.7%
7	New Jersey	2,865	4.2%	30	Arkansas	447	0.7%
36	New Mexico	356	0.5%	31	Kansas	442	0.7%
2	New York	7,215	10.7%	31	Oklahoma	442	0.7%
12	North Carolina	1,891	2.8%	33	Mississippi	421	0.6%
49	North Dakota	76	0.1%	34	Rhode Island	399	0.6%
6	Ohio	2,880	4.3%	35	Hawaii	380	0.6%
31	Oklahoma	442	0.7%	36	New Mexico	356	0.5%
28	Oregon	639	0.9%	37	Iowa	355	0.5%
8	Pennsylvania	2,810	4.2%	38	Nebraska	314	0.5%
34	Rhode Island	399	0.6%	38	West Virginia	314	0.5%
27	South Carolina	773	1.1%	40	Nevada	300	0.4%
48	South Dakota	90	0.1%	41	New Hampshire	282	0.4%
15	Tennessee	1,389	2.1%	42	Maine	258	0.4%
3	Texas	4,229	6.3%	43	Delaware	249	0.4%
29	Utah	496	0.7%	44	Vermont	188	0.3%
44	Vermont	188	0.3%	45	Alaska	113	0.2%
13	Virginia	1,786	2.6%	45	Idaho	113	0.2%
17	Washington	1,214	1.8%	47	Montana	112	0.2%
38	West Virginia	314	0.5%	48	South Dakota	90	0.1%
20	Wisconsin	1,061	1.6%	49	North Dakota	76	0.1%
50	Wyoming	53	0.1%	50	Wyoming	53	0.1%
					District of Columbia	407	0.6%

Source: American Medical Association (Chicago, Illinois)
    "Physician Characteristics and Distribution in the U.S." (2005 Edition)
*As of December 31, 2003. Total does not include 1,095 physicians in U.S. territories and possessions. Pediatrics includes Adolescent Medicine, Neonatal-Perinatal, Pediatric Allergy, Pediatric Endocrinology, Pediatric Pulmonology, Pediatric Hematology-Oncology and Pediatric Nephrology.

Rate of Physicians in Pediatrics in 2003

National Rate = 93 Physicians per 100,000 Population 17 Years and Younger*

ALPHA ORDER

RANK	STATE	RATE
34	Alabama	71
41	Alaska	60
36	Arizona	67
38	Arkansas	66
21	California	88
22	Colorado	83
7	Connecticut	131
9	Delaware	126
19	Florida	90
29	Georgia	77
8	Hawaii	129
50	Idaho	31
15	Illinois	93
40	Indiana	64
43	Iowa	52
39	Kansas	65
22	Kentucky	83
14	Louisiana	94
17	Maine	91
4	Maryland	159
1	Massachusetts	170
26	Michigan	81
22	Minnesota	83
42	Mississippi	56
19	Missouri	90
43	Montana	52
32	Nebraska	72
43	Nevada	52
15	New Hampshire	93
6	New Jersey	135
32	New Mexico	72
3	New York	160
17	North Carolina	91
43	North Dakota	52
10	Ohio	103
47	Oklahoma	50
30	Oregon	76
11	Pennsylvania	100
2	Rhode Island	164
30	South Carolina	76
48	South Dakota	47
11	Tennessee	100
35	Texas	68
36	Utah	67
5	Vermont	138
11	Virginia	100
25	Washington	82
26	West Virginia	81
28	Wisconsin	80
49	Wyoming	44

RANK ORDER

RANK	STATE	RATE
1	Massachusetts	170
2	Rhode Island	164
3	New York	160
4	Maryland	159
5	Vermont	138
6	New Jersey	135
7	Connecticut	131
8	Hawaii	129
9	Delaware	126
10	Ohio	103
11	Pennsylvania	100
11	Tennessee	100
11	Virginia	100
14	Louisiana	94
15	Illinois	93
15	New Hampshire	93
17	Maine	91
17	North Carolina	91
19	Florida	90
19	Missouri	90
21	California	88
22	Colorado	83
22	Kentucky	83
22	Minnesota	83
25	Washington	82
26	Michigan	81
26	West Virginia	81
28	Wisconsin	80
29	Georgia	77
30	Oregon	76
30	South Carolina	76
32	Nebraska	72
32	New Mexico	72
34	Alabama	71
35	Texas	68
36	Arizona	67
36	Utah	67
38	Arkansas	66
39	Kansas	65
40	Indiana	64
41	Alaska	60
42	Mississippi	56
43	Iowa	52
43	Montana	52
43	Nevada	52
43	North Dakota	52
47	Oklahoma	50
48	South Dakota	47
49	Wyoming	44
50	Idaho	31

District of Columbia   379

Source: Morgan Quitno Press using data from American Medical Association (Chicago, Illinois)
"Physician Characteristics and Distribution in the U.S." (2005 Edition)
*As of December 31, 2003. National rate does not include physicians in U.S. territories and possessions. Pediatrics includes Adolescent Medicine, Neonatal-Perinatal, Pediatric Allergy, Pediatric Endocrinology, Pediatric Pulmonology, Pediatric Hematology-Oncology and Pediatric Nephrology.

Physicians in Surgical Specialties in 2003

National Total = 158,813 Physicians*

ALPHA ORDER

RANK	STATE	PHYSICIANS	% of USA
25	Alabama	2,277	1.4%
48	Alaska	307	0.2%
23	Arizona	2,441	1.5%
32	Arkansas	1,164	0.7%
1	California	18,417	11.6%
24	Colorado	2,394	1.5%
22	Connecticut	2,563	1.6%
46	Delaware	420	0.3%
4	Florida	9,165	5.8%
12	Georgia	4,390	2.8%
38	Hawaii	850	0.5%
43	Idaho	588	0.4%
6	Illinois	6,577	4.1%
20	Indiana	2,713	1.7%
33	Iowa	1,160	0.7%
31	Kansas	1,268	0.8%
27	Kentucky	2,065	1.3%
18	Louisiana	2,879	1.8%
42	Maine	692	0.4%
14	Maryland	4,240	2.7%
10	Massachusetts	4,720	3.0%
9	Michigan	4,937	3.1%
21	Minnesota	2,587	1.6%
30	Mississippi	1,318	0.8%
17	Missouri	2,957	1.9%
44	Montana	508	0.3%
36	Nebraska	930	0.6%
37	Nevada	891	0.6%
41	New Hampshire	732	0.5%
8	New Jersey	5,442	3.4%
39	New Mexico	812	0.5%
2	New York	14,022	8.8%
11	North Carolina	4,614	2.9%
49	North Dakota	306	0.2%
7	Ohio	6,058	3.8%
29	Oklahoma	1,327	0.8%
28	Oregon	1,963	1.2%
5	Pennsylvania	7,378	4.6%
40	Rhode Island	754	0.5%
26	South Carolina	2,211	1.4%
47	South Dakota	360	0.2%
15	Tennessee	3,455	2.2%
3	Texas	10,229	6.4%
34	Utah	1,109	0.7%
45	Vermont	436	0.3%
13	Virginia	4,316	2.7%
16	Washington	3,131	2.0%
35	West Virginia	931	0.6%
19	Wisconsin	2,722	1.7%
50	Wyoming	235	0.1%

RANK ORDER

RANK	STATE	PHYSICIANS	% of USA
1	California	18,417	11.6%
2	New York	14,022	8.8%
3	Texas	10,229	6.4%
4	Florida	9,165	5.8%
5	Pennsylvania	7,378	4.6%
6	Illinois	6,577	4.1%
7	Ohio	6,058	3.8%
8	New Jersey	5,442	3.4%
9	Michigan	4,937	3.1%
10	Massachusetts	4,720	3.0%
11	North Carolina	4,614	2.9%
12	Georgia	4,390	2.8%
13	Virginia	4,316	2.7%
14	Maryland	4,240	2.7%
15	Tennessee	3,455	2.2%
16	Washington	3,131	2.0%
17	Missouri	2,957	1.9%
18	Louisiana	2,879	1.8%
19	Wisconsin	2,722	1.7%
20	Indiana	2,713	1.7%
21	Minnesota	2,587	1.6%
22	Connecticut	2,563	1.6%
23	Arizona	2,441	1.5%
24	Colorado	2,394	1.5%
25	Alabama	2,277	1.4%
26	South Carolina	2,211	1.4%
27	Kentucky	2,065	1.3%
28	Oregon	1,963	1.2%
29	Oklahoma	1,327	0.8%
30	Mississippi	1,318	0.8%
31	Kansas	1,268	0.8%
32	Arkansas	1,164	0.7%
33	Iowa	1,160	0.7%
34	Utah	1,109	0.7%
35	West Virginia	931	0.6%
36	Nebraska	930	0.6%
37	Nevada	891	0.6%
38	Hawaii	850	0.5%
39	New Mexico	812	0.5%
40	Rhode Island	754	0.5%
41	New Hampshire	732	0.5%
42	Maine	692	0.4%
43	Idaho	588	0.4%
44	Montana	508	0.3%
45	Vermont	436	0.3%
46	Delaware	420	0.3%
47	South Dakota	360	0.2%
48	Alaska	307	0.2%
49	North Dakota	306	0.2%
50	Wyoming	235	0.1%
	District of Columbia	852	0.5%

Source: American Medical Association (Chicago, Illinois)
  "Physician Characteristics and Distribution in the U.S." (2005 Edition)
*As of December 31, 2003. Total does not include 1,754 physicians in U.S. territories and possessions. Surgical Specialties include Colon and Rectal, General, Neurological, Obstetrics & Gynecology, Ophthalmology, Orthopedic, Otolaryngology, Plastic, Thoracic and Urological Surgeries.

Rate of Physicians in Surgical Specialties in 2003

National Rate = 55 Physicians per 100,000 Population*

ALPHA ORDER

RANK	STATE	RATE
26	Alabama	51
36	Alaska	47
43	Arizona	44
45	Arkansas	43
23	California	52
19	Colorado	53
2	Connecticut	74
26	Delaware	51
17	Florida	54
26	Georgia	51
7	Hawaii	68
45	Idaho	43
23	Illinois	52
43	Indiana	44
49	Iowa	39
36	Kansas	47
32	Kentucky	50
8	Louisiana	64
19	Maine	53
1	Maryland	77
2	Massachusetts	74
34	Michigan	49
26	Minnesota	51
41	Mississippi	46
23	Missouri	52
14	Montana	55
17	Nebraska	54
48	Nevada	40
13	New Hampshire	57
9	New Jersey	63
45	New Mexico	43
4	New York	73
14	North Carolina	55
35	North Dakota	48
19	Ohio	53
50	Oklahoma	38
14	Oregon	55
10	Pennsylvania	60
5	Rhode Island	70
19	South Carolina	53
36	South Dakota	47
11	Tennessee	59
41	Texas	46
36	Utah	47
5	Vermont	70
11	Virginia	59
26	Washington	51
26	West Virginia	51
32	Wisconsin	50
36	Wyoming	47

RANK ORDER

RANK	STATE	RATE
1	Maryland	77
2	Connecticut	74
2	Massachusetts	74
4	New York	73
5	Rhode Island	70
5	Vermont	70
7	Hawaii	68
8	Louisiana	64
9	New Jersey	63
10	Pennsylvania	60
11	Tennessee	59
11	Virginia	59
13	New Hampshire	57
14	Montana	55
14	North Carolina	55
14	Oregon	55
17	Florida	54
17	Nebraska	54
19	Colorado	53
19	Maine	53
19	Ohio	53
19	South Carolina	53
23	California	52
23	Illinois	52
23	Missouri	52
26	Alabama	51
26	Delaware	51
26	Georgia	51
26	Minnesota	51
26	Washington	51
26	West Virginia	51
32	Kentucky	50
32	Wisconsin	50
34	Michigan	49
35	North Dakota	48
36	Alaska	47
36	Kansas	47
36	South Dakota	47
36	Utah	47
36	Wyoming	47
41	Mississippi	46
41	Texas	46
43	Arizona	44
43	Indiana	44
45	Arkansas	43
45	Idaho	43
45	New Mexico	43
48	Nevada	40
49	Iowa	39
50	Oklahoma	38

	District of Columbia	153

Source: Morgan Quitno Press using data from American Medical Association (Chicago, Illinois)
    "Physician Characteristics and Distribution in the U.S." (2005 Edition)
*As of December 31, 2003. National rate does not include physicians in U.S. territories and possessions. Surgical Specialties include Colon and Rectal, General, Neurological, Obstetrics & Gynecology, Ophthalmology, Orthopedic, Otolaryngology, Plastic, Thoracic and Urological Surgeries.

Average Annual Wages of Surgeons in 2003

National Average = $182,690*

ALPHA ORDER

RANK	STATE	WAGES
14	Alabama	$194,840
4	Alaska	198,820
38	Arizona	177,970
27	Arkansas	185,200
41	California	170,520
8	Colorado	197,690
40	Connecticut	171,860
24	Delaware	188,220
47	Florida	158,770
23	Georgia	189,380
NA	Hawaii**	NA
15	Idaho	194,040
43	Illinois	169,600
25	Indiana	186,600
16	Iowa	193,630
35	Kansas	179,350
45	Kentucky	167,220
21	Louisiana	190,240
5	Maine	198,590
34	Maryland	179,580
28	Massachusetts	184,530
7	Michigan	198,190
10	Minnesota	196,480
42	Mississippi	169,850
12	Missouri	195,270
46	Montana	165,670
3	Nebraska	200,060
11	Nevada	195,850
1	New Hampshire	201,720
20	New Jersey	190,460
39	New Mexico	174,110
32	New York	180,850
22	North Carolina	189,800
33	North Dakota	180,240
9	Ohio	196,670
2	Oklahoma	201,580
NA	Oregon**	NA
44	Pennsylvania	167,820
6	Rhode Island	198,470
17	South Carolina	193,370
31	South Dakota	182,990
29	Tennessee	184,290
36	Texas	178,740
37	Utah	178,110
18	Vermont	191,550
26	Virginia	185,940
19	Washington	190,780
30	West Virginia	184,010
13	Wisconsin	195,150
NA	Wyoming**	NA

RANK ORDER

RANK	STATE	WAGES
1	New Hampshire	$201,720
2	Oklahoma	201,580
3	Nebraska	200,060
4	Alaska	198,820
5	Maine	198,590
6	Rhode Island	198,470
7	Michigan	198,190
8	Colorado	197,690
9	Ohio	196,670
10	Minnesota	196,480
11	Nevada	195,850
12	Missouri	195,270
13	Wisconsin	195,150
14	Alabama	194,840
15	Idaho	194,040
16	Iowa	193,630
17	South Carolina	193,370
18	Vermont	191,550
19	Washington	190,780
20	New Jersey	190,460
21	Louisiana	190,240
22	North Carolina	189,800
23	Georgia	189,380
24	Delaware	188,220
25	Indiana	186,600
26	Virginia	185,940
27	Arkansas	185,200
28	Massachusetts	184,530
29	Tennessee	184,290
30	West Virginia	184,010
31	South Dakota	182,990
32	New York	180,850
33	North Dakota	180,240
34	Maryland	179,580
35	Kansas	179,350
36	Texas	178,740
37	Utah	178,110
38	Arizona	177,970
39	New Mexico	174,110
40	Connecticut	171,860
41	California	170,520
42	Mississippi	169,850
43	Illinois	169,600
44	Pennsylvania	167,820
45	Kentucky	167,220
46	Montana	165,670
47	Florida	158,770
NA	Hawaii**	NA
NA	Oregon**	NA
NA	Wyoming**	NA
	District of Columbia	130,740

Source: U.S. Department of Labor, Bureau of Labor Statistics
   "Occupational Employment and Wages, 2003" (http://www.bls.gov/oes/)
*Does not include self-employed.
**Not available.

Physicians in General Surgery in 2003

National Total = 37,288 Physicians*

ALPHA ORDER

RANK ORDER

RANK	STATE	PHYSICIANS	% of USA
24	Alabama	550	1.5%
49	Alaska	71	0.2%
23	Arizona	577	1.5%
33	Arkansas	278	0.7%
1	California	3,949	10.6%
25	Colorado	546	1.5%
20	Connecticut	591	1.6%
45	Delaware	110	0.3%
5	Florida	1,888	5.1%
12	Georgia	1,011	2.7%
38	Hawaii	200	0.5%
43	Idaho	137	0.4%
6	Illinois	1,581	4.2%
21	Indiana	585	1.6%
30	Iowa	305	0.8%
29	Kansas	319	0.9%
26	Kentucky	533	1.4%
18	Louisiana	659	1.8%
40	Maine	188	0.5%
13	Maryland	970	2.6%
10	Massachusetts	1,249	3.3%
9	Michigan	1,276	3.4%
21	Minnesota	585	1.6%
32	Mississippi	301	0.8%
17	Missouri	684	1.8%
45	Montana	110	0.3%
35	Nebraska	249	0.7%
39	Nevada	199	0.5%
42	New Hampshire	182	0.5%
8	New Jersey	1,283	3.4%
37	New Mexico	205	0.5%
2	New York	3,475	9.3%
11	North Carolina	1,074	2.9%
48	North Dakota	84	0.2%
7	Ohio	1,530	4.1%
30	Oklahoma	305	0.8%
28	Oregon	466	1.2%
4	Pennsylvania	1,897	5.1%
41	Rhode Island	187	0.5%
27	South Carolina	529	1.4%
47	South Dakota	94	0.3%
15	Tennessee	856	2.3%
3	Texas	2,211	5.9%
36	Utah	216	0.6%
44	Vermont	132	0.4%
14	Virginia	966	2.6%
16	Washington	711	1.9%
34	West Virginia	263	0.7%
19	Wisconsin	630	1.7%
50	Wyoming	52	0.1%

RANK	STATE	PHYSICIANS	% of USA
1	California	3,949	10.6%
2	New York	3,475	9.3%
3	Texas	2,211	5.9%
4	Pennsylvania	1,897	5.1%
5	Florida	1,888	5.1%
6	Illinois	1,581	4.2%
7	Ohio	1,530	4.1%
8	New Jersey	1,283	3.4%
9	Michigan	1,276	3.4%
10	Massachusetts	1,249	3.3%
11	North Carolina	1,074	2.9%
12	Georgia	1,011	2.7%
13	Maryland	970	2.6%
14	Virginia	966	2.6%
15	Tennessee	856	2.3%
16	Washington	711	1.9%
17	Missouri	684	1.8%
18	Louisiana	659	1.8%
19	Wisconsin	630	1.7%
20	Connecticut	591	1.6%
21	Indiana	585	1.6%
21	Minnesota	585	1.6%
23	Arizona	577	1.5%
24	Alabama	550	1.5%
25	Colorado	546	1.5%
26	Kentucky	533	1.4%
27	South Carolina	529	1.4%
28	Oregon	466	1.2%
29	Kansas	319	0.9%
30	Iowa	305	0.8%
30	Oklahoma	305	0.8%
32	Mississippi	301	0.8%
33	Arkansas	278	0.7%
34	West Virginia	263	0.7%
35	Nebraska	249	0.7%
36	Utah	216	0.6%
37	New Mexico	205	0.5%
38	Hawaii	200	0.5%
39	Nevada	199	0.5%
40	Maine	188	0.5%
41	Rhode Island	187	0.5%
42	New Hampshire	182	0.5%
43	Idaho	137	0.4%
44	Vermont	132	0.4%
45	Delaware	110	0.3%
45	Montana	110	0.3%
47	South Dakota	94	0.3%
48	North Dakota	84	0.2%
49	Alaska	71	0.2%
50	Wyoming	52	0.1%
	District of Columbia	239	0.6%

Source: American Medical Association (Chicago, Illinois)
   "Physician Characteristics and Distribution in the U.S." (2005 Edition)
*As of December 31, 2003. Total does not include 470 physicians in U.S. territories and possessions. General Surgery includes Abdominal, Cardiovascular, Hand, Head and Neck, Pediatric, Traumatic and Vascular Surgeries.

Rate of Physicians in General Surgery in 2003

National Rate = 13 Physicians per 100,000 Population*

ALPHA ORDER

RANK ORDER

RANK	STATE	RATE	RANK	STATE	RATE
25	Alabama	12	1	Vermont	21
36	Alaska	11	2	Massachusetts	19
40	Arizona	10	3	Maryland	18
40	Arkansas	10	3	New York	18
36	California	11	5	Connecticut	17
25	Colorado	12	5	Rhode Island	17
5	Connecticut	17	7	Hawaii	16
16	Delaware	13	8	Louisiana	15
36	Florida	11	8	New Jersey	15
25	Georgia	12	8	Pennsylvania	15
7	Hawaii	16	8	Tennessee	15
40	Idaho	10	8	West Virginia	15
25	Illinois	12	13	Maine	14
47	Indiana	9	13	Nebraska	14
40	Iowa	10	13	New Hampshire	14
25	Kansas	12	16	Delaware	13
16	Kentucky	13	16	Kentucky	13
8	Louisiana	15	16	Michigan	13
13	Maine	14	16	North Carolina	13
3	Maryland	18	16	North Dakota	13
2	Massachusetts	19	16	Ohio	13
16	Michigan	13	16	Oregon	13
25	Minnesota	12	16	South Carolina	13
40	Mississippi	10	16	Virginia	13
25	Missouri	12	25	Alabama	12
25	Montana	12	25	Colorado	12
13	Nebraska	14	25	Georgia	12
47	Nevada	9	25	Illinois	12
13	New Hampshire	14	25	Kansas	12
8	New Jersey	15	25	Minnesota	12
36	New Mexico	11	25	Missouri	12
3	New York	18	25	Montana	12
16	North Carolina	13	25	South Dakota	12
16	North Dakota	13	25	Washington	12
16	Ohio	13	25	Wisconsin	12
47	Oklahoma	9	36	Alaska	11
16	Oregon	13	36	California	11
8	Pennsylvania	15	36	Florida	11
5	Rhode Island	17	36	New Mexico	11
16	South Carolina	13	40	Arizona	10
25	South Dakota	12	40	Arkansas	10
8	Tennessee	15	40	Idaho	10
40	Texas	10	40	Iowa	10
47	Utah	9	40	Mississippi	10
1	Vermont	21	40	Texas	10
16	Virginia	13	40	Wyoming	10
25	Washington	12	47	Indiana	9
8	West Virginia	15	47	Nevada	9
25	Wisconsin	12	47	Oklahoma	9
40	Wyoming	10	47	Utah	9
				District of Columbia	43

Source: Morgan Quitno Press using data from American Medical Association (Chicago, Illinois)
    "Physician Characteristics and Distribution in the U.S." (2005 Edition)
*As of December 31, 2003. National rate does not include physicians in U.S. territories and possessions. General
Surgery includes Abdominal, Cardiovascular, Hand, Head and Neck, Pediatric, Traumatic and Vascular Surgeries.

Physicians in Obstetrics and Gynecology in 2003

National Total = 41,312 Physicians*

ALPHA ORDER

RANK	STATE	PHYSICIANS	% of USA
26	Alabama	583	1.4%
47	Alaska	76	0.2%
21	Arizona	646	1.6%
34	Arkansas	258	0.6%
1	California	4,887	11.8%
22	Colorado	628	1.5%
19	Connecticut	711	1.7%
45	Delaware	109	0.3%
4	Florida	2,177	5.3%
9	Georgia	1,374	3.3%
35	Hawaii	252	0.6%
43	Idaho	134	0.3%
5	Illinois	1,870	4.5%
20	Indiana	709	1.7%
36	Iowa	223	0.5%
31	Kansas	287	0.7%
28	Kentucky	499	1.2%
17	Louisiana	733	1.8%
42	Maine	153	0.4%
14	Maryland	1,126	2.7%
13	Massachusetts	1,159	2.8%
10	Michigan	1,363	3.3%
25	Minnesota	585	1.4%
29	Mississippi	339	0.8%
18	Missouri	730	1.8%
44	Montana	112	0.3%
41	Nebraska	198	0.5%
32	Nevada	267	0.6%
38	New Hampshire	207	0.5%
7	New Jersey	1,586	3.8%
39	New Mexico	200	0.5%
2	New York	3,771	9.1%
11	North Carolina	1,266	3.1%
50	North Dakota	51	0.1%
8	Ohio	1,538	3.7%
30	Oklahoma	316	0.8%
27	Oregon	501	1.2%
6	Pennsylvania	1,724	4.2%
39	Rhode Island	200	0.5%
23	South Carolina	590	1.4%
48	South Dakota	67	0.2%
15	Tennessee	848	2.1%
3	Texas	2,845	6.9%
32	Utah	267	0.6%
46	Vermont	106	0.3%
12	Virginia	1,213	2.9%
16	Washington	739	1.8%
37	West Virginia	210	0.5%
23	Wisconsin	590	1.4%
49	Wyoming	57	0.1%

RANK ORDER

RANK	STATE	PHYSICIANS	% of USA
1	California	4,887	11.8%
2	New York	3,771	9.1%
3	Texas	2,845	6.9%
4	Florida	2,177	5.3%
5	Illinois	1,870	4.5%
6	Pennsylvania	1,724	4.2%
7	New Jersey	1,586	3.8%
8	Ohio	1,538	3.7%
9	Georgia	1,374	3.3%
10	Michigan	1,363	3.3%
11	North Carolina	1,266	3.1%
12	Virginia	1,213	2.9%
13	Massachusetts	1,159	2.8%
14	Maryland	1,126	2.7%
15	Tennessee	848	2.1%
16	Washington	739	1.8%
17	Louisiana	733	1.8%
18	Missouri	730	1.8%
19	Connecticut	711	1.7%
20	Indiana	709	1.7%
21	Arizona	646	1.6%
22	Colorado	628	1.5%
23	South Carolina	590	1.4%
23	Wisconsin	590	1.4%
25	Minnesota	585	1.4%
26	Alabama	583	1.4%
27	Oregon	501	1.2%
28	Kentucky	499	1.2%
29	Mississippi	339	0.8%
30	Oklahoma	316	0.8%
31	Kansas	287	0.7%
32	Nevada	267	0.6%
32	Utah	267	0.6%
34	Arkansas	258	0.6%
35	Hawaii	252	0.6%
36	Iowa	223	0.5%
37	West Virginia	210	0.5%
38	New Hampshire	207	0.5%
39	New Mexico	200	0.5%
39	Rhode Island	200	0.5%
41	Nebraska	198	0.5%
42	Maine	153	0.4%
43	Idaho	134	0.3%
44	Montana	112	0.3%
45	Delaware	109	0.3%
46	Vermont	106	0.3%
47	Alaska	76	0.2%
48	South Dakota	67	0.2%
49	Wyoming	57	0.1%
50	North Dakota	51	0.1%
	District of Columbia	232	0.6%

Source: American Medical Association (Chicago, Illinois)
    "Physician Characteristics and Distribution in the U.S." (2005 Edition)
*As of December 31, 2003. Total does not include 604 physicians in U.S. territories and possessions. Obstetrics and Gynecology includes Gynecology and Oncology, Maternal and Fetal Medicine and Reproductive Endocrinology.

Rate of Physicians in Obstetrics and Gynecology in 2003

National Rate = 29 Physicians per 100,000 Female Population*

ALPHA ORDER

RANK	STATE	RATE
22	Alabama	27
34	Alaska	23
34	Arizona	23
46	Arkansas	19
18	California	28
22	Colorado	27
1	Connecticut	42
22	Delaware	27
25	Florida	26
12	Georgia	32
4	Hawaii	40
45	Idaho	20
14	Illinois	30
34	Indiana	23
50	Iowa	15
44	Kansas	21
28	Kentucky	25
9	Louisiana	34
29	Maine	24
1	Maryland	42
7	Massachusetts	37
18	Michigan	28
34	Minnesota	23
29	Mississippi	24
25	Missouri	26
29	Montana	24
34	Nebraska	23
34	Nevada	23
10	New Hampshire	33
6	New Jersey	38
42	New Mexico	22
3	New York	41
13	North Carolina	31
49	North Dakota	16
18	Ohio	28
47	Oklahoma	18
18	Oregon	28
16	Pennsylvania	29
5	Rhode Island	39
16	South Carolina	29
47	South Dakota	18
14	Tennessee	30
25	Texas	26
34	Utah	23
8	Vermont	35
10	Virginia	33
29	Washington	24
29	West Virginia	24
42	Wisconsin	22
34	Wyoming	23

RANK ORDER

RANK	STATE	RATE
1	Connecticut	42
1	Maryland	42
3	New York	41
4	Hawaii	40
5	Rhode Island	39
6	New Jersey	38
7	Massachusetts	37
8	Vermont	35
9	Louisiana	34
10	New Hampshire	33
10	Virginia	33
12	Georgia	32
13	North Carolina	31
14	Illinois	30
14	Tennessee	30
16	Pennsylvania	29
16	South Carolina	29
18	California	28
18	Michigan	28
18	Ohio	28
18	Oregon	28
22	Alabama	27
22	Colorado	27
22	Delaware	27
25	Florida	26
25	Missouri	26
25	Texas	26
28	Kentucky	25
29	Maine	24
29	Mississippi	24
29	Montana	24
29	Washington	24
29	West Virginia	24
34	Alaska	23
34	Arizona	23
34	Indiana	23
34	Minnesota	23
34	Nebraska	23
34	Nevada	23
34	Utah	23
34	Wyoming	23
42	New Mexico	22
42	Wisconsin	22
44	Kansas	21
45	Idaho	20
46	Arkansas	19
47	Oklahoma	18
47	South Dakota	18
49	North Dakota	16
50	Iowa	15

District of Columbia 87

*Source: Morgan Quitno Press using data from American Medical Association (Chicago, Illinois)
"Physician Characteristics and Distribution in the U.S." (2005 Edition)*
As of December 31, 2003. National rate does not include physicians in U.S. territories and possessions. Obstetrics and Gynecology includes Gynecology and Oncology, Maternal and Fetal Medicine and Reproductive Endocrinology.

Physicians in Ophthalmology in 2003

National Total = 18,543 Physicians*

ALPHA ORDER

RANK	STATE	PHYSICIANS	% of USA
27	Alabama	221	1.2%
49	Alaska	27	0.1%
22	Arizona	285	1.5%
33	Arkansas	140	0.8%
1	California	2,267	12.2%
24	Colorado	268	1.4%
21	Connecticut	317	1.7%
46	Delaware	41	0.2%
3	Florida	1,223	6.6%
14	Georgia	426	2.3%
37	Hawaii	99	0.5%
43	Idaho	62	0.3%
6	Illinois	738	4.0%
23	Indiana	283	1.5%
29	Iowa	164	0.9%
30	Kansas	155	0.8%
28	Kentucky	199	1.1%
18	Louisiana	343	1.8%
41	Maine	77	0.4%
10	Maryland	559	3.0%
11	Massachusetts	551	3.0%
9	Michigan	582	3.1%
20	Minnesota	322	1.7%
31	Mississippi	147	0.8%
17	Missouri	354	1.9%
44	Montana	56	0.3%
35	Nebraska	100	0.5%
38	Nevada	93	0.5%
42	New Hampshire	74	0.4%
8	New Jersey	636	3.4%
39	New Mexico	85	0.5%
2	New York	1,808	9.8%
13	North Carolina	448	2.4%
48	North Dakota	37	0.2%
7	Ohio	650	3.5%
32	Oklahoma	145	0.8%
26	Oregon	228	1.2%
5	Pennsylvania	896	4.8%
40	Rhode Island	84	0.5%
25	South Carolina	252	1.4%
46	South Dakota	41	0.2%
16	Tennessee	358	1.9%
4	Texas	1,119	6.0%
34	Utah	123	0.7%
45	Vermont	50	0.3%
12	Virginia	468	2.5%
15	Washington	382	2.1%
35	West Virginia	100	0.5%
18	Wisconsin	343	1.8%
50	Wyoming	18	0.1%

RANK ORDER

RANK	STATE	PHYSICIANS	% of USA
1	California	2,267	12.2%
2	New York	1,808	9.8%
3	Florida	1,223	6.6%
4	Texas	1,119	6.0%
5	Pennsylvania	896	4.8%
6	Illinois	738	4.0%
7	Ohio	650	3.5%
8	New Jersey	636	3.4%
9	Michigan	582	3.1%
10	Maryland	559	3.0%
11	Massachusetts	551	3.0%
12	Virginia	468	2.5%
13	North Carolina	448	2.4%
14	Georgia	426	2.3%
15	Washington	382	2.1%
16	Tennessee	358	1.9%
17	Missouri	354	1.9%
18	Louisiana	343	1.8%
18	Wisconsin	343	1.8%
20	Minnesota	322	1.7%
21	Connecticut	317	1.7%
22	Arizona	285	1.5%
23	Indiana	283	1.5%
24	Colorado	268	1.4%
25	South Carolina	252	1.4%
26	Oregon	228	1.2%
27	Alabama	221	1.2%
28	Kentucky	199	1.1%
29	Iowa	164	0.9%
30	Kansas	155	0.8%
31	Mississippi	147	0.8%
32	Oklahoma	145	0.8%
33	Arkansas	140	0.8%
34	Utah	123	0.7%
35	Nebraska	100	0.5%
35	West Virginia	100	0.5%
37	Hawaii	99	0.5%
38	Nevada	93	0.5%
39	New Mexico	85	0.5%
40	Rhode Island	84	0.5%
41	Maine	77	0.4%
42	New Hampshire	74	0.4%
43	Idaho	62	0.3%
44	Montana	56	0.3%
45	Vermont	50	0.3%
46	Delaware	41	0.2%
46	South Dakota	41	0.2%
48	North Dakota	37	0.2%
49	Alaska	27	0.1%
50	Wyoming	18	0.1%
	District of Columbia	99	0.5%

Source: American Medical Association (Chicago, Illinois)
    "Physician Characteristics and Distribution in the U.S." (2005 Edition)
*As of December 31, 2003. Total does not include 190 physicians in U.S. territories and possessions.
Ophthalmology is the branch of medicine dealing with the anatomy, functions and diseases of the eye.

Rate of Physicians in Ophthalmology in 2003

National Rate = 6 Physicians per 100,000 Population*

<u>ALPHA ORDER</u>

RANK	STATE	RATE
33	Alabama	5
47	Alaska	4
33	Arizona	5
33	Arkansas	5
12	California	6
12	Colorado	6
2	Connecticut	9
33	Delaware	5
9	Florida	7
33	Georgia	5
5	Hawaii	8
33	Idaho	5
12	Illinois	6
33	Indiana	5
12	Iowa	6
12	Kansas	6
33	Kentucky	5
5	Louisiana	8
12	Maine	6
1	Maryland	10
2	Massachusetts	9
12	Michigan	6
12	Minnesota	6
33	Mississippi	5
12	Missouri	6
12	Montana	6
12	Nebraska	6
47	Nevada	4
12	New Hampshire	6
9	New Jersey	7
33	New Mexico	5
2	New York	9
33	North Carolina	5
12	North Dakota	6
12	Ohio	6
47	Oklahoma	4
12	Oregon	6
9	Pennsylvania	7
5	Rhode Island	8
12	South Carolina	6
33	South Dakota	5
12	Tennessee	6
33	Texas	5
33	Utah	5
5	Vermont	8
12	Virginia	6
12	Washington	6
12	West Virginia	6
12	Wisconsin	6
47	Wyoming	4

<u>RANK ORDER</u>

RANK	STATE	RATE
1	Maryland	10
2	Connecticut	9
2	Massachusetts	9
2	New York	9
5	Hawaii	8
5	Louisiana	8
5	Rhode Island	8
5	Vermont	8
9	Florida	7
9	New Jersey	7
9	Pennsylvania	7
12	California	6
12	Colorado	6
12	Illinois	6
12	Iowa	6
12	Kansas	6
12	Maine	6
12	Michigan	6
12	Minnesota	6
12	Missouri	6
12	Montana	6
12	Nebraska	6
12	New Hampshire	6
12	North Dakota	6
12	Ohio	6
12	Oregon	6
12	South Carolina	6
12	Tennessee	6
12	Virginia	6
12	Washington	6
12	West Virginia	6
12	Wisconsin	6
33	Alabama	5
33	Arizona	5
33	Arkansas	5
33	Delaware	5
33	Georgia	5
33	Idaho	5
33	Indiana	5
33	Kentucky	5
33	Mississippi	5
33	New Mexico	5
33	North Carolina	5
33	South Dakota	5
33	Texas	5
33	Utah	5
47	Alaska	4
47	Nevada	4
47	Oklahoma	4
47	Wyoming	4

District of Columbia   18

Source: Morgan Quitno Press using data from American Medical Association (Chicago, Illinois)
   "Physician Characteristics and Distribution in the U.S." (2005 Edition)
*As of December 31, 2003. National rate does not include physicians in U.S. territories and possessions.
Ophthalmology is the branch of medicine dealing with the anatomy, functions and diseases of the eye.

Physicians in Orthopedic Surgery in 2003

National Total = 23,329 Physicians*

ALPHA ORDER

RANK	STATE	PHYSICIANS	% of USA
26	Alabama	348	1.5%
46	Alaska	66	0.3%
25	Arizona	350	1.5%
33	Arkansas	188	0.8%
1	California	2,823	12.1%
21	Colorado	413	1.8%
23	Connecticut	373	1.6%
47	Delaware	63	0.3%
4	Florida	1,308	5.6%
13	Georgia	591	2.5%
42	Hawaii	117	0.5%
43	Idaho	116	0.5%
7	Illinois	869	3.7%
19	Indiana	448	1.9%
32	Iowa	189	0.8%
30	Kansas	202	0.9%
28	Kentucky	296	1.3%
22	Louisiana	402	1.7%
37	Maine	127	0.5%
14	Maryland	584	2.5%
8	Massachusetts	718	3.1%
12	Michigan	603	2.6%
18	Minnesota	452	1.9%
34	Mississippi	184	0.8%
20	Missouri	430	1.8%
44	Montana	106	0.5%
35	Nebraska	165	0.7%
38	Nevada	121	0.5%
39	New Hampshire	120	0.5%
9	New Jersey	712	3.1%
36	New Mexico	145	0.6%
2	New York	1,782	7.6%
10	North Carolina	691	3.0%
50	North Dakota	46	0.2%
6	Ohio	873	3.7%
29	Oklahoma	214	0.9%
27	Oregon	310	1.3%
5	Pennsylvania	1,071	4.6%
41	Rhode Island	118	0.5%
24	South Carolina	356	1.5%
48	South Dakota	62	0.3%
16	Tennessee	522	2.2%
3	Texas	1,473	6.3%
30	Utah	202	0.9%
45	Vermont	72	0.3%
11	Virginia	619	2.7%
15	Washington	533	2.3%
39	West Virginia	120	0.5%
17	Wisconsin	470	2.0%
49	Wyoming	61	0.3%

RANK ORDER

RANK	STATE	PHYSICIANS	% of USA
1	California	2,823	12.1%
2	New York	1,782	7.6%
3	Texas	1,473	6.3%
4	Florida	1,308	5.6%
5	Pennsylvania	1,071	4.6%
6	Ohio	873	3.7%
7	Illinois	869	3.7%
8	Massachusetts	718	3.1%
9	New Jersey	712	3.1%
10	North Carolina	691	3.0%
11	Virginia	619	2.7%
12	Michigan	603	2.6%
13	Georgia	591	2.5%
14	Maryland	584	2.5%
15	Washington	533	2.3%
16	Tennessee	522	2.2%
17	Wisconsin	470	2.0%
18	Minnesota	452	1.9%
19	Indiana	448	1.9%
20	Missouri	430	1.8%
21	Colorado	413	1.8%
22	Louisiana	402	1.7%
23	Connecticut	373	1.6%
24	South Carolina	356	1.5%
25	Arizona	350	1.5%
26	Alabama	348	1.5%
27	Oregon	310	1.3%
28	Kentucky	296	1.3%
29	Oklahoma	214	0.9%
30	Kansas	202	0.9%
30	Utah	202	0.9%
32	Iowa	189	0.8%
33	Arkansas	188	0.8%
34	Mississippi	184	0.8%
35	Nebraska	165	0.7%
36	New Mexico	145	0.6%
37	Maine	127	0.5%
38	Nevada	121	0.5%
39	New Hampshire	120	0.5%
39	West Virginia	120	0.5%
41	Rhode Island	118	0.5%
42	Hawaii	117	0.5%
43	Idaho	116	0.5%
44	Montana	106	0.5%
45	Vermont	72	0.3%
46	Alaska	66	0.3%
47	Delaware	63	0.3%
48	South Dakota	62	0.3%
49	Wyoming	61	0.3%
50	North Dakota	46	0.2%
	District of Columbia	105	0.5%

Source: American Medical Association (Chicago, Illinois)
    "Physician Characteristics and Distribution in the U.S." (2005 Edition)
As of December 31, 2003. Total does not include 175 physicians in U.S. territories and possessions.
Orthopedics is the branch of medicine dealing with the skeletal system.

Rate of Physicians in Orthopedic Surgery in 2003

National Rate = 8 Physicians per 100,000 Population*

ALPHA ORDER

RANK	STATE	RATE
24	Alabama	8
8	Alaska	10
45	Arizona	6
36	Arkansas	7
24	California	8
10	Colorado	9
4	Connecticut	11
24	Delaware	8
24	Florida	8
36	Georgia	7
10	Hawaii	9
24	Idaho	8
36	Illinois	7
36	Indiana	7
45	Iowa	6
36	Kansas	7
36	Kentucky	7
10	Louisiana	9
8	Maine	10
4	Maryland	11
4	Massachusetts	11
45	Michigan	6
10	Minnesota	9
45	Mississippi	6
24	Missouri	8
1	Montana	12
10	Nebraska	9
50	Nevada	5
10	New Hampshire	9
24	New Jersey	8
24	New Mexico	8
10	New York	9
24	North Carolina	8
36	North Dakota	7
24	Ohio	8
45	Oklahoma	6
10	Oregon	9
10	Pennsylvania	9
4	Rhode Island	11
10	South Carolina	9
24	South Dakota	8
10	Tennessee	9
36	Texas	7
10	Utah	9
1	Vermont	12
24	Virginia	8
10	Washington	9
36	West Virginia	7
10	Wisconsin	9
1	Wyoming	12

RANK ORDER

RANK	STATE	RATE
1	Montana	12
1	Vermont	12
1	Wyoming	12
4	Connecticut	11
4	Maryland	11
4	Massachusetts	11
4	Rhode Island	11
8	Alaska	10
8	Maine	10
10	Colorado	9
10	Hawaii	9
10	Louisiana	9
10	Minnesota	9
10	Nebraska	9
10	New Hampshire	9
10	New York	9
10	Oregon	9
10	Pennsylvania	9
10	South Carolina	9
10	Tennessee	9
10	Utah	9
10	Washington	9
10	Wisconsin	9
24	Alabama	8
24	California	8
24	Delaware	8
24	Florida	8
24	Idaho	8
24	Missouri	8
24	New Jersey	8
24	New Mexico	8
24	North Carolina	8
24	Ohio	8
24	South Dakota	8
24	Virginia	8
36	Arkansas	7
36	Georgia	7
36	Illinois	7
36	Indiana	7
36	Kansas	7
36	Kentucky	7
36	North Dakota	7
36	Texas	7
36	West Virginia	7
45	Arizona	6
45	Iowa	6
45	Michigan	6
45	Mississippi	6
45	Oklahoma	6
50	Nevada	5

District of Columbia   19

Source: Morgan Quitno Press using data from American Medical Association (Chicago, Illinois)
"Physician Characteristics and Distribution in the U.S." (2005 Edition)
As of December 31, 2003. National rate does not include physicians in U.S. territories and possessions.
Orthopedics is the branch of medicine dealing with the skeletal system.

Physicians in Plastic Surgery in 2003

National Total = 6,670 Physicians*

ALPHA ORDER

RANK	STATE	PHYSICIANS	% of USA
26	Alabama	78	1.2%
49	Alaska	8	0.1%
17	Arizona	132	2.0%
34	Arkansas	35	0.5%
1	California	993	14.9%
21	Colorado	94	1.4%
20	Connecticut	96	1.4%
43	Delaware	19	0.3%
3	Florida	540	8.1%
13	Georgia	168	2.5%
34	Hawaii	35	0.5%
41	Idaho	23	0.3%
6	Illinois	247	3.7%
19	Indiana	102	1.5%
40	Iowa	25	0.4%
30	Kansas	59	0.9%
22	Kentucky	91	1.4%
24	Louisiana	86	1.3%
45	Maine	13	0.2%
12	Maryland	170	2.5%
10	Massachusetts	180	2.7%
9	Michigan	197	3.0%
22	Minnesota	91	1.4%
33	Mississippi	42	0.6%
16	Missouri	134	2.0%
44	Montana	17	0.3%
38	Nebraska	27	0.4%
31	Nevada	44	0.7%
42	New Hampshire	21	0.3%
7	New Jersey	219	3.3%
39	New Mexico	26	0.4%
2	New York	614	9.2%
14	North Carolina	165	2.5%
45	North Dakota	13	0.2%
8	Ohio	210	3.1%
32	Oklahoma	43	0.6%
29	Oregon	65	1.0%
5	Pennsylvania	257	3.9%
37	Rhode Island	29	0.4%
28	South Carolina	69	1.0%
47	South Dakota	10	0.1%
15	Tennessee	148	2.2%
4	Texas	506	7.6%
27	Utah	70	1.0%
47	Vermont	10	0.1%
11	Virginia	176	2.6%
18	Washington	121	1.8%
36	West Virginia	30	0.4%
24	Wisconsin	86	1.3%
50	Wyoming	3	0.0%

RANK ORDER

RANK	STATE	PHYSICIANS	% of USA
1	California	993	14.9%
2	New York	614	9.2%
3	Florida	540	8.1%
4	Texas	506	7.6%
5	Pennsylvania	257	3.9%
6	Illinois	247	3.7%
7	New Jersey	219	3.3%
8	Ohio	210	3.1%
9	Michigan	197	3.0%
10	Massachusetts	180	2.7%
11	Virginia	176	2.6%
12	Maryland	170	2.5%
13	Georgia	168	2.5%
14	North Carolina	165	2.5%
15	Tennessee	148	2.2%
16	Missouri	134	2.0%
17	Arizona	132	2.0%
18	Washington	121	1.8%
19	Indiana	102	1.5%
20	Connecticut	96	1.4%
21	Colorado	94	1.4%
22	Kentucky	91	1.4%
22	Minnesota	91	1.4%
24	Louisiana	86	1.3%
24	Wisconsin	86	1.3%
26	Alabama	78	1.2%
27	Utah	70	1.0%
28	South Carolina	69	1.0%
29	Oregon	65	1.0%
30	Kansas	59	0.9%
31	Nevada	44	0.7%
32	Oklahoma	43	0.6%
33	Mississippi	42	0.6%
34	Arkansas	35	0.5%
34	Hawaii	35	0.5%
36	West Virginia	30	0.4%
37	Rhode Island	29	0.4%
38	Nebraska	27	0.4%
39	New Mexico	26	0.4%
40	Iowa	25	0.4%
41	Idaho	23	0.3%
42	New Hampshire	21	0.3%
43	Delaware	19	0.3%
44	Montana	17	0.3%
45	Maine	13	0.2%
45	North Dakota	13	0.2%
47	South Dakota	10	0.1%
47	Vermont	10	0.1%
49	Alaska	8	0.1%
50	Wyoming	3	0.0%
	District of Columbia	33	0.5%

Source: American Medical Association (Chicago, Illinois)
   "Physician Characteristics and Distribution in the U.S." (2005 Edition)
As of December 31, 2003. Total does not include 36 physicians in U.S. territories and possessions.

Rate of Physicians in Plastic Surgery in 2003

National Rate = 2 Physicians per 100,000 Population*

ALPHA ORDER

RANK	STATE	RATE
12	Alabama	2
42	Alaska	1
12	Arizona	2
42	Arkansas	1
1	California	3
12	Colorado	2
1	Connecticut	3
12	Delaware	2
1	Florida	3
12	Georgia	2
1	Hawaii	3
12	Idaho	2
12	Illinois	2
12	Indiana	2
42	Iowa	1
12	Kansas	2
12	Kentucky	2
12	Louisiana	2
42	Maine	1
1	Maryland	3
1	Massachusetts	3
12	Michigan	2
12	Minnesota	2
42	Mississippi	1
12	Missouri	2
12	Montana	2
12	Nebraska	2
12	Nevada	2
12	New Hampshire	2
1	New Jersey	3
42	New Mexico	1
1	New York	3
12	North Carolina	2
12	North Dakota	2
12	Ohio	2
42	Oklahoma	1
12	Oregon	2
12	Pennsylvania	2
1	Rhode Island	3
12	South Carolina	2
42	South Dakota	1
1	Tennessee	3
12	Texas	2
1	Utah	3
12	Vermont	2
12	Virginia	2
12	Washington	2
12	West Virginia	2
12	Wisconsin	2
42	Wyoming	1

RANK ORDER

RANK	STATE	RATE
1	California	3
1	Connecticut	3
1	Florida	3
1	Hawaii	3
1	Maryland	3
1	Massachusetts	3
1	New Jersey	3
1	New York	3
1	Rhode Island	3
1	Tennessee	3
1	Utah	3
12	Alabama	2
12	Arizona	2
12	Colorado	2
12	Delaware	2
12	Georgia	2
12	Idaho	2
12	Illinois	2
12	Indiana	2
12	Kansas	2
12	Kentucky	2
12	Louisiana	2
12	Michigan	2
12	Minnesota	2
12	Missouri	2
12	Montana	2
12	Nebraska	2
12	Nevada	2
12	New Hampshire	2
12	North Carolina	2
12	North Dakota	2
12	Ohio	2
12	Oregon	2
12	Pennsylvania	2
12	South Carolina	2
12	Texas	2
12	Vermont	2
12	Virginia	2
12	Washington	2
12	West Virginia	2
12	Wisconsin	2
42	Alaska	1
42	Arkansas	1
42	Iowa	1
42	Maine	1
42	Mississippi	1
42	New Mexico	1
42	Oklahoma	1
42	South Dakota	1
42	Wyoming	1

District of Columbia   6

Source: Morgan Quitno Press using data from American Medical Association (Chicago, Illinois)
    "Physician Characteristics and Distribution in the U.S." (2005 Edition)
*As of December 31, 2003. National rate does not include physicians in U.S. territories and possessions.

Physicians in Other Specialties in 2003

National Total = 204,613 Physicians*

ALPHA ORDER

RANK	STATE	PHYSICIANS	% of USA
28	Alabama	2,258	1.1%
47	Alaska	391	0.2%
22	Arizona	3,352	1.6%
33	Arkansas	1,357	0.7%
1	California	25,152	12.3%
23	Colorado	3,279	1.6%
20	Connecticut	3,475	1.7%
46	Delaware	542	0.3%
4	Florida	10,855	5.3%
14	Georgia	4,986	2.4%
37	Hawaii	1,085	0.5%
44	Idaho	576	0.3%
6	Illinois	8,890	4.3%
18	Indiana	3,652	1.8%
32	Iowa	1,379	0.7%
29	Kansas	1,549	0.8%
27	Kentucky	2,379	1.2%
24	Louisiana	2,905	1.4%
39	Maine	1,004	0.5%
10	Maryland	6,452	3.2%
7	Massachusetts	8,211	4.0%
11	Michigan	6,204	3.0%
21	Minnesota	3,444	1.7%
35	Mississippi	1,246	0.6%
19	Missouri	3,494	1.7%
45	Montana	545	0.3%
40	Nebraska	1,002	0.5%
36	Nevada	1,172	0.6%
42	New Hampshire	929	0.5%
9	New Jersey	6,684	3.3%
34	New Mexico	1,247	0.6%
2	New York	19,729	9.6%
12	North Carolina	5,499	2.7%
49	North Dakota	357	0.2%
8	Ohio	7,399	3.6%
30	Oklahoma	1,507	0.7%
25	Oregon	2,589	1.3%
5	Pennsylvania	10,002	4.9%
41	Rhode Island	933	0.5%
26	South Carolina	2,425	1.2%
48	South Dakota	381	0.2%
17	Tennessee	3,655	1.8%
3	Texas	12,282	6.0%
31	Utah	1,392	0.7%
43	Vermont	641	0.3%
13	Virginia	5,345	2.6%
15	Washington	4,544	2.2%
38	West Virginia	1,016	0.5%
16	Wisconsin	3,742	1.8%
50	Wyoming	249	0.1%

RANK ORDER

RANK	STATE	PHYSICIANS	% of USA
1	California	25,152	12.3%
2	New York	19,729	9.6%
3	Texas	12,282	6.0%
4	Florida	10,855	5.3%
5	Pennsylvania	10,002	4.9%
6	Illinois	8,890	4.3%
7	Massachusetts	8,211	4.0%
8	Ohio	7,399	3.6%
9	New Jersey	6,684	3.3%
10	Maryland	6,452	3.2%
11	Michigan	6,204	3.0%
12	North Carolina	5,499	2.7%
13	Virginia	5,345	2.6%
14	Georgia	4,986	2.4%
15	Washington	4,544	2.2%
16	Wisconsin	3,742	1.8%
17	Tennessee	3,655	1.8%
18	Indiana	3,652	1.8%
19	Missouri	3,494	1.7%
20	Connecticut	3,475	1.7%
21	Minnesota	3,444	1.7%
22	Arizona	3,352	1.6%
23	Colorado	3,279	1.6%
24	Louisiana	2,905	1.4%
25	Oregon	2,589	1.3%
26	South Carolina	2,425	1.2%
27	Kentucky	2,379	1.2%
28	Alabama	2,258	1.1%
29	Kansas	1,549	0.8%
30	Oklahoma	1,507	0.7%
31	Utah	1,392	0.7%
32	Iowa	1,379	0.7%
33	Arkansas	1,357	0.7%
34	New Mexico	1,247	0.6%
35	Mississippi	1,246	0.6%
36	Nevada	1,172	0.6%
37	Hawaii	1,085	0.5%
38	West Virginia	1,016	0.5%
39	Maine	1,004	0.5%
40	Nebraska	1,002	0.5%
41	Rhode Island	933	0.5%
42	New Hampshire	929	0.5%
43	Vermont	641	0.3%
44	Idaho	576	0.3%
45	Montana	545	0.3%
46	Delaware	542	0.3%
47	Alaska	391	0.2%
48	South Dakota	381	0.2%
49	North Dakota	357	0.2%
50	Wyoming	249	0.1%
	District of Columbia	1,230	0.6%

Source: American Medical Association (Chicago, Illinois)
    "Physician Characteristics and Distribution in the U.S." (2005 Edition)
*As of December 31, 2003. Total does not include 2,459 physicians in U.S. territories and possessions. Other Specialties include Aerospace Medicine, Anesthesiology, Child Psychiatry, Diagnostic Radiology, Emergency Medicine, Forensic Pathology, Nuclear Medicine, Occupational Medicine, Neurology, Psychiatry, Public Health, Anatomic/Clinical Pathology, Radiology, Radiation Oncology and other specialties.

Rate of Physicians in Other Specialties in 2003

National Rate = 70 Physicians per 100,000 Population*

ALPHA ORDER

RANK	STATE	RATE
43	Alabama	50
29	Alaska	60
29	Arizona	60
43	Arkansas	50
16	California	71
14	Colorado	72
5	Connecticut	100
20	Delaware	66
25	Florida	64
37	Georgia	57
6	Hawaii	87
50	Idaho	42
17	Illinois	70
31	Indiana	59
47	Iowa	47
37	Kansas	57
34	Kentucky	58
22	Louisiana	65
9	Maine	77
2	Maryland	117
1	Massachusetts	128
27	Michigan	62
18	Minnesota	68
48	Mississippi	43
28	Missouri	61
31	Montana	59
34	Nebraska	58
42	Nevada	52
14	New Hampshire	72
9	New Jersey	77
20	New Mexico	66
3	New York	103
22	North Carolina	65
39	North Dakota	56
22	Ohio	65
48	Oklahoma	43
12	Oregon	73
8	Pennsylvania	81
6	Rhode Island	87
34	South Carolina	58
43	South Dakota	50
26	Tennessee	63
39	Texas	56
31	Utah	59
3	Vermont	103
12	Virginia	73
11	Washington	74
39	West Virginia	56
18	Wisconsin	68
43	Wyoming	50

RANK ORDER

RANK	STATE	RATE
1	Massachusetts	128
2	Maryland	117
3	New York	103
3	Vermont	103
5	Connecticut	100
6	Hawaii	87
6	Rhode Island	87
8	Pennsylvania	81
9	Maine	77
9	New Jersey	77
11	Washington	74
12	Oregon	73
12	Virginia	73
14	Colorado	72
14	New Hampshire	72
16	California	71
17	Illinois	70
18	Minnesota	68
18	Wisconsin	68
20	Delaware	66
20	New Mexico	66
22	Louisiana	65
22	North Carolina	65
22	Ohio	65
25	Florida	64
26	Tennessee	63
27	Michigan	62
28	Missouri	61
29	Alaska	60
29	Arizona	60
31	Indiana	59
31	Montana	59
31	Utah	59
34	Kentucky	58
34	Nebraska	58
34	South Carolina	58
37	Georgia	57
37	Kansas	57
39	North Dakota	56
39	Texas	56
39	West Virginia	56
42	Nevada	52
43	Alabama	50
43	Arkansas	50
43	South Dakota	50
43	Wyoming	50
47	Iowa	47
48	Mississippi	43
48	Oklahoma	43
50	Idaho	42

	District of Columbia	221

Source: Morgan Quitno Press using data from American Medical Association (Chicago, Illinois)
"Physician Characteristics and Distribution in the U.S." (2005 Edition)
*As of December 31, 2003. National rate does not include physicians in U.S. territories and possessions. Other Specialties include Aerospace Medicine, Anesthesiology, Child Psychiatry, Diagnostic Radiology, Emergency Medicine, Forensic Pathology, Nuclear Medicine, Occupational Medicine, Neurology, Psychiatry, Public Health, Anatomic/Clinical Pathology, Radiology, Radiation Oncology and other specialties.

Physicians in Anesthesiology in 2003

National Total = 38,229 Physicians*

ALPHA ORDER

RANK	STATE	PHYSICIANS	% of USA
27	Alabama	438	1.1%
46	Alaska	83	0.2%
18	Arizona	772	2.0%
34	Arkansas	274	0.7%
1	California	4,747	12.4%
20	Colorado	650	1.7%
24	Connecticut	514	1.3%
47	Delaware	81	0.2%
4	Florida	2,358	6.2%
15	Georgia	879	2.3%
41	Hawaii	143	0.4%
44	Idaho	104	0.3%
5	Illinois	1,782	4.7%
16	Indiana	869	2.3%
31	Iowa	312	0.8%
33	Kansas	299	0.8%
26	Kentucky	485	1.3%
25	Louisiana	502	1.3%
40	Maine	168	0.4%
10	Maryland	985	2.6%
9	Massachusetts	1,329	3.5%
12	Michigan	925	2.4%
22	Minnesota	555	1.5%
35	Mississippi	246	0.6%
21	Missouri	646	1.7%
42	Montana	126	0.3%
36	Nebraska	217	0.6%
32	Nevada	307	0.8%
39	New Hampshire	170	0.4%
7	New Jersey	1,408	3.7%
37	New Mexico	211	0.6%
2	New York	3,201	8.4%
11	North Carolina	935	2.4%
49	North Dakota	51	0.1%
8	Ohio	1,383	3.6%
29	Oklahoma	337	0.9%
23	Oregon	516	1.3%
6	Pennsylvania	1,634	4.3%
43	Rhode Island	106	0.3%
28	South Carolina	435	1.1%
48	South Dakota	59	0.2%
19	Tennessee	729	1.9%
3	Texas	2,882	7.5%
30	Utah	313	0.8%
45	Vermont	93	0.2%
13	Virginia	924	2.4%
14	Washington	920	2.4%
38	West Virginia	174	0.5%
17	Wisconsin	787	2.1%
50	Wyoming	49	0.1%

RANK ORDER

RANK	STATE	PHYSICIANS	% of USA
1	California	4,747	12.4%
2	New York	3,201	8.4%
3	Texas	2,882	7.5%
4	Florida	2,358	6.2%
5	Illinois	1,782	4.7%
6	Pennsylvania	1,634	4.3%
7	New Jersey	1,408	3.7%
8	Ohio	1,383	3.6%
9	Massachusetts	1,329	3.5%
10	Maryland	985	2.6%
11	North Carolina	935	2.4%
12	Michigan	925	2.4%
13	Virginia	924	2.4%
14	Washington	920	2.4%
15	Georgia	879	2.3%
16	Indiana	869	2.3%
17	Wisconsin	787	2.1%
18	Arizona	772	2.0%
19	Tennessee	729	1.9%
20	Colorado	650	1.7%
21	Missouri	646	1.7%
22	Minnesota	555	1.5%
23	Oregon	516	1.3%
24	Connecticut	514	1.3%
25	Louisiana	502	1.3%
26	Kentucky	485	1.3%
27	Alabama	438	1.1%
28	South Carolina	435	1.1%
29	Oklahoma	337	0.9%
30	Utah	313	0.8%
31	Iowa	312	0.8%
32	Nevada	307	0.8%
33	Kansas	299	0.8%
34	Arkansas	274	0.7%
35	Mississippi	246	0.6%
36	Nebraska	217	0.6%
37	New Mexico	211	0.6%
38	West Virginia	174	0.5%
39	New Hampshire	170	0.4%
40	Maine	168	0.4%
41	Hawaii	143	0.4%
42	Montana	126	0.3%
43	Rhode Island	106	0.3%
44	Idaho	104	0.3%
45	Vermont	93	0.2%
46	Alaska	83	0.2%
47	Delaware	81	0.2%
48	South Dakota	59	0.2%
49	North Dakota	51	0.1%
50	Wyoming	49	0.1%
	District of Columbia	116	0.3%

Source: American Medical Association (Chicago, Illinois)
"Physician Characteristics and Distribution in the U.S." (2005 Edition)
*As of December 31, 2003. Total does not include 249 physicians in U.S. territories and possessions.

Rate of Physicians in Anesthesiology in 2003

National Rate = 13 Physicians per 100,000 Population*

ALPHA ORDER

RANK	STATE	RATE
37	Alabama	10
17	Alaska	13
8	Arizona	14
37	Arkansas	10
17	California	13
8	Colorado	14
5	Connecticut	15
37	Delaware	10
8	Florida	14
37	Georgia	10
29	Hawaii	11
48	Idaho	8
8	Illinois	14
8	Indiana	14
29	Iowa	11
29	Kansas	11
25	Kentucky	12
29	Louisiana	11
17	Maine	13
2	Maryland	18
1	Massachusetts	21
46	Michigan	9
29	Minnesota	11
46	Mississippi	9
29	Missouri	11
8	Montana	14
25	Nebraska	12
8	Nevada	14
17	New Hampshire	13
4	New Jersey	16
29	New Mexico	11
3	New York	17
29	North Carolina	11
48	North Dakota	8
25	Ohio	12
37	Oklahoma	10
8	Oregon	14
17	Pennsylvania	13
37	Rhode Island	10
37	South Carolina	10
48	South Dakota	8
25	Tennessee	12
17	Texas	13
17	Utah	13
5	Vermont	15
17	Virginia	13
5	Washington	15
37	West Virginia	10
8	Wisconsin	14
37	Wyoming	10

RANK ORDER

RANK	STATE	RATE
1	Massachusetts	21
2	Maryland	18
3	New York	17
4	New Jersey	16
5	Connecticut	15
5	Vermont	15
5	Washington	15
8	Arizona	14
8	Colorado	14
8	Florida	14
8	Illinois	14
8	Indiana	14
8	Montana	14
8	Nevada	14
8	Oregon	14
8	Wisconsin	14
17	Alaska	13
17	California	13
17	Maine	13
17	New Hampshire	13
17	Pennsylvania	13
17	Texas	13
17	Utah	13
17	Virginia	13
25	Kentucky	12
25	Nebraska	12
25	Ohio	12
25	Tennessee	12
29	Hawaii	11
29	Iowa	11
29	Kansas	11
29	Louisiana	11
29	Minnesota	11
29	Missouri	11
29	New Mexico	11
29	North Carolina	11
37	Alabama	10
37	Arkansas	10
37	Delaware	10
37	Georgia	10
37	Oklahoma	10
37	Rhode Island	10
37	South Carolina	10
37	West Virginia	10
37	Wyoming	10
46	Michigan	9
46	Mississippi	9
48	Idaho	8
48	North Dakota	8
48	South Dakota	8

District of Columbia   21

Source: Morgan Quitno Press using data from American Medical Association (Chicago, Illinois)
    "Physician Characteristics and Distribution in the U.S." (2005 Edition)
*As of December 31, 2003. National rate does not include physicians in U.S. territories and possessions.

Physicians in Psychiatry in 2003

National Total = 39,897 Physicians*

ALPHA ORDER

RANK	STATE	PHYSICIANS	% of USA
28	Alabama	340	0.9%
46	Alaska	73	0.2%
20	Arizona	559	1.4%
35	Arkansas	215	0.5%
2	California	5,464	13.7%
17	Colorado	583	1.5%
14	Connecticut	906	2.3%
44	Delaware	89	0.2%
6	Florida	1,703	4.3%
15	Georgia	875	2.2%
34	Hawaii	238	0.6%
47	Idaho	70	0.2%
7	Illinois	1,555	3.9%
24	Indiana	504	1.3%
35	Iowa	215	0.5%
29	Kansas	308	0.8%
27	Kentucky	393	1.0%
22	Louisiana	524	1.3%
32	Maine	242	0.6%
9	Maryland	1,358	3.4%
3	Massachusetts	2,117	5.3%
11	Michigan	1,084	2.7%
23	Minnesota	519	1.3%
39	Mississippi	194	0.5%
19	Missouri	575	1.4%
45	Montana	75	0.2%
41	Nebraska	169	0.4%
43	Nevada	162	0.4%
38	New Hampshire	196	0.5%
8	New Jersey	1,422	3.6%
31	New Mexico	260	0.7%
1	New York	5,538	13.9%
13	North Carolina	995	2.5%
48	North Dakota	67	0.2%
10	Ohio	1,211	3.0%
30	Oklahoma	265	0.7%
26	Oregon	445	1.1%
4	Pennsylvania	1,967	4.9%
33	Rhode Island	239	0.6%
25	South Carolina	463	1.2%
48	South Dakota	67	0.2%
21	Tennessee	550	1.4%
5	Texas	1,781	4.5%
37	Utah	203	0.5%
40	Vermont	171	0.4%
12	Virginia	1,039	2.6%
16	Washington	782	2.0%
42	West Virginia	166	0.4%
18	Wisconsin	580	1.5%
50	Wyoming	38	0.1%

RANK ORDER

RANK	STATE	PHYSICIANS	% of USA
1	New York	5,538	13.9%
2	California	5,464	13.7%
3	Massachusetts	2,117	5.3%
4	Pennsylvania	1,967	4.9%
5	Texas	1,781	4.5%
6	Florida	1,703	4.3%
7	Illinois	1,555	3.9%
8	New Jersey	1,422	3.6%
9	Maryland	1,358	3.4%
10	Ohio	1,211	3.0%
11	Michigan	1,084	2.7%
12	Virginia	1,039	2.6%
13	North Carolina	995	2.5%
14	Connecticut	906	2.3%
15	Georgia	875	2.2%
16	Washington	782	2.0%
17	Colorado	583	1.5%
18	Wisconsin	580	1.5%
19	Missouri	575	1.4%
20	Arizona	559	1.4%
21	Tennessee	550	1.4%
22	Louisiana	524	1.3%
23	Minnesota	519	1.3%
24	Indiana	504	1.3%
25	South Carolina	463	1.2%
26	Oregon	445	1.1%
27	Kentucky	393	1.0%
28	Alabama	340	0.9%
29	Kansas	308	0.8%
30	Oklahoma	265	0.7%
31	New Mexico	260	0.7%
32	Maine	242	0.6%
33	Rhode Island	239	0.6%
34	Hawaii	238	0.6%
35	Arkansas	215	0.5%
35	Iowa	215	0.5%
37	Utah	203	0.5%
38	New Hampshire	196	0.5%
39	Mississippi	194	0.5%
40	Vermont	171	0.4%
41	Nebraska	169	0.4%
42	West Virginia	166	0.4%
43	Nevada	162	0.4%
44	Delaware	89	0.2%
45	Montana	75	0.2%
46	Alaska	73	0.2%
47	Idaho	70	0.2%
48	North Dakota	67	0.2%
48	South Dakota	67	0.2%
50	Wyoming	38	0.1%
	District of Columbia	343	0.9%

Source: American Medical Association (Chicago, Illinois)
   "Physician Characteristics and Distribution in the U.S." (2005 Edition)
*As of December 31, 2003. Total does not include 437 physicians in U.S. territories and possessions. Psychiatry includes psychoanalysis.

Rate of Physicians in Psychiatry in 2003

National Rate = 14 Physicians per 100,000 Population*

ALPHA ORDER

RANK	STATE	RATE
40	Alabama	8
21	Alaska	11
29	Arizona	10
40	Arkansas	8
11	California	15
15	Colorado	13
4	Connecticut	26
21	Delaware	11
29	Florida	10
29	Georgia	10
7	Hawaii	19
50	Idaho	5
17	Illinois	12
40	Indiana	8
47	Iowa	7
21	Kansas	11
29	Kentucky	10
17	Louisiana	12
8	Maine	18
5	Maryland	25
1	Massachusetts	33
21	Michigan	11
29	Minnesota	10
47	Mississippi	7
29	Missouri	10
40	Montana	8
29	Nebraska	10
47	Nevada	7
11	New Hampshire	15
9	New Jersey	16
13	New Mexico	14
2	New York	29
17	North Carolina	12
21	North Dakota	11
21	Ohio	11
40	Oklahoma	8
17	Oregon	12
9	Pennsylvania	16
6	Rhode Island	22
21	South Carolina	11
36	South Dakota	9
36	Tennessee	9
40	Texas	8
36	Utah	9
3	Vermont	28
13	Virginia	14
15	Washington	13
36	West Virginia	9
21	Wisconsin	11
40	Wyoming	8

RANK ORDER

RANK	STATE	RATE
1	Massachusetts	33
2	New York	29
3	Vermont	28
4	Connecticut	26
5	Maryland	25
6	Rhode Island	22
7	Hawaii	19
8	Maine	18
9	New Jersey	16
9	Pennsylvania	16
11	California	15
11	New Hampshire	15
13	New Mexico	14
13	Virginia	14
15	Colorado	13
15	Washington	13
17	Illinois	12
17	Louisiana	12
17	North Carolina	12
17	Oregon	12
21	Alaska	11
21	Delaware	11
21	Kansas	11
21	Michigan	11
21	North Dakota	11
21	Ohio	11
21	South Carolina	11
21	Wisconsin	11
29	Arizona	10
29	Florida	10
29	Georgia	10
29	Kentucky	10
29	Minnesota	10
29	Missouri	10
29	Nebraska	10
36	South Dakota	9
36	Tennessee	9
36	Utah	9
36	West Virginia	9
40	Alabama	8
40	Arkansas	8
40	Indiana	8
40	Montana	8
40	Oklahoma	8
40	Texas	8
40	Wyoming	8
47	Iowa	7
47	Mississippi	7
47	Nevada	7
50	Idaho	5

District of Columbia	62

Source: Morgan Quitno Press using data from American Medical Association (Chicago, Illinois)
    "Physician Characteristics and Distribution in the U.S." (2005 Edition)
*As of December 31, 2003. National rate does not include physicians in U.S. territories and possessions.
Psychiatry includes psychoanalysis.

Percent of Population Lacking Access to Mental Health Care in 2004

National Percent = 15.4% of Population*

ALPHA ORDER

RANK	STATE	PERCENT
3	Alabama	51.7
16	Alaska	31.6
31	Arizona	10.0
5	Arkansas	43.0
37	California	7.9
38	Colorado	7.8
48	Connecticut	1.2
50	Delaware	0.0
41	Florida	7.4
19	Georgia	22.5
36	Hawaii	8.0
2	Idaho	63.4
26	Illinois	18.3
44	Indiana	5.2
12	Iowa	34.8
15	Kansas	31.7
8	Kentucky	41.6
47	Louisiana	3.3
28	Maine	12.8
46	Maryland	3.9
48	Massachusetts	1.2
27	Michigan	17.4
24	Minnesota	18.8
23	Mississippi	18.9
25	Missouri	18.7
9	Montana	41.2
7	Nebraska	41.7
34	Nevada	9.0
40	New Hampshire	7.5
45	New Jersey	4.6
4	New Mexico	48.4
42	New York	5.7
33	North Carolina	9.3
11	North Dakota	36.4
35	Ohio	8.2
10	Oklahoma	36.5
22	Oregon	19.8
32	Pennsylvania	9.8
20	Rhode Island	21.4
14	South Carolina	33.7
6	South Dakota	41.8
13	Tennessee	34.7
18	Texas	24.5
17	Utah	26.5
30	Vermont	12.5
43	Virginia	5.4
29	Washington	12.7
39	West Virginia	7.7
21	Wisconsin	20.8
1	Wyoming	74.3

RANK ORDER

RANK	STATE	PERCENT
1	Wyoming	74.3
2	Idaho	63.4
3	Alabama	51.7
4	New Mexico	48.4
5	Arkansas	43.0
6	South Dakota	41.8
7	Nebraska	41.7
8	Kentucky	41.6
9	Montana	41.2
10	Oklahoma	36.5
11	North Dakota	36.4
12	Iowa	34.8
13	Tennessee	34.7
14	South Carolina	33.7
15	Kansas	31.7
16	Alaska	31.6
17	Utah	26.5
18	Texas	24.5
19	Georgia	22.5
20	Rhode Island	21.4
21	Wisconsin	20.8
22	Oregon	19.8
23	Mississippi	18.9
24	Minnesota	18.8
25	Missouri	18.7
26	Illinois	18.3
27	Michigan	17.4
28	Maine	12.8
29	Washington	12.7
30	Vermont	12.5
31	Arizona	10.0
32	Pennsylvania	9.8
33	North Carolina	9.3
34	Nevada	9.0
35	Ohio	8.2
36	Hawaii	8.0
37	California	7.9
38	Colorado	7.8
39	West Virginia	7.7
40	New Hampshire	7.5
41	Florida	7.4
42	New York	5.7
43	Virginia	5.4
44	Indiana	5.2
45	New Jersey	4.6
46	Maryland	3.9
47	Louisiana	3.3
48	Connecticut	1.2
48	Massachusetts	1.2
50	Delaware	0.0

District of Columbia 0.7

Source: Morgan Quitno Press using data from U.S. Dept. of Health and Human Services, Div. of Shortage Designation
"Selected Statistics on Health Professional Shortage Areas" (as of September 30, 2004)
*Percent of population considered under-served by mental health practitioners. An under-served population does
not have primary medical care within reasonable economic and geographic bounds.

International Medical School Graduates in 2003

National Total = 210,940 Nonfederal Physicians*

ALPHA ORDER

RANK	STATE	PHYSICIANS	% of USA
26	Alabama	1,621	0.8%
48	Alaska	102	0.0%
19	Arizona	2,553	1.2%
34	Arkansas	876	0.4%
2	California	23,239	11.0%
33	Colorado	891	0.4%
13	Connecticut	3,881	1.8%
38	Delaware	672	0.3%
3	Florida	17,606	8.3%
14	Georgia	3,791	1.8%
39	Hawaii	668	0.3%
50	Idaho	79	0.0%
5	Illinois	12,858	6.1%
16	Indiana	2,914	1.4%
31	Iowa	1,164	0.6%
28	Kansas	1,209	0.6%
22	Kentucky	2,163	1.0%
21	Louisiana	2,233	1.1%
41	Maine	515	0.2%
10	Maryland	6,698	3.2%
11	Massachusetts	6,487	3.1%
9	Michigan	8,680	4.1%
23	Minnesota	2,117	1.0%
37	Mississippi	709	0.3%
15	Missouri	3,214	1.5%
47	Montana	105	0.0%
40	Nebraska	612	0.3%
30	Nevada	1,183	0.6%
42	New Hampshire	510	0.2%
4	New Jersey	12,927	6.1%
36	New Mexico	768	0.4%
1	New York	34,164	16.2%
17	North Carolina	2,798	1.3%
44	North Dakota	409	0.2%
8	Ohio	8,979	4.3%
29	Oklahoma	1,194	0.6%
35	Oregon	839	0.4%
7	Pennsylvania	10,006	4.7%
32	Rhode Island	1,083	0.5%
27	South Carolina	1,275	0.6%
45	South Dakota	247	0.1%
20	Tennessee	2,494	1.2%
6	Texas	11,826	5.6%
43	Utah	410	0.2%
46	Vermont	217	0.1%
12	Virginia	4,553	2.2%
24	Washington	2,092	1.0%
25	West Virginia	1,645	0.8%
18	Wisconsin	2,650	1.3%
49	Wyoming	85	0.0%

RANK ORDER

RANK	STATE	PHYSICIANS	% of USA
1	New York	34,164	16.2%
2	California	23,239	11.0%
3	Florida	17,606	8.3%
4	New Jersey	12,927	6.1%
5	Illinois	12,858	6.1%
6	Texas	11,826	5.6%
7	Pennsylvania	10,006	4.7%
8	Ohio	8,979	4.3%
9	Michigan	8,680	4.1%
10	Maryland	6,698	3.2%
11	Massachusetts	6,487	3.1%
12	Virginia	4,553	2.2%
13	Connecticut	3,881	1.8%
14	Georgia	3,791	1.8%
15	Missouri	3,214	1.5%
16	Indiana	2,914	1.4%
17	North Carolina	2,798	1.3%
18	Wisconsin	2,650	1.3%
19	Arizona	2,553	1.2%
20	Tennessee	2,494	1.2%
21	Louisiana	2,233	1.1%
22	Kentucky	2,163	1.0%
23	Minnesota	2,117	1.0%
24	Washington	2,092	1.0%
25	West Virginia	1,645	0.8%
26	Alabama	1,621	0.8%
27	South Carolina	1,275	0.6%
28	Kansas	1,209	0.6%
29	Oklahoma	1,194	0.6%
30	Nevada	1,183	0.6%
31	Iowa	1,164	0.6%
32	Rhode Island	1,083	0.5%
33	Colorado	891	0.4%
34	Arkansas	876	0.4%
35	Oregon	839	0.4%
36	New Mexico	768	0.4%
37	Mississippi	709	0.3%
38	Delaware	672	0.3%
39	Hawaii	668	0.3%
40	Nebraska	612	0.3%
41	Maine	515	0.2%
42	New Hampshire	510	0.2%
43	Utah	410	0.2%
44	North Dakota	409	0.2%
45	South Dakota	247	0.1%
46	Vermont	217	0.1%
47	Montana	105	0.0%
48	Alaska	102	0.0%
49	Wyoming	85	0.0%
50	Idaho	79	0.0%
	District of Columbia	929	0.4%

Source: American Medical Association (Chicago, Illinois)
   "Physician Characteristics and Distribution in the U.S." (2005 Edition)
*As of December 31, 2003. Total does not include 6,295 physicians in U.S. territories and possessions.

International Medical School Graduates as a Percent of Physicians in 2003

National Percent = 24.6% of Physicians*

Source: Morgan Quitno Press using data from American Medical Association (Chicago, Illinois)
"Physician Characteristics and Distribution in the U.S." (2005 Edition)
*As of December 31, 2003. National percent does not include physicians in U.S. territories and possessions.

Osteopathic Physicians in 2004

National Total = 48,380 Osteopathic Physicians*

ALPHA ORDER

RANK ORDER

RANK	STATE	OSTEOPATHS	% of USA	RANK	STATE	OSTEOPATHS	% of USA
30	Alabama	333	0.7%	1	Pennsylvania	5,246	10.8%
44	Alaska	105	0.2%	2	Michigan	4,539	9.4%
12	Arizona	1,313	2.7%	3	Ohio	3,418	7.1%
36	Arkansas	200	0.4%	4	Florida	3,251	6.7%
6	California	2,997	6.2%	5	New York	3,187	6.6%
14	Colorado	776	1.6%	6	California	2,997	6.2%
30	Connecticut	333	0.7%	7	Texas	2,887	6.0%
35	Delaware	204	0.4%	8	New Jersey	2,705	5.6%
4	Florida	3,251	6.7%	9	Illinois	2,132	4.4%
17	Georgia	645	1.3%	10	Missouri	1,739	3.6%
41	Hawaii	160	0.3%	11	Oklahoma	1,366	2.8%
41	Idaho	160	0.3%	12	Arizona	1,313	2.7%
9	Illinois	2,132	4.4%	13	Iowa	993	2.1%
15	Indiana	673	1.4%	14	Colorado	776	1.6%
13	Iowa	993	2.1%	15	Indiana	673	1.4%
19	Kansas	575	1.2%	16	Virginia	648	1.3%
32	Kentucky	325	0.7%	17	Georgia	645	1.3%
45	Louisiana	102	0.2%	18	Washington	606	1.3%
23	Maine	547	1.1%	19	Kansas	575	1.2%
22	Maryland	553	1.1%	20	West Virginia	565	1.2%
25	Massachusetts	473	1.0%	21	Wisconsin	561	1.2%
2	Michigan	4,539	9.4%	22	Maryland	553	1.1%
29	Minnesota	338	0.7%	23	Maine	547	1.1%
34	Mississippi	279	0.6%	24	North Carolina	484	1.0%
10	Missouri	1,739	3.6%	25	Massachusetts	473	1.0%
46	Montana	100	0.2%	26	Oregon	462	1.0%
43	Nebraska	122	0.3%	27	Tennessee	428	0.9%
28	Nevada	342	0.7%	28	Nevada	342	0.7%
40	New Hampshire	172	0.4%	29	Minnesota	338	0.7%
8	New Jersey	2,705	5.6%	30	Alabama	333	0.7%
37	New Mexico	197	0.4%	30	Connecticut	333	0.7%
5	New York	3,187	6.6%	32	Kentucky	325	0.7%
24	North Carolina	484	1.0%	33	South Carolina	281	0.6%
48	North Dakota	51	0.1%	34	Mississippi	279	0.6%
3	Ohio	3,418	7.1%	35	Delaware	204	0.4%
11	Oklahoma	1,366	2.8%	36	Arkansas	200	0.4%
26	Oregon	462	1.0%	37	New Mexico	197	0.4%
1	Pennsylvania	5,246	10.8%	38	Rhode Island	196	0.4%
38	Rhode Island	196	0.4%	39	Utah	195	0.4%
33	South Carolina	281	0.6%	40	New Hampshire	172	0.4%
47	South Dakota	78	0.2%	41	Hawaii	160	0.3%
27	Tennessee	428	0.9%	41	Idaho	160	0.3%
7	Texas	2,887	6.0%	43	Nebraska	122	0.3%
39	Utah	195	0.4%	44	Alaska	105	0.2%
49	Vermont	49	0.1%	45	Louisiana	102	0.2%
16	Virginia	648	1.3%	46	Montana	100	0.2%
18	Washington	606	1.3%	47	South Dakota	78	0.2%
20	West Virginia	565	1.2%	48	North Dakota	51	0.1%
21	Wisconsin	561	1.2%	49	Vermont	49	0.1%
50	Wyoming	45	0.1%	50	Wyoming	45	0.1%
					District of Columbia	41	0.1%

Source: American Osteopathic Association
   "Fact Sheet 2004" (August 2004)
*Active osteopaths under age 65 as of June 1, 2004. Includes 203 not shown by state. Osteopaths practice a system of medicine based on the theory that disturbances in the musculoskeletal system affect other body parts, causing many disorders that can be corrected by various manipulative techniques in conjunction with conventional medical, surgical, pharmacological, and other therapeutic procedures.

443

Rate of Osteopathic Physicians in 2004

National Rate = 16 Osteopaths per 100,000 Population*

ALPHA ORDER

RANK ORDER

RANK	STATE	RATE		RANK	STATE	RATE
41	Alabama	7		1	Michigan	45
18	Alaska	16		2	Maine	42
11	Arizona	23		2	Pennsylvania	42
41	Arkansas	7		4	Oklahoma	39
36	California	8		5	Iowa	34
15	Colorado	17		6	New Jersey	31
27	Connecticut	10		6	West Virginia	31
10	Delaware	25		8	Missouri	30
13	Florida	19		8	Ohio	30
41	Georgia	7		10	Delaware	25
20	Hawaii	13		11	Arizona	23
24	Idaho	11		12	Kansas	21
15	Illinois	17		13	Florida	19
24	Indiana	11		14	Rhode Island	18
5	Iowa	34		15	Colorado	17
12	Kansas	21		15	Illinois	17
36	Kentucky	8		15	New York	17
50	Louisiana	2		18	Alaska	16
2	Maine	42		19	Nevada	15
27	Maryland	10		20	Hawaii	13
41	Massachusetts	7		20	New Hampshire	13
1	Michigan	45		20	Oregon	13
41	Minnesota	7		20	Texas	13
27	Mississippi	10		24	Idaho	11
8	Missouri	30		24	Indiana	11
24	Montana	11		24	Montana	11
41	Nebraska	7		27	Connecticut	10
19	Nevada	15		27	Maryland	10
20	New Hampshire	13		27	Mississippi	10
6	New Jersey	31		27	New Mexico	10
27	New Mexico	10		27	South Dakota	10
15	New York	17		27	Washington	10
49	North Carolina	6		27	Wisconsin	10
36	North Dakota	8		34	Virginia	9
8	Ohio	30		34	Wyoming	9
4	Oklahoma	39		36	California	8
20	Oregon	13		36	Kentucky	8
2	Pennsylvania	42		36	North Dakota	8
14	Rhode Island	18		36	Utah	8
41	South Carolina	7		36	Vermont	8
27	South Dakota	10		41	Alabama	7
41	Tennessee	7		41	Arkansas	7
20	Texas	13		41	Georgia	7
36	Utah	8		41	Massachusetts	7
36	Vermont	8		41	Minnesota	7
34	Virginia	9		41	Nebraska	7
27	Washington	10		41	South Carolina	7
6	West Virginia	31		41	Tennessee	7
27	Wisconsin	10		49	North Carolina	6
34	Wyoming	9		50	Louisiana	2

	District of Columbia	7

Source: Morgan Quitno Press using data from American Osteopathic Association
"Fact Sheet 2004" (August 2004)

Active osteopaths under age 65 as of June 1, 2004. Includes 203 not shown by state. Osteopaths practice a system of medicine based on the theory that disturbances in the musculoskeletal system affect other body parts, causing many disorders that can be corrected by various manipulative techniques in conjunction with conventional medical, surgical, pharmacological, and other therapeutic procedures.

444

Podiatric Physicians in 2003

National Total = 7,650 Podiatric Physicians*

ALPHA ORDER

RANK	STATE	PODIATRISTS	% of USA
23	Alabama	50	0.7%
NA	Alaska**	NA	NA
10	Arizona	190	2.5%
23	Arkansas	50	0.7%
2	California	580	7.6%
14	Colorado	140	1.8%
11	Connecticut	180	2.4%
NA	Delaware**	NA	NA
3	Florida	510	6.7%
17	Georgia	110	1.4%
NA	Hawaii**	NA	NA
NA	Idaho**	NA	NA
8	Illinois	240	3.1%
13	Indiana	160	2.1%
22	Iowa	70	0.9%
NA	Kansas**	NA	NA
NA	Kentucky**	NA	NA
NA	Louisiana**	NA	NA
23	Maine	50	0.7%
9	Maryland	210	2.7%
21	Massachusetts	90	1.2%
7	Michigan	310	4.1%
12	Minnesota	170	2.2%
NA	Mississippi**	NA	NA
15	Missouri	120	1.6%
27	Montana	30	0.4%
27	Nebraska	30	0.4%
NA	Nevada**	NA	NA
NA	New Hampshire**	NA	NA
6	New Jersey	330	4.3%
NA	New Mexico**	NA	NA
1	New York	1,050	13.7%
NA	North Carolina**	NA	NA
NA	North Dakota**	NA	NA
4	Ohio	420	5.5%
NA	Oklahoma**	NA	NA
NA	Oregon**	NA	NA
5	Pennsylvania	400	5.2%
NA	Rhode Island**	NA	NA
17	South Carolina	110	1.4%
NA	South Dakota**	NA	NA
20	Tennessee	100	1.3%
NA	Texas**	NA	NA
26	Utah	40	0.5%
NA	Vermont**	NA	NA
15	Virginia	120	1.6%
NA	Washington**	NA	NA
NA	West Virginia**	NA	NA
17	Wisconsin	110	1.4%
NA	Wyoming**	NA	NA

RANK ORDER

RANK	STATE	PODIATRISTS	% of USA
1	New York	1,050	13.7%
2	California	580	7.6%
3	Florida	510	6.7%
4	Ohio	420	5.5%
5	Pennsylvania	400	5.2%
6	New Jersey	330	4.3%
7	Michigan	310	4.1%
8	Illinois	240	3.1%
9	Maryland	210	2.7%
10	Arizona	190	2.5%
11	Connecticut	180	2.4%
12	Minnesota	170	2.2%
13	Indiana	160	2.1%
14	Colorado	140	1.8%
15	Missouri	120	1.6%
15	Virginia	120	1.6%
17	Georgia	110	1.4%
17	South Carolina	110	1.4%
17	Wisconsin	110	1.4%
20	Tennessee	100	1.3%
21	Massachusetts	90	1.2%
22	Iowa	70	0.9%
23	Alabama	50	0.7%
23	Arkansas	50	0.7%
23	Maine	50	0.7%
26	Utah	40	0.5%
27	Montana	30	0.4%
27	Nebraska	30	0.4%
NA	Alaska**	NA	NA
NA	Delaware**	NA	NA
NA	Hawaii**	NA	NA
NA	Idaho**	NA	NA
NA	Kansas**	NA	NA
NA	Kentucky**	NA	NA
NA	Louisiana**	NA	NA
NA	Mississippi**	NA	NA
NA	Nevada**	NA	NA
NA	New Hampshire**	NA	NA
NA	New Mexico**	NA	NA
NA	North Carolina**	NA	NA
NA	North Dakota**	NA	NA
NA	Oklahoma**	NA	NA
NA	Oregon**	NA	NA
NA	Rhode Island**	NA	NA
NA	South Dakota**	NA	NA
NA	Texas**	NA	NA
NA	Vermont**	NA	NA
NA	Washington**	NA	NA
NA	West Virginia**	NA	NA
NA	Wyoming**	NA	NA
	District of Columbia	50	0.7%

Source: U.S. Department of Labor, Bureau of Labor Statistics
"Occupational Employment and Wages, 2003" (http://www.bls.gov/oes/)
*Does not include self-employed.
**Not available.

Rate of Podiatric Physicians in 2003

National Rate = 3 Podiatric Physicians per 100,000 Population*

ALPHA ORDER

RANK	STATE	RATE
26	Alabama	1
NA	Alaska**	NA
7	Arizona	3
16	Arkansas	2
16	California	2
7	Colorado	3
1	Connecticut	5
NA	Delaware**	NA
7	Florida	3
26	Georgia	1
NA	Hawaii**	NA
NA	Idaho**	NA
16	Illinois	2
7	Indiana	3
16	Iowa	2
NA	Kansas**	NA
NA	Kentucky**	NA
NA	Louisiana**	NA
3	Maine	4
3	Maryland	4
26	Massachusetts	1
7	Michigan	3
7	Minnesota	3
NA	Mississippi**	NA
16	Missouri	2
7	Montana	3
16	Nebraska	2
NA	Nevada**	NA
NA	New Hampshire**	NA
3	New Jersey	4
NA	New Mexico**	NA
1	New York	5
NA	North Carolina**	NA
NA	North Dakota**	NA
3	Ohio	4
NA	Oklahoma**	NA
NA	Oregon**	NA
7	Pennsylvania	3
NA	Rhode Island**	NA
7	South Carolina	3
NA	South Dakota**	NA
16	Tennessee	2
NA	Texas**	NA
16	Utah	2
NA	Vermont**	NA
16	Virginia	2
NA	Washington**	NA
NA	West Virginia**	NA
16	Wisconsin	2
NA	Wyoming**	NA

RANK ORDER

RANK	STATE	RATE
1	Connecticut	5
1	New York	5
3	Maine	4
3	Maryland	4
3	New Jersey	4
3	Ohio	4
7	Arizona	3
7	Colorado	3
7	Florida	3
7	Indiana	3
7	Michigan	3
7	Minnesota	3
7	Montana	3
7	Pennsylvania	3
7	South Carolina	3
16	Arkansas	2
16	California	2
16	Illinois	2
16	Iowa	2
16	Missouri	2
16	Nebraska	2
16	Tennessee	2
16	Utah	2
16	Virginia	2
16	Wisconsin	2
26	Alabama	1
26	Georgia	1
26	Massachusetts	1
NA	Alaska**	NA
NA	Delaware**	NA
NA	Hawaii**	NA
NA	Idaho**	NA
NA	Kansas**	NA
NA	Kentucky**	NA
NA	Louisiana**	NA
NA	Mississippi**	NA
NA	Nevada**	NA
NA	New Hampshire**	NA
NA	New Mexico**	NA
NA	North Carolina**	NA
NA	North Dakota**	NA
NA	Oklahoma**	NA
NA	Oregon**	NA
NA	Rhode Island**	NA
NA	South Dakota**	NA
NA	Texas**	NA
NA	Vermont**	NA
NA	Washington**	NA
NA	West Virginia**	NA
NA	Wyoming**	NA

District of Columbia 9

Source: Morgan Quitno Press using data from U.S. Department of Labor, Bureau of Labor Statistics
"Occupational Employment and Wages, 2003" (http://www.bls.gov/oes/)
*Does not include self-employed.
**Not available.

Average Annual Wages of Podiatric Physicians in 2003

National Average = $107,390*

<u>ALPHA ORDER</u>

RANK	STATE	WAGES
4	Alabama	$139,460
NA	Alaska**	NA
17	Arizona	107,970
5	Arkansas	137,930
28	California	91,600
7	Colorado	131,700
15	Connecticut	109,580
NA	Delaware**	NA
20	Florida	104,550
9	Georgia	122,820
NA	Hawaii**	NA
NA	Idaho**	NA
21	Illinois	102,700
13	Indiana	113,810
25	Iowa	99,360
NA	Kansas**	NA
NA	Kentucky**	NA
NA	Louisiana**	NA
30	Maine	79,790
1	Maryland	159,490
10	Massachusetts	119,690
3	Michigan	145,160
11	Minnesota	119,300
NA	Mississippi**	NA
16	Missouri	108,600
24	Montana	99,860
2	Nebraska	146,520
NA	Nevada**	NA
NA	New Hampshire**	NA
27	New Jersey	96,040
NA	New Mexico**	NA
23	New York	101,680
NA	North Carolina**	NA
NA	North Dakota**	NA
22	Ohio	101,910
NA	Oklahoma**	NA
NA	Oregon**	NA
29	Pennsylvania	89,130
NA	Rhode Island**	NA
8	South Carolina	125,360
NA	South Dakota**	NA
14	Tennessee	110,020
25	Texas	99,360
19	Utah	105,580
NA	Vermont**	NA
6	Virginia	134,750
12	Washington	115,920
NA	West Virginia**	NA
18	Wisconsin	107,380
NA	Wyoming**	NA

<u>RANK ORDER</u>

RANK	STATE	WAGES
1	Maryland	$159,490
2	Nebraska	146,520
3	Michigan	145,160
4	Alabama	139,460
5	Arkansas	137,930
6	Virginia	134,750
7	Colorado	131,700
8	South Carolina	125,360
9	Georgia	122,820
10	Massachusetts	119,690
11	Minnesota	119,300
12	Washington	115,920
13	Indiana	113,810
14	Tennessee	110,020
15	Connecticut	109,580
16	Missouri	108,600
17	Arizona	107,970
18	Wisconsin	107,380
19	Utah	105,580
20	Florida	104,550
21	Illinois	102,700
22	Ohio	101,910
23	New York	101,680
24	Montana	99,860
25	Iowa	99,360
25	Texas	99,360
27	New Jersey	96,040
28	California	91,600
29	Pennsylvania	89,130
30	Maine	79,790
NA	Alaska**	NA
NA	Delaware**	NA
NA	Hawaii**	NA
NA	Idaho**	NA
NA	Kansas**	NA
NA	Kentucky**	NA
NA	Louisiana**	NA
NA	Mississippi**	NA
NA	Nevada**	NA
NA	New Hampshire**	NA
NA	New Mexico**	NA
NA	North Carolina**	NA
NA	North Dakota**	NA
NA	Oklahoma**	NA
NA	Oregon**	NA
NA	Rhode Island**	NA
NA	South Dakota**	NA
NA	Vermont**	NA
NA	West Virginia**	NA
NA	Wyoming**	NA
	District of Columbia	65,980

Source: U.S. Department of Labor, Bureau of Labor Statistics
   "Occupational Employment and Wages, 2003" (http://www.bls.gov/oes/)
Does not include self-employed.
**Not available.*

Doctors of Chiropractic in 2003

National Total = 83,690 Chiropractors*

ALPHA ORDER

RANK	STATE	CHIROPRACTORS	% of USA
30	Alabama	749	0.9%
48	Alaska	204	0.2%
10	Arizona	2,394	2.9%
33	Arkansas	557	0.7%
1	California	13,421	16.0%
11	Colorado	2,258	2.7%
27	Connecticut	982	1.2%
44	Delaware	268	0.3%
3	Florida	4,687	5.6%
8	Georgia	3,126	3.7%
NA	Hawaii**	NA	NA
37	Idaho	414	0.5%
6	Illinois	3,623	4.3%
24	Indiana	1,043	1.2%
21	Iowa	1,411	1.7%
26	Kansas	1,009	1.2%
23	Kentucky	1,065	1.3%
32	Louisiana	567	0.7%
39	Maine	357	0.4%
31	Maryland	658	0.8%
17	Massachusetts	1,768	2.1%
9	Michigan	2,815	3.4%
12	Minnesota	2,233	2.7%
41	Mississippi	331	0.4%
15	Missouri	1,948	2.3%
40	Montana	339	0.4%
38	Nebraska	369	0.4%
34	Nevada	549	0.7%
36	New Hampshire	431	0.5%
7	New Jersey	3,294	3.9%
35	New Mexico	471	0.6%
2	New York	6,240	7.5%
18	North Carolina	1,729	2.1%
46	North Dakota	248	0.3%
13	Ohio	2,194	2.6%
29	Oklahoma	768	0.9%
22	Oregon	1,091	1.3%
5	Pennsylvania	4,000	4.8%
45	Rhode Island	263	0.3%
19	South Carolina	1,455	1.7%
43	South Dakota	280	0.3%
16	Tennessee	1,775	2.1%
4	Texas	4,190	5.0%
28	Utah	809	1.0%
47	Vermont	242	0.3%
20	Virginia	1,414	1.7%
14	Washington	2,131	2.5%
42	West Virginia	299	0.4%
25	Wisconsin	1,029	1.2%
49	Wyoming	192	0.2%

RANK ORDER

RANK	STATE	CHIROPRACTORS	% of USA
1	California	13,421	16.0%
2	New York	6,240	7.5%
3	Florida	4,687	5.6%
4	Texas	4,190	5.0%
5	Pennsylvania	4,000	4.8%
6	Illinois	3,623	4.3%
7	New Jersey	3,294	3.9%
8	Georgia	3,126	3.7%
9	Michigan	2,815	3.4%
10	Arizona	2,394	2.9%
11	Colorado	2,258	2.7%
12	Minnesota	2,233	2.7%
13	Ohio	2,194	2.6%
14	Washington	2,131	2.5%
15	Missouri	1,948	2.3%
16	Tennessee	1,775	2.1%
17	Massachusetts	1,768	2.1%
18	North Carolina	1,729	2.1%
19	South Carolina	1,455	1.7%
20	Virginia	1,414	1.7%
21	Iowa	1,411	1.7%
22	Oregon	1,091	1.3%
23	Kentucky	1,065	1.3%
24	Indiana	1,043	1.2%
25	Wisconsin	1,029	1.2%
26	Kansas	1,009	1.2%
27	Connecticut	982	1.2%
28	Utah	809	1.0%
29	Oklahoma	768	0.9%
30	Alabama	749	0.9%
31	Maryland	658	0.8%
32	Louisiana	567	0.7%
33	Arkansas	557	0.7%
34	Nevada	549	0.7%
35	New Mexico	471	0.6%
36	New Hampshire	431	0.5%
37	Idaho	414	0.5%
38	Nebraska	369	0.4%
39	Maine	357	0.4%
40	Montana	339	0.4%
41	Mississippi	331	0.4%
42	West Virginia	299	0.4%
43	South Dakota	280	0.3%
44	Delaware	268	0.3%
45	Rhode Island	263	0.3%
46	North Dakota	248	0.3%
47	Vermont	242	0.3%
48	Alaska	204	0.2%
49	Wyoming	192	0.2%
NA	Hawaii**	NA	NA
	District of Columbia**	NA	NA

Source: Federation of Chiropractic Licensing Boards
"Official Directory" (http://www.fclb.org/directory/index.htm)
As of December 2003. Licensed active doctors. There is some duplication as some doctors are licensed in more than one state.
***Not available.*

Rate of Doctors of Chiropractic in 2003

National Rate = 29 Chiropractors per 100,000 Population*

ALPHA ORDER

RANK	STATE	RATE
44	Alabama	17
22	Alaska	31
4	Arizona	43
39	Arkansas	20
7	California	38
1	Colorado	50
27	Connecticut	28
18	Delaware	33
27	Florida	28
13	Georgia	36
NA	Hawaii**	NA
24	Idaho	30
26	Illinois	29
44	Indiana	17
2	Iowa	48
10	Kansas	37
32	Kentucky	26
47	Louisiana	13
31	Maine	27
48	Maryland	12
27	Massachusetts	28
27	Michigan	28
3	Minnesota	44
49	Mississippi	11
16	Missouri	34
10	Montana	37
37	Nebraska	21
34	Nevada	24
18	New Hampshire	33
7	New Jersey	38
33	New Mexico	25
20	New York	32
37	North Carolina	21
5	North Dakota	39
40	Ohio	19
36	Oklahoma	22
22	Oregon	31
20	Pennsylvania	32
34	Rhode Island	24
14	South Carolina	35
10	South Dakota	37
24	Tennessee	30
40	Texas	19
16	Utah	34
5	Vermont	39
40	Virginia	19
14	Washington	35
44	West Virginia	17
40	Wisconsin	19
7	Wyoming	38

RANK ORDER

RANK	STATE	RATE
1	Colorado	50
2	Iowa	48
3	Minnesota	44
4	Arizona	43
5	North Dakota	39
5	Vermont	39
7	California	38
7	New Jersey	38
7	Wyoming	38
10	Kansas	37
10	Montana	37
10	South Dakota	37
13	Georgia	36
14	South Carolina	35
14	Washington	35
16	Missouri	34
16	Utah	34
18	Delaware	33
18	New Hampshire	33
20	New York	32
20	Pennsylvania	32
22	Alaska	31
22	Oregon	31
24	Idaho	30
24	Tennessee	30
26	Illinois	29
27	Connecticut	28
27	Florida	28
27	Massachusetts	28
27	Michigan	28
31	Maine	27
32	Kentucky	26
33	New Mexico	25
34	Nevada	24
34	Rhode Island	24
36	Oklahoma	22
37	Nebraska	21
37	North Carolina	21
39	Arkansas	20
40	Ohio	19
40	Texas	19
40	Virginia	19
40	Wisconsin	19
44	Alabama	17
44	Indiana	17
44	West Virginia	17
47	Louisiana	13
48	Maryland	12
49	Mississippi	11
NA	Hawaii**	NA
	District of Columbia**	NA

Source: Morgan Quitno Press using data from Federation of Chiropractic Licensing Boards "Official Directory" (http://www.fclb.org/directory/index.htm)

*As of December 2003. Licensed active doctors. There is some duplication as some doctors are licensed in more than one state.

**Not available.

Average Annual Wages of Chiropractors in 2003

National Average = $83,230*

ALPHA ORDER				RANK ORDER		
RANK	**STATE**	**WAGES**		**RANK**	**STATE**	**WAGES**
27	Alabama	$74,680		1	Alaska	$172,200
1	Alaska	172,200		2	Illinois	131,680
4	Arizona	123,580		3	New Jersey	127,440
13	Arkansas	97,900		4	Arizona	123,580
33	California	65,060		5	West Virginia	120,190
38	Colorado	58,580		6	Virginia	115,680
19	Connecticut	90,640		7	Louisiana	113,730
NA	Delaware**	NA		8	Tennessee	113,270
30	Florida	72,280		9	Nevada	109,130
37	Georgia	61,710		10	Maryland	103,640
36	Hawaii	63,990		11	Indiana	103,390
NA	Idaho**	NA		12	South Dakota	101,150
2	Illinois	131,680		13	Arkansas	97,900
11	Indiana	103,390		14	Wisconsin	97,580
NA	Iowa**	NA		15	Oklahoma	96,430
32	Kansas	68,170		16	Ohio	96,130
39	Kentucky	56,740		17	South Carolina	95,740
7	Louisiana	113,730		18	Texas	91,870
42	Maine	51,240		19	Connecticut	90,640
10	Maryland	103,640		20	Massachusetts	89,890
20	Massachusetts	89,890		21	Missouri	89,770
22	Michigan	85,270		22	Michigan	85,270
31	Minnesota	69,180		23	New Mexico	82,490
41	Mississippi	52,800		24	New Hampshire	77,700
21	Missouri	89,770		25	North Dakota	75,780
45	Montana	39,360		26	North Carolina	75,680
34	Nebraska	64,670		27	Alabama	74,680
9	Nevada	109,130		28	New York	74,200
24	New Hampshire	77,700		29	Washington	72,860
3	New Jersey	127,440		30	Florida	72,280
23	New Mexico	82,490		31	Minnesota	69,180
28	New York	74,200		32	Kansas	68,170
26	North Carolina	75,680		33	California	65,060
25	North Dakota	75,780		34	Nebraska	64,670
16	Ohio	96,130		35	Pennsylvania	64,250
15	Oklahoma	96,430		36	Hawaii	63,990
44	Oregon	48,270		37	Georgia	61,710
35	Pennsylvania	64,250		38	Colorado	58,580
NA	Rhode Island**	NA		39	Kentucky	56,740
17	South Carolina	95,740		40	Utah	53,960
12	South Dakota	101,150		41	Mississippi	52,800
8	Tennessee	113,270		42	Maine	51,240
18	Texas	91,870		43	Wyoming	49,950
40	Utah	53,960		44	Oregon	48,270
NA	Vermont**	NA		45	Montana	39,360
6	Virginia	115,680		NA	Delaware**	NA
29	Washington	72,860		NA	Idaho**	NA
5	West Virginia	120,190		NA	Iowa**	NA
14	Wisconsin	97,580		NA	Rhode Island**	NA
43	Wyoming	49,950		NA	Vermont**	NA
				District of Columbia**		NA

Source: U.S. Department of Labor, Bureau of Labor Statistics
   "Occupational Employment and Wages, 2003" (http://www.bls.gov/oes/)
Does not include self-employed.
**Not available.*

Physician Assistants in Clinical Practice in 2005

National Total = 53,667 Physician Assistants*

ALPHA ORDER

RANK	STATE	PAs	% of USA
40	Alabama	288	0.5%
41	Alaska	283	0.5%
16	Arizona	1,106	2.1%
49	Arkansas	61	0.1%
2	California	5,324	9.9%
13	Colorado	1,318	2.5%
17	Connecticut	1,066	2.0%
46	Delaware	156	0.3%
4	Florida	3,119	5.8%
8	Georgia	1,725	3.2%
48	Hawaii	128	0.2%
36	Idaho	352	0.7%
12	Illinois	1,356	2.5%
32	Indiana	449	0.8%
25	Iowa	599	1.1%
24	Kansas	605	1.1%
23	Kentucky	657	1.2%
35	Louisiana	368	0.7%
33	Maine	437	0.8%
9	Maryland	1,488	2.8%
14	Massachusetts	1,186	2.2%
7	Michigan	2,260	4.2%
20	Minnesota	813	1.5%
50	Mississippi	59	0.1%
31	Missouri	464	0.9%
42	Montana	269	0.5%
26	Nebraska	581	1.1%
38	Nevada	311	0.6%
39	New Hampshire	289	0.5%
19	New Jersey	890	1.7%
34	New Mexico	418	0.8%
1	New York	6,277	11.7%
6	North Carolina	2,611	4.9%
43	North Dakota	212	0.4%
11	Ohio	1,458	2.7%
21	Oklahoma	774	1.4%
27	Oregon	563	1.0%
5	Pennsylvania	3,117	5.8%
44	Rhode Island	187	0.3%
29	South Carolina	516	1.0%
37	South Dakota	316	0.6%
22	Tennessee	681	1.3%
3	Texas	3,365	6.3%
30	Utah	485	0.9%
45	Vermont	182	0.3%
18	Virginia	1,019	1.9%
10	Washington	1,475	2.7%
28	West Virginia	544	1.0%
15	Wisconsin	1,136	2.1%
47	Wyoming	133	0.2%

RANK ORDER

RANK	STATE	PAs	% of USA
1	New York	6,277	11.7%
2	California	5,324	9.9%
3	Texas	3,365	6.3%
4	Florida	3,119	5.8%
5	Pennsylvania	3,117	5.8%
6	North Carolina	2,611	4.9%
7	Michigan	2,260	4.2%
8	Georgia	1,725	3.2%
9	Maryland	1,488	2.8%
10	Washington	1,475	2.7%
11	Ohio	1,458	2.7%
12	Illinois	1,356	2.5%
13	Colorado	1,318	2.5%
14	Massachusetts	1,186	2.2%
15	Wisconsin	1,136	2.1%
16	Arizona	1,106	2.1%
17	Connecticut	1,066	2.0%
18	Virginia	1,019	1.9%
19	New Jersey	890	1.7%
20	Minnesota	813	1.5%
21	Oklahoma	774	1.4%
22	Tennessee	681	1.3%
23	Kentucky	657	1.2%
24	Kansas	605	1.1%
25	Iowa	599	1.1%
26	Nebraska	581	1.1%
27	Oregon	563	1.0%
28	West Virginia	544	1.0%
29	South Carolina	516	1.0%
30	Utah	485	0.9%
31	Missouri	464	0.9%
32	Indiana	449	0.8%
33	Maine	437	0.8%
34	New Mexico	418	0.8%
35	Louisiana	368	0.7%
36	Idaho	352	0.7%
37	South Dakota	316	0.6%
38	Nevada	311	0.6%
39	New Hampshire	289	0.5%
40	Alabama	288	0.5%
41	Alaska	283	0.5%
42	Montana	269	0.5%
43	North Dakota	212	0.4%
44	Rhode Island	187	0.3%
45	Vermont	182	0.3%
46	Delaware	156	0.3%
47	Wyoming	133	0.2%
48	Hawaii	128	0.2%
49	Arkansas	61	0.1%
50	Mississippi	59	0.1%
	District of Columbia	191	0.4%

Source: The American Academy of Physician Assistants
   "Projected Number of PAs in Clinical Practice as of January 1, 2005"
      (http://www.aapa.org/research/04-05num-clin-prac.pdf)
*Projected. National total does not include 1,396 physician assistants who work outside the United States or whose location is unknown.

Rate of Physician Assistants in Clinical Practice in 2005

National Rate = 18 PAs per 100,000 Population*

ALPHA ORDER

RANK	STATE	RATE
48	Alabama	6
1	Alaska	43
27	Arizona	19
49	Arkansas	2
35	California	15
10	Colorado	29
8	Connecticut	30
27	Delaware	19
29	Florida	18
24	Georgia	20
43	Hawaii	10
15	Idaho	25
42	Illinois	11
47	Indiana	7
24	Iowa	20
18	Kansas	22
32	Kentucky	16
45	Louisiana	8
3	Maine	33
13	Maryland	27
29	Massachusetts	18
18	Michigan	22
32	Minnesota	16
49	Mississippi	2
45	Missouri	8
10	Montana	29
3	Nebraska	33
38	Nevada	13
18	New Hampshire	22
43	New Jersey	10
18	New Mexico	22
3	New York	33
7	North Carolina	31
3	North Dakota	33
38	Ohio	13
18	Oklahoma	22
32	Oregon	16
15	Pennsylvania	25
31	Rhode Island	17
40	South Carolina	12
2	South Dakota	41
40	Tennessee	12
35	Texas	15
24	Utah	20
10	Vermont	29
37	Virginia	14
17	Washington	24
8	West Virginia	30
23	Wisconsin	21
14	Wyoming	26

RANK ORDER

RANK	STATE	RATE
1	Alaska	43
2	South Dakota	41
3	Maine	33
3	Nebraska	33
3	New York	33
3	North Dakota	33
7	North Carolina	31
8	Connecticut	30
8	West Virginia	30
10	Colorado	29
10	Montana	29
10	Vermont	29
13	Maryland	27
14	Wyoming	26
15	Idaho	25
15	Pennsylvania	25
17	Washington	24
18	Kansas	22
18	Michigan	22
18	New Hampshire	22
18	New Mexico	22
18	Oklahoma	22
23	Wisconsin	21
24	Georgia	20
24	Iowa	20
24	Utah	20
27	Arizona	19
27	Delaware	19
29	Florida	18
29	Massachusetts	18
31	Rhode Island	17
32	Kentucky	16
32	Minnesota	16
32	Oregon	16
35	California	15
35	Texas	15
37	Virginia	14
38	Nevada	13
38	Ohio	13
40	South Carolina	12
40	Tennessee	12
42	Illinois	11
43	Hawaii	10
43	New Jersey	10
45	Louisiana	8
45	Missouri	8
47	Indiana	7
48	Alabama	6
49	Arkansas	2
49	Mississippi	2
	District of Columbia	35

Source: Morgan Quitno Press using data from The American Academy of Physician Assistants
"Projected Number of PAs in Clinical Practice as of January 1, 2005"
(http://www.aapa.org/research/04-05num-clin-prac.pdf)
*Projected. Rates calculated using 2004 Census population figures.

Average Annual Wages of Physician Assistants in 2003

National Average = $66,600*

ALPHA ORDER

RANK	STATE	WAGES
40	Alabama	$59,590
1	Alaska	84,950
41	Arizona	59,120
2	Arkansas	84,000
3	California	79,110
38	Colorado	60,520
13	Connecticut	72,510
5	Delaware	76,600
31	Florida	63,610
7	Georgia	75,460
50	Hawaii	40,870
29	Idaho	64,700
47	Illinois	45,990
35	Indiana	61,380
24	Iowa	67,520
21	Kansas	69,020
42	Kentucky	58,820
45	Louisiana	49,250
4	Maine	78,410
27	Maryland	65,300
22	Massachusetts	68,960
8	Michigan	75,270
14	Minnesota	72,190
49	Mississippi	43,460
43	Missouri	58,160
34	Montana	61,470
12	Nebraska	72,630
46	Nevada	46,480
32	New Hampshire	63,070
20	New Jersey	69,290
39	New Mexico	59,620
19	New York	69,760
16	North Carolina	71,030
33	North Dakota	61,510
15	Ohio	71,730
48	Oklahoma	44,570
11	Oregon	72,910
37	Pennsylvania	60,530
17	Rhode Island	69,890
44	South Carolina	53,120
26	South Dakota	65,640
36	Tennessee	61,220
6	Texas	76,290
17	Utah	69,890
23	Vermont	68,510
10	Virginia	73,580
9	Washington	74,550
30	West Virginia	64,060
25	Wisconsin	67,020
28	Wyoming	65,200

RANK ORDER

RANK	STATE	WAGES
1	Alaska	$84,950
2	Arkansas	84,000
3	California	79,110
4	Maine	78,410
5	Delaware	76,600
6	Texas	76,290
7	Georgia	75,460
8	Michigan	75,270
9	Washington	74,550
10	Virginia	73,580
11	Oregon	72,910
12	Nebraska	72,630
13	Connecticut	72,510
14	Minnesota	72,190
15	Ohio	71,730
16	North Carolina	71,030
17	Rhode Island	69,890
17	Utah	69,890
19	New York	69,760
20	New Jersey	69,290
21	Kansas	69,020
22	Massachusetts	68,960
23	Vermont	68,510
24	Iowa	67,520
25	Wisconsin	67,020
26	South Dakota	65,640
27	Maryland	65,300
28	Wyoming	65,200
29	Idaho	64,700
30	West Virginia	64,060
31	Florida	63,610
32	New Hampshire	63,070
33	North Dakota	61,510
34	Montana	61,470
35	Indiana	61,380
36	Tennessee	61,220
37	Pennsylvania	60,530
38	Colorado	60,520
39	New Mexico	59,620
40	Alabama	59,590
41	Arizona	59,120
42	Kentucky	58,820
43	Missouri	58,160
44	South Carolina	53,120
45	Louisiana	49,250
46	Nevada	46,480
47	Illinois	45,990
48	Oklahoma	44,570
49	Mississippi	43,460
50	Hawaii	40,870
	District of Columbia	62,230

Source: U.S. Department of Labor, Bureau of Labor Statistics
   "Occupational Employment and Wages, 2003" (http://www.bls.gov/oes/)
Does not include self-employed.

Registered Nurses in 2003

National Total = 2,280,170 Registered Nurses*

ALPHA ORDER

RANK	STATE	NURSES	% of USA
22	Alabama	36,970	1.6%
49	Alaska	5,200	0.2%
24	Arizona	33,810	1.5%
33	Arkansas	19,360	0.8%
1	California	213,630	9.4%
27	Colorado	29,400	1.3%
25	Connecticut	32,180	1.4%
46	Delaware	6,550	0.3%
4	Florida	134,530	5.9%
12	Georgia	58,210	2.6%
44	Hawaii	7,860	0.3%
42	Idaho	9,890	0.4%
7	Illinois	100,390	4.4%
17	Indiana	47,940	2.1%
28	Iowa	28,550	1.3%
30	Kansas	24,960	1.1%
23	Kentucky	36,780	1.6%
21	Louisiana	38,590	1.7%
38	Maine	12,560	0.6%
19	Maryland	47,050	2.1%
9	Massachusetts	75,770	3.3%
8	Michigan	76,740	3.4%
15	Minnesota	51,440	2.3%
31	Mississippi	24,840	1.1%
13	Missouri	53,430	2.3%
45	Montana	7,840	0.3%
34	Nebraska	16,880	0.7%
36	Nevada	14,240	0.6%
39	New Hampshire	11,630	0.5%
10	New Jersey	73,270	3.2%
40	New Mexico	11,330	0.5%
2	New York	163,710	7.2%
11	North Carolina	67,700	3.0%
47	North Dakota	6,350	0.3%
6	Ohio	102,030	4.5%
32	Oklahoma	22,100	1.0%
29	Oregon	26,020	1.1%
5	Pennsylvania	120,230	5.3%
41	Rhode Island	10,480	0.5%
26	South Carolina	30,720	1.3%
43	South Dakota	8,840	0.4%
16	Tennessee	49,730	2.2%
3	Texas	139,910	6.1%
37	Utah	12,960	0.6%
48	Vermont	5,590	0.2%
14	Virginia	52,600	2.3%
20	Washington	44,430	1.9%
35	West Virginia	16,370	0.7%
18	Wisconsin	47,210	2.1%
50	Wyoming	3,710	0.2%

RANK ORDER

RANK	STATE	NURSES	% of USA
1	California	213,630	9.4%
2	New York	163,710	7.2%
3	Texas	139,910	6.1%
4	Florida	134,530	5.9%
5	Pennsylvania	120,230	5.3%
6	Ohio	102,030	4.5%
7	Illinois	100,390	4.4%
8	Michigan	76,740	3.4%
9	Massachusetts	75,770	3.3%
10	New Jersey	73,270	3.2%
11	North Carolina	67,700	3.0%
12	Georgia	58,210	2.6%
13	Missouri	53,430	2.3%
14	Virginia	52,600	2.3%
15	Minnesota	51,440	2.3%
16	Tennessee	49,730	2.2%
17	Indiana	47,940	2.1%
18	Wisconsin	47,210	2.1%
19	Maryland	47,050	2.1%
20	Washington	44,430	1.9%
21	Louisiana	38,590	1.7%
22	Alabama	36,970	1.6%
23	Kentucky	36,780	1.6%
24	Arizona	33,810	1.5%
25	Connecticut	32,180	1.4%
26	South Carolina	30,720	1.3%
27	Colorado	29,400	1.3%
28	Iowa	28,550	1.3%
29	Oregon	26,020	1.1%
30	Kansas	24,960	1.1%
31	Mississippi	24,840	1.1%
32	Oklahoma	22,100	1.0%
33	Arkansas	19,360	0.8%
34	Nebraska	16,880	0.7%
35	West Virginia	16,370	0.7%
36	Nevada	14,240	0.6%
37	Utah	12,960	0.6%
38	Maine	12,560	0.6%
39	New Hampshire	11,630	0.5%
40	New Mexico	11,330	0.5%
41	Rhode Island	10,480	0.5%
42	Idaho	9,890	0.4%
43	South Dakota	8,840	0.4%
44	Hawaii	7,860	0.3%
45	Montana	7,840	0.3%
46	Delaware	6,550	0.3%
47	North Dakota	6,350	0.3%
48	Vermont	5,590	0.2%
49	Alaska	5,200	0.2%
50	Wyoming	3,710	0.2%
	District of Columbia	7,660	0.3%

Source: U.S. Department of Labor, Bureau of Labor Statistics
"Occupational Employment and Wages, 2002" (http://www.bls.gov/oes/)
Does not include self-employed.

Rate of Registered Nurses in 2003

National Rate = 784 Nurses per 100,000 Population*

ALPHA ORDER

RANK	STATE	RATE
26	Alabama	821
28	Alaska	802
47	Arizona	606
40	Arkansas	710
49	California	602
42	Colorado	646
11	Connecticut	923
29	Delaware	801
31	Florida	791
41	Georgia	671
46	Hawaii	629
38	Idaho	723
30	Illinois	794
32	Indiana	773
8	Iowa	970
12	Kansas	916
16	Kentucky	893
20	Louisiana	859
9	Maine	959
21	Maryland	854
1	Massachusetts	1,180
33	Michigan	761
3	Minnesota	1,016
18	Mississippi	862
10	Missouri	934
21	Montana	854
6	Nebraska	972
43	Nevada	635
15	New Hampshire	902
25	New Jersey	848
48	New Mexico	603
23	New York	852
27	North Carolina	804
4	North Dakota	1,003
17	Ohio	892
45	Oklahoma	630
36	Oregon	730
6	Pennsylvania	972
5	Rhode Island	974
34	South Carolina	740
2	South Dakota	1,156
24	Tennessee	851
44	Texas	633
50	Utah	551
14	Vermont	903
39	Virginia	714
37	Washington	725
13	West Virginia	904
18	Wisconsin	862
35	Wyoming	739

RANK ORDER

RANK	STATE	RATE
1	Massachusetts	1,180
2	South Dakota	1,156
3	Minnesota	1,016
4	North Dakota	1,003
5	Rhode Island	974
6	Nebraska	972
6	Pennsylvania	972
8	Iowa	970
9	Maine	959
10	Missouri	934
11	Connecticut	923
12	Kansas	916
13	West Virginia	904
14	Vermont	903
15	New Hampshire	902
16	Kentucky	893
17	Ohio	892
18	Mississippi	862
18	Wisconsin	862
20	Louisiana	859
21	Maryland	854
21	Montana	854
23	New York	852
24	Tennessee	851
25	New Jersey	848
26	Alabama	821
27	North Carolina	804
28	Alaska	802
29	Delaware	801
30	Illinois	794
31	Florida	791
32	Indiana	773
33	Michigan	761
34	South Carolina	740
35	Wyoming	739
36	Oregon	730
37	Washington	725
38	Idaho	723
39	Virginia	714
40	Arkansas	710
41	Georgia	671
42	Colorado	646
43	Nevada	635
44	Texas	633
45	Oklahoma	630
46	Hawaii	629
47	Arizona	606
48	New Mexico	603
49	California	602
50	Utah	551
	District of Columbia	1,374

Source: Morgan Quitno Press using data from U.S. Department of Labor, Bureau of Labor Statistics
   "Occupational Employment and Wages, 2002" (http://www.bls.gov/oes/)
*Does not include self-employed.

Average Annual Wages of Registered Nurses in 2003

National Average = $52,810*

ALPHA ORDER

RANK	STATE	WAGES
41	Alabama	$44,870
6	Alaska	59,060
17	Arizona	51,730
42	Arkansas	44,810
1	California	65,100
16	Colorado	52,110
7	Connecticut	59,030
8	Delaware	57,870
26	Florida	49,260
31	Georgia	48,750
4	Hawaii	59,570
37	Idaho	46,590
28	Illinois	49,180
38	Indiana	46,240
50	Iowa	42,140
48	Kansas	43,730
36	Kentucky	46,720
32	Louisiana	48,150
23	Maine	50,040
2	Maryland	63,070
3	Massachusetts	59,890
15	Michigan	52,630
12	Minnesota	55,310
40	Mississippi	45,590
35	Missouri	46,890
49	Montana	43,110
39	Nebraska	45,730
11	Nevada	57,130
30	New Hampshire	48,800
9	New Jersey	57,820
21	New Mexico	50,080
5	New York	59,370
29	North Carolina	48,870
47	North Dakota	43,850
26	Ohio	49,260
46	Oklahoma	44,200
13	Oregon	54,320
18	Pennsylvania	51,410
14	Rhode Island	54,260
25	South Carolina	49,510
45	South Dakota	44,340
33	Tennessee	47,980
19	Texas	51,040
22	Utah	50,050
34	Vermont	47,060
24	Virginia	49,770
10	Washington	57,670
44	West Virginia	44,450
20	Wisconsin	50,840
43	Wyoming	44,670

RANK ORDER

RANK	STATE	WAGES
1	California	$65,100
2	Maryland	63,070
3	Massachusetts	59,890
4	Hawaii	59,570
5	New York	59,370
6	Alaska	59,060
7	Connecticut	59,030
8	Delaware	57,870
9	New Jersey	57,820
10	Washington	57,670
11	Nevada	57,130
12	Minnesota	55,310
13	Oregon	54,320
14	Rhode Island	54,260
15	Michigan	52,630
16	Colorado	52,110
17	Arizona	51,730
18	Pennsylvania	51,410
19	Texas	51,040
20	Wisconsin	50,840
21	New Mexico	50,080
22	Utah	50,050
23	Maine	50,040
24	Virginia	49,770
25	South Carolina	49,510
26	Florida	49,260
26	Ohio	49,260
28	Illinois	49,180
29	North Carolina	48,870
30	New Hampshire	48,800
31	Georgia	48,750
32	Louisiana	48,150
33	Tennessee	47,980
34	Vermont	47,060
35	Missouri	46,890
36	Kentucky	46,720
37	Idaho	46,590
38	Indiana	46,240
39	Nebraska	45,730
40	Mississippi	45,590
41	Alabama	44,870
42	Arkansas	44,810
43	Wyoming	44,670
44	West Virginia	44,450
45	South Dakota	44,340
46	Oklahoma	44,200
47	North Dakota	43,850
48	Kansas	43,730
49	Montana	43,110
50	Iowa	42,140
	District of Columbia	57,000

Source: U.S. Department of Labor, Bureau of Labor Statistics
"Occupational Employment and Wages, 2003" (http://www.bls.gov/oes/)
*Does not include self-employed.

Licensed Practical and Licensed Vocational Nurses in 2003

National Total = 691,110 LPN/LVNs*

ALPHA ORDER

RANK	STATE	NURSES	% of USA
19	Alabama	15,580	2.3%
49	Alaska	470	0.1%
27	Arizona	8,310	1.2%
21	Arkansas	12,730	1.8%
2	California	51,040	7.4%
34	Colorado	6,130	0.9%
29	Connecticut	7,660	1.1%
41	Delaware	2,330	0.3%
4	Florida	46,390	6.7%
7	Georgia	22,560	3.3%
42	Hawaii	2,310	0.3%
36	Idaho	3,100	0.4%
9	Illinois	20,530	3.0%
11	Indiana	18,830	2.7%
30	Iowa	7,030	1.0%
31	Kansas	7,020	1.0%
22	Kentucky	12,510	1.8%
10	Louisiana	19,020	2.8%
44	Maine	2,250	0.3%
28	Maryland	8,140	1.2%
17	Massachusetts	16,640	2.4%
16	Michigan	16,960	2.5%
14	Minnesota	17,150	2.5%
26	Mississippi	9,870	1.4%
17	Missouri	16,640	2.4%
40	Montana	2,400	0.3%
33	Nebraska	6,370	0.9%
43	Nevada	2,260	0.3%
46	New Hampshire	1,950	0.3%
15	New Jersey	16,970	2.5%
35	New Mexico	3,440	0.5%
3	New York	47,990	6.9%
13	North Carolina	17,240	2.5%
38	North Dakota	2,760	0.4%
5	Ohio	35,550	5.1%
20	Oklahoma	13,050	1.9%
37	Oregon	2,910	0.4%
6	Pennsylvania	35,430	5.1%
NA	Rhode Island**	NA	NA
24	South Carolina	10,700	1.5%
45	South Dakota	1,980	0.3%
8	Tennessee	21,830	3.2%
1	Texas	61,400	8.9%
39	Utah	2,600	0.4%
47	Vermont	1,540	0.2%
12	Virginia	18,250	2.6%
25	Washington	9,960	1.4%
32	West Virginia	6,870	1.0%
23	Wisconsin	11,140	1.6%
48	Wyoming	900	0.1%

RANK ORDER

RANK	STATE	NURSES	% of USA
1	Texas	61,400	8.9%
2	California	51,040	7.4%
3	New York	47,990	6.9%
4	Florida	46,390	6.7%
5	Ohio	35,550	5.1%
6	Pennsylvania	35,430	5.1%
7	Georgia	22,560	3.3%
8	Tennessee	21,830	3.2%
9	Illinois	20,530	3.0%
10	Louisiana	19,020	2.8%
11	Indiana	18,830	2.7%
12	Virginia	18,250	2.6%
13	North Carolina	17,240	2.5%
14	Minnesota	17,150	2.5%
15	New Jersey	16,970	2.5%
16	Michigan	16,960	2.5%
17	Massachusetts	16,640	2.4%
17	Missouri	16,640	2.4%
19	Alabama	15,580	2.3%
20	Oklahoma	13,050	1.9%
21	Arkansas	12,730	1.8%
22	Kentucky	12,510	1.8%
23	Wisconsin	11,140	1.6%
24	South Carolina	10,700	1.5%
25	Washington	9,960	1.4%
26	Mississippi	9,870	1.4%
27	Arizona	8,310	1.2%
28	Maryland	8,140	1.2%
29	Connecticut	7,660	1.1%
30	Iowa	7,030	1.0%
31	Kansas	7,020	1.0%
32	West Virginia	6,870	1.0%
33	Nebraska	6,370	0.9%
34	Colorado	6,130	0.9%
35	New Mexico	3,440	0.5%
36	Idaho	3,100	0.4%
37	Oregon	2,910	0.4%
38	North Dakota	2,760	0.4%
39	Utah	2,600	0.4%
40	Montana	2,400	0.3%
41	Delaware	2,330	0.3%
42	Hawaii	2,310	0.3%
43	Nevada	2,260	0.3%
44	Maine	2,250	0.3%
45	South Dakota	1,980	0.3%
46	New Hampshire	1,950	0.3%
47	Vermont	1,540	0.2%
48	Wyoming	900	0.1%
49	Alaska	470	0.1%
NA	Rhode Island**	NA	NA
	District of Columbia	2,450	0.4%

Source: U.S. Department of Labor, Bureau of Labor Statistics
     "Occupational Employment and Wages, 2003" (http://www.bls.gov/oes/)
*Does not include self-employed.
**Not available.

Rate of Licensed Practical and Licensed Vocational Nurses in 2003

National Rate = 238 LPN/LVNs per 100,000 Population*

<u>ALPHA ORDER</u>

RANK	STATE	RATE
8	Alabama	346
49	Alaska	72
42	Arizona	149
1	Arkansas	467
44	California	144
45	Colorado	135
30	Connecticut	220
16	Delaware	285
18	Florida	273
20	Georgia	260
34	Hawaii	185
29	Idaho	227
39	Illinois	162
12	Indiana	304
28	Iowa	239
23	Kansas	258
12	Kentucky	304
3	Louisiana	423
37	Maine	172
43	Maryland	148
21	Massachusetts	259
38	Michigan	168
10	Minnesota	339
9	Mississippi	342
14	Missouri	291
19	Montana	261
7	Nebraska	367
47	Nevada	101
41	New Hampshire	151
33	New Jersey	196
35	New Mexico	183
25	New York	250
31	North Carolina	205
2	North Dakota	436
11	Ohio	311
6	Oklahoma	372
48	Oregon	82
15	Pennsylvania	286
NA	Rhode Island**	NA
23	South Carolina	258
21	South Dakota	259
5	Tennessee	373
17	Texas	278
46	Utah	111
26	Vermont	249
27	Virginia	248
39	Washington	162
4	West Virginia	379
32	Wisconsin	203
36	Wyoming	179

<u>RANK ORDER</u>

RANK	STATE	RATE
1	Arkansas	467
2	North Dakota	436
3	Louisiana	423
4	West Virginia	379
5	Tennessee	373
6	Oklahoma	372
7	Nebraska	367
8	Alabama	346
9	Mississippi	342
10	Minnesota	339
11	Ohio	311
12	Indiana	304
12	Kentucky	304
14	Missouri	291
15	Pennsylvania	286
16	Delaware	285
17	Texas	278
18	Florida	273
19	Montana	261
20	Georgia	260
21	Massachusetts	259
21	South Dakota	259
23	Kansas	258
23	South Carolina	258
25	New York	250
26	Vermont	249
27	Virginia	248
28	Iowa	239
29	Idaho	227
30	Connecticut	220
31	North Carolina	205
32	Wisconsin	203
33	New Jersey	196
34	Hawaii	185
35	New Mexico	183
36	Wyoming	179
37	Maine	172
38	Michigan	168
39	Illinois	162
39	Washington	162
41	New Hampshire	151
42	Arizona	149
43	Maryland	148
44	California	144
45	Colorado	135
46	Utah	111
47	Nevada	101
48	Oregon	82
49	Alaska	72
NA	Rhode Island**	NA
	District of Columbia	439

*Source: Morgan Quitno Press using data from U.S. Department of Labor, Bureau of Labor Statistics
"Occupational Employment and Wages, 2003" (http://www.bls.gov/oes/)*
Does not include self-employed.
***Not available.*

Average Annual Wages of Licensed Practical and Licensed Vocational Nurses in 2003
National Average = $33,930*

ALPHA ORDER

RANK	STATE	WAGES
47	Alabama	$27,340
9	Alaska	37,860
15	Arizona	35,370
46	Arkansas	27,860
7	California	39,990
12	Colorado	35,880
1	Connecticut	45,880
3	Delaware	42,300
24	Florida	33,620
38	Georgia	29,770
20	Hawaii	34,420
33	Idaho	30,930
22	Illinois	33,810
26	Indiana	33,290
39	Iowa	29,660
37	Kansas	30,230
34	Kentucky	30,890
42	Louisiana	29,040
31	Maine	31,860
5	Maryland	41,790
2	Massachusetts	42,580
16	Michigan	35,280
25	Minnesota	33,380
50	Mississippi	26,070
41	Missouri	29,490
45	Montana	27,980
36	Nebraska	30,370
8	Nevada	38,220
13	New Hampshire	35,590
4	New Jersey	42,020
21	New Mexico	34,220
17	New York	35,210
28	North Carolina	32,940
44	North Dakota	28,050
19	Ohio	34,750
43	Oklahoma	28,480
10	Oregon	36,650
14	Pennsylvania	35,400
6	Rhode Island	41,690
23	South Carolina	33,690
48	South Dakota	27,290
40	Tennessee	29,620
27	Texas	32,980
32	Utah	31,720
30	Vermont	31,870
29	Virginia	32,570
11	Washington	36,560
49	West Virginia	26,800
18	Wisconsin	34,940
35	Wyoming	30,500

RANK ORDER

RANK	STATE	WAGES
1	Connecticut	$45,880
2	Massachusetts	42,580
3	Delaware	42,300
4	New Jersey	42,020
5	Maryland	41,790
6	Rhode Island	41,690
7	California	39,990
8	Nevada	38,220
9	Alaska	37,860
10	Oregon	36,650
11	Washington	36,560
12	Colorado	35,880
13	New Hampshire	35,590
14	Pennsylvania	35,400
15	Arizona	35,370
16	Michigan	35,280
17	New York	35,210
18	Wisconsin	34,940
19	Ohio	34,750
20	Hawaii	34,420
21	New Mexico	34,220
22	Illinois	33,810
23	South Carolina	33,690
24	Florida	33,620
25	Minnesota	33,380
26	Indiana	33,290
27	Texas	32,980
28	North Carolina	32,940
29	Virginia	32,570
30	Vermont	31,870
31	Maine	31,860
32	Utah	31,720
33	Idaho	30,930
34	Kentucky	30,890
35	Wyoming	30,500
36	Nebraska	30,370
37	Kansas	30,230
38	Georgia	29,770
39	Iowa	29,660
40	Tennessee	29,620
41	Missouri	29,490
42	Louisiana	29,040
43	Oklahoma	28,480
44	North Dakota	28,050
45	Montana	27,980
46	Arkansas	27,860
47	Alabama	27,340
48	South Dakota	27,290
49	West Virginia	26,800
50	Mississippi	26,070
	District of Columbia	44,130

Source: U.S. Department of Labor, Bureau of Labor Statistics
   "Occupational Employment and Wages, 2003" (http://www.bls.gov/oes/)
*Does not include self-employed.

Dentists in 2001

National Total = 168,556 Dentists*

RANK	STATE	DENTISTS	% of USA
27	Alabama	1,904	1.1%
45	Alaska	458	0.3%
23	Arizona	2,421	1.4%
35	Arkansas	1,083	0.6%
1	California	23,536	14.0%
20	Colorado	2,839	1.7%
22	Connecticut	2,666	1.6%
48	Delaware	345	0.2%
4	Florida	8,424	5.0%
14	Georgia	3,681	2.2%
36	Hawaii	991	0.6%
41	Idaho	706	0.4%
5	Illinois	8,196	4.9%
19	Indiana	2,921	1.7%
30	Iowa	1,558	0.9%
32	Kansas	1,380	0.8%
25	Kentucky	2,274	1.3%
26	Louisiana	2,078	1.2%
42	Maine	605	0.4%
12	Maryland	4,057	2.4%
10	Massachusetts	5,207	3.1%
9	Michigan	5,952	3.5%
18	Minnesota	2,986	1.8%
33	Mississippi	1,119	0.7%
21	Missouri	2,758	1.6%
44	Montana	507	0.3%
34	Nebraska	1,098	0.7%
39	Nevada	781	0.5%
40	New Hampshire	727	0.4%
7	New Jersey	6,632	3.9%
38	New Mexico	810	0.5%
2	New York	15,244	9.0%
15	North Carolina	3,459	2.1%
49	North Dakota	306	0.2%
8	Ohio	6,060	3.6%
29	Oklahoma	1,693	1.0%
24	Oregon	2,323	1.4%
6	Pennsylvania	8,050	4.8%
43	Rhode Island	592	0.4%
28	South Carolina	1,833	1.1%
46	South Dakota	366	0.2%
17	Tennessee	3,003	1.8%
3	Texas	9,989	5.9%
31	Utah	1,441	0.9%
47	Vermont	357	0.2%
11	Virginia	4,128	2.4%
13	Washington	3,962	2.4%
37	West Virginia	839	0.5%
16	Wisconsin	3,163	1.9%
50	Wyoming	261	0.2%

RANK	STATE	DENTISTS	% of USA
1	California	23,536	14.0%
2	New York	15,244	9.0%
3	Texas	9,989	5.9%
4	Florida	8,424	5.0%
5	Illinois	8,196	4.9%
6	Pennsylvania	8,050	4.8%
7	New Jersey	6,632	3.9%
8	Ohio	6,060	3.6%
9	Michigan	5,952	3.5%
10	Massachusetts	5,207	3.1%
11	Virginia	4,128	2.4%
12	Maryland	4,057	2.4%
13	Washington	3,962	2.4%
14	Georgia	3,681	2.2%
15	North Carolina	3,459	2.1%
16	Wisconsin	3,163	1.9%
17	Tennessee	3,003	1.8%
18	Minnesota	2,986	1.8%
19	Indiana	2,921	1.7%
20	Colorado	2,839	1.7%
21	Missouri	2,758	1.6%
22	Connecticut	2,666	1.6%
23	Arizona	2,421	1.4%
24	Oregon	2,323	1.4%
25	Kentucky	2,274	1.3%
26	Louisiana	2,078	1.2%
27	Alabama	1,904	1.1%
28	South Carolina	1,833	1.1%
29	Oklahoma	1,693	1.0%
30	Iowa	1,558	0.9%
31	Utah	1,441	0.9%
32	Kansas	1,380	0.8%
33	Mississippi	1,119	0.7%
34	Nebraska	1,098	0.7%
35	Arkansas	1,083	0.6%
36	Hawaii	991	0.6%
37	West Virginia	839	0.5%
38	New Mexico	810	0.5%
39	Nevada	781	0.5%
40	New Hampshire	727	0.4%
41	Idaho	706	0.4%
42	Maine	605	0.4%
43	Rhode Island	592	0.4%
44	Montana	507	0.3%
45	Alaska	458	0.3%
46	South Dakota	366	0.2%
47	Vermont	357	0.2%
48	Delaware	345	0.2%
49	North Dakota	306	0.2%
50	Wyoming	261	0.2%
	District of Columbia	721	0.4%

Source: American Dental Association
"Distribution of Dentists, by Region and State, 2001"
Professionally active dentists. Total includes 66 dentists for whom state is not known. Total does not include 2,233 dentists in territories nor dentists in the Armed Forces stationed overseas.

Rate of Dentists in 2001

National Rate = 59 Dentists per 100,000 Population*

ALPHA ORDER

RANK	STATE	RATE
45	Alabama	43
7	Alaska	72
41	Arizona	46
48	Arkansas	40
8	California	68
13	Colorado	64
4	Connecticut	78
45	Delaware	43
29	Florida	52
43	Georgia	44
1	Hawaii	81
25	Idaho	53
11	Illinois	65
34	Indiana	48
25	Iowa	53
31	Kansas	51
22	Kentucky	56
37	Louisiana	47
37	Maine	47
6	Maryland	75
1	Massachusetts	81
17	Michigan	59
16	Minnesota	60
49	Mississippi	39
32	Missouri	49
22	Montana	56
13	Nebraska	64
50	Nevada	37
19	New Hampshire	58
4	New Jersey	78
43	New Mexico	44
3	New York	80
47	North Carolina	42
34	North Dakota	48
25	Ohio	53
32	Oklahoma	49
9	Oregon	67
11	Pennsylvania	65
22	Rhode Island	56
42	South Carolina	45
34	South Dakota	48
29	Tennessee	52
37	Texas	47
15	Utah	63
19	Vermont	58
21	Virginia	57
10	Washington	66
37	West Virginia	47
17	Wisconsin	59
25	Wyoming	53

RANK ORDER

RANK	STATE	RATE
1	Hawaii	81
1	Massachusetts	81
3	New York	80
4	Connecticut	78
4	New Jersey	78
6	Maryland	75
7	Alaska	72
8	California	68
9	Oregon	67
10	Washington	66
11	Illinois	65
11	Pennsylvania	65
13	Colorado	64
13	Nebraska	64
15	Utah	63
16	Minnesota	60
17	Michigan	59
17	Wisconsin	59
19	New Hampshire	58
19	Vermont	58
21	Virginia	57
22	Kentucky	56
22	Montana	56
22	Rhode Island	56
25	Idaho	53
25	Iowa	53
25	Ohio	53
25	Wyoming	53
29	Florida	52
29	Tennessee	52
31	Kansas	51
32	Missouri	49
32	Oklahoma	49
34	Indiana	48
34	North Dakota	48
34	South Dakota	48
37	Louisiana	47
37	Maine	47
37	Texas	47
37	West Virginia	47
41	Arizona	46
42	South Carolina	45
43	Georgia	44
43	New Mexico	44
45	Alabama	43
45	Delaware	43
47	North Carolina	42
48	Arkansas	40
49	Mississippi	39
50	Nevada	37

District of Columbia — 126

Source: Morgan Quitno Press using data from American Dental Association
"Distribution of Dentists, by Region and State, 2001"
*Professionally active dentists. National rate includes dentists for whom state is not known. National rate does not include dentists in territories nor dentists in the Armed Forces stationed overseas.

Average Annual Wages of Dentists in 2003

National Average = $129,040*

ALPHA ORDER

RANK	STATE	WAGES
8	Alabama	$156,350
4	Alaska	160,130
18	Arizona	141,660
44	Arkansas	92,910
28	California	130,410
2	Colorado	162,830
31	Connecticut	128,660
23	Delaware	134,290
37	Florida	119,420
13	Georgia	153,150
22	Hawaii	136,420
25	Idaho	131,710
47	Illinois	82,610
16	Indiana	145,380
10	Iowa	154,880
42	Kansas	101,840
32	Kentucky	128,060
36	Louisiana	124,560
40	Maine	106,040
24	Maryland	133,450
21	Massachusetts	139,270
29	Michigan	129,620
14	Minnesota	149,950
48	Mississippi	74,780
35	Missouri	126,570
43	Montana	95,300
17	Nebraska	142,470
15	Nevada	146,310
11	New Hampshire	154,520
27	New Jersey	130,490
38	New Mexico	118,400
34	New York	127,150
5	North Carolina	158,950
9	North Dakota	155,490
1	Ohio	168,550
3	Oklahoma	160,300
NA	Oregon**	NA
33	Pennsylvania	127,530
NA	Rhode Island**	NA
19	South Carolina	140,180
39	South Dakota	117,120
46	Tennessee	83,810
26	Texas	130,820
7	Utah	156,540
6	Vermont	157,000
12	Virginia	153,170
20	Washington	139,830
45	West Virginia	92,900
41	Wisconsin	104,610
30	Wyoming	129,540

RANK ORDER

RANK	STATE	WAGES
1	Ohio	$168,550
2	Colorado	162,830
3	Oklahoma	160,300
4	Alaska	160,130
5	North Carolina	158,950
6	Vermont	157,000
7	Utah	156,540
8	Alabama	156,350
9	North Dakota	155,490
10	Iowa	154,880
11	New Hampshire	154,520
12	Virginia	153,170
13	Georgia	153,150
14	Minnesota	149,950
15	Nevada	146,310
16	Indiana	145,380
17	Nebraska	142,470
18	Arizona	141,660
19	South Carolina	140,180
20	Washington	139,830
21	Massachusetts	139,270
22	Hawaii	136,420
23	Delaware	134,290
24	Maryland	133,450
25	Idaho	131,710
26	Texas	130,820
27	New Jersey	130,490
28	California	130,410
29	Michigan	129,620
30	Wyoming	129,540
31	Connecticut	128,660
32	Kentucky	128,060
33	Pennsylvania	127,530
34	New York	127,150
35	Missouri	126,570
36	Louisiana	124,560
37	Florida	119,420
38	New Mexico	118,400
39	South Dakota	117,120
40	Maine	106,040
41	Wisconsin	104,610
42	Kansas	101,840
43	Montana	95,300
44	Arkansas	92,910
45	West Virginia	92,900
46	Tennessee	83,810
47	Illinois	82,610
48	Mississippi	74,780
NA	Oregon**	NA
NA	Rhode Island**	NA
	District of Columbia	108,120

Source: U.S. Department of Labor, Bureau of Labor Statistics
"Occupational Employment and Wages, 2003" (http://www.bls.gov/oes/)
*Does not include self-employed.
**Not available.

Percent of Population Lacking Access to Dental Care in 2004

National Percent = 9.3% of Population*

ALPHA ORDER

RANK ORDER

RANK	STATE	PERCENT	RANK	STATE	PERCENT
1	Alabama	32.3	1	Alabama	32.3
14	Alaska	13.7	2	New Mexico	26.6
30	Arizona	8.2	3	Montana	23.6
41	Arkansas	5.2	4	South Carolina	23.1
48	California	3.2	5	Missouri	21.4
44	Colorado	4.5	6	Maine	21.1
38	Connecticut	5.4	7	Tennessee	20.3
12	Delaware	15.8	8	Kansas	19.2
18	Florida	11.6	9	Idaho	17.8
25	Georgia	9.3	10	Utah	17.0
28	Hawaii	8.7	11	Iowa	16.9
9	Idaho	17.8	12	Delaware	15.8
29	Illinois	8.3	13	Oregon	14.8
45	Indiana	4.0	14	Alaska	13.7
11	Iowa	16.9	15	North Carolina	12.9
8	Kansas	19.2	16	Nevada	11.8
36	Kentucky	6.2	17	Wyoming	11.7
35	Louisiana	6.5	18	Florida	11.6
6	Maine	21.1	19	Michigan	11.4
38	Maryland	5.4	20	Texas	11.3
37	Massachusetts	5.6	21	Wisconsin	11.1
19	Michigan	11.4	22	Mississippi	10.5
45	Minnesota	4.0	23	Pennsylvania	10.4
22	Mississippi	10.5	24	South Dakota	10.3
5	Missouri	21.4	25	Georgia	9.3
3	Montana	23.6	26	Washington	9.2
50	Nebraska	1.2	27	Rhode Island	8.8
16	Nevada	11.8	28	Hawaii	8.7
41	New Hampshire	5.2	29	Illinois	8.3
49	New Jersey	1.8	30	Arizona	8.2
2	New Mexico	26.6	31	West Virginia	7.7
43	New York	5.1	32	Ohio	7.4
15	North Carolina	12.9	33	North Dakota	7.1
33	North Dakota	7.1	34	Virginia	6.7
32	Ohio	7.4	35	Louisiana	6.5
38	Oklahoma	5.4	36	Kentucky	6.2
13	Oregon	14.8	37	Massachusetts	5.6
23	Pennsylvania	10.4	38	Connecticut	5.4
27	Rhode Island	8.8	38	Maryland	5.4
4	South Carolina	23.1	38	Oklahoma	5.4
24	South Dakota	10.3	41	Arkansas	5.2
7	Tennessee	20.3	41	New Hampshire	5.2
20	Texas	11.3	43	New York	5.1
10	Utah	17.0	44	Colorado	4.5
47	Vermont	3.3	45	Indiana	4.0
34	Virginia	6.7	45	Minnesota	4.0
26	Washington	9.2	47	Vermont	3.3
31	West Virginia	7.7	48	California	3.2
21	Wisconsin	11.1	49	New Jersey	1.8
17	Wyoming	11.7	50	Nebraska	1.2

District of Columbia   7.8

Source: Morgan Quitno Press using data from U.S. Dept. of Health and Human Services, Div. of Shortage Designation
"Selected Statistics on Health Professional Shortage Areas" (as of September 30, 2004)
*Percent of population considered under-served by dental practitioners. An under-served population does not have primary medical care within reasonable economic and geographic bounds.

Pharmacists in 2003

National Total = 219,790 Pharmacists*

<u>ALPHA ORDER</u>

RANK	STATE	PHARMACISTS	% of USA
21	Alabama	3,980	1.8%
50	Alaska	380	0.2%
24	Arizona	3,280	1.5%
31	Arkansas	2,370	1.1%
1	California	22,710	10.3%
26	Colorado	3,090	1.4%
30	Connecticut	2,440	1.1%
46	Delaware	570	0.3%
4	Florida	12,380	5.6%
10	Georgia	6,530	3.0%
40	Hawaii	1,000	0.5%
39	Idaho	1,040	0.5%
5	Illinois	11,080	5.0%
12	Indiana	5,330	2.4%
29	Iowa	2,450	1.1%
32	Kansas	2,180	1.0%
23	Kentucky	3,730	1.7%
17	Louisiana	4,560	2.1%
42	Maine	900	0.4%
19	Maryland	4,290	2.0%
15	Massachusetts	4,850	2.2%
8	Michigan	7,580	3.4%
22	Minnesota	3,870	1.8%
33	Mississippi	2,140	1.0%
16	Missouri	4,580	2.1%
43	Montana	730	0.3%
34	Nebraska	1,910	0.9%
35	Nevada	1,790	0.8%
41	New Hampshire	960	0.4%
9	New Jersey	6,660	3.0%
38	New Mexico	1,390	0.6%
3	New York	12,620	5.7%
11	North Carolina	5,870	2.7%
47	North Dakota	520	0.2%
7	Ohio	10,610	4.8%
28	Oklahoma	2,610	1.2%
25	Oregon	3,170	1.4%
6	Pennsylvania	10,820	4.9%
45	Rhode Island	620	0.3%
27	South Carolina	3,080	1.4%
43	South Dakota	730	0.3%
13	Tennessee	5,280	2.4%
2	Texas	14,790	6.7%
36	Utah	1,740	0.8%
49	Vermont	430	0.2%
14	Virginia	5,130	2.3%
18	Washington	4,360	2.0%
37	West Virginia	1,680	0.8%
20	Wisconsin	4,100	1.9%
48	Wyoming	460	0.2%

<u>RANK ORDER</u>

RANK	STATE	PHARMACISTS	% of USA
1	California	22,710	10.3%
2	Texas	14,790	6.7%
3	New York	12,620	5.7%
4	Florida	12,380	5.6%
5	Illinois	11,080	5.0%
6	Pennsylvania	10,820	4.9%
7	Ohio	10,610	4.8%
8	Michigan	7,580	3.4%
9	New Jersey	6,660	3.0%
10	Georgia	6,530	3.0%
11	North Carolina	5,870	2.7%
12	Indiana	5,330	2.4%
13	Tennessee	5,280	2.4%
14	Virginia	5,130	2.3%
15	Massachusetts	4,850	2.2%
16	Missouri	4,580	2.1%
17	Louisiana	4,560	2.1%
18	Washington	4,360	2.0%
19	Maryland	4,290	2.0%
20	Wisconsin	4,100	1.9%
21	Alabama	3,980	1.8%
22	Minnesota	3,870	1.8%
23	Kentucky	3,730	1.7%
24	Arizona	3,280	1.5%
25	Oregon	3,170	1.4%
26	Colorado	3,090	1.4%
27	South Carolina	3,080	1.4%
28	Oklahoma	2,610	1.2%
29	Iowa	2,450	1.1%
30	Connecticut	2,440	1.1%
31	Arkansas	2,370	1.1%
32	Kansas	2,180	1.0%
33	Mississippi	2,140	1.0%
34	Nebraska	1,910	0.9%
35	Nevada	1,790	0.8%
36	Utah	1,740	0.8%
37	West Virginia	1,680	0.8%
38	New Mexico	1,390	0.6%
39	Idaho	1,040	0.5%
40	Hawaii	1,000	0.5%
41	New Hampshire	960	0.4%
42	Maine	900	0.4%
43	Montana	730	0.3%
43	South Dakota	730	0.3%
45	Rhode Island	620	0.3%
46	Delaware	570	0.3%
47	North Dakota	520	0.2%
48	Wyoming	460	0.2%
49	Vermont	430	0.2%
50	Alaska	380	0.2%
	District of Columbia	430	0.2%

Source: U.S. Department of Labor, Bureau of Labor Statistics
   "Occupational Employment and Wages, 2003" (http://www.bls.gov/oes/)
*Does not include self-employed.
**Not available.

Rate of Pharmacists in 2003

National Rate = 76 Pharmacists per 100,000 Population*

ALPHA ORDER

RANK	STATE	RATE
10	Alabama	88
48	Alaska	59
48	Arizona	59
12	Arkansas	87
47	California	64
44	Colorado	68
38	Connecticut	70
38	Delaware	70
36	Florida	73
27	Georgia	75
17	Hawaii	80
24	Idaho	76
10	Illinois	88
14	Indiana	86
15	Iowa	83
17	Kansas	80
7	Kentucky	91
2	Louisiana	101
42	Maine	69
22	Maryland	78
24	Massachusetts	76
27	Michigan	75
24	Minnesota	76
30	Mississippi	74
17	Missouri	80
17	Montana	80
1	Nebraska	110
17	Nevada	80
30	New Hampshire	74
23	New Jersey	77
30	New Mexico	74
46	New York	66
38	North Carolina	70
16	North Dakota	82
4	Ohio	93
30	Oklahoma	74
9	Oregon	89
12	Pennsylvania	87
50	Rhode Island	58
30	South Carolina	74
3	South Dakota	95
8	Tennessee	90
45	Texas	67
30	Utah	74
42	Vermont	69
38	Virginia	70
37	Washington	71
4	West Virginia	93
27	Wisconsin	75
6	Wyoming	92

RANK ORDER

RANK	STATE	RATE
1	Nebraska	110
2	Louisiana	101
3	South Dakota	95
4	Ohio	93
4	West Virginia	93
6	Wyoming	92
7	Kentucky	91
8	Tennessee	90
9	Oregon	89
10	Alabama	88
10	Illinois	88
12	Arkansas	87
12	Pennsylvania	87
14	Indiana	86
15	Iowa	83
16	North Dakota	82
17	Hawaii	80
17	Kansas	80
17	Missouri	80
17	Montana	80
17	Nevada	80
22	Maryland	78
23	New Jersey	77
24	Idaho	76
24	Massachusetts	76
24	Minnesota	76
27	Georgia	75
27	Michigan	75
27	Wisconsin	75
30	Mississippi	74
30	New Hampshire	74
30	New Mexico	74
30	Oklahoma	74
30	South Carolina	74
30	Utah	74
36	Florida	73
37	Washington	71
38	Connecticut	70
38	Delaware	70
38	North Carolina	70
38	Virginia	70
42	Maine	69
42	Vermont	69
44	Colorado	68
45	Texas	67
46	New York	66
47	California	64
48	Alaska	59
48	Arizona	59
50	Rhode Island	58

	District of Columbia	77

Source: Morgan Quitno Press using data from U.S. Department of Labor, Bureau of Labor Statistics
    "Occupational Employment and Wages, 2003" (http://www.bls.gov/oes/)
*Does not include self-employed.
**Not available.

Average Annual Wages of Pharmacists in 2003

National Average = $81,180*

ALPHA ORDER

RANK	STATE	WAGES
24	Alabama	$79,640
4	Alaska	86,070
15	Arizona	81,630
45	Arkansas	72,340
1	California	93,610
10	Colorado	82,460
14	Connecticut	81,690
12	Delaware	81,800
8	Florida	84,020
34	Georgia	77,640
32	Hawaii	78,420
40	Idaho	74,710
2	Illinois	87,060
31	Indiana	78,860
36	Iowa	77,000
43	Kansas	72,980
7	Kentucky	84,090
39	Louisiana	75,490
9	Maine	82,750
27	Maryland	79,340
37	Massachusetts	76,990
21	Michigan	80,030
5	Minnesota	84,170
49	Mississippi	67,300
22	Missouri	79,940
47	Montana	70,690
46	Nebraska	71,660
3	Nevada	86,220
11	New Hampshire	82,080
20	New Jersey	80,080
38	New Mexico	76,600
18	New York	80,590
19	North Carolina	80,120
50	North Dakota	66,750
26	Ohio	79,500
42	Oklahoma	74,050
12	Oregon	81,800
41	Pennsylvania	74,150
25	Rhode Island	79,560
35	South Carolina	77,030
44	South Dakota	72,890
16	Tennessee	81,510
17	Texas	80,970
28	Utah	79,290
23	Vermont	79,690
30	Virginia	78,900
33	Washington	78,280
29	West Virginia	79,000
6	Wisconsin	84,120
48	Wyoming	69,000

RANK ORDER

RANK	STATE	WAGES
1	California	$93,610
2	Illinois	87,060
3	Nevada	86,220
4	Alaska	86,070
5	Minnesota	84,170
6	Wisconsin	84,120
7	Kentucky	84,090
8	Florida	84,020
9	Maine	82,750
10	Colorado	82,460
11	New Hampshire	82,080
12	Delaware	81,800
12	Oregon	81,800
14	Connecticut	81,690
15	Arizona	81,630
16	Tennessee	81,510
17	Texas	80,970
18	New York	80,590
19	North Carolina	80,120
20	New Jersey	80,080
21	Michigan	80,030
22	Missouri	79,940
23	Vermont	79,690
24	Alabama	79,640
25	Rhode Island	79,560
26	Ohio	79,500
27	Maryland	79,340
28	Utah	79,290
29	West Virginia	79,000
30	Virginia	78,900
31	Indiana	78,860
32	Hawaii	78,420
33	Washington	78,280
34	Georgia	77,640
35	South Carolina	77,030
36	Iowa	77,000
37	Massachusetts	76,990
38	New Mexico	76,600
39	Louisiana	75,490
40	Idaho	74,710
41	Pennsylvania	74,150
42	Oklahoma	74,050
43	Kansas	72,980
44	South Dakota	72,890
45	Arkansas	72,340
46	Nebraska	71,660
47	Montana	70,690
48	Wyoming	69,000
49	Mississippi	67,300
50	North Dakota	66,750
	District of Columbia	61,640

Source: U.S. Department of Labor, Bureau of Labor Statistics
"Occupational Employment and Wages, 2003" (http://www.bls.gov/oes/)
Does not include self-employed.
**Not available.*

Optometrists in 2003

National Total = 22,760 Optometrists*

ALPHA ORDER

RANK	STATE	OPTOMETRISTS	% of USA
24	Alabama	280	1.2%
47	Alaska	40	0.2%
24	Arizona	280	1.2%
33	Arkansas	200	0.9%
1	California	1,870	8.2%
27	Colorado	260	1.1%
26	Connecticut	270	1.2%
33	Delaware	200	0.9%
10	Florida	740	3.3%
21	Georgia	380	1.7%
44	Hawaii	90	0.4%
39	Idaho	140	0.6%
4	Illinois	1,390	6.1%
12	Indiana	550	2.4%
22	Iowa	340	1.5%
18	Kansas	420	1.8%
23	Kentucky	290	1.3%
30	Louisiana	220	1.0%
38	Maine	150	0.7%
27	Maryland	260	1.1%
9	Massachusetts	760	3.3%
6	Michigan	910	4.0%
17	Minnesota	430	1.9%
44	Mississippi	90	0.4%
20	Missouri	390	1.7%
41	Montana	130	0.6%
29	Nebraska	240	1.1%
30	Nevada	220	1.0%
36	New Hampshire	170	0.7%
6	New Jersey	910	4.0%
NA	New Mexico**	NA	NA
2	New York	1,860	8.2%
11	North Carolina	560	2.5%
43	North Dakota	100	0.4%
8	Ohio	900	4.0%
13	Oklahoma	540	2.4%
NA	Oregon**	NA	NA
5	Pennsylvania	1,040	4.6%
NA	Rhode Island**	NA	NA
33	South Carolina	200	0.9%
39	South Dakota	140	0.6%
15	Tennessee	470	2.1%
3	Texas	1,590	7.0%
32	Utah	210	0.9%
46	Vermont	70	0.3%
14	Virginia	500	2.2%
15	Washington	470	2.1%
37	West Virginia	160	0.7%
18	Wisconsin	420	1.8%
42	Wyoming	110	0.5%

RANK ORDER

RANK	STATE	OPTOMETRISTS	% of USA
1	California	1,870	8.2%
2	New York	1,860	8.2%
3	Texas	1,590	7.0%
4	Illinois	1,390	6.1%
5	Pennsylvania	1,040	4.6%
6	Michigan	910	4.0%
6	New Jersey	910	4.0%
8	Ohio	900	4.0%
9	Massachusetts	760	3.3%
10	Florida	740	3.3%
11	North Carolina	560	2.5%
12	Indiana	550	2.4%
13	Oklahoma	540	2.4%
14	Virginia	500	2.2%
15	Tennessee	470	2.1%
15	Washington	470	2.1%
17	Minnesota	430	1.9%
18	Kansas	420	1.8%
18	Wisconsin	420	1.8%
20	Missouri	390	1.7%
21	Georgia	380	1.7%
22	Iowa	340	1.5%
23	Kentucky	290	1.3%
24	Alabama	280	1.2%
24	Arizona	280	1.2%
26	Connecticut	270	1.2%
27	Colorado	260	1.1%
27	Maryland	260	1.1%
29	Nebraska	240	1.1%
30	Louisiana	220	1.0%
30	Nevada	220	1.0%
32	Utah	210	0.9%
33	Arkansas	200	0.9%
33	Delaware	200	0.9%
33	South Carolina	200	0.9%
36	New Hampshire	170	0.7%
37	West Virginia	160	0.7%
38	Maine	150	0.7%
39	Idaho	140	0.6%
39	South Dakota	140	0.6%
41	Montana	130	0.6%
42	Wyoming	110	0.5%
43	North Dakota	100	0.4%
44	Hawaii	90	0.4%
44	Mississippi	90	0.4%
46	Vermont	70	0.3%
47	Alaska	40	0.2%
NA	New Mexico**	NA	NA
NA	Oregon**	NA	NA
NA	Rhode Island**	NA	NA
	District of Columbia	170	0.7%

Source: U.S. Department of Labor, Bureau of Labor Statistics
  "Occupational Employment and Wages, 2003" (http://www.bls.gov/oes/)
*Does not include self-employed.
**Not available.

Rate of Optometrists in 2003

National Rate = 8 Optometrists per 100,000 Population*

ALPHA ORDER

RANK	STATE	RATE
37	Alabama	6
37	Alaska	6
40	Arizona	5
30	Arkansas	7
40	California	5
37	Colorado	6
23	Connecticut	8
1	Delaware	24
45	Florida	4
45	Georgia	4
30	Hawaii	7
16	Idaho	10
12	Illinois	11
19	Indiana	9
10	Iowa	12
5	Kansas	15
30	Kentucky	7
40	Louisiana	5
12	Maine	11
40	Maryland	5
10	Massachusetts	12
19	Michigan	9
23	Minnesota	8
47	Mississippi	3
30	Missouri	7
7	Montana	14
7	Nebraska	14
16	Nevada	10
9	New Hampshire	13
12	New Jersey	11
NA	New Mexico**	NA
16	New York	10
30	North Carolina	7
4	North Dakota	16
23	Ohio	8
5	Oklahoma	15
NA	Oregon**	NA
23	Pennsylvania	8
NA	Rhode Island**	NA
40	South Carolina	5
3	South Dakota	18
23	Tennessee	8
30	Texas	7
19	Utah	9
12	Vermont	11
30	Virginia	7
23	Washington	8
19	West Virginia	9
23	Wisconsin	8
2	Wyoming	22

RANK ORDER

RANK	STATE	RATE
1	Delaware	24
2	Wyoming	22
3	South Dakota	18
4	North Dakota	16
5	Kansas	15
5	Oklahoma	15
7	Montana	14
7	Nebraska	14
9	New Hampshire	13
10	Iowa	12
10	Massachusetts	12
12	Illinois	11
12	Maine	11
12	New Jersey	11
12	Vermont	11
16	Idaho	10
16	Nevada	10
16	New York	10
19	Indiana	9
19	Michigan	9
19	Utah	9
19	West Virginia	9
23	Connecticut	8
23	Minnesota	8
23	Ohio	8
23	Pennsylvania	8
23	Tennessee	8
23	Washington	8
23	Wisconsin	8
30	Arkansas	7
30	Hawaii	7
30	Kentucky	7
30	Missouri	7
30	North Carolina	7
30	Texas	7
30	Virginia	7
37	Alabama	6
37	Alaska	6
37	Colorado	6
40	Arizona	5
40	California	5
40	Louisiana	5
40	Maryland	5
40	South Carolina	5
45	Florida	4
45	Georgia	4
47	Mississippi	3
NA	New Mexico**	NA
NA	Oregon**	NA
NA	Rhode Island**	NA

District of Columbia   30

*Source: Morgan Quitno Press using data from U.S. Department of Labor, Bureau of Labor Statistics
"Occupational Employment and Wages, 2003" (http://www.bls.gov/oes/)*
Does not include self-employed.
***Not available.*

Average Annual Wages of Optometrists in 2003

National Average = $96,610 Optometrists*

ALPHA ORDER

RANK	STATE	WAGES
39	Alabama	$83,240
3	Alaska	135,020
36	Arizona	84,550
4	Arkansas	121,820
13	California	106,980
31	Colorado	90,630
27	Connecticut	94,590
30	Delaware	90,770
29	Florida	93,410
41	Georgia	81,180
33	Hawaii	89,340
45	Idaho	73,360
35	Illinois	88,260
10	Indiana	111,710
28	Iowa	94,120
21	Kansas	98,250
38	Kentucky	83,810
18	Louisiana	99,990
42	Maine	79,650
21	Maryland	98,250
17	Massachusetts	100,700
25	Michigan	95,380
12	Minnesota	109,330
8	Mississippi	112,340
14	Missouri	106,880
48	Montana	60,170
9	Nebraska	112,020
23	Nevada	97,430
2	New Hampshire	144,780
34	New Jersey	88,950
46	New Mexico	69,580
43	New York	78,840
5	North Carolina	115,040
16	North Dakota	103,140
7	Ohio	112,380
37	Oklahoma	83,910
NA	Oregon**	NA
40	Pennsylvania	83,050
NA	Rhode Island**	NA
26	South Carolina	94,600
1	South Dakota	154,340
15	Tennessee	103,670
10	Texas	111,710
47	Utah	63,720
24	Vermont	97,200
20	Virginia	98,280
6	Washington	113,220
44	West Virginia	74,640
32	Wisconsin	90,400
19	Wyoming	98,330

RANK ORDER

RANK	STATE	WAGES
1	South Dakota	$154,340
2	New Hampshire	144,780
3	Alaska	135,020
4	Arkansas	121,820
5	North Carolina	115,040
6	Washington	113,220
7	Ohio	112,380
8	Mississippi	112,340
9	Nebraska	112,020
10	Indiana	111,710
10	Texas	111,710
12	Minnesota	109,330
13	California	106,980
14	Missouri	106,880
15	Tennessee	103,670
16	North Dakota	103,140
17	Massachusetts	100,700
18	Louisiana	99,990
19	Wyoming	98,330
20	Virginia	98,280
21	Kansas	98,250
21	Maryland	98,250
23	Nevada	97,430
24	Vermont	97,200
25	Michigan	95,380
26	South Carolina	94,600
27	Connecticut	94,590
28	Iowa	94,120
29	Florida	93,410
30	Delaware	90,770
31	Colorado	90,630
32	Wisconsin	90,400
33	Hawaii	89,340
34	New Jersey	88,950
35	Illinois	88,260
36	Arizona	84,550
37	Oklahoma	83,910
38	Kentucky	83,810
39	Alabama	83,240
40	Pennsylvania	83,050
41	Georgia	81,180
42	Maine	79,650
43	New York	78,840
44	West Virginia	74,640
45	Idaho	73,360
46	New Mexico	69,580
47	Utah	63,720
48	Montana	60,170
NA	Oregon**	NA
NA	Rhode Island**	NA
	District of Columbia	71,020

Source: U.S. Department of Labor, Bureau of Labor Statistics
     "Occupational Employment and Wages, 2003" (http://www.bls.gov/oes/)
*Does not include self-employed.
**Not available.

Emergency Medical Technicians and Paramedics in 2003

National Total = 186,110 Technicians and Paramedics*

RANK	STATE	PARAMEDICS	% of USA
25	Alabama	2,620	1.4%
49	Alaska	260	0.1%
29	Arizona	2,280	1.2%
28	Arkansas	2,330	1.3%
2	California	12,270	6.6%
22	Colorado	3,130	1.7%
27	Connecticut	2,500	1.3%
48	Delaware	330	0.2%
7	Florida	8,380	4.5%
9	Georgia	6,720	3.6%
43	Hawaii	580	0.3%
37	Idaho	1,000	0.5%
5	Illinois	9,860	5.3%
16	Indiana	4,540	2.4%
30	Iowa	2,160	1.2%
20	Kansas	3,340	1.8%
17	Kentucky	4,350	2.3%
23	Louisiana	2,890	1.6%
35	Maine	1,470	0.8%
21	Maryland	3,160	1.7%
13	Massachusetts	5,120	2.8%
12	Michigan	5,530	3.0%
19	Minnesota	3,400	1.8%
33	Mississippi	1,670	0.9%
15	Missouri	5,070	2.7%
45	Montana	550	0.3%
NA	Nebraska**	NA	NA
38	Nevada	990	0.5%
39	New Hampshire	910	0.5%
14	New Jersey	5,110	2.7%
40	New Mexico	840	0.5%
4	New York	10,100	5.4%
8	North Carolina	7,090	3.8%
42	North Dakota	710	0.4%
5	Ohio	9,860	5.3%
31	Oklahoma	2,040	1.1%
36	Oregon	1,350	0.7%
3	Pennsylvania	11,670	6.3%
41	Rhode Island	780	0.4%
18	South Carolina	3,640	2.0%
44	South Dakota	570	0.3%
11	Tennessee	5,790	3.1%
1	Texas	12,420	6.7%
34	Utah	1,510	0.8%
47	Vermont	350	0.2%
24	Virginia	2,660	1.4%
26	Washington	2,610	1.4%
32	West Virginia	1,890	1.0%
10	Wisconsin	6,360	3.4%
46	Wyoming	420	0.2%

RANK	STATE	PARAMEDICS	% of USA
1	Texas	12,420	6.7%
2	California	12,270	6.6%
3	Pennsylvania	11,670	6.3%
4	New York	10,100	5.4%
5	Illinois	9,860	5.3%
5	Ohio	9,860	5.3%
7	Florida	8,380	4.5%
8	North Carolina	7,090	3.8%
9	Georgia	6,720	3.6%
10	Wisconsin	6,360	3.4%
11	Tennessee	5,790	3.1%
12	Michigan	5,530	3.0%
13	Massachusetts	5,120	2.8%
14	New Jersey	5,110	2.7%
15	Missouri	5,070	2.7%
16	Indiana	4,540	2.4%
17	Kentucky	4,350	2.3%
18	South Carolina	3,640	2.0%
19	Minnesota	3,400	1.8%
20	Kansas	3,340	1.8%
21	Maryland	3,160	1.7%
22	Colorado	3,130	1.7%
23	Louisiana	2,890	1.6%
24	Virginia	2,660	1.4%
25	Alabama	2,620	1.4%
26	Washington	2,610	1.4%
27	Connecticut	2,500	1.3%
28	Arkansas	2,330	1.3%
29	Arizona	2,280	1.2%
30	Iowa	2,160	1.2%
31	Oklahoma	2,040	1.1%
32	West Virginia	1,890	1.0%
33	Mississippi	1,670	0.9%
34	Utah	1,510	0.8%
35	Maine	1,470	0.8%
36	Oregon	1,350	0.7%
37	Idaho	1,000	0.5%
38	Nevada	990	0.5%
39	New Hampshire	910	0.5%
40	New Mexico	840	0.5%
41	Rhode Island	780	0.4%
42	North Dakota	710	0.4%
43	Hawaii	580	0.3%
44	South Dakota	570	0.3%
45	Montana	550	0.3%
46	Wyoming	420	0.2%
47	Vermont	350	0.2%
48	Delaware	330	0.2%
49	Alaska	260	0.1%
NA	Nebraska**	NA	NA
	District of Columbia**	NA	NA

Source: U.S. Department of Labor, Bureau of Labor Statistics
   "Occupational Employment and Wages, 2003" (http://www.bls.gov/oes/)
Does not include self-employed. National total includes EMTs and Paramedics in U.S. territories.
**Not available.*

Rate of Emergency Medical Technicians and Paramedics in 2003

National Rate = 64 Technicians and Paramedics per 100,000 Population*

ALPHA ORDER

RANK	STATE	RATE
31	Alabama	58
45	Alaska	40
44	Arizona	41
12	Arkansas	85
49	California	35
25	Colorado	69
22	Connecticut	72
45	Delaware	40
39	Florida	49
17	Georgia	77
40	Hawaii	46
19	Idaho	73
16	Illinois	78
19	Indiana	73
19	Iowa	73
1	Kansas	123
5	Kentucky	106
27	Louisiana	64
3	Maine	112
34	Maryland	57
15	Massachusetts	80
37	Michigan	55
26	Minnesota	67
31	Mississippi	58
9	Missouri	89
29	Montana	60
NA	Nebraska**	NA
42	Nevada	44
24	New Hampshire	71
30	New Jersey	59
41	New Mexico	45
38	New York	53
13	North Carolina	84
3	North Dakota	112
11	Ohio	86
31	Oklahoma	58
47	Oregon	38
8	Pennsylvania	94
22	Rhode Island	72
10	South Carolina	88
18	South Dakota	75
7	Tennessee	99
36	Texas	56
27	Utah	64
34	Vermont	57
48	Virginia	36
43	Washington	43
6	West Virginia	104
2	Wisconsin	116
13	Wyoming	84

RANK ORDER

RANK	STATE	RATE
1	Kansas	123
2	Wisconsin	116
3	Maine	112
3	North Dakota	112
5	Kentucky	106
6	West Virginia	104
7	Tennessee	99
8	Pennsylvania	94
9	Missouri	89
10	South Carolina	88
11	Ohio	86
12	Arkansas	85
13	North Carolina	84
13	Wyoming	84
15	Massachusetts	80
16	Illinois	78
17	Georgia	77
18	South Dakota	75
19	Idaho	73
19	Indiana	73
19	Iowa	73
22	Connecticut	72
22	Rhode Island	72
24	New Hampshire	71
25	Colorado	69
26	Minnesota	67
27	Louisiana	64
27	Utah	64
29	Montana	60
30	New Jersey	59
31	Alabama	58
31	Mississippi	58
31	Oklahoma	58
34	Maryland	57
34	Vermont	57
36	Texas	56
37	Michigan	55
38	New York	53
39	Florida	49
40	Hawaii	46
41	New Mexico	45
42	Nevada	44
43	Washington	43
44	Arizona	41
45	Alaska	40
45	Delaware	40
47	Oregon	38
48	Virginia	36
49	California	35
NA	Nebraska**	NA
	District of Columbia**	NA

Source: U.S. Department of Labor, Bureau of Labor Statistics
"Occupational Employment and Wages, 2003" (http://www.bls.gov/oes/)
*Does not include self-employed.
**Not available.

Average Annual Wages of
Emergency Medical Technicians and Paramedics in 2003
National Average = $27,080*

ALPHA ORDER

RANK	STATE	WAGES
46	Alabama	$21,420
1	Alaska	37,230
14	Arizona	30,120
41	Arkansas	23,150
20	California	27,950
8	Colorado	31,300
9	Connecticut	31,170
16	Delaware	29,550
24	Florida	26,560
28	Georgia	25,460
6	Hawaii	31,970
11	Idaho	30,860
15	Illinois	29,830
32	Indiana	24,840
42	Iowa	22,610
48	Kansas	20,260
44	Kentucky	21,630
26	Louisiana	26,160
36	Maine	23,660
3	Maryland	34,730
5	Massachusetts	32,590
19	Michigan	28,090
17	Minnesota	29,240
29	Mississippi	25,340
18	Missouri	28,250
45	Montana	21,460
39	Nebraska	23,340
23	Nevada	26,580
21	New Hampshire	27,830
12	New Jersey	30,830
10	New Mexico	30,940
4	New York	34,100
22	North Carolina	26,670
49	North Dakota	19,520
25	Ohio	26,460
35	Oklahoma	24,390
13	Oregon	30,650
34	Pennsylvania	24,670
7	Rhode Island	31,770
27	South Carolina	25,670
43	South Dakota	22,530
37	Tennessee	23,490
33	Texas	24,710
31	Utah	25,000
38	Vermont	23,370
30	Virginia	25,020
2	Washington	35,220
50	West Virginia	18,250
40	Wisconsin	23,260
47	Wyoming	21,280

RANK ORDER

RANK	STATE	WAGES
1	Alaska	$37,230
2	Washington	35,220
3	Maryland	34,730
4	New York	34,100
5	Massachusetts	32,590
6	Hawaii	31,970
7	Rhode Island	31,770
8	Colorado	31,300
9	Connecticut	31,170
10	New Mexico	30,940
11	Idaho	30,860
12	New Jersey	30,830
13	Oregon	30,650
14	Arizona	30,120
15	Illinois	29,830
16	Delaware	29,550
17	Minnesota	29,240
18	Missouri	28,250
19	Michigan	28,090
20	California	27,950
21	New Hampshire	27,830
22	North Carolina	26,670
23	Nevada	26,580
24	Florida	26,560
25	Ohio	26,460
26	Louisiana	26,160
27	South Carolina	25,670
28	Georgia	25,460
29	Mississippi	25,340
30	Virginia	25,020
31	Utah	25,000
32	Indiana	24,840
33	Texas	24,710
34	Pennsylvania	24,670
35	Oklahoma	24,390
36	Maine	23,660
37	Tennessee	23,490
38	Vermont	23,370
39	Nebraska	23,340
40	Wisconsin	23,260
41	Arkansas	23,150
42	Iowa	22,610
43	South Dakota	22,530
44	Kentucky	21,630
45	Montana	21,460
46	Alabama	21,420
47	Wyoming	21,280
48	Kansas	20,260
49	North Dakota	19,520
50	West Virginia	18,250

District of Columbia**   NA

Source: U.S. Department of Labor, Bureau of Labor Statistics
    "Occupational Employment and Wages, 2003" (http://www.bls.gov/oes/)
*Does not include self-employed.
**Not available.

Employment in Health Care Support Industries in 2003

National Total = 3,235,840 Aides and Assistants*

ALPHA ORDER

RANK	STATE	EMPLOYEES	% of USA
26	Alabama	43,540	1.3%
49	Alaska	6,260	0.2%
20	Arizona	55,350	1.7%
32	Arkansas	27,730	0.9%
1	California	311,360	9.6%
28	Colorado	39,940	1.2%
23	Connecticut	48,010	1.5%
47	Delaware	8,950	0.3%
4	Florida	177,240	5.5%
13	Georgia	75,700	2.3%
43	Hawaii	12,550	0.4%
41	Idaho	14,370	0.4%
7	Illinois	123,170	3.8%
18	Indiana	63,600	2.0%
30	Iowa	39,140	1.2%
29	Kansas	39,720	1.2%
24	Kentucky	47,970	1.5%
21	Louisiana	52,770	1.6%
37	Maine	19,240	0.6%
22	Maryland	50,620	1.6%
11	Massachusetts	87,780	2.7%
8	Michigan	115,820	3.6%
15	Minnesota	70,650	2.2%
33	Mississippi	27,610	0.9%
14	Missouri	73,770	2.3%
44	Montana	11,090	0.3%
34	Nebraska	25,170	0.8%
39	Nevada	16,420	0.5%
42	New Hampshire	13,060	0.4%
10	New Jersey	99,870	3.1%
38	New Mexico	18,950	0.6%
2	New York	282,340	8.7%
9	North Carolina	103,050	3.2%
46	North Dakota	10,000	0.3%
5	Ohio	157,290	4.9%
25	Oklahoma	44,050	1.4%
31	Oregon	34,690	1.1%
6	Pennsylvania	154,630	4.8%
40	Rhode Island	16,290	0.5%
27	South Carolina	42,780	1.3%
45	South Dakota	10,310	0.3%
19	Tennessee	59,890	1.9%
3	Texas	229,310	7.1%
35	Utah	21,330	0.7%
48	Vermont	8,180	0.3%
16	Virginia	67,910	2.1%
17	Washington	64,560	2.0%
36	West Virginia	20,660	0.6%
12	Wisconsin	79,100	2.4%
50	Wyoming	5,480	0.2%

RANK ORDER

RANK	STATE	EMPLOYEES	% of USA
1	California	311,360	9.6%
2	New York	282,340	8.7%
3	Texas	229,310	7.1%
4	Florida	177,240	5.5%
5	Ohio	157,290	4.9%
6	Pennsylvania	154,630	4.8%
7	Illinois	123,170	3.8%
8	Michigan	115,820	3.6%
9	North Carolina	103,050	3.2%
10	New Jersey	99,870	3.1%
11	Massachusetts	87,780	2.7%
12	Wisconsin	79,100	2.4%
13	Georgia	75,700	2.3%
14	Missouri	73,770	2.3%
15	Minnesota	70,650	2.2%
16	Virginia	67,910	2.1%
17	Washington	64,560	2.0%
18	Indiana	63,600	2.0%
19	Tennessee	59,890	1.9%
20	Arizona	55,350	1.7%
21	Louisiana	52,770	1.6%
22	Maryland	50,620	1.6%
23	Connecticut	48,010	1.5%
24	Kentucky	47,970	1.5%
25	Oklahoma	44,050	1.4%
26	Alabama	43,540	1.3%
27	South Carolina	42,780	1.3%
28	Colorado	39,940	1.2%
29	Kansas	39,720	1.2%
30	Iowa	39,140	1.2%
31	Oregon	34,690	1.1%
32	Arkansas	27,730	0.9%
33	Mississippi	27,610	0.9%
34	Nebraska	25,170	0.8%
35	Utah	21,330	0.7%
36	West Virginia	20,660	0.6%
37	Maine	19,240	0.6%
38	New Mexico	18,950	0.6%
39	Nevada	16,420	0.5%
40	Rhode Island	16,290	0.5%
41	Idaho	14,370	0.4%
42	New Hampshire	13,060	0.4%
43	Hawaii	12,550	0.4%
44	Montana	11,090	0.3%
45	South Dakota	10,310	0.3%
46	North Dakota	10,000	0.3%
47	Delaware	8,950	0.3%
48	Vermont	8,180	0.3%
49	Alaska	6,260	0.2%
50	Wyoming	5,480	0.2%
	District of Columbia	6,570	0.2%

Source: U.S. Department of Labor, Bureau of Labor Statistics
    "Occupational Employment and Wages, 2003" (http://www.bls.gov/oes/)
*Does not include self-employed. Includes various health care assistants and aides not included in the category of health care practitioners and technicians. Among the included occupations are home health aides, nursing aides, psychiatric aides, dental assistants and pharmacy aides.

Rate of Employees in Health Care Support Industries in 2003

National Rate = 1,113 Aides and Assistants per 100,000 Population*

<u>ALPHA ORDER</u>

RANK	STATE	RATE
41	Alabama	967
42	Alaska	966
38	Arizona	992
34	Arkansas	1,017
47	California	878
47	Colorado	878
9	Connecticut	1,377
25	Delaware	1,094
29	Florida	1,043
49	Georgia	872
37	Hawaii	1,005
28	Idaho	1,051
39	Illinois	974
32	Indiana	1,026
13	Iowa	1,330
5	Kansas	1,458
21	Kentucky	1,165
20	Louisiana	1,174
3	Maine	1,470
45	Maryland	918
11	Massachusetts	1,367
23	Michigan	1,149
8	Minnesota	1,395
43	Mississippi	958
15	Missouri	1,290
19	Montana	1,208
6	Nebraska	1,449
50	Nevada	732
35	New Hampshire	1,013
22	New Jersey	1,156
36	New Mexico	1,009
3	New York	1,470
18	North Carolina	1,224
1	North Dakota	1,579
10	Ohio	1,375
16	Oklahoma	1,256
40	Oregon	973
17	Pennsylvania	1,250
2	Rhode Island	1,514
31	South Carolina	1,031
12	South Dakota	1,348
33	Tennessee	1,025
30	Texas	1,037
46	Utah	907
14	Vermont	1,321
44	Virginia	922
27	Washington	1,053
24	West Virginia	1,141
7	Wisconsin	1,445
26	Wyoming	1,091

<u>RANK ORDER</u>

RANK	STATE	RATE
1	North Dakota	1,579
2	Rhode Island	1,514
3	Maine	1,470
3	New York	1,470
5	Kansas	1,458
6	Nebraska	1,449
7	Wisconsin	1,445
8	Minnesota	1,395
9	Connecticut	1,377
10	Ohio	1,375
11	Massachusetts	1,367
12	South Dakota	1,348
13	Iowa	1,330
14	Vermont	1,321
15	Missouri	1,290
16	Oklahoma	1,256
17	Pennsylvania	1,250
18	North Carolina	1,224
19	Montana	1,208
20	Louisiana	1,174
21	Kentucky	1,165
22	New Jersey	1,156
23	Michigan	1,149
24	West Virginia	1,141
25	Delaware	1,094
26	Wyoming	1,091
27	Washington	1,053
28	Idaho	1,051
29	Florida	1,043
30	Texas	1,037
31	South Carolina	1,031
32	Indiana	1,026
33	Tennessee	1,025
34	Arkansas	1,017
35	New Hampshire	1,013
36	New Mexico	1,009
37	Hawaii	1,005
38	Arizona	992
39	Illinois	974
40	Oregon	973
41	Alabama	967
42	Alaska	966
43	Mississippi	958
44	Virginia	922
45	Maryland	918
46	Utah	907
47	California	878
47	Colorado	878
49	Georgia	872
50	Nevada	732

District of Columbia 1,178

Source: Morgan Quitno Press using data from U.S. Department of Labor, Bureau of Labor Statistics "Occupational Employment and Wages, 2003" (http://www.bls.gov/oes/)
Does not include self-employed. Includes various health care assistants and aides not included in the category of health care practitioners and technicians. Among the included occupations are home health aides, nursing aides, psychiatric aides, dental assistants and pharmacy aides.

Average Annual Wages of Employees in Health Care Support Industries in 2003

National Average = $22,960*

ALPHA ORDER

RANK	STATE	WAGES
46	Alabama	$18,740
1	Alaska	29,430
20	Arizona	23,030
47	Arkansas	18,500
5	California	26,130
6	Colorado	26,050
2	Connecticut	27,670
15	Delaware	24,550
25	Florida	22,020
30	Georgia	21,510
8	Hawaii	25,660
38	Idaho	20,870
21	Illinois	22,880
24	Indiana	22,280
29	Iowa	21,560
34	Kansas	21,050
32	Kentucky	21,240
50	Louisiana	17,660
26	Maine	22,010
11	Maryland	24,980
4	Massachusetts	26,980
17	Michigan	23,650
13	Minnesota	24,740
49	Mississippi	18,100
40	Missouri	20,510
43	Montana	20,020
28	Nebraska	21,570
3	Nevada	27,380
9	New Hampshire	25,340
14	New Jersey	24,690
37	New Mexico	20,980
12	New York	24,760
36	North Carolina	21,020
42	North Dakota	20,310
22	Ohio	22,540
45	Oklahoma	19,570
16	Oregon	24,450
19	Pennsylvania	23,150
10	Rhode Island	25,260
39	South Carolina	20,620
41	South Dakota	20,390
31	Tennessee	21,440
44	Texas	19,600
35	Utah	21,030
23	Vermont	22,480
27	Virginia	21,970
7	Washington	25,860
48	West Virginia	18,340
18	Wisconsin	23,490
33	Wyoming	21,190

RANK ORDER

RANK	STATE	WAGES
1	Alaska	$29,430
2	Connecticut	27,670
3	Nevada	27,380
4	Massachusetts	26,980
5	California	26,130
6	Colorado	26,050
7	Washington	25,860
8	Hawaii	25,660
9	New Hampshire	25,340
10	Rhode Island	25,260
11	Maryland	24,980
12	New York	24,760
13	Minnesota	24,740
14	New Jersey	24,690
15	Delaware	24,550
16	Oregon	24,450
17	Michigan	23,650
18	Wisconsin	23,490
19	Pennsylvania	23,150
20	Arizona	23,030
21	Illinois	22,880
22	Ohio	22,540
23	Vermont	22,480
24	Indiana	22,280
25	Florida	22,020
26	Maine	22,010
27	Virginia	21,970
28	Nebraska	21,570
29	Iowa	21,560
30	Georgia	21,510
31	Tennessee	21,440
32	Kentucky	21,240
33	Wyoming	21,190
34	Kansas	21,050
35	Utah	21,030
36	North Carolina	21,020
37	New Mexico	20,980
38	Idaho	20,870
39	South Carolina	20,620
40	Missouri	20,510
41	South Dakota	20,390
42	North Dakota	20,310
43	Montana	20,020
44	Texas	19,600
45	Oklahoma	19,570
46	Alabama	18,740
47	Arkansas	18,500
48	West Virginia	18,340
49	Mississippi	18,100
50	Louisiana	17,660
	District of Columbia	26,560

Source: U.S. Department of Labor, Bureau of Labor Statistics
   "Occupational Employment and Wages, 2003" (http://www.bls.gov/oes/)
*Does not include self-employed. Includes various health care assistants and aides not included in the category of health care practitioners and technicians. Among the included occupations are home health aides, nursing aides, psychiatric aides, dental assistants and pharmacy aides.

VII. PHYSICAL FITNESS

Users of Exercise Equipment in 2003

National Total = 48,631,000 Users

ALPHA ORDER

RANK	STATE	USERS	% of USA
23	Alabama	743,000	1.5%
NA	Alaska**	NA	NA
22	Arizona	748,000	1.5%
35	Arkansas	400,000	0.8%
1	California	6,229,000	12.8%
20	Colorado	804,000	1.7%
25	Connecticut	721,000	1.5%
41	Delaware	176,000	0.4%
3	Florida	3,244,000	6.7%
12	Georgia	1,252,000	2.6%
NA	Hawaii**	NA	NA
36	Idaho	304,000	0.6%
5	Illinois	2,350,000	4.8%
14	Indiana	1,147,000	2.4%
27	Iowa	567,000	1.2%
30	Kansas	457,000	0.9%
24	Kentucky	737,000	1.5%
26	Louisiana	621,000	1.3%
44	Maine	156,000	0.3%
16	Maryland	1,028,000	2.1%
13	Massachusetts	1,210,000	2.5%
11	Michigan	1,457,000	3.0%
19	Minnesota	893,000	1.8%
34	Mississippi	417,000	0.9%
18	Missouri	938,000	1.9%
39	Montana	221,000	0.5%
31	Nebraska	442,000	0.9%
37	Nevada	281,000	0.6%
47	New Hampshire	104,000	0.2%
9	New Jersey	1,601,000	3.3%
43	New Mexico	164,000	0.3%
2	New York	3,274,000	6.7%
8	North Carolina	1,678,000	3.5%
45	North Dakota	150,000	0.3%
6	Ohio	2,196,000	4.5%
29	Oklahoma	537,000	1.1%
33	Oregon	427,000	0.9%
7	Pennsylvania	1,907,000	3.9%
42	Rhode Island	166,000	0.3%
28	South Carolina	559,000	1.1%
40	South Dakota	198,000	0.4%
21	Tennessee	773,000	1.6%
4	Texas	2,766,000	5.7%
32	Utah	439,000	0.9%
46	Vermont	130,000	0.3%
10	Virginia	1,557,000	3.2%
15	Washington	1,063,000	2.2%
38	West Virginia	267,000	0.5%
17	Wisconsin	979,000	2.0%
48	Wyoming	90,000	0.2%

RANK ORDER

RANK	STATE	USERS	% of USA
1	California	6,229,000	12.8%
2	New York	3,274,000	6.7%
3	Florida	3,244,000	6.7%
4	Texas	2,766,000	5.7%
5	Illinois	2,350,000	4.8%
6	Ohio	2,196,000	4.5%
7	Pennsylvania	1,907,000	3.9%
8	North Carolina	1,678,000	3.5%
9	New Jersey	1,601,000	3.3%
10	Virginia	1,557,000	3.2%
11	Michigan	1,457,000	3.0%
12	Georgia	1,252,000	2.6%
13	Massachusetts	1,210,000	2.5%
14	Indiana	1,147,000	2.4%
15	Washington	1,063,000	2.2%
16	Maryland	1,028,000	2.1%
17	Wisconsin	979,000	2.0%
18	Missouri	938,000	1.9%
19	Minnesota	893,000	1.8%
20	Colorado	804,000	1.7%
21	Tennessee	773,000	1.6%
22	Arizona	748,000	1.5%
23	Alabama	743,000	1.5%
24	Kentucky	737,000	1.5%
25	Connecticut	721,000	1.5%
26	Louisiana	621,000	1.3%
27	Iowa	567,000	1.2%
28	South Carolina	559,000	1.1%
29	Oklahoma	537,000	1.1%
30	Kansas	457,000	0.9%
31	Nebraska	442,000	0.9%
32	Utah	439,000	0.9%
33	Oregon	427,000	0.9%
34	Mississippi	417,000	0.9%
35	Arkansas	400,000	0.8%
36	Idaho	304,000	0.6%
37	Nevada	281,000	0.6%
38	West Virginia	267,000	0.5%
39	Montana	221,000	0.5%
40	South Dakota	198,000	0.4%
41	Delaware	176,000	0.4%
42	Rhode Island	166,000	0.3%
43	New Mexico	164,000	0.3%
44	Maine	156,000	0.3%
45	North Dakota	150,000	0.3%
46	Vermont	130,000	0.3%
47	New Hampshire	104,000	0.2%
48	Wyoming	90,000	0.2%
NA	Alaska**	NA	NA
NA	Hawaii**	NA	NA
	District of Columbia**	NA	NA

Source: The National Sporting Goods Association
"NSGA Sports Participation Survey, January-December 2003 (Copyright 2004, reprinted with permission)
*Not available.

Participants in Golf in 2003

National Total = 25,650,000 Golfers

ALPHA ORDER

RANK	STATE	GOLFERS	% of USA
22	Alabama	338,000	1.3%
NA	Alaska**	NA	NA
25	Arizona	316,000	1.2%
29	Arkansas	272,000	1.1%
1	California	3,023,000	11.8%
23	Colorado	322,000	1.3%
32	Connecticut	235,000	0.9%
40	Delaware	113,000	0.4%
6	Florida	1,101,000	4.3%
16	Georgia	478,000	1.9%
NA	Hawaii**	NA	NA
39	Idaho	115,000	0.4%
4	Illinois	1,655,000	6.5%
15	Indiana	552,000	2.2%
20	Iowa	379,000	1.5%
30	Kansas	238,000	0.9%
17	Kentucky	476,000	1.9%
36	Louisiana	142,000	0.6%
43	Maine	88,000	0.3%
24	Maryland	317,000	1.2%
14	Massachusetts	621,000	2.4%
2	Michigan	2,034,000	7.9%
12	Minnesota	770,000	3.0%
35	Mississippi	151,000	0.6%
19	Missouri	384,000	1.5%
37	Montana	130,000	0.5%
33	Nebraska	182,000	0.7%
34	Nevada	164,000	0.6%
45	New Hampshire	80,000	0.3%
8	New Jersey	1,028,000	4.0%
44	New Mexico	85,000	0.3%
3	New York	1,717,000	6.7%
11	North Carolina	775,000	3.0%
42	North Dakota	93,000	0.4%
7	Ohio	1,070,000	4.2%
26	Oklahoma	299,000	1.2%
28	Oregon	288,000	1.1%
10	Pennsylvania	784,000	3.1%
41	Rhode Island	105,000	0.4%
27	South Carolina	290,000	1.1%
38	South Dakota	126,000	0.5%
21	Tennessee	372,000	1.5%
5	Texas	1,428,000	5.6%
31	Utah	237,000	0.9%
NA	Vermont**	NA	NA
13	Virginia	744,000	2.9%
18	Washington	464,000	1.8%
47	West Virginia	38,000	0.1%
9	Wisconsin	967,000	3.8%
46	Wyoming	65,000	0.3%

RANK ORDER

RANK	STATE	GOLFERS	% of USA
1	California	3,023,000	11.8%
2	Michigan	2,034,000	7.9%
3	New York	1,717,000	6.7%
4	Illinois	1,655,000	6.5%
5	Texas	1,428,000	5.6%
6	Florida	1,101,000	4.3%
7	Ohio	1,070,000	4.2%
8	New Jersey	1,028,000	4.0%
9	Wisconsin	967,000	3.8%
10	Pennsylvania	784,000	3.1%
11	North Carolina	775,000	3.0%
12	Minnesota	770,000	3.0%
13	Virginia	744,000	2.9%
14	Massachusetts	621,000	2.4%
15	Indiana	552,000	2.2%
16	Georgia	478,000	1.9%
17	Kentucky	476,000	1.9%
18	Washington	464,000	1.8%
19	Missouri	384,000	1.5%
20	Iowa	379,000	1.5%
21	Tennessee	372,000	1.5%
22	Alabama	338,000	1.3%
23	Colorado	322,000	1.3%
24	Maryland	317,000	1.2%
25	Arizona	316,000	1.2%
26	Oklahoma	299,000	1.2%
27	South Carolina	290,000	1.1%
28	Oregon	288,000	1.1%
29	Arkansas	272,000	1.1%
30	Kansas	238,000	0.9%
31	Utah	237,000	0.9%
32	Connecticut	235,000	0.9%
33	Nebraska	182,000	0.7%
34	Nevada	164,000	0.6%
35	Mississippi	151,000	0.6%
36	Louisiana	142,000	0.6%
37	Montana	130,000	0.5%
38	South Dakota	126,000	0.5%
39	Idaho	115,000	0.4%
40	Delaware	113,000	0.4%
41	Rhode Island	105,000	0.4%
42	North Dakota	93,000	0.4%
43	Maine	88,000	0.3%
44	New Mexico	85,000	0.3%
45	New Hampshire	80,000	0.3%
46	Wyoming	65,000	0.3%
47	West Virginia	38,000	0.1%
NA	Alaska**	NA	NA
NA	Hawaii**	NA	NA
NA	Vermont**	NA	NA
	District of Columbia**	NA	NA

Source: The National Sporting Goods Association
 "NSGA Sports Participation Survey, January-December 2003 (Copyright 2004, reprinted with permission)
*Not available.

Participants in Running/Jogging in 2003

National Total = 22,937,000 Runners/Joggers

ALPHA ORDER

RANK	STATE	RUNNERS	% of USA
31	Alabama	212,000	0.9%
NA	Alaska**	NA	NA
18	Arizona	441,000	1.9%
46	Arkansas	22,000	0.1%
1	California	3,818,000	16.6%
27	Colorado	254,000	1.1%
32	Connecticut	194,000	0.8%
37	Delaware	141,000	0.6%
8	Florida	901,000	3.9%
12	Georgia	620,000	2.7%
NA	Hawaii**	NA	NA
33	Idaho	182,000	0.8%
4	Illinois	1,137,000	5.0%
21	Indiana	330,000	1.4%
26	Iowa	278,000	1.2%
30	Kansas	216,000	0.9%
29	Kentucky	221,000	1.0%
19	Louisiana	387,000	1.7%
35	Maine	157,000	0.7%
17	Maryland	455,000	2.0%
15	Massachusetts	482,000	2.1%
5	Michigan	1,105,000	4.8%
20	Minnesota	371,000	1.6%
47	Mississippi	19,000	0.1%
24	Missouri	313,000	1.4%
40	Montana	96,000	0.4%
36	Nebraska	155,000	0.7%
43	Nevada	79,000	0.3%
45	New Hampshire	24,000	0.1%
10	New Jersey	726,000	3.2%
38	New Mexico	140,000	0.6%
2	New York	1,468,000	6.4%
7	North Carolina	950,000	4.1%
39	North Dakota	133,000	0.6%
6	Ohio	954,000	4.2%
22	Oklahoma	327,000	1.4%
25	Oregon	280,000	1.2%
11	Pennsylvania	713,000	3.1%
42	Rhode Island	87,000	0.4%
28	South Carolina	240,000	1.0%
44	South Dakota	76,000	0.3%
16	Tennessee	469,000	2.0%
3	Texas	1,269,000	5.5%
23	Utah	323,000	1.4%
41	Vermont	88,000	0.4%
9	Virginia	744,000	3.2%
13	Washington	570,000	2.5%
34	West Virginia	177,000	0.8%
14	Wisconsin	506,000	2.2%
48	Wyoming	12,000	0.1%

RANK ORDER

RANK	STATE	RUNNERS	% of USA
1	California	3,818,000	16.6%
2	New York	1,468,000	6.4%
3	Texas	1,269,000	5.5%
4	Illinois	1,137,000	5.0%
5	Michigan	1,105,000	4.8%
6	Ohio	954,000	4.2%
7	North Carolina	950,000	4.1%
8	Florida	901,000	3.9%
9	Virginia	744,000	3.2%
10	New Jersey	726,000	3.2%
11	Pennsylvania	713,000	3.1%
12	Georgia	620,000	2.7%
13	Washington	570,000	2.5%
14	Wisconsin	506,000	2.2%
15	Massachusetts	482,000	2.1%
16	Tennessee	469,000	2.0%
17	Maryland	455,000	2.0%
18	Arizona	441,000	1.9%
19	Louisiana	387,000	1.7%
20	Minnesota	371,000	1.6%
21	Indiana	330,000	1.4%
22	Oklahoma	327,000	1.4%
23	Utah	323,000	1.4%
24	Missouri	313,000	1.4%
25	Oregon	280,000	1.2%
26	Iowa	278,000	1.2%
27	Colorado	254,000	1.1%
28	South Carolina	240,000	1.0%
29	Kentucky	221,000	1.0%
30	Kansas	216,000	0.9%
31	Alabama	212,000	0.9%
32	Connecticut	194,000	0.8%
33	Idaho	182,000	0.8%
34	West Virginia	177,000	0.8%
35	Maine	157,000	0.7%
36	Nebraska	155,000	0.7%
37	Delaware	141,000	0.6%
38	New Mexico	140,000	0.6%
39	North Dakota	133,000	0.6%
40	Montana	96,000	0.4%
41	Vermont	88,000	0.4%
42	Rhode Island	87,000	0.4%
43	Nevada	79,000	0.3%
44	South Dakota	76,000	0.3%
45	New Hampshire	24,000	0.1%
46	Arkansas	22,000	0.1%
47	Mississippi	19,000	0.1%
48	Wyoming	12,000	0.1%
NA	Alaska**	NA	NA
NA	Hawaii**	NA	NA
	District of Columbia**	NA	NA

Source: The National Sporting Goods Association
"NSGA Sports Participation Survey, January-December 2003 (Copyright 2004, reprinted with permission)
*Not available.

Participants in Swimming in 2003

National Total = 47,027,000 Swimmers

ALPHA ORDER

RANK	STATE	SWIMMERS	% of USA
24	Alabama	606,000	1.3%
NA	Alaska*	NA	NA
17	Arizona	907,000	1.9%
35	Arkansas	334,000	0.7%
1	California	5,458,000	11.6%
23	Colorado	674,000	1.4%
25	Connecticut	581,000	1.2%
43	Delaware	140,000	0.3%
2	Florida	3,557,000	7.6%
14	Georgia	1,019,000	2.2%
NA	Hawaii*	NA	NA
37	Idaho	263,000	0.6%
7	Illinois	2,181,000	4.6%
12	Indiana	1,214,000	2.6%
31	Iowa	398,000	0.8%
38	Kansas	259,000	0.6%
34	Kentucky	340,000	0.7%
27	Louisiana	561,000	1.2%
29	Maine	467,000	1.0%
21	Maryland	727,000	1.5%
20	Massachusetts	739,000	1.6%
8	Michigan	2,050,000	4.4%
22	Minnesota	712,000	1.5%
40	Mississippi	201,000	0.4%
15	Missouri	976,000	2.1%
44	Montana	138,000	0.3%
36	Nebraska	297,000	0.6%
30	Nevada	405,000	0.9%
42	New Hampshire	152,000	0.3%
9	New Jersey	1,900,000	4.0%
45	New Mexico	121,000	0.3%
3	New York	3,538,000	7.5%
10	North Carolina	1,538,000	3.3%
39	North Dakota	203,000	0.4%
5	Ohio	2,270,000	4.8%
25	Oklahoma	581,000	1.2%
32	Oregon	378,000	0.8%
6	Pennsylvania	2,186,000	4.6%
46	Rhode Island	69,000	0.1%
16	South Carolina	966,000	2.1%
48	South Dakota	65,000	0.1%
17	Tennessee	907,000	1.9%
4	Texas	2,661,000	5.7%
28	Utah	479,000	1.0%
41	Vermont	199,000	0.4%
11	Virginia	1,398,000	3.0%
19	Washington	764,000	1.6%
33	West Virginia	353,000	0.8%
13	Wisconsin	1,027,000	2.2%
47	Wyoming	68,000	0.1%

RANK ORDER

RANK	STATE	SWIMMERS	% of USA
1	California	5,458,000	11.6%
2	Florida	3,557,000	7.6%
3	New York	3,538,000	7.5%
4	Texas	2,661,000	5.7%
5	Ohio	2,270,000	4.8%
6	Pennsylvania	2,186,000	4.6%
7	Illinois	2,181,000	4.6%
8	Michigan	2,050,000	4.4%
9	New Jersey	1,900,000	4.0%
10	North Carolina	1,538,000	3.3%
11	Virginia	1,398,000	3.0%
12	Indiana	1,214,000	2.6%
13	Wisconsin	1,027,000	2.2%
14	Georgia	1,019,000	2.2%
15	Missouri	976,000	2.1%
16	South Carolina	966,000	2.1%
17	Arizona	907,000	1.9%
17	Tennessee	907,000	1.9%
19	Washington	764,000	1.6%
20	Massachusetts	739,000	1.6%
21	Maryland	727,000	1.5%
22	Minnesota	712,000	1.5%
23	Colorado	674,000	1.4%
24	Alabama	606,000	1.3%
25	Connecticut	581,000	1.2%
25	Oklahoma	581,000	1.2%
27	Louisiana	561,000	1.2%
28	Utah	479,000	1.0%
29	Maine	467,000	1.0%
30	Nevada	405,000	0.9%
31	Iowa	398,000	0.8%
32	Oregon	378,000	0.8%
33	West Virginia	353,000	0.8%
34	Kentucky	340,000	0.7%
35	Arkansas	334,000	0.7%
36	Nebraska	297,000	0.6%
37	Idaho	263,000	0.6%
38	Kansas	259,000	0.6%
39	North Dakota	203,000	0.4%
40	Mississippi	201,000	0.4%
41	Vermont	199,000	0.4%
42	New Hampshire	152,000	0.3%
43	Delaware	140,000	0.3%
44	Montana	138,000	0.3%
45	New Mexico	121,000	0.3%
46	Rhode Island	69,000	0.1%
47	Wyoming	68,000	0.1%
48	South Dakota	65,000	0.1%
NA	Alaska*	NA	NA
NA	Hawaii*	NA	NA
	District of Columbia*	NA	NA

Source: The National Sporting Goods Association
"NSGA Sports Participation Survey, January-December 2003 (Copyright 2004, reprinted with permission)
*Not available.

Participants in Tennis in 2003

National Total = 9,572,000 Tennis Players

ALPHA ORDER

RANK	STATE	PLAYERS	% of USA
32	Alabama	58,000	0.6%
NA	Alaska*	NA	NA
24	Arizona	137,000	1.4%
35	Arkansas	30,000	0.3%
1	California	1,286,000	13.4%
23	Colorado	138,000	1.4%
22	Connecticut	154,000	1.6%
35	Delaware	30,000	0.3%
12	Florida	351,000	3.7%
11	Georgia	352,000	3.7%
NA	Hawaii*	NA	NA
38	Idaho	17,000	0.2%
3	Illinois	536,000	5.6%
13	Indiana	334,000	3.5%
27	Iowa	127,000	1.3%
NA	Kansas*	NA	NA
26	Kentucky	131,000	1.4%
17	Louisiana	206,000	2.2%
31	Maine	60,000	0.6%
19	Maryland	186,000	1.9%
29	Massachusetts	82,000	0.9%
9	Michigan	374,000	3.9%
16	Minnesota	253,000	2.6%
25	Mississippi	132,000	1.4%
20	Missouri	167,000	1.7%
NA	Montana*	NA	NA
40	Nebraska	13,000	0.1%
38	Nevada	17,000	0.2%
NA	New Hampshire*	NA	NA
10	New Jersey	366,000	3.8%
NA	New Mexico*	NA	NA
5	New York	469,000	4.9%
7	North Carolina	400,000	4.2%
33	North Dakota	56,000	0.6%
2	Ohio	623,000	6.5%
40	Oklahoma	13,000	0.1%
28	Oregon	92,000	1.0%
15	Pennsylvania	261,000	2.7%
37	Rhode Island	22,000	0.2%
14	South Carolina	322,000	3.4%
NA	South Dakota*	NA	NA
6	Tennessee	402,000	4.2%
4	Texas	521,000	5.4%
30	Utah	69,000	0.7%
NA	Vermont*	NA	NA
8	Virginia	390,000	4.1%
18	Washington	205,000	2.1%
34	West Virginia	32,000	0.3%
21	Wisconsin	158,000	1.7%
NA	Wyoming*	NA	NA

RANK ORDER

RANK	STATE	PLAYERS	% of USA
1	California	1,286,000	13.4%
2	Ohio	623,000	6.5%
3	Illinois	536,000	5.6%
4	Texas	521,000	5.4%
5	New York	469,000	4.9%
6	Tennessee	402,000	4.2%
7	North Carolina	400,000	4.2%
8	Virginia	390,000	4.1%
9	Michigan	374,000	3.9%
10	New Jersey	366,000	3.8%
11	Georgia	352,000	3.7%
12	Florida	351,000	3.7%
13	Indiana	334,000	3.5%
14	South Carolina	322,000	3.4%
15	Pennsylvania	261,000	2.7%
16	Minnesota	253,000	2.6%
17	Louisiana	206,000	2.2%
18	Washington	205,000	2.1%
19	Maryland	186,000	1.9%
20	Missouri	167,000	1.7%
21	Wisconsin	158,000	1.7%
22	Connecticut	154,000	1.6%
23	Colorado	138,000	1.4%
24	Arizona	137,000	1.4%
25	Mississippi	132,000	1.4%
26	Kentucky	131,000	1.4%
27	Iowa	127,000	1.3%
28	Oregon	92,000	1.0%
29	Massachusetts	82,000	0.9%
30	Utah	69,000	0.7%
31	Maine	60,000	0.6%
32	Alabama	58,000	0.6%
33	North Dakota	56,000	0.6%
34	West Virginia	32,000	0.3%
35	Arkansas	30,000	0.3%
35	Delaware	30,000	0.3%
37	Rhode Island	22,000	0.2%
38	Idaho	17,000	0.2%
38	Nevada	17,000	0.2%
40	Nebraska	13,000	0.1%
40	Oklahoma	13,000	0.1%
NA	Alaska*	NA	NA
NA	Hawaii*	NA	NA
NA	Kansas*	NA	NA
NA	Montana*	NA	NA
NA	New Hampshire*	NA	NA
NA	New Mexico*	NA	NA
NA	South Dakota*	NA	NA
NA	Vermont*	NA	NA
NA	Wyoming*	NA	NA
	District of Columbia*	NA	NA

Source: The National Sporting Goods Association
"NSGA Sports Participation Survey, January-December 2003 (Copyright 2004, reprinted with permission)
Not available.

480

Alcohol Consumption in 2000

National Total = 492,521,000 Gallons*

RANK	STATE	GALLONS	% of USA
25	Alabama	6,734,000	1.4%
47	Alaska	1,267,000	0.3%
16	Arizona	10,218,000	2.1%
35	Arkansas	3,749,000	0.8%
1	California	58,545,000	11.9%
20	Colorado	9,022,000	1.8%
27	Connecticut	5,982,000	1.2%
45	Delaware	1,836,000	0.4%
3	Florida	33,694,000	6.8%
10	Georgia	14,153,000	2.9%
41	Hawaii	2,285,000	0.5%
40	Idaho	2,360,000	0.5%
5	Illinois	22,161,000	4.5%
18	Indiana	9,629,000	2.0%
32	Iowa	4,690,000	1.0%
34	Kansas	3,898,000	0.8%
29	Kentucky	5,717,000	1.2%
22	Louisiana	8,585,000	1.7%
39	Maine	2,406,000	0.5%
21	Maryland	8,869,000	1.8%
11	Massachusetts	13,225,000	2.7%
8	Michigan	16,827,000	3.4%
19	Minnesota	9,338,000	1.9%
30	Mississippi	4,791,000	1.0%
17	Missouri	10,138,000	2.1%
44	Montana	1,851,000	0.4%
37	Nebraska	3,055,000	0.6%
28	Nevada	5,901,000	1.2%
33	New Hampshire	4,007,000	0.8%
9	New Jersey	14,888,000	3.0%
36	New Mexico	3,414,000	0.7%
4	New York	28,777,000	5.8%
12	North Carolina	12,651,000	2.6%
48	North Dakota	1,254,000	0.3%
7	Ohio	18,173,000	3.7%
31	Oklahoma	4,698,000	1.0%
26	Oregon	6,329,000	1.3%
6	Pennsylvania	19,043,000	3.9%
43	Rhode Island	1,981,000	0.4%
24	South Carolina	7,688,000	1.6%
46	South Dakota	1,368,000	0.3%
23	Tennessee	8,584,000	1.7%
2	Texas	36,767,000	7.5%
42	Utah	2,148,000	0.4%
49	Vermont	1,165,000	0.2%
14	Virginia	11,330,000	2.3%
15	Washington	10,256,000	2.1%
38	West Virginia	2,457,000	0.5%
13	Wisconsin	11,941,000	2.4%
50	Wyoming	981,000	0.2%

RANK	STATE	GALLONS	% of USA
1	California	58,545,000	11.9%
2	Texas	36,767,000	7.5%
3	Florida	33,694,000	6.8%
4	New York	28,777,000	5.8%
5	Illinois	22,161,000	4.5%
6	Pennsylvania	19,043,000	3.9%
7	Ohio	18,173,000	3.7%
8	Michigan	16,827,000	3.4%
9	New Jersey	14,888,000	3.0%
10	Georgia	14,153,000	2.9%
11	Massachusetts	13,225,000	2.7%
12	North Carolina	12,651,000	2.6%
13	Wisconsin	11,941,000	2.4%
14	Virginia	11,330,000	2.3%
15	Washington	10,256,000	2.1%
16	Arizona	10,218,000	2.1%
17	Missouri	10,138,000	2.1%
18	Indiana	9,629,000	2.0%
19	Minnesota	9,338,000	1.9%
20	Colorado	9,022,000	1.8%
21	Maryland	8,869,000	1.8%
22	Louisiana	8,585,000	1.7%
23	Tennessee	8,584,000	1.7%
24	South Carolina	7,688,000	1.6%
25	Alabama	6,734,000	1.4%
26	Oregon	6,329,000	1.3%
27	Connecticut	5,982,000	1.2%
28	Nevada	5,901,000	1.2%
29	Kentucky	5,717,000	1.2%
30	Mississippi	4,791,000	1.0%
31	Oklahoma	4,698,000	1.0%
32	Iowa	4,690,000	1.0%
33	New Hampshire	4,007,000	0.8%
34	Kansas	3,898,000	0.8%
35	Arkansas	3,749,000	0.8%
36	New Mexico	3,414,000	0.7%
37	Nebraska	3,055,000	0.6%
38	West Virginia	2,457,000	0.5%
39	Maine	2,406,000	0.5%
40	Idaho	2,360,000	0.5%
41	Hawaii	2,285,000	0.5%
42	Utah	2,148,000	0.4%
43	Rhode Island	1,981,000	0.4%
44	Montana	1,851,000	0.4%
45	Delaware	1,836,000	0.4%
46	South Dakota	1,368,000	0.3%
47	Alaska	1,267,000	0.3%
48	North Dakota	1,254,000	0.3%
49	Vermont	1,165,000	0.2%
50	Wyoming	981,000	0.2%
	District of Columbia	1,693,000	0.3%

Source: U.S. Department of Health and Human Services, National Institute on Alcohol Abuse and Alcoholism
"Volume Beverage and Ethanol Consumption for States" (http://www.niaaa.nih.gov/databases/consum02.txt)
*This is apparent consumption of actual alcohol, not entire volume of an alcoholic beverage (e.g. wine is roughly 11% absolute alcohol content). Apparent consumption is based on several sources which together approximate sales but do not actually measure consumption. Accordingly, figures for some states may be skewed by purchases by nonresidents.

Adult Per Capita Alcohol Consumption in 2000

National Per Capita = 2.5 Gallons Consumed per Adult 21 Years and Older*

ALPHA ORDER				RANK ORDER		
RANK	STATE	PER CAPITA		RANK	STATE	PER CAPITA
39	Alabama	2.2		1	New Hampshire	4.6
5	Alaska	3.1		2	Nevada	4.2
7	Arizona	2.9		3	Delaware	3.3
46	Arkansas	2.0		4	Wisconsin	3.2
28	California	2.5		5	Alaska	3.1
6	Colorado	3.0		6	Colorado	3.0
28	Connecticut	2.5		7	Arizona	2.9
3	Delaware	3.3		7	Florida	2.9
7	Florida	2.9		7	Massachusetts	2.9
28	Georgia	2.5		7	Montana	2.9
20	Hawaii	2.6		7	Wyoming	2.9
15	Idaho	2.7		12	Louisiana	2.8
20	Illinois	2.6		12	New Mexico	2.8
36	Indiana	2.3		12	North Dakota	2.8
36	Iowa	2.3		15	Idaho	2.7
43	Kansas	2.1		15	Minnesota	2.7
46	Kentucky	2.0		15	South Carolina	2.7
12	Louisiana	2.8		15	South Dakota	2.7
20	Maine	2.6		15	Vermont	2.7
34	Maryland	2.4		20	Hawaii	2.6
7	Massachusetts	2.9		20	Illinois	2.6
34	Michigan	2.4		20	Maine	2.6
15	Minnesota	2.7		20	Missouri	2.6
28	Mississippi	2.5		20	Nebraska	2.6
20	Missouri	2.6		20	Oregon	2.6
7	Montana	2.9		20	Rhode Island	2.6
20	Nebraska	2.6		20	Texas	2.6
2	Nevada	4.2		28	California	2.5
1	New Hampshire	4.6		28	Connecticut	2.5
28	New Jersey	2.5		28	Georgia	2.5
12	New Mexico	2.8		28	Mississippi	2.5
43	New York	2.1		28	New Jersey	2.5
39	North Carolina	2.2		28	Washington	2.5
12	North Dakota	2.8		34	Maryland	2.4
36	Ohio	2.3		34	Michigan	2.4
46	Oklahoma	2.0		36	Indiana	2.3
20	Oregon	2.6		36	Iowa	2.3
39	Pennsylvania	2.2		36	Ohio	2.3
20	Rhode Island	2.6		39	Alabama	2.2
15	South Carolina	2.7		39	North Carolina	2.2
15	South Dakota	2.7		39	Pennsylvania	2.2
43	Tennessee	2.1		39	Virginia	2.2
20	Texas	2.6		43	Kansas	2.1
50	Utah	1.6		43	New York	2.1
15	Vermont	2.7		43	Tennessee	2.1
39	Virginia	2.2		46	Arkansas	2.0
28	Washington	2.5		46	Kentucky	2.0
49	West Virginia	1.9		46	Oklahoma	2.0
4	Wisconsin	3.2		49	West Virginia	1.9
7	Wyoming	2.9		50	Utah	1.6

District of Columbia   4.0

Source: Morgan Quitno Press using data from U.S. Dept. of HHS, National Institute on Alcohol Abuse and Alcoholism "Volume Beverage and Ethanol Consumption for States" (http://www.niaaa.nih.gov/databases/consum02.txt)
*This is apparent consumption of actual alcohol, not entire volume of an alcoholic beverage (e.g. wine is roughly 11% absolute alcohol content). Apparent consumption is based on several sources which together approximate sales but do not actually measure consumption. Accordingly, figures for some states may be skewed by purchases by nonresidents.

Apparent Beer Consumption in 2000

National Total = 6,139,957,000 Gallons of Beer Consumed*

ALPHA ORDER

RANK	STATE	GALLONS	% of USA
25	Alabama	94,530,000	1.5%
48	Alaska	14,373,000	0.2%
15	Arizona	134,336,000	2.2%
34	Arkansas	52,053,000	0.8%
1	California	637,080,000	10.4%
23	Colorado	103,734,000	1.7%
32	Connecticut	57,491,000	0.9%
46	Delaware	19,156,000	0.3%
3	Florida	388,796,000	6.3%
9	Georgia	177,061,000	2.9%
39	Hawaii	29,065,000	0.5%
42	Idaho	26,257,000	0.4%
5	Illinois	282,189,000	4.6%
17	Indiana	125,490,000	2.0%
29	Iowa	71,323,000	1.2%
33	Kansas	54,832,000	0.9%
26	Kentucky	78,055,000	1.3%
19	Louisiana	117,937,000	1.9%
41	Maine	27,370,000	0.4%
24	Maryland	97,754,000	1.6%
16	Massachusetts	133,990,000	2.2%
8	Michigan	209,608,000	3.4%
21	Minnesota	108,478,000	1.8%
28	Mississippi	71,823,000	1.2%
14	Missouri	135,246,000	2.2%
43	Montana	25,257,000	0.4%
36	Nebraska	43,943,000	0.7%
31	Nevada	64,055,000	1.0%
38	New Hampshire	39,001,000	0.6%
13	New Jersey	144,883,000	2.4%
35	New Mexico	48,624,000	0.8%
4	New York	313,158,000	5.1%
10	North Carolina	173,293,000	2.8%
47	North Dakota	17,018,000	0.3%
7	Ohio	263,287,000	4.3%
30	Oklahoma	69,346,000	1.1%
27	Oregon	74,313,000	1.2%
6	Pennsylvania	270,006,000	4.4%
44	Rhode Island	21,988,000	0.4%
22	South Carolina	104,116,000	1.7%
45	South Dakota	19,349,000	0.3%
18	Tennessee	124,041,000	2.0%
2	Texas	556,051,000	9.1%
40	Utah	28,797,000	0.5%
49	Vermont	13,656,000	0.2%
11	Virginia	148,362,000	2.4%
20	Washington	115,148,000	1.9%
37	West Virginia	39,513,000	0.6%
12	Wisconsin	147,700,000	2.4%
50	Wyoming	12,595,000	0.2%

RANK ORDER

RANK	STATE	GALLONS	% of USA
1	California	637,080,000	10.4%
2	Texas	556,051,000	9.1%
3	Florida	388,796,000	6.3%
4	New York	313,158,000	5.1%
5	Illinois	282,189,000	4.6%
6	Pennsylvania	270,006,000	4.4%
7	Ohio	263,287,000	4.3%
8	Michigan	209,608,000	3.4%
9	Georgia	177,061,000	2.9%
10	North Carolina	173,293,000	2.8%
11	Virginia	148,362,000	2.4%
12	Wisconsin	147,700,000	2.4%
13	New Jersey	144,883,000	2.4%
14	Missouri	135,246,000	2.2%
15	Arizona	134,336,000	2.2%
16	Massachusetts	133,990,000	2.2%
17	Indiana	125,490,000	2.0%
18	Tennessee	124,041,000	2.0%
19	Louisiana	117,937,000	1.9%
20	Washington	115,148,000	1.9%
21	Minnesota	108,478,000	1.8%
22	South Carolina	104,116,000	1.7%
23	Colorado	103,734,000	1.7%
24	Maryland	97,754,000	1.6%
25	Alabama	94,530,000	1.5%
26	Kentucky	78,055,000	1.3%
27	Oregon	74,313,000	1.2%
28	Mississippi	71,823,000	1.2%
29	Iowa	71,323,000	1.2%
30	Oklahoma	69,346,000	1.1%
31	Nevada	64,055,000	1.0%
32	Connecticut	57,491,000	0.9%
33	Kansas	54,832,000	0.9%
34	Arkansas	52,053,000	0.8%
35	New Mexico	48,624,000	0.8%
36	Nebraska	43,943,000	0.7%
37	West Virginia	39,513,000	0.6%
38	New Hampshire	39,001,000	0.6%
39	Hawaii	29,065,000	0.5%
40	Utah	28,797,000	0.5%
41	Maine	27,370,000	0.4%
42	Idaho	26,257,000	0.4%
43	Montana	25,257,000	0.4%
44	Rhode Island	21,988,000	0.4%
45	South Dakota	19,349,000	0.3%
46	Delaware	19,156,000	0.3%
47	North Dakota	17,018,000	0.3%
48	Alaska	14,373,000	0.2%
49	Vermont	13,656,000	0.2%
50	Wyoming	12,595,000	0.2%
	District of Columbia	14,428,000	0.2%

Source: U.S. Department of Health and Human Services, National Institute on Alcohol Abuse and Alcoholism "Volume Beverage and Ethanol Consumption for States" (http://www.niaaa.nih.gov/databases/consum02.txt)
This is apparent consumption and is based on several sources which together approximate sales but do not actually measure consumption. Reported state volumes reflect only in-state purchases. Accordingly, figures for some states may be skewed by purchases by nonresidents.

Adult Per Capita Beer Consumption in 2000

National Per Capita = 31.2 Gallons Consumed per Adult 21 Years and Older*

ALPHA ORDER

RANK	STATE	PER CAPITA
31	Alabama	30.3
15	Alaska	35.0
9	Arizona	38.0
43	Arkansas	27.8
44	California	27.5
19	Colorado	34.4
48	Connecticut	23.6
17	Delaware	34.6
21	Florida	33.1
26	Georgia	31.4
20	Hawaii	33.5
29	Idaho	30.5
23	Illinois	32.7
35	Indiana	29.7
16	Iowa	34.8
35	Kansas	29.7
45	Kentucky	27.2
7	Louisiana	38.9
37	Maine	29.6
46	Maryland	26.2
40	Massachusetts	29.2
31	Michigan	30.3
24	Minnesota	31.8
11	Mississippi	37.3
18	Missouri	34.5
3	Montana	40.0
12	Nebraska	37.2
1	Nevada	45.4
2	New Hampshire	44.5
47	New Jersey	24.0
5	New Mexico	39.6
49	New York	23.2
33	North Carolina	30.2
8	North Dakota	38.1
22	Ohio	33.0
41	Oklahoma	29.0
28	Oregon	30.6
29	Pennsylvania	30.5
38	Rhode Island	29.4
13	South Carolina	37.0
10	South Dakota	37.6
27	Tennessee	30.7
4	Texas	39.8
50	Utah	20.9
25	Vermont	31.5
38	Virginia	29.4
42	Washington	27.9
34	West Virginia	29.8
6	Wisconsin	39.4
13	Wyoming	37.0

RANK ORDER

RANK	STATE	PER CAPITA
1	Nevada	45.4
2	New Hampshire	44.5
3	Montana	40.0
4	Texas	39.8
5	New Mexico	39.6
6	Wisconsin	39.4
7	Louisiana	38.9
8	North Dakota	38.1
9	Arizona	38.0
10	South Dakota	37.6
11	Mississippi	37.3
12	Nebraska	37.2
13	South Carolina	37.0
13	Wyoming	37.0
15	Alaska	35.0
16	Iowa	34.8
17	Delaware	34.6
18	Missouri	34.5
19	Colorado	34.4
20	Hawaii	33.5
21	Florida	33.1
22	Ohio	33.0
23	Illinois	32.7
24	Minnesota	31.8
25	Vermont	31.5
26	Georgia	31.4
27	Tennessee	30.7
28	Oregon	30.6
29	Idaho	30.5
29	Pennsylvania	30.5
31	Alabama	30.3
31	Michigan	30.3
33	North Carolina	30.2
34	West Virginia	29.8
35	Indiana	29.7
35	Kansas	29.7
37	Maine	29.6
38	Rhode Island	29.4
38	Virginia	29.4
40	Massachusetts	29.2
41	Oklahoma	29.0
42	Washington	27.9
43	Arkansas	27.8
44	California	27.5
45	Kentucky	27.2
46	Maryland	26.2
47	New Jersey	24.0
48	Connecticut	23.6
49	New York	23.2
50	Utah	20.9

District of Columbia   33.9

Source: Morgan Quitno Press using data from U.S. Dept. of HHS, National Institute on Alcohol Abuse and Alcoholism "Volume Beverage and Ethanol Consumption for States" (http://www.niaaa.nih.gov/databases/consum02.txt)
*This is apparent consumption and is based on several sources which together approximate sales but do not actually measure consumption. Reported state volumes reflect only in-state purchases. Accordingly, figures for some states may be skewed by purchases by nonresidents.

Wine Consumption in 2000

National Total = 546,540,000 Gallons of Wine Consumed*

ALPHA ORDER

RANK	STATE	GALLONS	% of USA
29	Alabama	4,934,000	0.9%
46	Alaska	1,379,000	0.3%
17	Arizona	9,869,000	1.8%
40	Arkansas	1,993,000	0.4%
1	California	99,930,000	18.3%
18	Colorado	9,845,000	1.8%
15	Connecticut	10,521,000	1.9%
38	Delaware	2,382,000	0.4%
3	Florida	41,383,000	7.6%
13	Georgia	12,902,000	2.4%
34	Hawaii	3,002,000	0.5%
28	Idaho	5,142,000	0.9%
5	Illinois	24,663,000	4.5%
24	Indiana	7,738,000	1.4%
39	Iowa	2,353,000	0.4%
37	Kansas	2,516,000	0.5%
31	Kentucky	3,460,000	0.6%
25	Louisiana	6,159,000	1.1%
32	Maine	3,179,000	0.6%
16	Maryland	10,009,000	1.8%
7	Massachusetts	20,635,000	3.8%
10	Michigan	14,757,000	2.7%
22	Minnesota	7,918,000	1.4%
44	Mississippi	1,657,000	0.3%
21	Missouri	8,144,000	1.5%
43	Montana	1,671,000	0.3%
42	Nebraska	1,791,000	0.3%
23	Nevada	7,745,000	1.4%
30	New Hampshire	4,373,000	0.8%
6	New Jersey	24,472,000	4.5%
35	New Mexico	2,771,000	0.5%
2	New York	44,840,000	8.2%
14	North Carolina	11,486,000	2.1%
49	North Dakota	591,000	0.1%
12	Ohio	13,693,000	2.5%
36	Oklahoma	2,672,000	0.5%
19	Oregon	9,409,000	1.7%
8	Pennsylvania	16,553,000	3.0%
33	Rhode Island	3,033,000	0.6%
26	South Carolina	5,611,000	1.0%
48	South Dakota	680,000	0.1%
27	Tennessee	5,290,000	1.0%
4	Texas	27,653,000	5.1%
45	Utah	1,416,000	0.3%
41	Vermont	1,824,000	0.3%
11	Virginia	14,010,000	2.6%
9	Washington	15,125,000	2.8%
47	West Virginia	1,135,000	0.2%
20	Wisconsin	9,085,000	1.7%
50	Wyoming	547,000	0.1%

RANK ORDER

RANK	STATE	GALLONS	% of USA
1	California	99,930,000	18.3%
2	New York	44,840,000	8.2%
3	Florida	41,383,000	7.6%
4	Texas	27,653,000	5.1%
5	Illinois	24,663,000	4.5%
6	New Jersey	24,472,000	4.5%
7	Massachusetts	20,635,000	3.8%
8	Pennsylvania	16,553,000	3.0%
9	Washington	15,125,000	2.8%
10	Michigan	14,757,000	2.7%
11	Virginia	14,010,000	2.6%
12	Ohio	13,693,000	2.5%
13	Georgia	12,902,000	2.4%
14	North Carolina	11,486,000	2.1%
15	Connecticut	10,521,000	1.9%
16	Maryland	10,009,000	1.8%
17	Arizona	9,869,000	1.8%
18	Colorado	9,845,000	1.8%
19	Oregon	9,409,000	1.7%
20	Wisconsin	9,085,000	1.7%
21	Missouri	8,144,000	1.5%
22	Minnesota	7,918,000	1.4%
23	Nevada	7,745,000	1.4%
24	Indiana	7,738,000	1.4%
25	Louisiana	6,159,000	1.1%
26	South Carolina	5,611,000	1.0%
27	Tennessee	5,290,000	1.0%
28	Idaho	5,142,000	0.9%
29	Alabama	4,934,000	0.9%
30	New Hampshire	4,373,000	0.8%
31	Kentucky	3,460,000	0.6%
32	Maine	3,179,000	0.6%
33	Rhode Island	3,033,000	0.6%
34	Hawaii	3,002,000	0.5%
35	New Mexico	2,771,000	0.5%
36	Oklahoma	2,672,000	0.5%
37	Kansas	2,516,000	0.5%
38	Delaware	2,382,000	0.4%
39	Iowa	2,353,000	0.4%
40	Arkansas	1,993,000	0.4%
41	Vermont	1,824,000	0.3%
42	Nebraska	1,791,000	0.3%
43	Montana	1,671,000	0.3%
44	Mississippi	1,657,000	0.3%
45	Utah	1,416,000	0.3%
46	Alaska	1,379,000	0.3%
47	West Virginia	1,135,000	0.2%
48	South Dakota	680,000	0.1%
49	North Dakota	591,000	0.1%
50	Wyoming	547,000	0.1%
	District of Columbia	2,597,000	0.5%

Source: U.S. Department of Health and Human Services, National Institute on Alcohol Abuse and Alcoholism
"Volume Beverage and Ethanol Consumption for States" (http://www.niaaa.nih.gov/databases/consum02.txt)
This is apparent consumption and is based on several sources which together approximate sales but do not actually measure consumption. Reported state volumes reflect only in-state purchases. Accordingly, figures for some states may be skewed by purchases by nonresidents.

Adult Per Capita Wine Consumption in 2000

National Per Capita = 2.8 Gallons Consumed per Adult 21 Years and Older

ALPHA ORDER

RANK	STATE	PER CAPITA
37	Alabama	1.6
15	Alaska	3.4
20	Arizona	2.8
45	Arkansas	1.1
5	California	4.3
17	Colorado	3.3
5	Connecticut	4.3
5	Delaware	4.3
13	Florida	3.5
25	Georgia	2.3
13	Hawaii	3.5
1	Idaho	6.0
19	Illinois	2.9
35	Indiana	1.8
45	Iowa	1.1
40	Kansas	1.4
44	Kentucky	1.2
30	Louisiana	2.0
15	Maine	3.4
22	Maryland	2.7
4	Massachusetts	4.5
28	Michigan	2.1
25	Minnesota	2.3
49	Mississippi	0.9
28	Missouri	2.1
23	Montana	2.6
39	Nebraska	1.5
2	Nevada	5.5
3	New Hampshire	5.0
9	New Jersey	4.1
25	New Mexico	2.3
17	New York	3.3
30	North Carolina	2.0
41	North Dakota	1.3
36	Ohio	1.7
45	Oklahoma	1.1
11	Oregon	3.9
34	Pennsylvania	1.9
9	Rhode Island	4.1
30	South Carolina	2.0
41	South Dakota	1.3
41	Tennessee	1.3
30	Texas	2.0
48	Utah	1.0
8	Vermont	4.2
20	Virginia	2.8
12	Washington	3.7
49	West Virginia	0.9
24	Wisconsin	2.4
37	Wyoming	1.6

RANK ORDER

RANK	STATE	PER CAPITA
1	Idaho	6.0
2	Nevada	5.5
3	New Hampshire	5.0
4	Massachusetts	4.5
5	California	4.3
5	Connecticut	4.3
5	Delaware	4.3
8	Vermont	4.2
9	New Jersey	4.1
9	Rhode Island	4.1
11	Oregon	3.9
12	Washington	3.7
13	Florida	3.5
13	Hawaii	3.5
15	Alaska	3.4
15	Maine	3.4
17	Colorado	3.3
17	New York	3.3
19	Illinois	2.9
20	Arizona	2.8
20	Virginia	2.8
22	Maryland	2.7
23	Montana	2.6
24	Wisconsin	2.4
25	Georgia	2.3
25	Minnesota	2.3
25	New Mexico	2.3
28	Michigan	2.1
28	Missouri	2.1
30	Louisiana	2.0
30	North Carolina	2.0
30	South Carolina	2.0
30	Texas	2.0
34	Pennsylvania	1.9
35	Indiana	1.8
36	Ohio	1.7
37	Alabama	1.6
37	Wyoming	1.6
39	Nebraska	1.5
40	Kansas	1.4
41	North Dakota	1.3
41	South Dakota	1.3
41	Tennessee	1.3
44	Kentucky	1.2
45	Arkansas	1.1
45	Iowa	1.1
45	Oklahoma	1.1
48	Utah	1.0
49	Mississippi	0.9
49	West Virginia	0.9
	District of Columbia	6.1

*Source: Morgan Quitno Press using data from U.S. Dept. of HHS, National Institute on Alcohol Abuse and Alcoholism
"Volume Beverage and Ethanol Consumption for States" (http://www.niaaa.nih.gov/databases/consum02.txt)
*This is apparent consumption and is based on several sources which together approximate sales but do not
actually measure consumption. Reported state volumes reflect only in-state purchases. Accordingly, figures for
some states may be skewed by purchases by nonresidents.*

Distilled Spirits Consumption in 2000

National Total = 354,548,000 Gallons of Distilled Spirits Consumed*

ALPHA ORDER

RANK	STATE	GALLONS	% of USA
27	Alabama	4,485,000	1.3%
46	Alaska	1,076,000	0.3%
20	Arizona	7,055,000	2.0%
34	Arkansas	2,796,000	0.8%
1	California	41,327,000	11.7%
17	Colorado	7,503,000	2.1%
25	Connecticut	4,959,000	1.4%
40	Delaware	1,622,000	0.5%
2	Florida	26,422,000	7.5%
11	Georgia	10,999,000	3.1%
42	Hawaii	1,434,000	0.4%
44	Idaho	1,253,000	0.4%
5	Illinois	15,281,000	4.3%
19	Indiana	7,261,000	2.0%
33	Iowa	2,863,000	0.8%
35	Kansas	2,692,000	0.8%
29	Kentucky	4,278,000	1.2%
22	Louisiana	6,043,000	1.7%
38	Maine	1,861,000	0.5%
15	Maryland	7,735,000	2.2%
10	Massachusetts	11,031,000	3.1%
6	Michigan	13,360,000	3.8%
13	Minnesota	8,359,000	2.4%
31	Mississippi	3,273,000	0.9%
18	Missouri	7,302,000	2.1%
45	Montana	1,213,000	0.3%
37	Nebraska	2,061,000	0.6%
26	Nevada	4,913,000	1.4%
30	New Hampshire	4,107,000	1.2%
7	New Jersey	12,681,000	3.6%
36	New Mexico	2,113,000	0.6%
3	New York	21,657,000	6.1%
14	North Carolina	8,204,000	2.3%
47	North Dakota	1,003,000	0.3%
9	Ohio	11,091,000	3.1%
32	Oklahoma	2,998,000	0.8%
28	Oregon	4,309,000	1.2%
8	Pennsylvania	11,576,000	3.3%
41	Rhode Island	1,461,000	0.4%
24	South Carolina	5,545,000	1.6%
48	South Dakota	996,000	0.3%
23	Tennessee	5,644,000	1.6%
4	Texas	19,897,000	5.6%
39	Utah	1,629,000	0.5%
50	Vermont	767,000	0.2%
21	Virginia	6,925,000	2.0%
16	Washington	7,599,000	2.1%
43	West Virginia	1,297,000	0.4%
12	Wisconsin	10,032,000	2.8%
49	Wyoming	837,000	0.2%

RANK ORDER

RANK	STATE	GALLONS	% of USA
1	California	41,327,000	11.7%
2	Florida	26,422,000	7.5%
3	New York	21,657,000	6.1%
4	Texas	19,897,000	5.6%
5	Illinois	15,281,000	4.3%
6	Michigan	13,360,000	3.8%
7	New Jersey	12,681,000	3.6%
8	Pennsylvania	11,576,000	3.3%
9	Ohio	11,091,000	3.1%
10	Massachusetts	11,031,000	3.1%
11	Georgia	10,999,000	3.1%
12	Wisconsin	10,032,000	2.8%
13	Minnesota	8,359,000	2.4%
14	North Carolina	8,204,000	2.3%
15	Maryland	7,735,000	2.2%
16	Washington	7,599,000	2.1%
17	Colorado	7,503,000	2.1%
18	Missouri	7,302,000	2.1%
19	Indiana	7,261,000	2.0%
20	Arizona	7,055,000	2.0%
21	Virginia	6,925,000	2.0%
22	Louisiana	6,043,000	1.7%
23	Tennessee	5,644,000	1.6%
24	South Carolina	5,545,000	1.6%
25	Connecticut	4,959,000	1.4%
26	Nevada	4,913,000	1.4%
27	Alabama	4,485,000	1.3%
28	Oregon	4,309,000	1.2%
29	Kentucky	4,278,000	1.2%
30	New Hampshire	4,107,000	1.2%
31	Mississippi	3,273,000	0.9%
32	Oklahoma	2,998,000	0.8%
33	Iowa	2,863,000	0.8%
34	Arkansas	2,796,000	0.8%
35	Kansas	2,692,000	0.8%
36	New Mexico	2,113,000	0.6%
37	Nebraska	2,061,000	0.6%
38	Maine	1,861,000	0.5%
39	Utah	1,629,000	0.5%
40	Delaware	1,622,000	0.5%
41	Rhode Island	1,461,000	0.4%
42	Hawaii	1,434,000	0.4%
43	West Virginia	1,297,000	0.4%
44	Idaho	1,253,000	0.4%
45	Montana	1,213,000	0.3%
46	Alaska	1,076,000	0.3%
47	North Dakota	1,003,000	0.3%
48	South Dakota	996,000	0.3%
49	Wyoming	837,000	0.2%
50	Vermont	767,000	0.2%
	District of Columbia	1,724,000	0.5%

Source: U.S. Department of Health and Human Services, National Institute on Alcohol Abuse and Alcoholism
"Volume Beverage and Ethanol Consumption for States" (http://www.niaaa.nih.gov/databases/consum02.txt)
*This is apparent consumption and is based on several sources which together approximate sales but do not actually measure consumption. Reported state volumes reflect only in-state purchases. Accordingly, figures for some states may be skewed by purchases by nonresidents.

Adult Per Capita Distilled Spirits Consumption in 2000

National Per Capita = 1.8 Gallons Consumed per Adult 21 Years and Older*

ALPHA ORDER

RANK ORDER

RANK	STATE	PER CAPITA		RANK	STATE	PER CAPITA
40	Alabama	1.4		1	New Hampshire	4.7
5	Alaska	2.6		2	Nevada	3.5
14	Arizona	2.0		3	Delaware	2.9
36	Arkansas	1.5		4	Wisconsin	2.7
25	California	1.8		5	Alaska	2.6
6	Colorado	2.5		6	Colorado	2.5
14	Connecticut	2.0		6	Wyoming	2.5
3	Delaware	2.9		8	Massachusetts	2.4
10	Florida	2.3		8	Minnesota	2.4
20	Georgia	1.9		10	Florida	2.3
30	Hawaii	1.7		11	North Dakota	2.2
36	Idaho	1.5		12	Maryland	2.1
25	Illinois	1.8		12	New Jersey	2.1
30	Indiana	1.7		14	Arizona	2.0
40	Iowa	1.4		14	Connecticut	2.0
36	Kansas	1.5		14	Louisiana	2.0
36	Kentucky	1.5		14	Maine	2.0
14	Louisiana	2.0		14	Rhode Island	2.0
14	Maine	2.0		14	South Carolina	2.0
12	Maryland	2.1		20	Georgia	1.9
8	Massachusetts	2.4		20	Michigan	1.9
20	Michigan	1.9		20	Missouri	1.9
8	Minnesota	2.4		20	Montana	1.9
30	Mississippi	1.7		20	South Dakota	1.9
20	Missouri	1.9		25	California	1.8
20	Montana	1.9		25	Illinois	1.8
30	Nebraska	1.7		25	Oregon	1.8
2	Nevada	3.5		25	Vermont	1.8
1	New Hampshire	4.7		25	Washington	1.8
12	New Jersey	2.1		30	Hawaii	1.7
30	New Mexico	1.7		30	Indiana	1.7
35	New York	1.6		30	Mississippi	1.7
40	North Carolina	1.4		30	Nebraska	1.7
11	North Dakota	2.2		30	New Mexico	1.7
40	Ohio	1.4		35	New York	1.6
47	Oklahoma	1.3		36	Arkansas	1.5
25	Oregon	1.8		36	Idaho	1.5
47	Pennsylvania	1.3		36	Kansas	1.5
14	Rhode Island	2.0		36	Kentucky	1.5
14	South Carolina	2.0		40	Alabama	1.4
20	South Dakota	1.9		40	Iowa	1.4
40	Tennessee	1.4		40	North Carolina	1.4
40	Texas	1.4		40	Ohio	1.4
49	Utah	1.2		40	Tennessee	1.4
25	Vermont	1.8		40	Texas	1.4
40	Virginia	1.4		40	Virginia	1.4
25	Washington	1.8		47	Oklahoma	1.3
50	West Virginia	1.0		47	Pennsylvania	1.3
4	Wisconsin	2.7		49	Utah	1.2
6	Wyoming	2.5		50	West Virginia	1.0

District of Columbia   4.1

Source: Morgan Quitno Press using data from U.S. Dept. of HHS, National Institute on Alcohol Abuse and Alcoholism "Volume Beverage and Ethanol Consumption for States" (http://www.niaaa.nih.gov/databases/consum02.txt)
*This is apparent consumption and is based on several sources which together approximate sales but do not actually measure consumption. Reported state volumes reflect only in-state purchases. Accordingly, figures for some states may be skewed by purchases by nonresidents.

Average Alcohol Consumption per Drinker in 1999

National Average = 4.21 Gallons*

ALPHA ORDER

RANK	STATE	GALLONS
19	Alabama	4.74
10	Alaska	5.06
1	Arizona	7.76
17	Arkansas	4.75
46	California	3.64
33	Colorado	4.00
40	Connecticut	3.81
12	Delaware	4.94
14	Florida	4.82
16	Georgia	4.76
17	Hawaii	4.75
13	Idaho	4.88
32	Illinois	4.04
47	Indiana	3.62
48	Iowa	3.59
35	Kansas	3.95
11	Kentucky	5.03
8	Louisiana	5.51
41	Maine	3.79
44	Maryland	3.65
34	Massachusetts	3.98
49	Michigan	3.56
20	Minnesota	4.72
7	Mississippi	5.67
28	Missouri	4.24
23	Montana	4.48
27	Nebraska	4.29
2	Nevada	6.44
4	New Hampshire	6.34
31	New Jersey	4.07
22	New Mexico	4.50
44	New York	3.65
15	North Carolina	4.79
25	North Dakota	4.43
21	Ohio	4.58
5	Oklahoma	6.01
39	Oregon	3.82
42	Pennsylvania	3.71
30	Rhode Island	4.14
6	South Carolina	5.74
35	South Dakota	3.95
3	Tennessee	6.41
29	Texas	4.18
23	Utah	4.48
38	Vermont	3.86
43	Virginia	3.67
49	Washington	3.56
9	West Virginia	5.08
37	Wisconsin	3.87
25	Wyoming	4.43

RANK ORDER

RANK	STATE	GALLONS
1	Arizona	7.76
2	Nevada	6.44
3	Tennessee	6.41
4	New Hampshire	6.34
5	Oklahoma	6.01
6	South Carolina	5.74
7	Mississippi	5.67
8	Louisiana	5.51
9	West Virginia	5.08
10	Alaska	5.06
11	Kentucky	5.03
12	Delaware	4.94
13	Idaho	4.88
14	Florida	4.82
15	North Carolina	4.79
16	Georgia	4.76
17	Arkansas	4.75
17	Hawaii	4.75
19	Alabama	4.74
20	Minnesota	4.72
21	Ohio	4.58
22	New Mexico	4.50
23	Montana	4.48
23	Utah	4.48
25	North Dakota	4.43
25	Wyoming	4.43
27	Nebraska	4.29
28	Missouri	4.24
29	Texas	4.18
30	Rhode Island	4.14
31	New Jersey	4.07
32	Illinois	4.04
33	Colorado	4.00
34	Massachusetts	3.98
35	Kansas	3.95
35	South Dakota	3.95
37	Wisconsin	3.87
38	Vermont	3.86
39	Oregon	3.82
40	Connecticut	3.81
41	Maine	3.79
42	Pennsylvania	3.71
43	Virginia	3.67
44	Maryland	3.65
44	New York	3.65
46	California	3.64
47	Indiana	3.62
48	Iowa	3.59
49	Michigan	3.56
49	Washington	3.56

District of Columbia   7.43

Source: U.S. Department of Health and Human Services, National Institute on Alcohol Abuse and Alcoholism
"Per Capita and Per Drinker Ethanol Consumption for States" (http://www.niaaa.nih.gov/databases/consum04.txt)
*National percent calculated by the editors. This is consumption of actual alcohol, not entire volume of an alcoholic beverage (e.g. wine is roughly 11% absolute alcohol content).

Percent of Adults Who Do Not Drink Alcohol: 2003

National Median = 40.8% of Adults*

ALPHA ORDER

RANK	STATE	PERCENT
7	Alabama	58.5
36	Alaska	38.4
23	Arizona	41.9
9	Arkansas	55.6
28	California	40.1
45	Colorado	33.1
49	Connecticut	31.4
31	Delaware	39.3
22	Florida	42.5
15	Georgia	49.1
13	Hawaii	50.6
14	Idaho	49.5
24	Illinois	41.4
16	Indiana	47.9
29	Iowa	40.0
10	Kansas	54.3
3	Kentucky	66.3
11	Louisiana	52.2
37	Maine	38.3
32	Maryland	39.2
48	Massachusetts	31.9
30	Michigan	39.5
47	Minnesota	32.5
5	Mississippi	59.1
17	Missouri	46.5
41	Montana	36.8
27	Nebraska	40.4
34	Nevada	38.9
43	New Hampshire	33.5
40	New Jersey	37.6
21	New Mexico	42.6
37	New York	38.3
6	North Carolina	58.6
42	North Dakota	34.8
20	Ohio	43.4
8	Oklahoma	56.6
35	Oregon	38.7
26	Pennsylvania	40.6
45	Rhode Island	33.1
12	South Carolina	51.3
32	South Dakota	39.2
2	Tennessee	68.0
18	Texas	46.0
1	Utah	68.6
44	Vermont	33.4
19	Virginia	45.1
39	Washington	38.2
4	West Virginia	66.0
50	Wisconsin	28.7
25	Wyoming	40.9

RANK ORDER

RANK	STATE	PERCENT
1	Utah	68.6
2	Tennessee	68.0
3	Kentucky	66.3
4	West Virginia	66.0
5	Mississippi	59.1
6	North Carolina	58.6
7	Alabama	58.5
8	Oklahoma	56.6
9	Arkansas	55.6
10	Kansas	54.3
11	Louisiana	52.2
12	South Carolina	51.3
13	Hawaii	50.6
14	Idaho	49.5
15	Georgia	49.1
16	Indiana	47.9
17	Missouri	46.5
18	Texas	46.0
19	Virginia	45.1
20	Ohio	43.4
21	New Mexico	42.6
22	Florida	42.5
23	Arizona	41.9
24	Illinois	41.4
25	Wyoming	40.9
26	Pennsylvania	40.6
27	Nebraska	40.4
28	California	40.1
29	Iowa	40.0
30	Michigan	39.5
31	Delaware	39.3
32	Maryland	39.2
32	South Dakota	39.2
34	Nevada	38.9
35	Oregon	38.7
36	Alaska	38.4
37	Maine	38.3
37	New York	38.3
39	Washington	38.2
40	New Jersey	37.6
41	Montana	36.8
42	North Dakota	34.8
43	New Hampshire	33.5
44	Vermont	33.4
45	Colorado	33.1
45	Rhode Island	33.1
47	Minnesota	32.5
48	Massachusetts	31.9
49	Connecticut	31.4
50	Wisconsin	28.7

	District of Columbia	37.4

Source: U.S. Department of Health and Human Services, Centers for Disease Control and Prevention
   "2003 Behavioral Risk Factor Surveillance Summary Prevalence Data" (http://apps.nccd.cdc.gov/brfss/)
*Persons 18 and older reporting not having at least one drink of alcohol in the past 30 days.

Percent of Adults Who Are Binge Drinkers: 2003

National Median = 16.5% of Adults*

ALPHA ORDER

RANK	STATE	PERCENT
44	Alabama	12.1
9	Alaska	18.4
24	Arizona	16.6
43	Arkansas	12.5
29	California	15.9
10	Colorado	18.3
25	Connecticut	16.5
8	Delaware	18.6
30	Florida	15.5
42	Georgia	13.0
40	Hawaii	13.3
30	Idaho	15.5
18	Illinois	17.3
35	Indiana	15.1
4	Iowa	19.4
39	Kansas	13.9
48	Kentucky	9.3
26	Louisiana	16.4
22	Maine	16.8
37	Maryland	15.0
10	Massachusetts	18.3
5	Michigan	19.1
3	Minnesota	19.7
45	Mississippi	11.4
20	Missouri	17.2
5	Montana	19.1
14	Nebraska	18.0
16	Nevada	17.9
17	New Hampshire	17.7
28	New Jersey	16.0
33	New Mexico	15.3
21	New York	16.9
49	North Carolina	8.6
2	North Dakota	21.4
23	Ohio	16.7
40	Oklahoma	13.3
30	Oregon	15.5
14	Pennsylvania	18.0
13	Rhode Island	18.2
38	South Carolina	14.4
7	South Dakota	19.0
50	Tennessee	6.6
27	Texas	16.3
47	Utah	10.2
18	Vermont	17.3
35	Virginia	15.1
34	Washington	15.2
46	West Virginia	11.1
1	Wisconsin	24.2
10	Wyoming	18.3

RANK ORDER

RANK	STATE	PERCENT
1	Wisconsin	24.2
2	North Dakota	21.4
3	Minnesota	19.7
4	Iowa	19.4
5	Michigan	19.1
5	Montana	19.1
7	South Dakota	19.0
8	Delaware	18.6
9	Alaska	18.4
10	Colorado	18.3
10	Massachusetts	18.3
10	Wyoming	18.3
13	Rhode Island	18.2
14	Nebraska	18.0
14	Pennsylvania	18.0
16	Nevada	17.9
17	New Hampshire	17.7
18	Illinois	17.3
18	Vermont	17.3
20	Missouri	17.2
21	New York	16.9
22	Maine	16.8
23	Ohio	16.7
24	Arizona	16.6
25	Connecticut	16.5
26	Louisiana	16.4
27	Texas	16.3
28	New Jersey	16.0
29	California	15.9
30	Florida	15.5
30	Idaho	15.5
30	Oregon	15.5
33	New Mexico	15.3
34	Washington	15.2
35	Indiana	15.1
35	Virginia	15.1
37	Maryland	15.0
38	South Carolina	14.4
39	Kansas	13.9
40	Hawaii	13.3
40	Oklahoma	13.3
42	Georgia	13.0
43	Arkansas	12.5
44	Alabama	12.1
45	Mississippi	11.4
46	West Virginia	11.1
47	Utah	10.2
48	Kentucky	9.3
49	North Carolina	8.6
50	Tennessee	6.6
	District of Columbia	18.6

Source: U.S. Department of Health and Human Services, Centers for Disease Control and Prevention
"2003 Behavioral Risk Factor Surveillance Summary Prevalence Data" (http://apps.nccd.cdc.gov/brfss/)
*Persons 18 and older reporting consumption of five or more alcoholic drinks on one or more occasions during the previous month.

Percent of Adults Who Smoke: 2003

National Median = 22.1% of Adults*

ALPHA ORDER

RANK	STATE	PERCENT
13	Alabama	25.3
5	Alaska	26.3
35	Arizona	21.0
16	Arkansas	24.8
49	California	16.8
47	Colorado	18.5
46	Connecticut	18.7
29	Delaware	21.9
20	Florida	23.9
22	Georgia	22.8
48	Hawaii	17.3
45	Idaho	19.0
19	Illinois	24.3
7	Indiana	26.1
30	Iowa	21.7
38	Kansas	20.4
1	Kentucky	30.8
4	Louisiana	26.6
21	Maine	23.6
39	Maryland	20.2
44	Massachusetts	19.2
6	Michigan	26.2
34	Minnesota	21.1
9	Mississippi	25.6
3	Missouri	27.3
40	Montana	19.9
32	Nebraska	21.3
14	Nevada	25.2
33	New Hampshire	21.2
42	New Jersey	19.5
28	New Mexico	22.0
31	New York	21.6
16	North Carolina	24.8
37	North Dakota	20.5
12	Ohio	25.4
14	Oklahoma	25.2
35	Oregon	21.0
10	Pennsylvania	25.5
24	Rhode Island	22.4
10	South Carolina	25.5
23	South Dakota	22.7
8	Tennessee	25.7
25	Texas	22.1
50	Utah	12.0
41	Vermont	19.6
25	Virginia	22.1
42	Washington	19.5
2	West Virginia	27.4
25	Wisconsin	22.1
18	Wyoming	24.6

RANK ORDER

RANK	STATE	PERCENT
1	Kentucky	30.8
2	West Virginia	27.4
3	Missouri	27.3
4	Louisiana	26.6
5	Alaska	26.3
6	Michigan	26.2
7	Indiana	26.1
8	Tennessee	25.7
9	Mississippi	25.6
10	Pennsylvania	25.5
10	South Carolina	25.5
12	Ohio	25.4
13	Alabama	25.3
14	Nevada	25.2
14	Oklahoma	25.2
16	Arkansas	24.8
16	North Carolina	24.8
18	Wyoming	24.6
19	Illinois	24.3
20	Florida	23.9
21	Maine	23.6
22	Georgia	22.8
23	South Dakota	22.7
24	Rhode Island	22.4
25	Texas	22.1
25	Virginia	22.1
25	Wisconsin	22.1
28	New Mexico	22.0
29	Delaware	21.9
30	Iowa	21.7
31	New York	21.6
32	Nebraska	21.3
33	New Hampshire	21.2
34	Minnesota	21.1
35	Arizona	21.0
35	Oregon	21.0
37	North Dakota	20.5
38	Kansas	20.4
39	Maryland	20.2
40	Montana	19.9
41	Vermont	19.6
42	New Jersey	19.5
42	Washington	19.5
44	Massachusetts	19.2
45	Idaho	19.0
46	Connecticut	18.7
47	Colorado	18.5
48	Hawaii	17.3
49	California	16.8
50	Utah	12.0

District of Columbia   22.3

Source: U.S. Department of Health and Human Services, Centers for Disease Control and Prevention
"2003 Behavioral Risk Factor Surveillance System" (Morbidity Mortality Weekly Report, Vol. 53, No. 44, 11/12/04)
*Persons 18 and older who have smoked more than 100 cigarettes during their lifetime and who currently smoke everyday or some days.

Percent of Men Who Smoke: 2003

National Median = 24.8% of Men*

ALPHA ORDER

RANK ORDER

RANK	STATE	PERCENT		RANK	STATE	PERCENT
9	Alabama	28.5		1	Kentucky	33.8
4	Alaska	30.3		2	Missouri	31.2
28	Arizona	23.8		3	Mississippi	31.1
14	Arkansas	27.6		4	Alaska	30.3
42	California	20.5		4	Louisiana	30.3
47	Colorado	19.6		6	Michigan	30.2
46	Connecticut	19.7		7	Nevada	29.0
21	Delaware	26.0		8	Indiana	28.6
21	Florida	26.0		9	Alabama	28.5
23	Georgia	25.8		9	South Carolina	28.5
43	Hawaii	20.1		11	Illinois	28.3
48	Idaho	19.5		12	North Carolina	28.0
11	Illinois	28.3		13	Oklahoma	27.8
8	Indiana	28.6		14	Arkansas	27.6
35	Iowa	22.8		14	West Virginia	27.6
40	Kansas	21.0		16	Tennessee	27.3
1	Kentucky	33.8		17	Pennsylvania	27.1
4	Louisiana	30.3		18	Ohio	26.9
32	Maine	23.1		19	Texas	26.7
34	Maryland	23.0		20	Virginia	26.4
44	Massachusetts	20.0		21	Delaware	26.0
6	Michigan	30.2		21	Florida	26.0
36	Minnesota	22.4		23	Georgia	25.8
3	Mississippi	31.1		24	Wyoming	25.2
2	Missouri	31.2		25	New York	24.8
48	Montana	19.5		26	South Dakota	24.7
30	Nebraska	23.6		27	Wisconsin	24.0
7	Nevada	29.0		28	Arizona	23.8
36	New Hampshire	22.4		28	Rhode Island	23.8
39	New Jersey	21.2		30	Nebraska	23.6
30	New Mexico	23.6		30	New Mexico	23.6
25	New York	24.8		32	Maine	23.1
12	North Carolina	28.0		32	Oregon	23.1
38	North Dakota	22.0		34	Maryland	23.0
18	Ohio	26.9		35	Iowa	22.8
13	Oklahoma	27.8		36	Minnesota	22.4
32	Oregon	23.1		36	New Hampshire	22.4
17	Pennsylvania	27.1		38	North Dakota	22.0
28	Rhode Island	23.8		39	New Jersey	21.2
9	South Carolina	28.5		40	Kansas	21.0
26	South Dakota	24.7		41	Washington	20.9
16	Tennessee	27.3		42	California	20.5
19	Texas	26.7		43	Hawaii	20.1
50	Utah	14.0		44	Massachusetts	20.0
45	Vermont	19.8		45	Vermont	19.8
20	Virginia	26.4		46	Connecticut	19.7
41	Washington	20.9		47	Colorado	19.6
14	West Virginia	27.6		48	Idaho	19.5
27	Wisconsin	24.0		48	Montana	19.5
24	Wyoming	25.2		50	Utah	14.0

District of Columbia   26.2

Source: U.S. Department of Health and Human Services, Centers for Disease Control and Prevention
    "2003 Behavioral Risk Factor Surveillance System" (Morbidity Mortality Weekly Report, Vol. 53, No. 44, 11/12/04)
*Persons 18 and older who have smoked more than 100 cigarettes during their lifetime and who currently smoke everyday or some days.

Percent of Women Who Smoke: 2003

National Median = 20.3% of Women*

RANK	STATE	PERCENT	RANK	STATE	PERCENT
13	Alabama	22.4	1	Kentucky	28.1
17	Alaska	21.9	2	West Virginia	27.2
39	Arizona	18.2	3	Tennessee	24.2
14	Arkansas	22.3	4	Pennsylvania	24.1
49	California	13.2	4	Wyoming	24.1
47	Colorado	17.5	6	Maine	24.0
43	Connecticut	17.9	6	Ohio	24.0
39	Delaware	18.2	8	Indiana	23.8
16	Florida	22.1	8	Missouri	23.8
29	Georgia	20.0	10	Louisiana	23.2
48	Hawaii	14.4	11	South Carolina	22.8
37	Idaho	18.5	12	Oklahoma	22.7
24	Illinois	20.5	13	Alabama	22.4
8	Indiana	23.8	14	Arkansas	22.3
21	Iowa	20.7	14	Michigan	22.3
31	Kansas	19.7	16	Florida	22.1
1	Kentucky	28.1	17	Alaska	21.9
10	Louisiana	23.2	17	North Carolina	21.9
6	Maine	24.0	19	Nevada	21.3
45	Maryland	17.7	20	Rhode Island	21.1
38	Massachusetts	18.4	21	Iowa	20.7
14	Michigan	22.3	21	Mississippi	20.7
30	Minnesota	19.9	21	South Dakota	20.7
21	Mississippi	20.7	24	Illinois	20.5
8	Missouri	23.8	24	New Mexico	20.5
26	Montana	20.3	26	Montana	20.3
33	Nebraska	19.0	26	Wisconsin	20.3
19	Nevada	21.3	28	New Hampshire	20.2
28	New Hampshire	20.2	29	Georgia	20.0
43	New Jersey	17.9	30	Minnesota	19.9
24	New Mexico	20.5	31	Kansas	19.7
36	New York	18.8	32	Vermont	19.4
17	North Carolina	21.9	33	Nebraska	19.0
33	North Dakota	19.0	33	North Dakota	19.0
6	Ohio	24.0	35	Oregon	18.9
12	Oklahoma	22.7	36	New York	18.8
35	Oregon	18.9	37	Idaho	18.5
4	Pennsylvania	24.1	38	Massachusetts	18.4
20	Rhode Island	21.1	39	Arizona	18.2
11	South Carolina	22.8	39	Delaware	18.2
21	South Dakota	20.7	39	Washington	18.2
3	Tennessee	24.2	42	Virginia	18.0
46	Texas	17.6	43	Connecticut	17.9
50	Utah	9.9	43	New Jersey	17.9
32	Vermont	19.4	45	Maryland	17.7
42	Virginia	18.0	46	Texas	17.6
39	Washington	18.2	47	Colorado	17.5
2	West Virginia	27.2	48	Hawaii	14.4
26	Wisconsin	20.3	49	California	13.2
4	Wyoming	24.1	50	Utah	9.9

				District of Columbia	19.0

Source: U.S. Department of Health and Human Services, Centers for Disease Control and Prevention
   "2003 Behavioral Risk Factor Surveillance System" (Morbidity Mortality Weekly Report, Vol. 53, No. 44, 11/12/04)
Persons 18 and older who have smoked more than 100 cigarettes during their lifetime and who currently smoke everyday or some days.

Percent of Adults Who are Former Smokers: 2003

National Median = 25.2% of Adults*

ALPHA ORDER

RANK	STATE	PERCENT
36	Alabama	23.9
18	Alaska	26.1
15	Arizona	26.2
23	Arkansas	25.4
26	California	25.2
11	Colorado	27.2
1	Connecticut	31.2
9	Delaware	28.1
12	Florida	26.8
45	Georgia	21.7
33	Hawaii	24.1
39	Idaho	23.5
30	Illinois	24.4
30	Indiana	24.4
29	Iowa	24.5
41	Kansas	23.0
43	Kentucky	22.5
47	Louisiana	20.7
2	Maine	31.1
38	Maryland	23.7
3	Massachusetts	31.0
20	Michigan	25.8
8	Minnesota	28.3
47	Mississippi	20.7
32	Missouri	24.3
7	Montana	28.4
34	Nebraska	24.0
26	Nevada	25.2
3	New Hampshire	31.0
14	New Jersey	26.3
19	New Mexico	25.9
23	New York	25.4
40	North Carolina	23.2
22	North Dakota	25.6
37	Ohio	23.8
44	Oklahoma	22.1
13	Oregon	26.7
26	Pennsylvania	25.2
6	Rhode Island	29.1
41	South Carolina	23.0
25	South Dakota	25.3
49	Tennessee	18.9
46	Texas	21.6
50	Utah	16.6
5	Vermont	30.4
34	Virginia	24.0
15	Washington	26.2
20	West Virginia	25.8
10	Wisconsin	27.3
15	Wyoming	26.2

RANK ORDER

RANK	STATE	PERCENT
1	Connecticut	31.2
2	Maine	31.1
3	Massachusetts	31.0
3	New Hampshire	31.0
5	Vermont	30.4
6	Rhode Island	29.1
7	Montana	28.4
8	Minnesota	28.3
9	Delaware	28.1
10	Wisconsin	27.3
11	Colorado	27.2
12	Florida	26.8
13	Oregon	26.7
14	New Jersey	26.3
15	Arizona	26.2
15	Washington	26.2
15	Wyoming	26.2
18	Alaska	26.1
19	New Mexico	25.9
20	Michigan	25.8
20	West Virginia	25.8
22	North Dakota	25.6
23	Arkansas	25.4
23	New York	25.4
25	South Dakota	25.3
26	California	25.2
26	Nevada	25.2
26	Pennsylvania	25.2
29	Iowa	24.5
30	Illinois	24.4
30	Indiana	24.4
32	Missouri	24.3
33	Hawaii	24.1
34	Nebraska	24.0
34	Virginia	24.0
36	Alabama	23.9
37	Ohio	23.8
38	Maryland	23.7
39	Idaho	23.5
40	North Carolina	23.2
41	Kansas	23.0
41	South Carolina	23.0
43	Kentucky	22.5
44	Oklahoma	22.1
45	Georgia	21.7
46	Texas	21.6
47	Louisiana	20.7
47	Mississippi	20.7
49	Tennessee	18.9
50	Utah	16.6
	District of Columbia	22.2

Source: U.S. Department of Health and Human Services, Centers for Disease Control and Prevention
"2003 Behavioral Risk Factor Surveillance Summary Prevalence Data" (http://apps.nccd.cdc.gov/brfss/)
*Persons 18 and older who have smoked more than 100 cigarettes during their lifetime and who currently do not smoke.

Percent of Adults Who Have Never Smoked: 2003

National Median = 52.0% of Adults*

ALPHA ORDER

RANK	STATE	PERCENT
30	Alabama	50.8
47	Alaska	47.7
18	Arizona	53.0
37	Arkansas	49.8
3	California	58.0
12	Colorado	54.2
33	Connecticut	50.2
35	Delaware	50.0
41	Florida	49.3
8	Georgia	55.6
2	Hawaii	58.6
4	Idaho	57.6
23	Illinois	52.2
39	Indiana	49.5
16	Iowa	53.8
5	Kansas	56.6
49	Kentucky	46.7
20	Louisiana	52.7
50	Maine	45.2
7	Maryland	56.2
36	Massachusetts	49.9
45	Michigan	48.1
32	Minnesota	50.6
16	Mississippi	53.8
43	Missouri	48.5
27	Montana	51.6
10	Nebraska	54.7
38	Nevada	49.7
46	New Hampshire	47.8
11	New Jersey	54.3
24	New Mexico	52.1
18	New York	53.0
25	North Carolina	52.0
15	North Dakota	53.9
29	Ohio	51.0
20	Oklahoma	52.7
22	Oregon	52.4
40	Pennsylvania	49.4
43	Rhode Island	48.5
28	South Carolina	51.5
25	South Dakota	52.0
9	Tennessee	55.4
6	Texas	56.3
1	Utah	71.5
34	Vermont	50.1
14	Virginia	54.0
12	Washington	54.2
48	West Virginia	46.9
31	Wisconsin	50.7
42	Wyoming	49.1

RANK ORDER

RANK	STATE	PERCENT
1	Utah	71.5
2	Hawaii	58.6
3	California	58.0
4	Idaho	57.6
5	Kansas	56.6
6	Texas	56.3
7	Maryland	56.2
8	Georgia	55.6
9	Tennessee	55.4
10	Nebraska	54.7
11	New Jersey	54.3
12	Colorado	54.2
12	Washington	54.2
14	Virginia	54.0
15	North Dakota	53.9
16	Iowa	53.8
16	Mississippi	53.8
18	Arizona	53.0
18	New York	53.0
20	Louisiana	52.7
20	Oklahoma	52.7
22	Oregon	52.4
23	Illinois	52.2
24	New Mexico	52.1
25	North Carolina	52.0
25	South Dakota	52.0
27	Montana	51.6
28	South Carolina	51.5
29	Ohio	51.0
30	Alabama	50.8
31	Wisconsin	50.7
32	Minnesota	50.6
33	Connecticut	50.2
34	Vermont	50.1
35	Delaware	50.0
36	Massachusetts	49.9
37	Arkansas	49.8
38	Nevada	49.7
39	Indiana	49.5
40	Pennsylvania	49.4
41	Florida	49.3
42	Wyoming	49.1
43	Missouri	48.5
43	Rhode Island	48.5
45	Michigan	48.1
46	New Hampshire	47.8
47	Alaska	47.7
48	West Virginia	46.9
49	Kentucky	46.7
50	Maine	45.2

| | District of Columbia | 55.8 |

Source: U.S. Department of Health and Human Services, Centers for Disease Control and Prevention
  "2003 Behavioral Risk Factor Surveillance Summary Prevalence Data" (http://apps.nccd.cdc.gov/brfss/)
*Persons 18 and older who have not smoked more than 100 cigarettes during their lifetime.

Percent of Population Who are Illicit Drug Users: 2002

National Percent = 8.3% of Population*

ALPHA ORDER

RANK	STATE	PERCENT
46	Alabama	6.6
1	Alaska	12.2
21	Arizona	8.5
31	Arkansas	7.7
11	California	9.1
8	Colorado	10.2
11	Connecticut	9.1
11	Delaware	9.1
18	Florida	8.8
37	Georgia	7.1
11	Hawaii	9.1
40	Idaho	7.0
31	Illinois	7.7
21	Indiana	8.5
50	Iowa	6.1
44	Kansas	6.7
20	Kentucky	8.6
18	Louisiana	8.8
11	Maine	9.1
24	Maryland	8.3
21	Massachusetts	8.5
11	Michigan	9.1
29	Minnesota	8.0
37	Mississippi	7.1
17	Missouri	9.0
9	Montana	10.0
28	Nebraska	8.1
4	Nevada	10.8
2	New Hampshire	11.1
34	New Jersey	7.4
34	New Mexico	7.4
10	New York	9.4
25	North Carolina	8.2
37	North Dakota	7.1
25	Ohio	8.2
30	Oklahoma	7.9
7	Oregon	10.5
33	Pennsylvania	7.6
4	Rhode Island	10.8
48	South Carolina	6.5
40	South Dakota	7.0
43	Tennessee	6.9
44	Texas	6.7
49	Utah	6.2
3	Vermont	11.0
25	Virginia	8.2
4	Washington	10.8
46	West Virginia	6.6
36	Wisconsin	7.3
40	Wyoming	7.0

RANK ORDER

RANK	STATE	PERCENT
1	Alaska	12.2
2	New Hampshire	11.1
3	Vermont	11.0
4	Nevada	10.8
4	Rhode Island	10.8
4	Washington	10.8
7	Oregon	10.5
8	Colorado	10.2
9	Montana	10.0
10	New York	9.4
11	California	9.1
11	Connecticut	9.1
11	Delaware	9.1
11	Hawaii	9.1
11	Maine	9.1
11	Michigan	9.1
17	Missouri	9.0
18	Florida	8.8
18	Louisiana	8.8
20	Kentucky	8.6
21	Arizona	8.5
21	Indiana	8.5
21	Massachusetts	8.5
24	Maryland	8.3
25	North Carolina	8.2
25	Ohio	8.2
25	Virginia	8.2
28	Nebraska	8.1
29	Minnesota	8.0
30	Oklahoma	7.9
31	Arkansas	7.7
31	Illinois	7.7
33	Pennsylvania	7.6
34	New Jersey	7.4
34	New Mexico	7.4
36	Wisconsin	7.3
37	Georgia	7.1
37	Mississippi	7.1
37	North Dakota	7.1
40	Idaho	7.0
40	South Dakota	7.0
40	Wyoming	7.0
43	Tennessee	6.9
44	Kansas	6.7
44	Texas	6.7
46	Alabama	6.6
46	West Virginia	6.6
48	South Carolina	6.5
49	Utah	6.2
50	Iowa	6.1

	District of Columbia	12.4

Source: U.S. Department of Health and Human Services, Substance Abuse and Mental Health Services Administration
"2002 National Survey on Drug Use and Health" (July 2004)
*Population 12 years and older who used any illicit drug at least once within month of survey.

Percent of Adults Obese: 2003

National Median = 22.8% of Adults*

ALPHA ORDER

RANK	STATE	PERCENT
1	Alabama	28.4
23	Alaska	23.5
39	Arizona	20.1
6	Arkansas	25.2
24	California	23.2
50	Colorado	16.0
45	Connecticut	19.1
15	Delaware	24.0
42	Florida	19.9
6	Georgia	25.2
49	Hawaii	16.4
29	Idaho	21.8
20	Illinois	23.7
4	Indiana	26.0
17	Iowa	23.9
27	Kansas	22.6
5	Kentucky	25.6
11	Louisiana	24.8
42	Maine	19.9
28	Maryland	21.9
48	Massachusetts	16.8
6	Michigan	25.2
25	Minnesota	23.0
2	Mississippi	28.1
22	Missouri	23.6
46	Montana	18.8
17	Nebraska	23.9
33	Nevada	21.2
37	New Hampshire	20.2
39	New Jersey	20.1
37	New Mexico	20.2
34	New York	20.9
15	North Carolina	24.0
20	North Dakota	23.7
10	Ohio	24.9
14	Oklahoma	24.4
32	Oregon	21.5
19	Pennsylvania	23.8
47	Rhode Island	18.4
13	South Carolina	24.5
26	South Dakota	22.9
9	Tennessee	25.0
12	Texas	24.6
36	Utah	20.8
44	Vermont	19.6
30	Virginia	21.7
30	Washington	21.7
3	West Virginia	27.7
34	Wisconsin	20.9
39	Wyoming	20.1

RANK ORDER

RANK	STATE	PERCENT
1	Alabama	28.4
2	Mississippi	28.1
3	West Virginia	27.7
4	Indiana	26.0
5	Kentucky	25.6
6	Arkansas	25.2
6	Georgia	25.2
6	Michigan	25.2
9	Tennessee	25.0
10	Ohio	24.9
11	Louisiana	24.8
12	Texas	24.6
13	South Carolina	24.5
14	Oklahoma	24.4
15	Delaware	24.0
15	North Carolina	24.0
17	Iowa	23.9
17	Nebraska	23.9
19	Pennsylvania	23.8
20	Illinois	23.7
20	North Dakota	23.7
22	Missouri	23.6
23	Alaska	23.5
24	California	23.2
25	Minnesota	23.0
26	South Dakota	22.9
27	Kansas	22.6
28	Maryland	21.9
29	Idaho	21.8
30	Virginia	21.7
30	Washington	21.7
32	Oregon	21.5
33	Nevada	21.2
34	New York	20.9
34	Wisconsin	20.9
36	Utah	20.8
37	New Hampshire	20.2
37	New Mexico	20.2
39	Arizona	20.1
39	New Jersey	20.1
39	Wyoming	20.1
42	Florida	19.9
42	Maine	19.9
44	Vermont	19.6
45	Connecticut	19.1
46	Montana	18.8
47	Rhode Island	18.4
48	Massachusetts	16.8
49	Hawaii	16.4
50	Colorado	16.0

| | District of Columbia | 20.3 |

Source: U.S. Department of Health and Human Services, Centers for Disease Control and Prevention
"2003 Behavioral Risk Factor Surveillance Summary Prevalence Data" (http://apps.nccd.cdc.gov/brfss/)
*Persons 18 and older. Obese is defined as a Body Mass Index (BMI) of 30.0 or more regardless of sex. BMI is a ratio of height to weight. As an example, a person 5' 8" and weighing 197 pounds has a BMI of 30. See http://www.cdc.gov/nccdphp/dnpa/bmi/bmi-adult.htm.

Percent of Adults Overweight: 2003

National Median = 36.7% of Adults*

ALPHA ORDER

RANK	STATE	PERCENT
47	Alabama	34.8
14	Alaska	37.2
18	Arizona	37.0
23	Arkansas	36.8
32	California	36.2
43	Colorado	35.4
40	Connecticut	35.7
32	Delaware	36.2
3	Florida	38.7
43	Georgia	35.4
50	Hawaii	33.6
14	Idaho	37.2
10	Illinois	37.4
40	Indiana	35.7
9	Iowa	37.7
8	Kansas	37.8
10	Kentucky	37.4
30	Louisiana	36.3
5	Maine	38.3
14	Maryland	37.2
32	Massachusetts	36.2
28	Michigan	36.6
7	Minnesota	38.0
25	Mississippi	36.7
42	Missouri	35.6
6	Montana	38.1
18	Nebraska	37.0
12	Nevada	37.3
25	New Hampshire	36.7
14	New Jersey	37.2
29	New Mexico	36.4
46	New York	35.3
18	North Carolina	37.0
1	North Dakota	39.2
36	Ohio	36.0
35	Oklahoma	36.1
25	Oregon	36.7
30	Pennsylvania	36.3
4	Rhode Island	38.5
39	South Carolina	35.8
12	South Dakota	37.3
43	Tennessee	35.4
22	Texas	36.9
49	Utah	33.8
38	Vermont	35.9
36	Virginia	36.0
23	Washington	36.8
48	West Virginia	34.0
2	Wisconsin	39.1
18	Wyoming	37.0

RANK ORDER

RANK	STATE	PERCENT
1	North Dakota	39.2
2	Wisconsin	39.1
3	Florida	38.7
4	Rhode Island	38.5
5	Maine	38.3
6	Montana	38.1
7	Minnesota	38.0
8	Kansas	37.8
9	Iowa	37.7
10	Illinois	37.4
10	Kentucky	37.4
12	Nevada	37.3
12	South Dakota	37.3
14	Alaska	37.2
14	Idaho	37.2
14	Maryland	37.2
14	New Jersey	37.2
18	Arizona	37.0
18	Nebraska	37.0
18	North Carolina	37.0
18	Wyoming	37.0
22	Texas	36.9
23	Arkansas	36.8
23	Washington	36.8
25	Mississippi	36.7
25	New Hampshire	36.7
25	Oregon	36.7
28	Michigan	36.6
29	New Mexico	36.4
30	Louisiana	36.3
30	Pennsylvania	36.3
32	California	36.2
32	Delaware	36.2
32	Massachusetts	36.2
35	Oklahoma	36.1
36	Ohio	36.0
36	Virginia	36.0
38	Vermont	35.9
39	South Carolina	35.8
40	Connecticut	35.7
40	Indiana	35.7
42	Missouri	35.6
43	Colorado	35.4
43	Georgia	35.4
43	Tennessee	35.4
46	New York	35.3
47	Alabama	34.8
48	West Virginia	34.0
49	Utah	33.8
50	Hawaii	33.6

District of Columbia	31.9

Source: U.S. Department of Health and Human Services, Centers for Disease Control and Prevention
    "2003 Behavioral Risk Factor Surveillance Summary Prevalence Data" (http://apps.nccd.cdc.gov/brfss/)
*Persons 18 and older. Does not include obese adults. Overweight is defined as a Body Mass Index (BMI) of 25.0
to 29.9 regardless of sex. BMI is a ratio of height to weight. As an example, a person 5' 8" and weighing 171
pounds has a BMI of 26. See http://www.cdc.gov/nccdphp/dnpa/bmi/bmi-adult.htm.*

Percent of Adults at Risk for Health Problems
Because of Being Overweight: 2003
National Median = 60.1% of Adults*

RANK	STATE	PERCENT
2	Alabama	63.2
17	Alaska	60.7
38	Arizona	57.1
5	Arkansas	62.0
27	California	59.3
49	Colorado	51.4
46	Connecticut	54.8
22	Delaware	60.2
31	Florida	58.6
18	Georgia	60.6
50	Hawaii	50.0
29	Idaho	59.0
11	Illinois	61.1
7	Indiana	61.7
9	Iowa	61.6
19	Kansas	60.5
3	Kentucky	63.1
11	Louisiana	61.1
35	Maine	58.2
29	Maryland	59.0
48	Massachusetts	53.0
6	Michigan	61.8
14	Minnesota	60.9
1	Mississippi	64.9
28	Missouri	59.2
41	Montana	56.9
14	Nebraska	60.9
32	Nevada	58.5
40	New Hampshire	57.0
37	New Jersey	57.2
43	New Mexico	56.6
44	New York	56.3
13	North Carolina	61.0
4	North Dakota	63.0
14	Ohio	60.9
19	Oklahoma	60.5
34	Oregon	58.3
22	Pennsylvania	60.2
41	Rhode Island	56.9
22	South Carolina	60.2
25	South Dakota	60.1
21	Tennessee	60.4
10	Texas	61.5
47	Utah	54.7
45	Vermont	55.5
36	Virginia	57.7
32	Washington	58.5
7	West Virginia	61.7
26	Wisconsin	60.0
38	Wyoming	57.1

RANK	STATE	PERCENT
1	Mississippi	64.9
2	Alabama	63.2
3	Kentucky	63.1
4	North Dakota	63.0
5	Arkansas	62.0
6	Michigan	61.8
7	Indiana	61.7
7	West Virginia	61.7
9	Iowa	61.6
10	Texas	61.5
11	Illinois	61.1
11	Louisiana	61.1
13	North Carolina	61.0
14	Minnesota	60.9
14	Nebraska	60.9
14	Ohio	60.9
17	Alaska	60.7
18	Georgia	60.6
19	Kansas	60.5
19	Oklahoma	60.5
21	Tennessee	60.4
22	Delaware	60.2
22	Pennsylvania	60.2
22	South Carolina	60.2
25	South Dakota	60.1
26	Wisconsin	60.0
27	California	59.3
28	Missouri	59.2
29	Idaho	59.0
29	Maryland	59.0
31	Florida	58.6
32	Nevada	58.5
32	Washington	58.5
34	Oregon	58.3
35	Maine	58.2
36	Virginia	57.7
37	New Jersey	57.2
38	Arizona	57.1
38	Wyoming	57.1
40	New Hampshire	57.0
41	Montana	56.9
41	Rhode Island	56.9
43	New Mexico	56.6
44	New York	56.3
45	Vermont	55.5
46	Connecticut	54.8
47	Utah	54.7
48	Massachusetts	53.0
49	Colorado	51.4
50	Hawaii	50.0

	District of Columbia	52.1

Source: U.S. Department of Health and Human Services, Centers for Disease Control and Prevention
"2003 Behavioral Risk Factor Surveillance Summary Prevalence Data" (http://apps.nccd.cdc.gov/brfss/)
*Persons 18 and older. "At risk for health problems" is defined according to the NHANES II definition of a Body Mass Index (BMI) of 27.8 for men and 27.3 for women. BMI is a ratio of height to weight. As an example, a person 5' 8" and weighing 197 pounds has a BMI of 30. See http://www.cdc.gov/nccdphp/dnpa/bmi/bmi-adult.htm.

Percent of Adults Who Exercise Vigorously: 2003

National Median = 26.3% of Adults*

ALPHA ORDER

RANK	STATE	PERCENT
43	Alabama	21.3
2	Alaska	34.6
16	Arizona	29.1
36	Arkansas	23.3
19	California	28.6
4	Colorado	32.9
11	Connecticut	30.6
35	Delaware	23.4
42	Florida	21.4
32	Georgia	24.9
25	Hawaii	26.3
7	Idaho	31.8
34	Illinois	23.5
31	Indiana	25.3
44	Iowa	20.9
37	Kansas	22.8
50	Kentucky	16.3
41	Louisiana	21.5
16	Maine	29.1
18	Maryland	28.8
9	Massachusetts	31.1
23	Michigan	26.6
24	Minnesota	26.4
45	Mississippi	20.2
38	Missouri	22.5
3	Montana	33.2
40	Nebraska	21.6
13	Nevada	30.3
10	New Hampshire	31.0
30	New Jersey	25.4
19	New Mexico	28.6
33	New York	24.5
48	North Carolina	19.3
22	North Dakota	26.7
27	Ohio	26.1
47	Oklahoma	19.5
12	Oregon	30.4
25	Pennsylvania	26.3
15	Rhode Island	29.5
29	South Carolina	25.9
39	South Dakota	22.0
46	Tennessee	20.0
27	Texas	26.1
1	Utah	35.5
5	Vermont	32.3
21	Virginia	28.1
8	Washington	31.3
49	West Virginia	19.1
14	Wisconsin	30.2
6	Wyoming	32.1

RANK ORDER

RANK	STATE	PERCENT
1	Utah	35.5
2	Alaska	34.6
3	Montana	33.2
4	Colorado	32.9
5	Vermont	32.3
6	Wyoming	32.1
7	Idaho	31.8
8	Washington	31.3
9	Massachusetts	31.1
10	New Hampshire	31.0
11	Connecticut	30.6
12	Oregon	30.4
13	Nevada	30.3
14	Wisconsin	30.2
15	Rhode Island	29.5
16	Arizona	29.1
16	Maine	29.1
18	Maryland	28.8
19	California	28.6
19	New Mexico	28.6
21	Virginia	28.1
22	North Dakota	26.7
23	Michigan	26.6
24	Minnesota	26.4
25	Hawaii	26.3
25	Pennsylvania	26.3
27	Ohio	26.1
27	Texas	26.1
29	South Carolina	25.9
30	New Jersey	25.4
31	Indiana	25.3
32	Georgia	24.9
33	New York	24.5
34	Illinois	23.5
35	Delaware	23.4
36	Arkansas	23.3
37	Kansas	22.8
38	Missouri	22.5
39	South Dakota	22.0
40	Nebraska	21.6
41	Louisiana	21.5
42	Florida	21.4
43	Alabama	21.3
44	Iowa	20.9
45	Mississippi	20.2
46	Tennessee	20.0
47	Oklahoma	19.5
48	North Carolina	19.3
49	West Virginia	19.1
50	Kentucky	16.3

District of Columbia 32.9

Source: U.S. Department of Health and Human Services, Centers for Disease Control and Prevention
    "2003 Behavioral Risk Factor Surveillance Summary Prevalence Data" (http://apps.nccd.cdc.gov/brfss/)
*Persons 18 and older. Activity that caused large increases in breathing or heart rate at least 20 minutes three or more times per week (such as running, aerobics or heavy yard work).

Percent of Adults Reporting No Leisure Time
Physical Activities in Past Month: 2003
National Median = 23.1% of Adults*

ALPHA ORDER

RANK	STATE	PERCENT
5	Alabama	29.9
41	Alaska	19.2
34	Arizona	21.2
7	Arkansas	29.1
28	California	22.3
49	Colorado	16.8
36	Connecticut	21.0
13	Delaware	26.5
9	Florida	27.9
20	Georgia	24.5
46	Hawaii	18.3
45	Idaho	18.6
17	Illinois	25.7
15	Indiana	26.2
26	Iowa	22.7
16	Kansas	25.9
1	Kentucky	30.6
2	Louisiana	30.5
38	Maine	20.6
33	Maryland	21.3
32	Massachusetts	21.6
30	Michigan	21.8
50	Minnesota	15.0
4	Mississippi	30.3
21	Missouri	24.0
39	Montana	20.2
37	Nebraska	20.7
19	Nevada	24.7
40	New Hampshire	19.9
12	New Jersey	26.9
25	New Mexico	22.9
11	New York	27.1
18	North Carolina	25.0
22	North Dakota	23.7
14	Ohio	26.4
3	Oklahoma	30.4
42	Oregon	18.8
27	Pennsylvania	22.6
23	Rhode Island	23.3
23	South Carolina	23.3
31	South Dakota	21.7
6	Tennessee	29.8
10	Texas	27.6
48	Utah	17.3
44	Vermont	18.7
29	Virginia	22.1
47	Washington	17.7
8	West Virginia	28.0
42	Wisconsin	18.8
35	Wyoming	21.1

RANK ORDER

RANK	STATE	PERCENT
1	Kentucky	30.6
2	Louisiana	30.5
3	Oklahoma	30.4
4	Mississippi	30.3
5	Alabama	29.9
6	Tennessee	29.8
7	Arkansas	29.1
8	West Virginia	28.0
9	Florida	27.9
10	Texas	27.6
11	New York	27.1
12	New Jersey	26.9
13	Delaware	26.5
14	Ohio	26.4
15	Indiana	26.2
16	Kansas	25.9
17	Illinois	25.7
18	North Carolina	25.0
19	Nevada	24.7
20	Georgia	24.5
21	Missouri	24.0
22	North Dakota	23.7
23	Rhode Island	23.3
23	South Carolina	23.3
25	New Mexico	22.9
26	Iowa	22.7
27	Pennsylvania	22.6
28	California	22.3
29	Virginia	22.1
30	Michigan	21.8
31	South Dakota	21.7
32	Massachusetts	21.6
33	Maryland	21.3
34	Arizona	21.2
35	Wyoming	21.1
36	Connecticut	21.0
37	Nebraska	20.7
38	Maine	20.6
39	Montana	20.2
40	New Hampshire	19.9
41	Alaska	19.2
42	Oregon	18.8
42	Wisconsin	18.8
44	Vermont	18.7
45	Idaho	18.6
46	Hawaii	18.3
47	Washington	17.7
48	Utah	17.3
49	Colorado	16.8
50	Minnesota	15.0

| | District of Columbia | 22.5 |

Source: U.S. Department of Health and Human Services, Centers for Disease Control and Prevention
"2003 Behavioral Risk Factor Surveillance Summary Prevalence Data" (http://apps.nccd.cdc.gov/brfss/)
*Persons 18 and older who report no leisure time physical activity or exercise during the past 30 days other than the respondent's regular job.

Percent of Adults with High Blood Pressure: 2003

National Median = 24.8% of Adults*

ALPHA ORDER

RANK	STATE	PERCENT
3	Alabama	33.1
48	Alaska	20.8
43	Arizona	22.7
4	Arkansas	30.5
37	California	23.4
49	Colorado	19.8
29	Connecticut	24.2
14	Delaware	27.7
7	Florida	29.3
12	Georgia	28.0
39	Hawaii	23.2
40	Idaho	23.1
30	Illinois	24.1
16	Indiana	27.0
23	Iowa	25.1
38	Kansas	23.3
6	Kentucky	29.8
8	Louisiana	29.0
20	Maine	26.0
24	Maryland	25.0
40	Massachusetts	23.1
17	Michigan	26.8
45	Minnesota	22.2
2	Mississippi	33.4
15	Missouri	27.5
46	Montana	21.3
36	Nebraska	23.5
35	Nevada	23.6
44	New Hampshire	22.5
21	New Jersey	25.6
47	New Mexico	21.1
22	New York	25.3
11	North Carolina	28.6
31	North Dakota	24.0
19	Ohio	26.3
12	Oklahoma	28.0
31	Oregon	24.0
18	Pennsylvania	26.5
9	Rhode Island	28.9
10	South Carolina	28.8
25	South Dakota	24.8
5	Tennessee	30.3
26	Texas	24.6
50	Utah	18.8
40	Vermont	23.1
27	Virginia	24.4
33	Washington	23.8
1	West Virginia	33.6
28	Wisconsin	24.3
33	Wyoming	23.8

RANK ORDER

RANK	STATE	PERCENT
1	West Virginia	33.6
2	Mississippi	33.4
3	Alabama	33.1
4	Arkansas	30.5
5	Tennessee	30.3
6	Kentucky	29.8
7	Florida	29.3
8	Louisiana	29.0
9	Rhode Island	28.9
10	South Carolina	28.8
11	North Carolina	28.6
12	Georgia	28.0
12	Oklahoma	28.0
14	Delaware	27.7
15	Missouri	27.5
16	Indiana	27.0
17	Michigan	26.8
18	Pennsylvania	26.5
19	Ohio	26.3
20	Maine	26.0
21	New Jersey	25.6
22	New York	25.3
23	Iowa	25.1
24	Maryland	25.0
25	South Dakota	24.8
26	Texas	24.6
27	Virginia	24.4
28	Wisconsin	24.3
29	Connecticut	24.2
30	Illinois	24.1
31	North Dakota	24.0
31	Oregon	24.0
33	Washington	23.8
33	Wyoming	23.8
35	Nevada	23.6
36	Nebraska	23.5
37	California	23.4
38	Kansas	23.3
39	Hawaii	23.2
40	Idaho	23.1
40	Massachusetts	23.1
40	Vermont	23.1
43	Arizona	22.7
44	New Hampshire	22.5
45	Minnesota	22.2
46	Montana	21.3
47	New Mexico	21.1
48	Alaska	20.8
49	Colorado	19.8
50	Utah	18.8
	District of Columbia	25.2

Source: U.S. Department of Health and Human Services, Centers for Disease Control and Prevention
"2003 Behavioral Risk Factor Surveillance Summary Prevalence Data" (http://apps.nccd.cdc.gov/brfss/)
*Persons 18 and older who have been told by a doctor, nurse or other health professional that they have high blood pressure.

Percent of Adults with High Cholesterol: 2003

National Median = 33.1% of Adults*

ALPHA ORDER

RANK	STATE	PERCENT
4	Alabama	36.0
48	Alaska	27.6
13	Arizona	34.6
11	Arkansas	34.8
31	California	32.7
35	Colorado	31.9
40	Connecticut	30.8
12	Delaware	34.7
7	Florida	35.1
26	Georgia	33.2
50	Hawaii	27.0
38	Idaho	31.1
20	Illinois	33.6
7	Indiana	35.1
36	Iowa	31.7
46	Kansas	29.4
5	Kentucky	35.5
40	Louisiana	30.8
20	Maine	33.6
17	Maryland	33.9
33	Massachusetts	32.4
1	Michigan	38.2
40	Minnesota	30.8
27	Mississippi	33.1
20	Missouri	33.6
45	Montana	29.8
43	Nebraska	30.5
3	Nevada	36.8
23	New Hampshire	33.4
19	New Jersey	33.8
49	New Mexico	27.2
9	New York	34.9
16	North Carolina	34.0
32	North Dakota	32.6
17	Ohio	33.9
34	Oklahoma	32.0
15	Oregon	34.1
6	Pennsylvania	35.2
27	Rhode Island	33.1
23	South Carolina	33.4
37	South Dakota	31.2
44	Tennessee	30.1
14	Texas	34.3
47	Utah	27.8
39	Vermont	30.9
29	Virginia	32.9
25	Washington	33.3
2	West Virginia	38.1
30	Wisconsin	32.8
9	Wyoming	34.9

RANK ORDER

RANK	STATE	PERCENT
1	Michigan	38.2
2	West Virginia	38.1
3	Nevada	36.8
4	Alabama	36.0
5	Kentucky	35.5
6	Pennsylvania	35.2
7	Florida	35.1
7	Indiana	35.1
9	New York	34.9
9	Wyoming	34.9
11	Arkansas	34.8
12	Delaware	34.7
13	Arizona	34.6
14	Texas	34.3
15	Oregon	34.1
16	North Carolina	34.0
17	Maryland	33.9
17	Ohio	33.9
19	New Jersey	33.8
20	Illinois	33.6
20	Maine	33.6
20	Missouri	33.6
23	New Hampshire	33.4
23	South Carolina	33.4
25	Washington	33.3
26	Georgia	33.2
27	Mississippi	33.1
27	Rhode Island	33.1
29	Virginia	32.9
30	Wisconsin	32.8
31	California	32.7
32	North Dakota	32.6
33	Massachusetts	32.4
34	Oklahoma	32.0
35	Colorado	31.9
36	Iowa	31.7
37	South Dakota	31.2
38	Idaho	31.1
39	Vermont	30.9
40	Connecticut	30.8
40	Louisiana	30.8
40	Minnesota	30.8
43	Nebraska	30.5
44	Tennessee	30.1
45	Montana	29.8
46	Kansas	29.4
47	Utah	27.8
48	Alaska	27.6
49	New Mexico	27.2
50	Hawaii	27.0

District of Columbia	29.2

Source: U.S. Department of Health and Human Services, Centers for Disease Control and Prevention
   "2003 Behavioral Risk Factor Surveillance Summary Prevalence Data" (http://apps.nccd.cdc.gov/brfss/)
Persons 18 and older who have had their cholesterol checked and have been told that they have high blood cholesterol.

Percent of Adults Who Have Visited a Dentist or Dental Clinic: 2002

National Median = 69.2%*

ALPHA ORDER

RANK	STATE	PERCENT
31	Alabama	67.8
40	Alaska	65.5
29	Arizona	68.2
46	Arkansas	60.9
28	California	68.4
36	Colorado	67.3
1	Connecticut	80.2
11	Delaware	74.5
27	Florida	69.0
41	Georgia	65.3
43	Hawaii	65.2
35	Idaho	67.5
13	Illinois	73.7
33	Indiana	67.6
8	Iowa	75.3
17	Kansas	72.7
36	Kentucky	67.3
38	Louisiana	66.6
21	Maine	71.0
9	Maryland	74.9
4	Massachusetts	77.3
7	Michigan	75.9
6	Minnesota	76.0
48	Mississippi	60.1
44	Missouri	64.7
39	Montana	66.4
14	Nebraska	73.3
45	Nevada	62.6
5	New Hampshire	76.8
12	New Jersey	74.3
41	New Mexico	65.3
18	New York	71.7
33	North Carolina	67.6
25	North Dakota	69.2
16	Ohio	73.1
47	Oklahoma	60.5
30	Oregon	68.0
20	Pennsylvania	71.4
3	Rhode Island	77.5
25	South Carolina	69.2
19	South Dakota	71.5
23	Tennessee	70.1
50	Texas	60.0
15	Utah	73.2
10	Vermont	74.6
24	Virginia	69.6
22	Washington	70.4
48	West Virginia	60.1
2	Wisconsin	77.7
31	Wyoming	67.8

RANK ORDER

RANK	STATE	PERCENT
1	Connecticut	80.2
2	Wisconsin	77.7
3	Rhode Island	77.5
4	Massachusetts	77.3
5	New Hampshire	76.8
6	Minnesota	76.0
7	Michigan	75.9
8	Iowa	75.3
9	Maryland	74.9
10	Vermont	74.6
11	Delaware	74.5
12	New Jersey	74.3
13	Illinois	73.7
14	Nebraska	73.3
15	Utah	73.2
16	Ohio	73.1
17	Kansas	72.7
18	New York	71.7
19	South Dakota	71.5
20	Pennsylvania	71.4
21	Maine	71.0
22	Washington	70.4
23	Tennessee	70.1
24	Virginia	69.6
25	North Dakota	69.2
25	South Carolina	69.2
27	Florida	69.0
28	California	68.4
29	Arizona	68.2
30	Oregon	68.0
31	Alabama	67.8
31	Wyoming	67.8
33	Indiana	67.6
33	North Carolina	67.6
35	Idaho	67.5
36	Colorado	67.3
36	Kentucky	67.3
38	Louisiana	66.6
39	Montana	66.4
40	Alaska	65.5
41	Georgia	65.3
41	New Mexico	65.3
43	Hawaii	65.2
44	Missouri	64.7
45	Nevada	62.6
46	Arkansas	60.9
47	Oklahoma	60.5
48	Mississippi	60.1
48	West Virginia	60.1
50	Texas	60.0

| | District of Columbia | 73.7 |

Source: U.S. Department of Health and Human Services, Centers for Disease Control and Prevention
"2002 Behavioral Risk Factor Surveillance Summary Prevalence Data" (http://apps.nccd.cdc.gov/brfss/)
*Persons 18 and older who have visited a dentist within the past year for any reason.

Percent of Adults Who Have Lost 6 or More Teeth Due to Decay: 2002

National Median = 17.6%*

ALPHA ORDER

RANK	STATE	PERCENT
6	Alabama	24.8
42	Alaska	15.3
37	Arizona	15.8
5	Arkansas	24.9
49	California	11.2
48	Colorado	11.4
43	Connecticut	14.9
17	Delaware	19.2
16	Florida	19.5
15	Georgia	20.3
46	Hawaii	12.9
39	Idaho	15.4
35	Illinois	16.5
14	Indiana	20.5
25	Iowa	17.6
38	Kansas	15.7
3	Kentucky	26.6
13	Louisiana	20.8
7	Maine	24.3
39	Maryland	15.4
24	Massachusetts	17.7
28	Michigan	17.3
47	Minnesota	12.1
2	Mississippi	26.9
9	Missouri	21.8
27	Montana	17.4
32	Nebraska	16.8
32	Nevada	16.8
28	New Hampshire	17.3
25	New Jersey	17.6
39	New Mexico	15.4
20	New York	18.3
10	North Carolina	21.7
20	North Dakota	18.3
18	Ohio	18.8
8	Oklahoma	22.2
34	Oregon	16.7
10	Pennsylvania	21.7
30	Rhode Island	17.0
12	South Carolina	21.3
19	South Dakota	18.7
4	Tennessee	25.6
44	Texas	14.2
50	Utah	10.4
22	Vermont	18.1
36	Virginia	16.4
45	Washington	13.8
1	West Virginia	33.8
23	Wisconsin	17.9
30	Wyoming	17.0

RANK ORDER

RANK	STATE	PERCENT
1	West Virginia	33.8
2	Mississippi	26.9
3	Kentucky	26.6
4	Tennessee	25.6
5	Arkansas	24.9
6	Alabama	24.8
7	Maine	24.3
8	Oklahoma	22.2
9	Missouri	21.8
10	North Carolina	21.7
10	Pennsylvania	21.7
12	South Carolina	21.3
13	Louisiana	20.8
14	Indiana	20.5
15	Georgia	20.3
16	Florida	19.5
17	Delaware	19.2
18	Ohio	18.8
19	South Dakota	18.7
20	New York	18.3
20	North Dakota	18.3
22	Vermont	18.1
23	Wisconsin	17.9
24	Massachusetts	17.7
25	Iowa	17.6
25	New Jersey	17.6
27	Montana	17.4
28	Michigan	17.3
28	New Hampshire	17.3
30	Rhode Island	17.0
30	Wyoming	17.0
32	Nebraska	16.8
32	Nevada	16.8
34	Oregon	16.7
35	Illinois	16.5
36	Virginia	16.4
37	Arizona	15.8
38	Kansas	15.7
39	Idaho	15.4
39	Maryland	15.4
39	New Mexico	15.4
42	Alaska	15.3
43	Connecticut	14.9
44	Texas	14.2
45	Washington	13.8
46	Hawaii	12.9
47	Minnesota	12.1
48	Colorado	11.4
49	California	11.2
50	Utah	10.4
	District of Columbia	15.6

Source: U.S. Department of Health and Human Services, Centers for Disease Control and Prevention
   "2002 Behavioral Risk Factor Surveillance Summary Prevalence Data" (http://apps.nccd.cdc.gov/brfss/)
Persons 18 and older who have lost six or more teeth in their life due to decay or gum disease.

Percent of Adults 65 Years Old and Older
Who Have Lost All Their Natural Teeth: 2002
National Median = 22.8%*

ALPHA ORDER

RANK	STATE	PERCENT
11	Alabama	29.9
13	Alaska	26.3
37	Arizona	20.4
10	Arkansas	30.1
49	California	13.3
41	Colorado	19.2
46	Connecticut	16.0
14	Delaware	25.8
31	Florida	21.3
8	Georgia	32.6
50	Hawaii	13.1
27	Idaho	22.5
22	Illinois	24.0
19	Indiana	24.7
31	Iowa	21.3
26	Kansas	22.8
1	Kentucky	42.3
5	Louisiana	33.8
9	Maine	30.4
40	Maryland	19.3
25	Massachusetts	22.9
43	Michigan	18.8
47	Minnesota	14.8
4	Mississippi	35.1
12	Missouri	26.4
34	Montana	20.9
17	Nebraska	25.5
36	Nevada	20.5
29	New Hampshire	21.8
39	New Jersey	20.1
18	New Mexico	25.2
44	New York	18.7
6	North Carolina	33.3
24	North Dakota	23.2
23	Ohio	23.6
7	Oklahoma	33.2
42	Oregon	18.9
14	Pennsylvania	25.8
27	Rhode Island	22.5
21	South Carolina	24.4
19	South Dakota	24.7
3	Tennessee	36.0
37	Texas	20.4
48	Utah	14.7
30	Vermont	21.7
31	Virginia	21.3
45	Washington	16.8
2	West Virginia	41.9
35	Wisconsin	20.6
16	Wyoming	25.7

RANK ORDER

RANK	STATE	PERCENT
1	Kentucky	42.3
2	West Virginia	41.9
3	Tennessee	36.0
4	Mississippi	35.1
5	Louisiana	33.8
6	North Carolina	33.3
7	Oklahoma	33.2
8	Georgia	32.6
9	Maine	30.4
10	Arkansas	30.1
11	Alabama	29.9
12	Missouri	26.4
13	Alaska	26.3
14	Delaware	25.8
14	Pennsylvania	25.8
16	Wyoming	25.7
17	Nebraska	25.5
18	New Mexico	25.2
19	Indiana	24.7
19	South Dakota	24.7
21	South Carolina	24.4
22	Illinois	24.0
23	Ohio	23.6
24	North Dakota	23.2
25	Massachusetts	22.9
26	Kansas	22.8
27	Idaho	22.5
27	Rhode Island	22.5
29	New Hampshire	21.8
30	Vermont	21.7
31	Florida	21.3
31	Iowa	21.3
31	Virginia	21.3
34	Montana	20.9
35	Wisconsin	20.6
36	Nevada	20.5
37	Arizona	20.4
37	Texas	20.4
39	New Jersey	20.1
40	Maryland	19.3
41	Colorado	19.2
42	Oregon	18.9
43	Michigan	18.8
44	New York	18.7
45	Washington	16.8
46	Connecticut	16.0
47	Minnesota	14.8
48	Utah	14.7
49	California	13.3
50	Hawaii	13.1

District of Columbia 16.7

Source: U.S. Department of Health and Human Services, Centers for Disease Control and Prevention
"2002 Behavioral Risk Factor Surveillance Summary Prevalence Data" (http://apps.nccd.cdc.gov/brfss/)
*Age-adjusted percent of persons aged 65 years or more.

Percent of Adults Who Average Five or More Servings of Fruits and Vegetables Each Day: 2003
National Median = 22.6%*

ALPHA ORDER

RANK	STATE	PERCENT
24	Alabama	22.6
24	Alaska	22.6
22	Arizona	22.9
36	Arkansas	20.8
9	California	26.9
14	Colorado	24.2
2	Connecticut	29.8
31	Delaware	22.0
17	Florida	23.6
21	Georgia	23.0
6	Hawaii	27.6
37	Idaho	20.4
19	Illinois	23.1
31	Indiana	22.0
48	Iowa	17.1
43	Kansas	18.8
45	Kentucky	18.2
49	Louisiana	16.4
8	Maine	27.0
4	Maryland	28.9
3	Massachusetts	29.0
40	Michigan	20.1
14	Minnesota	24.2
46	Mississippi	17.9
39	Missouri	20.2
33	Montana	21.9
47	Nebraska	17.8
37	Nevada	20.4
5	New Hampshire	28.5
10	New Jersey	26.6
27	New Mexico	22.4
11	New York	25.8
19	North Carolina	23.1
34	North Dakota	21.5
23	Ohio	22.7
50	Oklahoma	15.4
16	Oregon	24.1
13	Pennsylvania	24.7
7	Rhode Island	27.1
28	South Carolina	22.3
42	South Dakota	19.0
29	Tennessee	22.2
26	Texas	22.5
41	Utah	19.5
1	Vermont	32.5
11	Virginia	25.8
18	Washington	23.3
44	West Virginia	18.7
34	Wisconsin	21.5
30	Wyoming	22.1

RANK ORDER

RANK	STATE	PERCENT
1	Vermont	32.5
2	Connecticut	29.8
3	Massachusetts	29.0
4	Maryland	28.9
5	New Hampshire	28.5
6	Hawaii	27.6
7	Rhode Island	27.1
8	Maine	27.0
9	California	26.9
10	New Jersey	26.6
11	New York	25.8
11	Virginia	25.8
13	Pennsylvania	24.7
14	Colorado	24.2
14	Minnesota	24.2
16	Oregon	24.1
17	Florida	23.6
18	Washington	23.3
19	Illinois	23.1
19	North Carolina	23.1
21	Georgia	23.0
22	Arizona	22.9
23	Ohio	22.7
24	Alabama	22.6
24	Alaska	22.6
26	Texas	22.5
27	New Mexico	22.4
28	South Carolina	22.3
29	Tennessee	22.2
30	Wyoming	22.1
31	Delaware	22.0
31	Indiana	22.0
33	Montana	21.9
34	North Dakota	21.5
34	Wisconsin	21.5
36	Arkansas	20.8
37	Idaho	20.4
37	Nevada	20.4
39	Missouri	20.2
40	Michigan	20.1
41	Utah	19.5
42	South Dakota	19.0
43	Kansas	18.8
44	West Virginia	18.7
45	Kentucky	18.2
46	Mississippi	17.9
47	Nebraska	17.8
48	Iowa	17.1
49	Louisiana	16.4
50	Oklahoma	15.4
	District of Columbia	29.6

Source: U.S. Department of Health and Human Services, Centers for Disease Control and Prevention
"2003 Behavioral Risk Factor Surveillance Summary Prevalence Data" (http://apps.nccd.cdc.gov/brfss/)
*Persons 18 and older.

Number of Days in Past Month When Physical Health was "Not Good": 2001

National Average = 3.5 Days*

ALPHA ORDER

RANK	STATE	DAYS
3	Alabama	4.2
18	Alaska	3.5
7	Arizona	3.9
2	Arkansas	4.5
18	California	3.5
27	Colorado	3.3
36	Connecticut	3.2
22	Delaware	3.4
18	Florida	3.5
27	Georgia	3.3
50	Hawaii	2.1
27	Idaho	3.3
43	Illinois	3.0
18	Indiana	3.5
43	Iowa	3.0
45	Kansas	2.9
6	Kentucky	4.0
36	Louisiana	3.2
10	Maine	3.7
40	Maryland	3.1
22	Massachusetts	3.4
10	Michigan	3.7
40	Minnesota	3.1
3	Mississippi	4.2
15	Missouri	3.6
22	Montana	3.4
48	Nebraska	2.8
15	Nevada	3.6
45	New Hampshire	2.9
27	New Jersey	3.3
10	New Mexico	3.7
10	New York	3.7
15	North Carolina	3.6
49	North Dakota	2.7
27	Ohio	3.3
5	Oklahoma	4.1
10	Oregon	3.7
22	Pennsylvania	3.4
8	Rhode Island	3.8
8	South Carolina	3.8
45	South Dakota	2.9
27	Tennessee	3.3
36	Texas	3.2
27	Utah	3.3
27	Vermont	3.3
27	Virginia	3.3
22	Washington	3.4
1	West Virginia	5.3
36	Wisconsin	3.2
40	Wyoming	3.1

RANK ORDER

RANK	STATE	DAYS
1	West Virginia	5.3
2	Arkansas	4.5
3	Alabama	4.2
3	Mississippi	4.2
5	Oklahoma	4.1
6	Kentucky	4.0
7	Arizona	3.9
8	Rhode Island	3.8
8	South Carolina	3.8
10	Maine	3.7
10	Michigan	3.7
10	New Mexico	3.7
10	New York	3.7
10	Oregon	3.7
15	Missouri	3.6
15	Nevada	3.6
15	North Carolina	3.6
18	Alaska	3.5
18	California	3.5
18	Florida	3.5
18	Indiana	3.5
22	Delaware	3.4
22	Massachusetts	3.4
22	Montana	3.4
22	Pennsylvania	3.4
22	Washington	3.4
27	Colorado	3.3
27	Georgia	3.3
27	Idaho	3.3
27	New Jersey	3.3
27	Ohio	3.3
27	Tennessee	3.3
27	Utah	3.3
27	Vermont	3.3
27	Virginia	3.3
36	Connecticut	3.2
36	Louisiana	3.2
36	Texas	3.2
36	Wisconsin	3.2
40	Maryland	3.1
40	Minnesota	3.1
40	Wyoming	3.1
43	Illinois	3.0
43	Iowa	3.0
45	Kansas	2.9
45	New Hampshire	2.9
45	South Dakota	2.9
48	Nebraska	2.8
49	North Dakota	2.7
50	Hawaii	2.1
	District of Columbia**	NA

Source: U.S. Department of Health and Human Services, Centers for Disease Control and Prevention
    "2001 Behavioral Risk Factor Surveillance Summary Prevalence Report" (August 9, 2002)
*Persons 18 and older.
**Not available.

Number of Days in Past Month When Mental Health was "Not Good": 2001

National Average = 3.4 Days*

ALPHA ORDER

RANK	STATE	DAYS
3	Alabama	4.3
29	Alaska	3.2
17	Arizona	3.4
4	Arkansas	3.8
14	California	3.5
8	Colorado	3.6
29	Connecticut	3.2
29	Delaware	3.2
34	Florida	3.1
5	Georgia	3.7
50	Hawaii	1.5
14	Idaho	3.5
41	Illinois	2.9
8	Indiana	3.6
44	Iowa	2.7
41	Kansas	2.9
1	Kentucky	4.7
41	Louisiana	2.9
26	Maine	3.3
29	Maryland	3.2
17	Massachusetts	3.4
5	Michigan	3.7
34	Minnesota	3.1
34	Mississippi	3.1
17	Missouri	3.4
48	Montana	2.5
44	Nebraska	2.7
5	Nevada	3.7
40	New Hampshire	3.0
17	New Jersey	3.4
17	New Mexico	3.4
14	New York	3.5
44	North Carolina	2.7
47	North Dakota	2.6
26	Ohio	3.3
17	Oklahoma	3.4
17	Oregon	3.4
8	Pennsylvania	3.6
8	Rhode Island	3.6
17	South Carolina	3.4
48	South Dakota	2.5
34	Tennessee	3.1
17	Texas	3.4
8	Utah	3.6
34	Vermont	3.1
8	Virginia	3.6
26	Washington	3.3
2	West Virginia	4.4
29	Wisconsin	3.2
34	Wyoming	3.1

RANK ORDER

RANK	STATE	DAYS
1	Kentucky	4.7
2	West Virginia	4.4
3	Alabama	4.3
4	Arkansas	3.8
5	Georgia	3.7
5	Michigan	3.7
5	Nevada	3.7
8	Colorado	3.6
8	Indiana	3.6
8	Pennsylvania	3.6
8	Rhode Island	3.6
8	Utah	3.6
8	Virginia	3.6
14	California	3.5
14	Idaho	3.5
14	New York	3.5
17	Arizona	3.4
17	Massachusetts	3.4
17	Missouri	3.4
17	New Jersey	3.4
17	New Mexico	3.4
17	Oklahoma	3.4
17	Oregon	3.4
17	South Carolina	3.4
17	Texas	3.4
26	Maine	3.3
26	Ohio	3.3
26	Washington	3.3
29	Alaska	3.2
29	Connecticut	3.2
29	Delaware	3.2
29	Maryland	3.2
29	Wisconsin	3.2
34	Florida	3.1
34	Minnesota	3.1
34	Mississippi	3.1
34	Tennessee	3.1
34	Vermont	3.1
34	Wyoming	3.1
40	New Hampshire	3.0
41	Illinois	2.9
41	Kansas	2.9
41	Louisiana	2.9
44	Iowa	2.7
44	Nebraska	2.7
44	North Carolina	2.7
47	North Dakota	2.6
48	Montana	2.5
48	South Dakota	2.5
50	Hawaii	1.5
	District of Columbia**	NA

Source: U.S. Department of Health and Human Services, Centers for Disease Control and Prevention
   "2001 Behavioral Risk Factor Surveillance Summary Prevalence Report" (August 9, 2002)
*Persons 18 and older.
**Not available.

Percent of Adults Rating Their Health as Fair or Poor in 2003

National Median = 15.0% of Adults*

ALPHA ORDER

RANK	STATE	PERCENT
4	Alabama	20.3
45	Alaska	11.8
20	Arizona	15.6
6	Arkansas	19.7
23	California	15.1
43	Colorado	12.0
37	Connecticut	12.6
27	Delaware	14.2
8	Florida	18.1
18	Georgia	16.3
41	Hawaii	12.2
31	Idaho	13.6
24	Illinois	15.0
16	Indiana	16.7
46	Iowa	11.7
32	Kansas	13.3
3	Kentucky	22.8
13	Louisiana	17.3
26	Maine	14.7
41	Maryland	12.2
38	Massachusetts	12.4
21	Michigan	15.2
48	Minnesota	11.2
2	Mississippi	23.1
12	Missouri	17.4
39	Montana	12.3
36	Nebraska	12.8
11	Nevada	17.5
49	New Hampshire	10.8
21	New Jersey	15.2
15	New Mexico	16.9
14	New York	17.2
7	North Carolina	18.9
33	North Dakota	13.2
27	Ohio	14.2
10	Oklahoma	17.8
19	Oregon	16.2
24	Pennsylvania	15.0
27	Rhode Island	14.2
16	South Carolina	16.7
34	South Dakota	13.0
8	Tennessee	18.1
5	Texas	20.2
47	Utah	11.3
50	Vermont	10.7
35	Virginia	12.9
30	Washington	13.8
1	West Virginia	25.3
43	Wisconsin	12.0
39	Wyoming	12.3

RANK ORDER

RANK	STATE	PERCENT
1	West Virginia	25.3
2	Mississippi	23.1
3	Kentucky	22.8
4	Alabama	20.3
5	Texas	20.2
6	Arkansas	19.7
7	North Carolina	18.9
8	Florida	18.1
8	Tennessee	18.1
10	Oklahoma	17.8
11	Nevada	17.5
12	Missouri	17.4
13	Louisiana	17.3
14	New York	17.2
15	New Mexico	16.9
16	Indiana	16.7
16	South Carolina	16.7
18	Georgia	16.3
19	Oregon	16.2
20	Arizona	15.6
21	Michigan	15.2
21	New Jersey	15.2
23	California	15.1
24	Illinois	15.0
24	Pennsylvania	15.0
26	Maine	14.7
27	Delaware	14.2
27	Ohio	14.2
27	Rhode Island	14.2
30	Washington	13.8
31	Idaho	13.6
32	Kansas	13.3
33	North Dakota	13.2
34	South Dakota	13.0
35	Virginia	12.9
36	Nebraska	12.8
37	Connecticut	12.6
38	Massachusetts	12.4
39	Montana	12.3
39	Wyoming	12.3
41	Hawaii	12.2
41	Maryland	12.2
43	Colorado	12.0
43	Wisconsin	12.0
45	Alaska	11.8
46	Iowa	11.7
47	Utah	11.3
48	Minnesota	11.2
49	New Hampshire	10.8
50	Vermont	10.7

District of Columbia	12.4

Source: U.S. Department of Health and Human Services, Centers for Disease Control and Prevention
    "2003 Behavioral Risk Factor Surveillance Summary Prevalence Data" (http://apps.nccd.cdc.gov/brfss/)
*Persons 18 and older.

Safety Belt Usage Rate in 2004

National Rate = 80.0% Use Safety Belts*

ALPHA ORDER

RANK	STATE	PERCENT
25	Alabama	80.0
30	Alaska	76.7
1	Arizona	95.3
47	Arkansas	64.2
6	California	90.4
28	Colorado	79.3
18	Connecticut	82.9
19	Delaware	82.3
31	Florida	76.3
9	Georgia	86.7
2	Hawaii	95.1
37	Idaho	74.0
17	Illinois	83.0
15	Indiana	83.4
11	Iowa	86.4
43	Kansas	68.3
45	Kentucky	66.0
35	Louisiana	75.0
39	Maine	72.3
8	Maryland	89.0
48	Massachusetts	63.3
5	Michigan	90.5
20	Minnesota	82.1
49	Mississippi	63.2
33	Missouri	75.9
23	Montana	80.9
29	Nebraska	79.2
10	Nevada	86.6
NA	New Hampshire**	NA
21	New Jersey	82.0
7	New Mexico	89.7
14	New York	85.0
12	North Carolina	86.1
44	North Dakota	67.4
36	Ohio	74.1
24	Oklahoma	80.3
4	Oregon	92.6
22	Pennsylvania	81.8
32	Rhode Island	76.2
46	South Carolina	65.7
42	South Dakota	69.4
40	Tennessee	72.0
16	Texas	83.2
13	Utah	85.7
26	Vermont	79.9
26	Virginia	79.9
3	Washington	94.2
34	West Virginia	75.8
38	Wisconsin	72.4
41	Wyoming	70.1

RANK ORDER

RANK	STATE	PERCENT
1	Arizona	95.3
2	Hawaii	95.1
3	Washington	94.2
4	Oregon	92.6
5	Michigan	90.5
6	California	90.4
7	New Mexico	89.7
8	Maryland	89.0
9	Georgia	86.7
10	Nevada	86.6
11	Iowa	86.4
12	North Carolina	86.1
13	Utah	85.7
14	New York	85.0
15	Indiana	83.4
16	Texas	83.2
17	Illinois	83.0
18	Connecticut	82.9
19	Delaware	82.3
20	Minnesota	82.1
21	New Jersey	82.0
22	Pennsylvania	81.8
23	Montana	80.9
24	Oklahoma	80.3
25	Alabama	80.0
26	Vermont	79.9
26	Virginia	79.9
28	Colorado	79.3
29	Nebraska	79.2
30	Alaska	76.7
31	Florida	76.3
32	Rhode Island	76.2
33	Missouri	75.9
34	West Virginia	75.8
35	Louisiana	75.0
36	Ohio	74.1
37	Idaho	74.0
38	Wisconsin	72.4
39	Maine	72.3
40	Tennessee	72.0
41	Wyoming	70.1
42	South Dakota	69.4
43	Kansas	68.3
44	North Dakota	67.4
45	Kentucky	66.0
46	South Carolina	65.7
47	Arkansas	64.2
48	Massachusetts	63.3
49	Mississippi	63.2
NA	New Hampshire**	NA

District of Columbia   87.1

Source: U.S. Department of Transportation, National Highway Traffic Safety Administration
   "Safety Belt Use in 2004" (http://www.nhtsa.dot.gov/people/injury/SafetyBelt/SafetyBeltUse_2004/index.html)
*National estimate is from the National Occupant Protection Use Survey (NOPUS) using a different methodology.
**Not available.

VIII. APPENDIX

Population Charts

Population in 2004

National Total = 293,655,404*

ALPHA ORDER

RANK	STATE	POPULATION	% of USA
23	Alabama	4,530,182	1.5%
47	Alaska	655,435	0.2%
18	Arizona	5,743,834	2.0%
32	Arkansas	2,752,629	0.9%
1	California	35,893,799	12.2%
22	Colorado	4,601,403	1.6%
29	Connecticut	3,503,604	1.2%
45	Delaware	830,364	0.3%
4	Florida	17,397,161	5.9%
9	Georgia	8,829,383	3.0%
42	Hawaii	1,262,840	0.4%
39	Idaho	1,393,262	0.5%
5	Illinois	12,713,634	4.3%
14	Indiana	6,237,569	2.1%
30	Iowa	2,954,451	1.0%
33	Kansas	2,735,502	0.9%
26	Kentucky	4,145,922	1.4%
24	Louisiana	4,515,770	1.5%
40	Maine	1,317,253	0.4%
19	Maryland	5,558,058	1.9%
13	Massachusetts	6,416,505	2.2%
8	Michigan	10,112,620	3.4%
21	Minnesota	5,100,958	1.7%
31	Mississippi	2,902,966	1.0%
17	Missouri	5,754,618	2.0%
44	Montana	926,865	0.3%
38	Nebraska	1,747,214	0.6%
35	Nevada	2,334,771	0.8%
41	New Hampshire	1,299,500	0.4%
10	New Jersey	8,698,879	3.0%
36	New Mexico	1,903,289	0.6%
3	New York	19,227,088	6.5%
11	North Carolina	8,541,221	2.9%
48	North Dakota	634,366	0.2%
7	Ohio	11,459,011	3.9%
28	Oklahoma	3,523,553	1.2%
27	Oregon	3,594,586	1.2%
6	Pennsylvania	12,406,292	4.2%
43	Rhode Island	1,080,632	0.4%
25	South Carolina	4,198,068	1.4%
46	South Dakota	770,883	0.3%
16	Tennessee	5,900,962	2.0%
2	Texas	22,490,022	7.7%
34	Utah	2,389,039	0.8%
49	Vermont	621,394	0.2%
12	Virginia	7,459,827	2.5%
15	Washington	6,203,788	2.1%
37	West Virginia	1,815,354	0.6%
20	Wisconsin	5,509,026	1.9%
50	Wyoming	506,529	0.2%

RANK ORDER

RANK	STATE	POPULATION	% of USA
1	California	35,893,799	12.2%
2	Texas	22,490,022	7.7%
3	New York	19,227,088	6.5%
4	Florida	17,397,161	5.9%
5	Illinois	12,713,634	4.3%
6	Pennsylvania	12,406,292	4.2%
7	Ohio	11,459,011	3.9%
8	Michigan	10,112,620	3.4%
9	Georgia	8,829,383	3.0%
10	New Jersey	8,698,879	3.0%
11	North Carolina	8,541,221	2.9%
12	Virginia	7,459,827	2.5%
13	Massachusetts	6,416,505	2.2%
14	Indiana	6,237,569	2.1%
15	Washington	6,203,788	2.1%
16	Tennessee	5,900,962	2.0%
17	Missouri	5,754,618	2.0%
18	Arizona	5,743,834	2.0%
19	Maryland	5,558,058	1.9%
20	Wisconsin	5,509,026	1.9%
21	Minnesota	5,100,958	1.7%
22	Colorado	4,601,403	1.6%
23	Alabama	4,530,182	1.5%
24	Louisiana	4,515,770	1.5%
25	South Carolina	4,198,068	1.4%
26	Kentucky	4,145,922	1.4%
27	Oregon	3,594,586	1.2%
28	Oklahoma	3,523,553	1.2%
29	Connecticut	3,503,604	1.2%
30	Iowa	2,954,451	1.0%
31	Mississippi	2,902,966	1.0%
32	Arkansas	2,752,629	0.9%
33	Kansas	2,735,502	0.9%
34	Utah	2,389,039	0.8%
35	Nevada	2,334,771	0.8%
36	New Mexico	1,903,289	0.6%
37	West Virginia	1,815,354	0.6%
38	Nebraska	1,747,214	0.6%
39	Idaho	1,393,262	0.5%
40	Maine	1,317,253	0.4%
41	New Hampshire	1,299,500	0.4%
42	Hawaii	1,262,840	0.4%
43	Rhode Island	1,080,632	0.4%
44	Montana	926,865	0.3%
45	Delaware	830,364	0.3%
46	South Dakota	770,883	0.3%
47	Alaska	655,435	0.2%
48	North Dakota	634,366	0.2%
49	Vermont	621,394	0.2%
50	Wyoming	506,529	0.2%
	District of Columbia	553,523	0.2%

Source: U.S. Bureau of the Census
   "Population Estimates" (January 7, 2005, http://www.census.gov/popest/estimates.php)
*Resident population.

Population in 2003

National Total = 290,788,976*

ALPHA ORDER

RANK	STATE	POPULATION	% of USA
23	Alabama	4,503,726	1.5%
47	Alaska	648,280	0.2%
18	Arizona	5,579,222	1.9%
32	Arkansas	2,727,774	0.9%
1	California	35,462,712	12.2%
22	Colorado	4,547,633	1.6%
29	Connecticut	3,486,960	1.2%
45	Delaware	818,166	0.3%
4	Florida	16,999,181	5.8%
9	Georgia	8,676,460	3.0%
42	Hawaii	1,248,755	0.4%
39	Idaho	1,367,034	0.5%
5	Illinois	12,649,087	4.3%
14	Indiana	6,199,571	2.1%
30	Iowa	2,941,976	1.0%
33	Kansas	2,724,786	0.9%
26	Kentucky	4,118,189	1.4%
24	Louisiana	4,493,665	1.5%
40	Maine	1,309,205	0.5%
19	Maryland	5,512,310	1.9%
13	Massachusetts	6,420,357	2.2%
8	Michigan	10,082,364	3.5%
21	Minnesota	5,064,172	1.7%
31	Mississippi	2,882,594	1.0%
17	Missouri	5,719,204	2.0%
44	Montana	918,157	0.3%
38	Nebraska	1,737,475	0.6%
35	Nevada	2,242,207	0.8%
41	New Hampshire	1,288,705	0.4%
10	New Jersey	8,642,412	3.0%
36	New Mexico	1,878,562	0.6%
3	New York	19,212,425	6.6%
11	North Carolina	8,421,190	2.9%
48	North Dakota	633,400	0.2%
7	Ohio	11,437,680	3.9%
28	Oklahoma	3,506,469	1.2%
27	Oregon	3,564,330	1.2%
6	Pennsylvania	12,370,761	4.3%
43	Rhode Island	1,076,084	0.4%
25	South Carolina	4,148,744	1.4%
46	South Dakota	764,905	0.3%
16	Tennessee	5,845,208	2.0%
2	Texas	22,103,374	7.6%
34	Utah	2,352,119	0.8%
49	Vermont	619,343	0.2%
12	Virginia	7,365,284	2.5%
15	Washington	6,131,298	2.1%
37	West Virginia	1,811,440	0.6%
20	Wisconsin	5,474,290	1.9%
50	Wyoming	502,111	0.2%

RANK ORDER

RANK	STATE	POPULATION	% of USA
1	California	35,462,712	12.2%
2	Texas	22,103,374	7.6%
3	New York	19,212,425	6.6%
4	Florida	16,999,181	5.8%
5	Illinois	12,649,087	4.3%
6	Pennsylvania	12,370,761	4.3%
7	Ohio	11,437,680	3.9%
8	Michigan	10,082,364	3.5%
9	Georgia	8,676,460	3.0%
10	New Jersey	8,642,412	3.0%
11	North Carolina	8,421,190	2.9%
12	Virginia	7,365,284	2.5%
13	Massachusetts	6,420,357	2.2%
14	Indiana	6,199,571	2.1%
15	Washington	6,131,298	2.1%
16	Tennessee	5,845,208	2.0%
17	Missouri	5,719,204	2.0%
18	Arizona	5,579,222	1.9%
19	Maryland	5,512,310	1.9%
20	Wisconsin	5,474,290	1.9%
21	Minnesota	5,064,172	1.7%
22	Colorado	4,547,633	1.6%
23	Alabama	4,503,726	1.5%
24	Louisiana	4,493,665	1.5%
25	South Carolina	4,148,744	1.4%
26	Kentucky	4,118,189	1.4%
27	Oregon	3,564,330	1.2%
28	Oklahoma	3,506,469	1.2%
29	Connecticut	3,486,960	1.2%
30	Iowa	2,941,976	1.0%
31	Mississippi	2,882,594	1.0%
32	Arkansas	2,727,774	0.9%
33	Kansas	2,724,786	0.9%
34	Utah	2,352,119	0.8%
35	Nevada	2,242,207	0.8%
36	New Mexico	1,878,562	0.6%
37	West Virginia	1,811,440	0.6%
38	Nebraska	1,737,475	0.6%
39	Idaho	1,367,034	0.5%
40	Maine	1,309,205	0.5%
41	New Hampshire	1,288,705	0.4%
42	Hawaii	1,248,755	0.4%
43	Rhode Island	1,076,084	0.4%
44	Montana	918,157	0.3%
45	Delaware	818,166	0.3%
46	South Dakota	764,905	0.3%
47	Alaska	648,280	0.2%
48	North Dakota	633,400	0.2%
49	Vermont	619,343	0.2%
50	Wyoming	502,111	0.2%
	District of Columbia	557,620	0.2%

Source: U.S. Bureau of the Census
"Population Estimates" (January 7, 2005, http://www.census.gov/popest/estimates.php)
Resident population. Revised estimates.

Male Population in 2003

National Total = 143,037,260 Males

ALPHA ORDER					RANK ORDER			

RANK	STATE	MALES	% of USA
24	Alabama	2,179,164	1.5%
47	Alaska	335,279	0.2%
17	Arizona	2,791,507	2.0%
33	Arkansas	1,333,876	0.9%
1	California	17,711,194	12.4%
22	Colorado	2,295,243	1.6%
29	Connecticut	1,691,205	1.2%
45	Delaware	398,119	0.3%
4	Florida	8,334,694	5.8%
9	Georgia	4,286,680	3.0%
42	Hawaii	630,517	0.4%
39	Idaho	684,815	0.5%
5	Illinois	6,209,639	4.3%
15	Indiana	3,046,727	2.1%
30	Iowa	1,447,808	1.0%
32	Kansas	1,350,243	0.9%
26	Kentucky	2,017,632	1.4%
23	Louisiana	2,182,332	1.5%
40	Maine	636,701	0.4%
20	Maryland	2,665,643	1.9%
13	Massachusetts	3,110,478	2.2%
8	Michigan	4,951,811	3.5%
21	Minnesota	2,509,132	1.8%
31	Mississippi	1,396,216	1.0%
18	Missouri	2,782,464	1.9%
44	Montana	457,537	0.3%
38	Nebraska	859,284	0.6%
35	Nevada	1,141,901	0.8%
41	New Hampshire	634,476	0.4%
10	New Jersey	4,203,612	2.9%
36	New Mexico	922,455	0.6%
3	New York	9,276,425	6.5%
11	North Carolina	4,130,447	2.9%
48	North Dakota	316,745	0.2%
7	Ohio	5,566,215	3.9%
28	Oklahoma	1,731,449	1.2%
27	Oregon	1,768,478	1.2%
6	Pennsylvania	5,988,280	4.2%
43	Rhode Island	518,415	0.4%
25	South Carolina	2,018,593	1.4%
46	South Dakota	379,867	0.3%
16	Tennessee	2,852,395	2.0%
2	Texas	11,009,394	7.7%
34	Utah	1,180,483	0.8%
49	Vermont	304,098	0.2%
12	Virginia	3,631,658	2.5%
14	Washington	3,057,063	2.1%
37	West Virginia	882,889	0.6%
19	Wisconsin	2,707,564	1.9%
50	Wyoming	252,342	0.2%

RANK ORDER

RANK	STATE	MALES	% of USA
1	California	17,711,194	12.4%
2	Texas	11,009,394	7.7%
3	New York	9,276,425	6.5%
4	Florida	8,334,694	5.8%
5	Illinois	6,209,639	4.3%
6	Pennsylvania	5,988,280	4.2%
7	Ohio	5,566,215	3.9%
8	Michigan	4,951,811	3.5%
9	Georgia	4,286,680	3.0%
10	New Jersey	4,203,612	2.9%
11	North Carolina	4,130,447	2.9%
12	Virginia	3,631,658	2.5%
13	Massachusetts	3,110,478	2.2%
14	Washington	3,057,063	2.1%
15	Indiana	3,046,727	2.1%
16	Tennessee	2,852,395	2.0%
17	Arizona	2,791,507	2.0%
18	Missouri	2,782,464	1.9%
19	Wisconsin	2,707,564	1.9%
20	Maryland	2,665,643	1.9%
21	Minnesota	2,509,132	1.8%
22	Colorado	2,295,243	1.6%
23	Louisiana	2,182,332	1.5%
24	Alabama	2,179,164	1.5%
25	South Carolina	2,018,593	1.4%
26	Kentucky	2,017,632	1.4%
27	Oregon	1,768,478	1.2%
28	Oklahoma	1,731,449	1.2%
29	Connecticut	1,691,205	1.2%
30	Iowa	1,447,808	1.0%
31	Mississippi	1,396,216	1.0%
32	Kansas	1,350,243	0.9%
33	Arkansas	1,333,876	0.9%
34	Utah	1,180,483	0.8%
35	Nevada	1,141,901	0.8%
36	New Mexico	922,455	0.6%
37	West Virginia	882,889	0.6%
38	Nebraska	859,284	0.6%
39	Idaho	684,815	0.5%
40	Maine	636,701	0.4%
41	New Hampshire	634,476	0.4%
42	Hawaii	630,517	0.4%
43	Rhode Island	518,415	0.4%
44	Montana	457,537	0.3%
45	Delaware	398,119	0.3%
46	South Dakota	379,867	0.3%
47	Alaska	335,279	0.2%
48	North Dakota	316,745	0.2%
49	Vermont	304,098	0.2%
50	Wyoming	252,342	0.2%
	District of Columbia	266,076	0.2%

Source: Morgan Quitno Press using data from U.S. Bureau of the Census
"SC-EST2003-race6 - State Characteristic Estimates" (September 30, 2004)

Female Population in 2003

National Total = 147,773,459 Females

ALPHA ORDER

RANK	STATE	FEMALES	% of USA
22	Alabama	2,321,588	1.6%
49	Alaska	313,539	0.2%
19	Arizona	2,789,304	1.9%
32	Arkansas	1,391,838	0.9%
1	California	17,773,259	12.0%
24	Colorado	2,255,445	1.5%
27	Connecticut	1,792,167	1.2%
45	Delaware	419,372	0.3%
4	Florida	8,684,374	5.9%
10	Georgia	4,398,035	3.0%
42	Hawaii	627,091	0.4%
39	Idaho	681,517	0.5%
5	Illinois	6,443,905	4.4%
14	Indiana	3,148,916	2.1%
30	Iowa	1,496,254	1.0%
33	Kansas	1,373,264	0.9%
26	Kentucky	2,100,195	1.4%
23	Louisiana	2,314,002	1.6%
40	Maine	669,027	0.5%
18	Maryland	2,843,266	1.9%
13	Massachusetts	3,322,944	2.2%
8	Michigan	5,128,174	3.5%
21	Minnesota	2,550,243	1.7%
31	Mississippi	1,485,065	1.0%
17	Missouri	2,922,020	2.0%
44	Montana	460,084	0.3%
38	Nebraska	880,007	0.6%
35	Nevada	1,099,253	0.7%
41	New Hampshire	653,211	0.4%
9	New Jersey	4,434,784	3.0%
36	New Mexico	952,159	0.6%
3	New York	9,913,690	6.7%
11	North Carolina	4,276,801	2.9%
47	North Dakota	317,092	0.2%
7	Ohio	5,869,583	4.0%
29	Oklahoma	1,780,083	1.2%
28	Oregon	1,791,118	1.2%
6	Pennsylvania	6,377,175	4.3%
43	Rhode Island	557,749	0.4%
25	South Carolina	2,128,559	1.4%
46	South Dakota	384,442	0.3%
16	Tennessee	2,989,353	2.0%
2	Texas	11,109,115	7.5%
34	Utah	1,170,984	0.8%
48	Vermont	315,009	0.2%
12	Virginia	3,754,672	2.5%
15	Washington	3,074,382	2.1%
37	West Virginia	927,465	0.6%
20	Wisconsin	2,764,735	1.9%
50	Wyoming	248,900	0.2%

RANK ORDER

RANK	STATE	FEMALES	% of USA
1	California	17,773,259	12.0%
2	Texas	11,109,115	7.5%
3	New York	9,913,690	6.7%
4	Florida	8,684,374	5.9%
5	Illinois	6,443,905	4.4%
6	Pennsylvania	6,377,175	4.3%
7	Ohio	5,869,583	4.0%
8	Michigan	5,128,174	3.5%
9	New Jersey	4,434,784	3.0%
10	Georgia	4,398,035	3.0%
11	North Carolina	4,276,801	2.9%
12	Virginia	3,754,672	2.5%
13	Massachusetts	3,322,944	2.2%
14	Indiana	3,148,916	2.1%
15	Washington	3,074,382	2.1%
16	Tennessee	2,989,353	2.0%
17	Missouri	2,922,020	2.0%
18	Maryland	2,843,266	1.9%
19	Arizona	2,789,304	1.9%
20	Wisconsin	2,764,735	1.9%
21	Minnesota	2,550,243	1.7%
22	Alabama	2,321,588	1.6%
23	Louisiana	2,314,002	1.6%
24	Colorado	2,255,445	1.5%
25	South Carolina	2,128,559	1.4%
26	Kentucky	2,100,195	1.4%
27	Connecticut	1,792,167	1.2%
28	Oregon	1,791,118	1.2%
29	Oklahoma	1,780,083	1.2%
30	Iowa	1,496,254	1.0%
31	Mississippi	1,485,065	1.0%
32	Arkansas	1,391,838	0.9%
33	Kansas	1,373,264	0.9%
34	Utah	1,170,984	0.8%
35	Nevada	1,099,253	0.7%
36	New Mexico	952,159	0.6%
37	West Virginia	927,465	0.6%
38	Nebraska	880,007	0.6%
39	Idaho	681,517	0.5%
40	Maine	669,027	0.5%
41	New Hampshire	653,211	0.4%
42	Hawaii	627,091	0.4%
43	Rhode Island	557,749	0.4%
44	Montana	460,084	0.3%
45	Delaware	419,372	0.3%
46	South Dakota	384,442	0.3%
47	North Dakota	317,092	0.2%
48	Vermont	315,009	0.2%
49	Alaska	313,539	0.2%
50	Wyoming	248,900	0.2%
	District of Columbia	298,250	0.2%

Source: Morgan Quitno Press using data from U.S. Bureau of the Census
"SC-EST2003-race6 - State Characteristic Estimates" (September 30, 2004)

IX. SOURCES

American Academy of Physicians Assistants
950 North Washington Street
Alexandria, VA 22314-1552
703-836-2272
www.aapa.org

American Cancer Society, Inc.
1599 Clifton Road, NE.
Atlanta, GA 30329-4251
800-227-2345
www.cancer.org

American Dental Association
211 E. Chicago Ave.
Chicago, IL 60611-2678
312-440-2500
www.ada.org

American Hospital Association
One North Franklin
Chicago, IL 60606-3421
312-422-3000
www.aha.org

American Medical Association
515 North State Street
Chicago, IL 60610
800-621-8335
www.ama-assn.org

American Osteopathic Association
142 East Ontario Street
Chicago, IL 60611
800-621-1773
www.osteopathic.org

American Podiatric Medical Association
9312 Old Georgetown Road
Bethesda, MD 20814-1621
301-581-9200
www.apma.org

Bureau of Labor Statistics
2 Massachusetts Ave., NE
Washington, DC 20212-0001
202-691-6175
www.bls.gov/iif/

Census Bureau
4700 Silver Hill Road
Washington, DC 20233-0001
301-457-2800
www.census.gov

Centers for Disease Control and Prevention
1600 Clifton Road, NE.
Atlanta, GA 30333
404-639-3311 (Public Affairs)
800-458-5231 (AIDS Clearinghouse)
www.cdc.gov

Centers for Medicare and Medicaid Services
7500 Security Boulevard
Baltimore, MD 21244-1850
877-267-2323
www.cms.gov

Federation of Chiropractic Licensing Boards
901 54th Ave., Ste. 101
Greeley, CO 80634-4400
970-356-3500
www.fclb.org

Health Resources and Services Admin
Division of Practitioner Data Banks
7519 Standish Place, Ste 300
Rockville MD 20857
800-767-6732
www.npdb-hipdb.com

InterStudy
P.O. Box 4366
St. Paul, MN 55104
800-844-3351
www.hmodata.com

Medical Expenditure Panel Survey
Agency for Healthcare Research and Quality
540 Gaither Road
Rockville MD 20850
301-427-1656
www.meps.ahrq.gov

National Center for Health Statistics
U.S. Department of Health and Human Services
3311 Toledo Road
Hyattsville, MD 20782-2003
301-458-4000
www.cdc.gov/nchs/

**National Institute on Alcohol Abuse
and Alcoholism**
National Institutes of Health
5635 Fishers Lane, MSC 9304
Bethesda, MD 20892-9304
301-443-9970
www.niaaa.nih.gov/

National Highway Traffic Safety Admin.
400 Seventh Street, SW
Washington, DC 20590
202-366-0123
www.nhtsa.dot.gov

National Sporting Goods Association
1601 Feehanville Drive, Ste 300
Mt. Prospect, IL 60056
847-296-6742
www.nsga.org

Smoking and Health Office
Centers for Disease Control and Prevention
4770 Buford Hwy, NE., Mail Stop K-50
Atlanta, GA 30341-3717
770-488-5705
www.cdc.gov/tobacco/

X. INDEX

X. INDEX (continued)

X. INDEX (continued)

CHAPTER INDEX

HOW TO USE THIS INDEX

Place left thumb on the outer edge of this page. To locate the desired entry, fold back the remaining page edges and align the index edge mark with the appropriate page edge mark.

Other books by Morgan Quitno Press:

- *State Rankings 2005 ($56.95)*
- *Crime State Rankings 2005 ($56.95)*
- *City Crime Rankings, 11th Edition ($44.95)*
- *Education State Rankings 2004-2005 ($49.95)*
- *State Trends, 1st Edition ($59.95)*

Call toll free: 1-800-457-0742 or
visit us at www.statestats.com

GREYSCALE

BIN TRAVELER FORM

Cut By: William J   Qty 28   Date 11-15-2024

Scanned By _____ Qty _____ Date _____

Scanned Batch IDs

_____   _____

Notes / Exception

_____

_____

_____

_____

_____